New Learning S

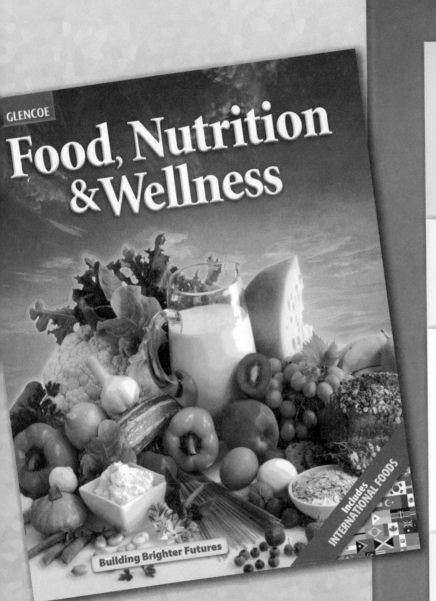

GLENCOE

Food, Nutrition & Wellness

Includes INTERNATIONAL FOODS

Building Brighter Futures

Improve Academic Performance
- National Academic Standards
- Academic Vocabulary
- Reading Guides
- Writing Tips and Activities
- Math and Science in Action
- Standardized Test Practice

Connect to the Real World
- Discover International Foods
- Financial Literacy
- Hot Jobs!

Hands-On Learning
- Interpersonal and Collaborative Skills Support FCCLA
- Nutrition and Wellness Tips
- Easy Recipes: Everyday Favorites and International Flavors
- Food Prep How To
- Unit Thematic Projects

Online Resources
- Online Student Edition
- Graphic Organizers
- Evaluation Rubrics
- Glossary/Spanish Glosario

Log on to the *Food, Nutrition & Wellness* Online Learning Center at **glencoe.com**

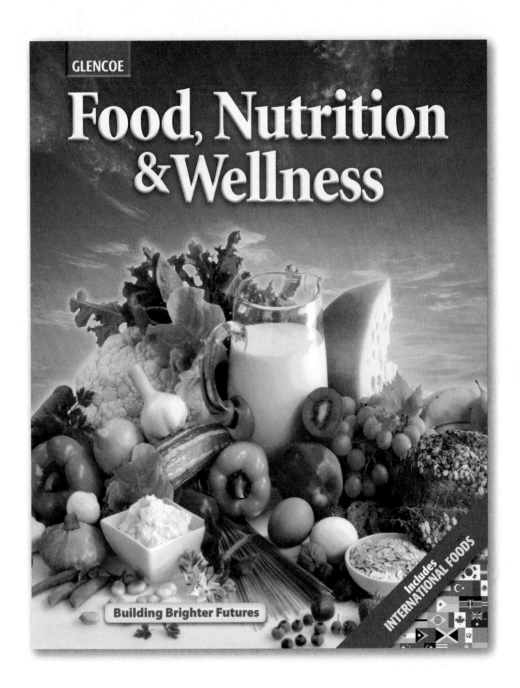

GLENCOE

Food, Nutrition & Wellness

Building Brighter Futures

Includes INTERNATIONAL FOODS

Roberta Larson Duyff

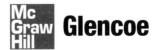

Glencoe

Author

About the Author Roberta Larson Duyff

Roberta Larson Duyff, MS, RD, FADA, CFCS, received her bachelor's degree in home economics education with a food emphasis from the University of Illinois and a master's degree in nutrition and education from Cornell University. She also spent an International Semester at Sea and is committed to global perspectives in food and nutrition. Roberta has written many books for teens, children, and adults, including the *American Dietetic Association Complete Food & Nutrition Guide, 365 Days of Healthy Eating,* and several children's books. Roberta writes about healthful eating for newspapers and national magazines and appears on radio, Webcasts, and TV. Her work includes recipe development and food styling, and she has worked on several cookbooks. Roberta has been a leader with in the American Association of Family and Consumer Sciences, the Society for Nutrition Education, the American Dietetic Association, and the International Association of Culinary Professionals. She is a National School Volunteer Program Award winner for her work with international youth exchange.

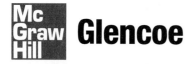

Glencoe

The *McGraw·Hill* Companies

Printed in the United States of America.

Send all inquiries to:
Glencoe/McGraw-Hill
21600 Oxnard Street, Suite 500
Woodland Hills, CA 91367

ISBN: 978-0-07-880663-6   (Student Edition)
MHID: 0-07-880663-1   (Student Edition)

1 2 3 4 5 6 7 8 9   043/079   13 12 11 10 09 08

Contributors and Reviewers

Contributors

Mary Etta Moorachian, Ph.D., RD, LD, CCP, CFCS
Charlotte, North Carolina

Margaret Cunningham RN, MSN
Battle Ground, Washington

Educational Reviewers

Suzi Beck
Trenton R-9 School
Trenton, Missouri

Dana Bertrand
Lake Arthur High School
Lake Arthur, Louisiana

Lori Black
Jacksonville High School
Jacksonville, Arkansas

Roxie V. Godfrey, Ed.D.
Mount Vernon High School
Alexandria, Virginia

Vikki Jackson
Kathleen Middle School
Lakeland, Florida

Tammy Lamparter
Smyrna High School
Smyrna, Tennessee

Dawn Lewis
Coffee High School Freshman
   Campus
Douglas, Georgia

Kimberley Myers
Aynor High School
Aynor, South Carolina

Holly Nix
Blacksburg High School
Blacksburg, South Carolina

Amanda Riggen
Walker Career Center
Indianapolis, Indiana

Patricia Sanchez
Preston Junior High School
Fort Collins, Colorado

Virginia Tate
East Forsyth High School
Kernsville, North Carolina

Nicole Thiel
Lake City High School
Coeur d' xvAlene, Idaho

Margaret E. Trione
Daphne High School
Daphne, Alabama

Linda Valiga, Med., CFCS
Waukesha South High School
Waukesha, Wisconsin

Carly Wassom
Nathan Hale High School
Tulsa, Oklahoma

Denise J. Watts Bowker
Capitol Hill High School
Oklahoma City, Oklahoma

Technical Reviewers

Judi Adams, M.S., RD
President
Grains Commission
Ridgway, Colorado

Joyce Armstrong, Ph.D.
Associate Professor
Texas Women's University
Denton, Texas

Keith Ayoob EdD, RD, FADA
Associate Professor of Pediatrics
Albert Einstein College of Medicine
New York City, New York

Betsy Hornick, M.S., RD
Food, Nutrition & Health
   Communications
Poplar Grove, Illinois

Reed Mangels, Ph.D., RN
Nutrition Advisor
The Vegetarian Resource Group
Amhurst, Massachusetts

Elaine McLaughlin, M.S., RD
Community Nutritionist
Alexandria, Virginia

Jeff Nelken, M.S., RD
Food Safety/HACCP Expert
Woodland Hills, California

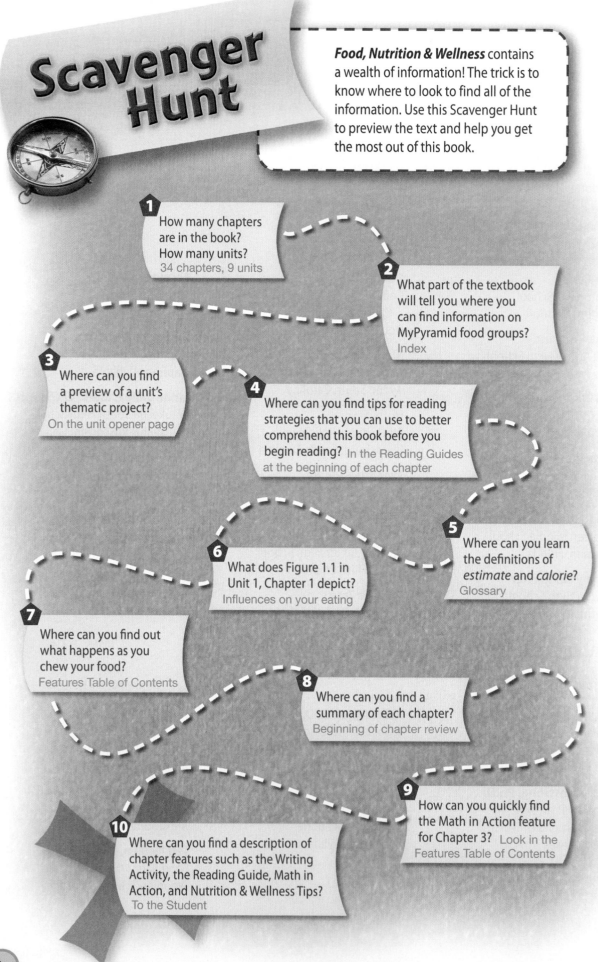

Scavenger Hunt

Food, Nutrition & Wellness contains a wealth of information! The trick is to know where to look to find all of the information. Use this Scavenger Hunt to preview the text and help you get the most out of this book.

1 How many chapters are in the book? How many units?
34 chapters, 9 units

2 What part of the textbook will tell you where you can find information on MyPyramid food groups?
Index

3 Where can you find a preview of a unit's thematic project?
On the unit opener page

4 Where can you find tips for reading strategies that you can use to better comprehend this book before you begin reading? In the Reading Guides at the beginning of each chapter

5 Where can you learn the definitions of *estimate* and *calorie*?
Glossary

6 What does Figure 1.1 in Unit 1, Chapter 1 depict?
Influences on your eating

7 Where can you find out what happens as you chew your food?
Features Table of Contents

8 Where can you find a summary of each chapter?
Beginning of chapter review

9 How can you quickly find the Math in Action feature for Chapter 3? Look in the Features Table of Contents

10 Where can you find a description of chapter features such as the Writing Activity, the Reading Guide, Math in Action, and Nutrition & Wellness Tips?
To the Student

Table of Contents

To the Student. . . . .**xviii**
National Academic Standards. . . .**xxviii**
Reading Skills Handbook . . . . **xxx**
How to Use Technology . . . . **xl**
Student Organizations and FCCLA. . **xlvi**

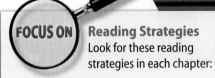

FOCUS ON Reading Strategies
Look for these reading
strategies in each chapter:

- Before You Read
- Graphic Organizer
- As You Read
- Reading Check
- After You Read

Unit 1 Choose Wellness 2

CHAPTER **1** Wellness and Food Choices 4
Writing Activity: Freewriting. 4
Reading Guide. 5
➤ *CHAPTER 1 Review and Applications* 15

CHAPTER **2** Physical Fitness
and Active Living 18
Writing Activity: Write About an Event . . .18
Reading Guide. 19
➤ *CHAPTER 2 Review and Applications* 29

Unit 1 Thematic Project Choose Wellness . . 32

Unit 2 The World of Food 34

CHAPTER **3** Food and Culture 36
Writing Activity: Journal Entry 36
Reading Guide. 37
➤ *CHAPTER 3 Review and Applications* 45

CHAPTER **4** Food and the Marketplace 48
Writing Activity: Write Using Details 48
Reading Guide. 49
➤ *CHAPTER 4 Review and Applications* 57

Unit 2 Thematic Project
Explore Ethnic Cuisines 60

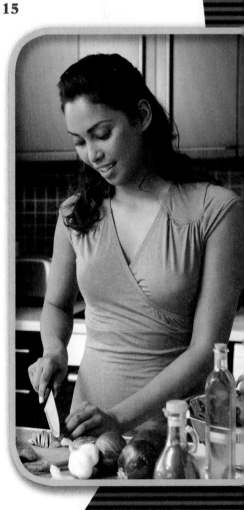

Table of Contents

Unit 3 Food and Kitchen Safety 62

CHAPTER **5** Food Safety and Sanitation 64

Writing Activity: Write a Paragraph **64**
Reading Guide. **65**
➤ *CHAPTER 5 Review and Applications* **77**

CHAPTER **6** Kitchen Safety 80

Writing Activity: Autobiographical Paragraph . . **80**
Reading Guide. **81**
➤ *CHAPTER 6 Review and Applications* **87**

Unit 3 Thematic Project Plan a Safe Kitchen 90

Unit 4 Food and Your Body 92

CHAPTER **7** Nutrients: From Food to You 94

Writing Activity: Write a Paragraph **94**
Reading Guide. **95**
➤ *CHAPTER 7 Review and Applications* **109**

CHAPTER **8** Dietary Guidelines 112

Writing Activity: Write a Letter **112**
Reading Guide. **113**
➤ *CHAPTER 8 Review and Applications* **121**

CHAPTER **9** MyPyramid and You 124

Writing Activity: Prewriting **124**
Reading Guide. **125**
➤ *CHAPTER 9 Review and Applications* **139**

Unit 4 Thematic Project
Investigate Food Trends **142**

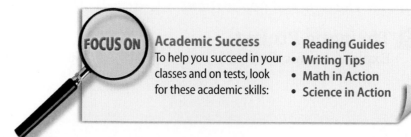

FOCUS ON

Academic Success
To help you succeed in your
classes and on tests, look
for these academic skills:

• Reading Guides
• Writing Tips
• Math in Action
• Science in Action

Table of Contents

Unit 5 Nutrition for Life 144

CHAPTER **10** Choices for Your Healthy Weight 146
  Writing Activity: Coherent Paragraph 146
  Reading Guide. 147
  ➤ *CHAPTER 10 Review and Applications* 157

CHAPTER **11** Fuel Up for Sports 160
  Writing Activity: Business Letter 160
  Reading Guide. 161
  ➤ *CHAPTER 11 Review and Applications* 167

CHAPTER **12** Nutrition Throughout
  the Life Cycle 170
  Writing Activity: Dialogue 170
  Reading Guide. 171
  ➤ *CHAPTER 12 Review and Applications* 181

CHAPTER **13** Vegetarian Choices 184
  Writing Activity: Descriptive Paragraph 184
  Reading Guide. 185
  ➤ *CHAPTER 13 Review and Applications* 191

CHAPTER **14** Special Health Concerns 194
  Writing Activity: Write an Explanation . . . 194
  Reading Guide. 195
  ➤ *CHAPTER 14 Review and Applications* 205

Unit 5 Thematic Project Plan a Healthy
  Lifestyle 208

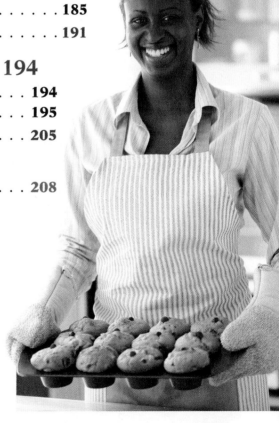

FOCUS ON Visuals
Images help you comprehend
key ideas. Answer the
questions for all:

• Unit and Chapter Openers
• Photos and Captions
• Figures and Tables

Table of Contents

Unit 6 **Smart Food Choices 210**

CHAPTER **15** **Consumer Issues: Fact vs. Fiction** **212**
　　Writing Activity: Step-by-Step Guide **212**
　　Reading Guide. **213**
➤ *CHAPTER 15 Review and Applications* **219**

CHAPTER **16** **Planning Nutritious Meals**
　　　　　　and Snacks **222**
　　Writing Activity: Character Analysis **222**
　　Reading Guide. **223**
➤ *CHAPTER 16 Review and Applications* **231**

CHAPTER **17** **Shopping for Food** **234**
　　Writing Activity: "How-To" Paper **234**
　　Reading Guide. **235**
➤ *CHAPTER 17 Review and Applications* **245**

CHAPTER **18** **Eating Well When Away from Home** **248**
　　Writing Activity: Cause-and-Effect Paragraph. . **248**
　　Reading Guide. **249**
➤ *CHAPTER 18 Review and Applications* **255**

Unit 6 Thematic Project Smart Food Choices . . **258**

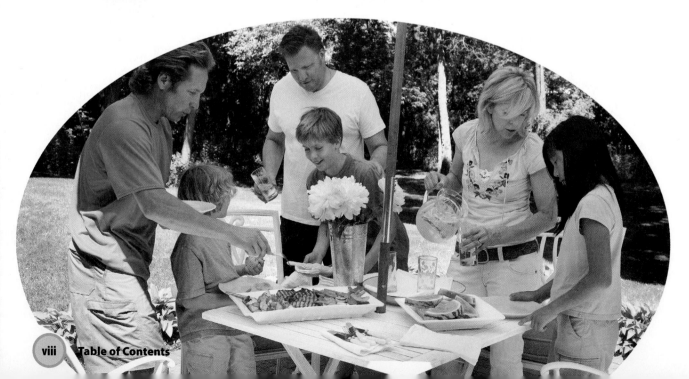

Table of Contents

Unit 7   From Kitchen to Table 260

CHAPTER **19**   Kitchen Equipment 262
   Writing Activity: Persuasive Paragraph 262
   Reading Guide. 263
➤ *CHAPTER 19 Review and Applications* 277

CHAPTER **20**   Skills for Preparing
   Flavorful Food   280
   Writing Activity: Write an Advertisement 280
   Reading Guide. 281
➤ *CHAPTER 20 Review and Applications* 297

CHAPTER **21**   Cooking Basics 300
   Writing Activity: Personal Narrative 300
   Reading Guide. 301
➤ *CHAPTER 21 Review and Applications* 313

CHAPTER **22**   Organizing the Kitchen   316
   Writing Activity: Identify Purpose and Audience . . 316
   Reading Guide. 317
➤ *CHAPTER 22 Review and Applications* 329

CHAPTER **23**   Serving a Meal 332
   Writing Activity: Compare
   and Contrast Paper 332
   Reading Guide. 333
➤ *CHAPTER 23 Review and Applications* . . .343

Unit 7   Thematic Project
   From Kitchen to Table 346

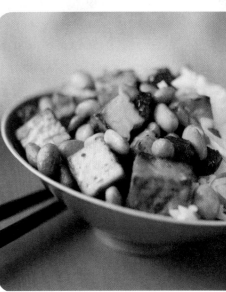

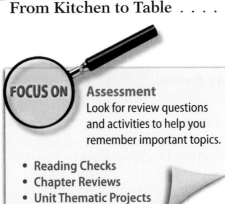

FOCUS ON   Assessment
Look for review questions
and activities to help you
remember important topics.

- Reading Checks
- Chapter Reviews
- Unit Thematic Projects

Table of Contents

Unit 8 Learning About Foods 348

CHAPTER 24 Grains 350

Writing Activity: First Draft 350
Reading Guide 351
➤ *CHAPTER 24 Review and Applications* 361

CHAPTER 25 Vegetables 364

Writing Activity: Edit a First Draft 364
Reading Guide 365
➤ *CHAPTER 25 Review and Applications* 375

CHAPTER 26 Fruit 378

Writing Activity: Essay Question and Answer . . 378
Reading Guide 379
➤ *CHAPTER 26 Review and Applications* 387

CHAPTER 27 Milk 390

Writing Activity: Write a Step-by-Step Guide 390
Reading Guide 391
➤ *CHAPTER 27 Review and Applications* 401

CHAPTER 28 Meat, Poultry, and Fish 404

Writing Activity: Persuasive Paragraph 404
Reading Guide 405
➤ *CHAPTER 28 Review and Applications* 419

CHAPTER 29 Eggs, Beans, and Nuts 422

Writing Activity: Descriptive Paragraph 422
Reading Guide 423
➤ *CHAPTER 29 Review and Applications* 433

CHAPTER 30 Fats and Oils 436

Writing Activity: Expository Essay 436
Reading Guide 437
➤ *CHAPTER 30 Review and Applications* 445

Unit 8 Thematic Project Discover Organic Foods . . . 448

Table of Contents

Unit 9 Combination Foods 450

CHAPTER 31 Salads 452

Writing Activity: Persuasive Essay 452
Reading Guide. 453
➤ *CHAPTER 31 Review and Applications* 461

CHAPTER 32 Quick and Yeast Breads 464

Writing Activity: Describe a Viewpoint 464
Reading Guide. 465
➤ *CHAPTER 32 Review and Applications* 477

CHAPTER 33 Mixed Foods and Snacks 480

Writing Activity: Step-by-Step Guide. 480
Reading Guide. 481
➤ *CHAPTER 33 Review and Applications* 497

CHAPTER 34 Desserts 500

Writing Activity: Expository Writing 500
Reading Guide. 501
➤ *CHAPTER 34 Review and Applications* 511

Unit 9 Thematic Project Food Industry Careers . 514

Food Group Equivalencies 516
Daily Value for Teens 517
Nutritive Values of Foods. 518
First Aid Appendix 526
Math Skills Appendix 535
Glossary. 557
Index. 566
Credits. 579

FOCUS ON Online Resources
Look for the online icon and go to the book's Online Learning Center at **glencoe.com** for:

- Graphic Organizers
- Practice Tests
- Evaluation Rubrics
- Career Resources
- Additional Activities

Academic Skills for Nutrition and Wellness!

How much time does it take to safely thaw a turkey? Can you increase the amount your favorite recipe makes? Do you know why beaten egg whites can make a cake fluffier? Use these academic features to succeed in school, on tests, and in life!

Math in Action

Increasing Recipes 11

Doubling Twice 41

Thaw a Turkey.................. 73

Daily Values.................... 107

Conversions.................... 128

Daily Allowance of Water........ 163

Healthy Amounts of Soy......... 187

Vitamin C from Food 215

Mental Math 243

Electricity Savings.............. 269

Altitude Boiling Chart 306

Choosing a Dining Table 335

Veggies-of-the-Month Club 369

Cream Cheese.................. 395

Egg Whites for a Pie 428

Salad Dressing Costs 455

The Right Pan for the Job........505

Science in Action

Weight Machines 23

New Approaches to Agriculture ... 52

Kitchen Fires 83

Compare Fat Content........... 116

Chew Your Food 152

Trail Mix 166

Growing Healthy Bones 176

Hidden Sodium 198

Calcium Loss and Soda 225

Evaluate Menu Options 251

Beating Egg Whites 293

Evaluate Green Methods 324

Germ vs. Germs 356

True Fruit 381

The Color of Meat 409

Fats and Cholesterol 440

Gluten-Free Baking 468

The Science of Cheese........... 492

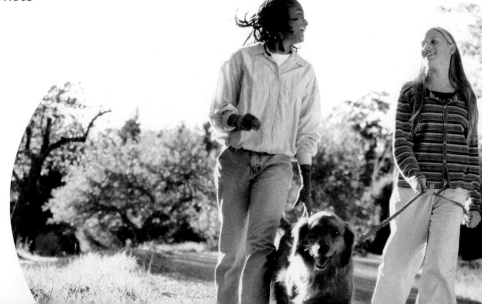

What Do You Want to Do?

What career options are open to you? What do professionals in the nutrition and wellness industries really do? Discover a world of possibilities!

HOT JOBS!

Family and Consumer Sciences Teacher 13

Fitness Trainer 22

Food Historian 43

Agricultural Manager 53

Food Service Manager 69

Cafeteria Cook 84

Food Scientist 99

Public Health Educator 115

Dietitian 133

Weight-Loss Counselor 151

Consultant Dietitian 165

Social and Human Services Assistant 173

Food Technologist 188

Community Health Nurse 197

Food and Nutrition Writer 216

Caterer 227

Grocery Store Worker 240

Server 252

Kitchen Designer 266

Cookbook Author 291

Product Demonstrator 311

Party Planner 325

Banquet Manager 337

Restaurant-Supply Salesperson 355

Agricultural Scientist 372

Food Stylist 383

Food Processing Occupations 393

Food Technician 415

Recipe Developer 431

Chef 442

Food Photographer 459

Baker 470

Restaurant Manager 484

Food Editor 491

Pastry Chef 507

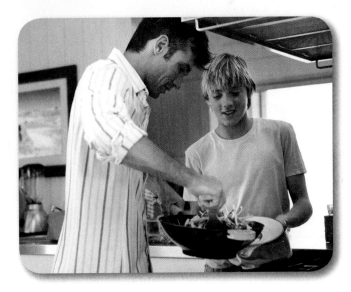

Features Table of Contents

Check Out These Useful Tips!

Do you know how to shop for your own meals? How can you make meals more nutritious? What appliances work best for making snacks? Find useful tips for everyday living here!

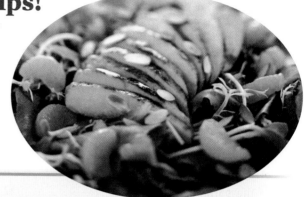

Nutrition & Wellness Tips

Healthy Skin 7

Cut the Salt 8

Snacks on Hand 12

Get Off the Couch! 24

Go Walking 27

Eat Japanese Style 39

Farmers' Market 50

Edible Garden 55

Healthy Shopping 97

Drink Nutrients 103

Healthy Alternatives 119

Variety and Balance 129

Moderation 134

Use Common Sense 153

No Salt Tablets 165

A Family Affair 174

Vegetarian Style 190

Medical Advice 199

Be Aware 200

Reliable Web Sites 214

Contact Food Companies 217

Save Time and Calories 226

Read Between the Lines 237

Smart Choices 252

Appliances for Snacks 268

Recipe Makeovers 292

Cook for Flavor and Nutrition 305

For Safety's Sake 322

Manners and Cleanliness 340

Shop for Convenience 358

Snack Attack 368

Shop Safely 371

Snack Ideas 382

Milk Safety 399

Lean Burgers and Hot Dogs! 414

Flavorful Meat, Poultry, and Fish 417

Go Nuts! 425

Fat Savvy 439

Take-Along Salads 457

Dress Lightly! 459

Bake with Less Fat 467

Soups and Stews—with Less Salt! 491

Give a Gift of Health 503

Discover a World of Flavors!

Do you know what people in other countries eat and how they cook their food? Can you make dishes from other cultures? These features will help you understand the wide world of food!

Discover International Foods

Spain 21
Peru 55
China 85
British Isles. 119
France 153
Greece 177
Italy 201
Mexico. 227
Vietnam 253

Egypt 289
North Africa 326
Russia. 354
Countries of the Caribbean 382
Argentina. 407
Canada 443
Germany. .470
India 493

EASY RECIPES International Flavors

Spain Gazpacho (cold vegetable soup) 28
Peru Lime Quinoa with Vegetables 56
China Asian Stir-Fried Vegetables 86
British Isles Beans and Chopped
        Vegetables on Toast 120
France Ratatouille (vegetable stew
        of France) 156
Greece Tzatziki (cucumber sauce) 180
Italy Quick Marinara Sauce 204
Mexico Chicken Quesadillas. 230

Vietnam Vietnamese Spring Rolls 254
Egypt Ful Mesdames (beans and eggs) 296
North Africa Orange-Mint Couscous. 328
Russia Blini (miniature pancakes). 359
The Carribean Roasted Pineapple 386
Argentina Chimichurri Sauce
        (olive oil and herbs) 418
Canada Pancakes with Maple Syrup 444
Germany Soft Pretzels 476
India Mulligatawny (spicy lentil soup) 496

What Will You Eat Today?

How much variety do you have in your diet? Do you know how to roast a chicken? Many tasty dishes pack a nutritional punch. Check out these recipes to get cooking!

EASY RECIPES   **Everyday Favorites**

Fruit, Granola, and Yogurt Parfait 14

Hummus 44

Pasta Salad 76

Italian-Style Chicken Strips 108

Balsamic Vinaigrette 138

Trail Mix 166

Southwest Salad 190

Cinnamon Baked Apples 218

Fruit Salad 244

New England Clam Chowder 276

Quick and Hearty Chili 312

Party Guacamole 342

Vegetable Cole Slaw 376

Egg Cream 400

Red Beans and Rice 432

Sunshine Salad 460

Apple Cobbler 510

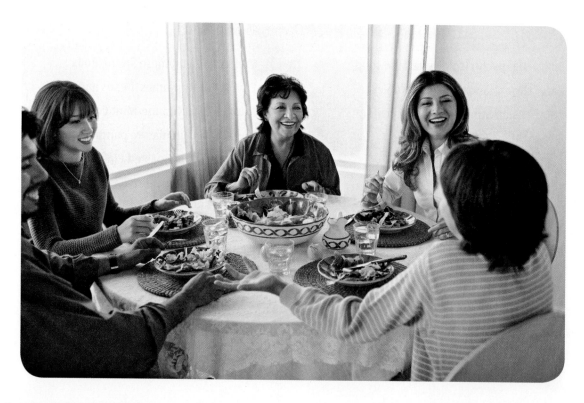

Sharpen Your Kitchen Skills

Do you know how to braise meat? Can you knead biscuit dough? You can improve your cooking and baking skills with these handy how-to hints!

Food Prep How To

Measure Dry Ingredients 286

Measure Liquid Ingredients 287

Cook Pasta 359

Simmer Vegetables 373

Make a Fruit Sauce 385

Make Yogurt Cheese 399

Braise Meat 416

Roast Meat 416

Break Eggs XX

Separate Eggs 429

Scramble Eggs 430

Cook Dry Beans 431

Make a Tossed Salad 456

Knead Biscuit Dough 473

Roll and Cut Biscuits 473

Prepare a Stir-Fry 495

Remove a Cake from the Pan 508

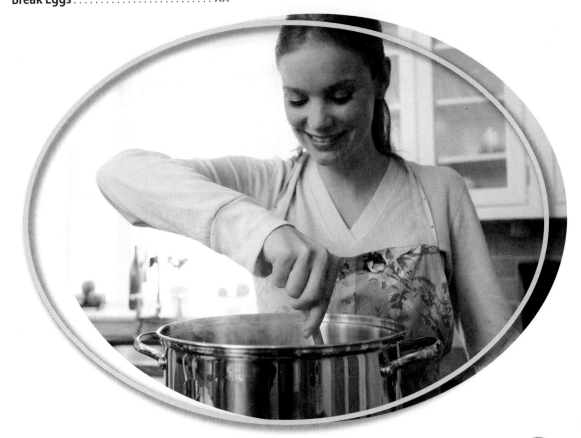

To the Student

Discover the World of Nutrition and Wellness

Successful readers first set a purpose for reading. *Food, Nutrition & Wellness* teaches skills you need to make healthful food choices, prepare nutritious meals, and bring activity into your daily life. Think about why you are reading this book. Use the unit opener to help you set a reading purpose and understand what you will learn in each unit. Consider how you might be able to use what you learn in your own life.

Read the Chapter Titles to find out what the topics will be.

Preview the Thematic Project at the end of the unit. A preview lets you know what is to come. Use the preview to think about how what you are learning applies to the project.

Unit 5
Nutrition for Life

Chapters in this Unit
Chapter 10 Choices for Your Healthy Weight
Chapter 11 Fuel Up for Sports
Chapter 12 Nutrition Throughout the Life Cycle
Chapter 13 Vegetarian Choices
Chapter 14 Special Health Concerns

Unit Thematic Project Preview
Plan a Healthy Lifestyle
In the unit thematic project at the end of this unit, you will choose and research a healthy lifestyle that appeals to you. You will plan an entire day's menu with foods from that lifestyle. Then, you will interview someone in your community who is qualified to discuss your choices. Last, you will make a presentation to your class to share what you have learned.

My Journal
Choosing a sensible diet and being physically active are important parts of becoming a healthy adult. There are many lifestyle options to choose from. Some are healthier than others. Write a journal entry that answers these questions:
• What healthy lifestyles appeal to you?
• How close or far are you from currently practicing your preferred lifestyle?
• How can you make better food choices?

144

EXPLORE THE PHOTO
You can learn to develop good eating habits by learning about nutrition. *Why might knowing how to evaluate information also be useful?*

145

Practice Your Writing in a personal journal. Your writing will help you prepare for the project at the end of the unit.

Use the Photo to Predict what the unit will be about. Answer the question to help focus on unit topics.

Close the Unit

What Did You Learn About Nutrition and Wellness?

Every unit ends with a Thematic Project that lets you explore an important issue from the unit. To complete each project, you will make decisions, do research, connect to your community, create a report, and present your project.

Read the Project Assignment
and numbered steps. The assignment explains what you will need to do.

Follow the Project Checklist
to make sure that you have done everything you need to complete your Thematic Project.

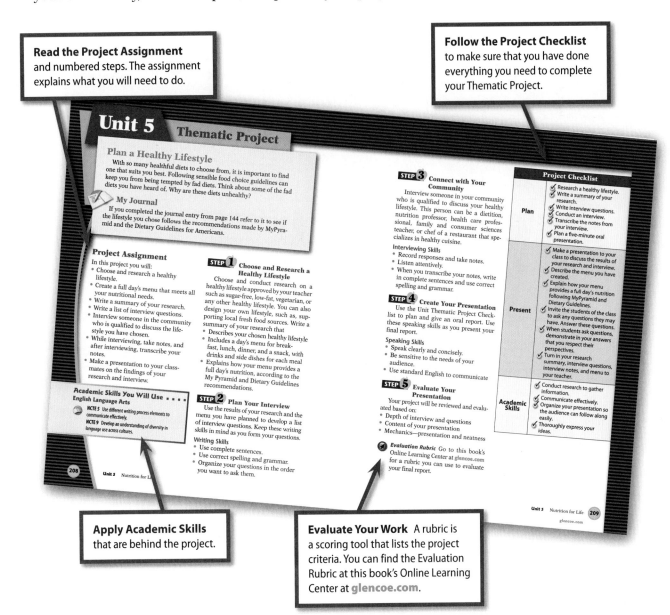

Unit 5   Thematic Project

Plan a Healthy Lifestyle

With so many healthful diets to choose from, it is important to find one that suits you best. Following sensible food choice guidelines can keep you from being tempted by fad diets. Think about some of the fad diets you have heard of. Why are these diets unhealthy?

My Journal
If you completed the journal entry from page 144 refer to it to see if the lifestyle you chose follows the recommendations made by MyPyramid and the Dietary Guidelines for Americans.

Project Assignment

In this project you will:
• Choose and research a healthy lifestyle.
• Create a full day's menu that meets all your nutritional needs.
• Write a summary of your research.
• Write a list of interview questions.
• Interview someone in the community who is qualified to discuss the lifestyle you have chosen.
• While interviewing, take notes, and after interviewing, transcribe your notes.
• Make a presentation to your classmates on the findings of your research and interview.

Academic Skills You Will Use
English Language Arts

NCTE 5 Use different writing process elements to communicate effectively.
NCTE 9 Develop an understanding of diversity in language use across cultures.

STEP 1 Choose and Research a Healthy Lifestyle
Choose and conduct research on a healthy lifestyle approved by your teacher such as sugar-free, low-fat, vegetarian, or any other healthy lifestyle. You can also design your own lifestyle, such as, supporting local fresh food sources. Write a summary of your research that
• Describes your chosen healthy lifestyle
• Includes a day's menu for breakfast, lunch, dinner, and a snack, with drinks and side dishes for each meal
• Explains how your menu provides a full day's nutrition, according to the My Pyramid and Dietary Guidelines recommendations.

STEP 2 Plan Your Interview
Use the results of your research and the menu you have planned to develop a list of interview questions. Keep these writing skills in mind as you form your questions.

Writing Skills
• Use complete sentences.
• Use correct spelling and grammar.
• Organize your questions in the order you want to ask them.

208   Unit 5   Nutrition for Li

STEP 3 Connect with Your Community
Interview someone in your community who is qualified to discuss your healthy lifestyle. This person can be a dietition, nutrition professor, health care professional, family and consumer sciences teacher, or chef of a restaurant that specializes in healthy cuisine.

Interviewing Skills
• Record responses and take notes.
• Listen attentively.
• When you transcribe your notes, write in complete sentences and use correct spelling and grammar.

STEP 4 Create Your Presentation
Use the Unit Thematic Project Checklist to plan and give an oral report. Use these speaking skills as you present your final report.

Speaking Skills
• Speak clearly and concisely.
• Be sensitive to the needs of your audience.
• Use standard English to communicate

STEP 5 Evaluate Your Presentation
Your project will be reviewed and evaluated based on:
• Depth of interview and questions
• Content of your presentation
• Mechanics—presentation and neatness

Evaluation Rubric Go to this book's Online Learning Center at **glencoe.com** for a rubric you can use to evaluate your final report.

Project Checklist

Plan
✓ Research a healthy lifestyle.
✓ Write a summary of your research.
✓ Write interview questions.
✓ Conduct an interview.
✓ Transcribe the notes from your interview.
✓ Plan a five-minute oral presentation.

Present
✓ Make a presentation to your class to discuss the results of your research and interview.
✓ Describe the menu you have created.
✓ Explain how your menu provides a full day's nutrition following MyPyramid and Dietary Guidelines.
✓ Invite the students of the class to ask any questions they may have. Answer these questions.
✓ When students ask questions, demonstrate in your answers that you respect their perspectives.
✓ Turn in your research summary, interview questions, interview notes, and menu to your teacher.

Academic Skills
✓ Conduct research to gather information.
✓ Communicate effectively.
✓ Organize your presentation so the audience can follow along easily.
✓ Thoroughly express your ideas.

Unit 5   Nutrition for Life   209
glencoe.com

Apply Academic Skills
that are behind the project.

Evaluate Your Work A rubric is a scoring tool that lists the project criteria. You can find the Evaluation Rubric at this book's Online Learning Center at **glencoe.com**.

To the Student

Begin the Chapter

Prepare to Read with Reading Guides

Use the chapter opener and Reading Guide at the beginning of each chapter to preview what you will learn in each chapter. See if you can predict events or outcomes by using clues and information that you already know.

Predict Before You Read what the section will be about.

Read the Key Concepts to preview the key ideas you will learn. Keep these in mind as you read the chapter.

CHAPTER 11
Fuel Up for Sports

Explore the Photo Whether you are preparing for tryouts, competing in a sports event, or being active for fun and fitness, smart eating can help you do your very best. Why is a smart eating plan important for peak performance in sports?

Writing Activity
Business Letter

Sports are a fun way to stay active and relax. What sports are available near you? Write a business letter to your local chamber of commerce or department of parks and recreation. Request information about sports programs near you. Also, suggest ideas for programs that interest you.

Writing Tips

1. Be clear, brief, and considerate.
2. Use correct form.
3. Proofread to correct errors in grammar, usage, spelling, and punctuation.

160 Unit 5   Nutrition for Life

Reading Guide

Before You Read
Look It Up Scan the vocabulary words in the chapter. If you see a word that you do not know, look it up in the glossary or the dictionary.

Read to Learn
Key Concepts
- **Describe** how physical activity affects your nutrient needs.
- **Discuss** smart food and fluid choices for before, during, and after physical activity.
- **Analyze** common myths about sports nutrition.

Main Idea
Rigorous physical activity requires smart food choices and more fluids—before, during, and after a workout or competition.

Content Vocabulary
- dehydration
- electrolyte
- steroid
- carbohydrate loading

Academic Vocabulary
You will find these words in your reading and on your tests. Use the glossary to look up their definitions if necessary.
- develop
- strategy

Graphic Organizer
As you read, write the main messages about eating for peak performance, supported by strategies for before, during, and after strenuous activity.

Eating for Peak Performance		
Before	During	After

Graphic Organizer Go to this book's Online Learning Center at glencoe.com to print out this graphic organizer.

Academic Standards

English Language Arts
NCTE 8 Use information resources to gather information and create and communicate knowledge.

Mathematics
NCTM Number and Operations Understand the meanings of operations and how they relate to one another.

NCTM Data Analysis and Probability Develop and evaluate inferences and predictions that are based on data.

Science
NSES Content Standard F Develop an understanding of personal and community health.

NCTE National Council of Teachers of English
NCTM National Council of Teachers of Mathematics
NSES National Science Education Standards
NCSS National Council of the Social Studies

Chapter 11   Fuel Up for Sports   161

Check Vocabulary lists for words you do not know. You can look them up in the glossary before you read the section.

Explore the Photo to jump-start your thinking about the chapter's main topics.

Take Notes and Study with graphic organizers. These help you find and identify relationships in the information you read.

Strengthen Your Writing Skills Use the writing tips to continue to develop your writing.

Look for Academic Standards throughout the text. You can apply what you learn to other subjects.

Review the Chapter

Make Sure You Know and Understand the Concepts

Review what you learned in the chapter and see how this learning applies to your other subjects and to real-world situations.

Review Vocabulary and Key Concepts to check your recall of important ideas.

Critical Thinking takes your knowledge of the chapter further. If you have difficulty answering these questions, go back and reread the related parts of the chapter.

Apply Real-World Skills to situations that you might find in your day-to-day life.

Read the Chapter Summary to review the most important ideas that you should have learned in this chapter.

Practice Academic Skills and connect what you learned to your knowledge of language arts, math, science, and social studies.

Succeed on Tests with test-taking tips and practice questions.

Find More Activities Online at this book's Online Learning Center at **glencoe.com**.

To the Student

As You Read

Use Reading Strategies and Visuals to Study Effectively

In addition to the Reading Guide at the beginning of each chapter, there are lots of reading strategies to help you comprehend the text.

Connect what you already know to the new ideas you learn as you read.

Keep a Vocabulary Journal Write down vocabulary words then find definitions in the text and in the glossary at the back of the book.

Reading Checks let you pause to respond to what you have read.

Skim the Headings to help identify the main idea and supporting details.

Examine Visuals to reinforce content. Answer the questions so you can better discuss topics in the section.

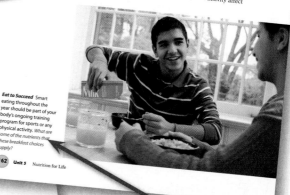

Nutrients for Active Living

As You Read

Connect What foods have you eaten recently that helped you to feel energetic?

Vocabulary
You can find definitions in the glossary at the back of this book.

All teens should follow MyPyramid when planning their meals and snacks. Eating the right amounts of foods from the five food groups will supply all the nutrients you need.

♦ **Carbohydrates** People who are very physically active need extra calories. Most of these calories should come from nutrient-dense foods high in starches, or complex carbohydrates. These include bread, cereal, rice, pasta, dry beans and peas, and starchy vegetables.

♦ **Protein** Eat 5 to 7 ounces daily from the Meat and Beans Group. Extra protein will not help you build bigger muscles. To build muscle, you need muscle-building physical activity, not more protein from food.

♦ **Vitamins and Minerals** Eat a variety of foods to get the vitamins and minerals you need. Iron-rich foods are good for your blood. Calcium-rich foods help develop, or promote the growth of, healthy bones. As an athlete, you do not need extra vitamins and minerals.

♦ **Water** During intense activity, your body heats up. To cool down, your body sweats. When you sweat, you must drink fluids to replace lost fluids.

Reading Check **Discuss** How does physical activity affect your nutrient needs?

Eat to Succeed Smart eating throughout the year should be part of your body's ongoing training program for sports or any physical activity. *What are some of the nutrients that these breakfast choices supply?*

162 Unit 5 Nutrition for Life

Choices for Peak Performance

Plan ahead to do your personal best at strenuous physical activity. During your workout, warm-up and cool-down properly. Performance also depends on what you eat and how much you drink before, during, and after activity.

Before You Are Active

About three to four hours before vigorous activity, enjoy a meal that is high in carbohydrates and low in fat and protein. This combination is easy to digest. Carbohydrates also provide energy for the activity. Carbohydrates also provide fuel for your working muscles. Eat until you are satisfied but not too full. These meals are great choices a few hours before physical activity:

♦ Orange juice, bagel, peanut butter, apple slices
♦ Apple juice, pancakes and syrup, low-fat yogurt, strawberries
♦ Tomato soup, grilled cheese sandwich, low-fat milk

Eat a light snack, such as some fruit, about a half hour before an activity if you are hungry. Sugary foods like candy may leave you feeling shaky or cause you to get tired quickly.

Drink at least 2 cups (500 mL) of water about two hours before the activity. Drink another 1 to 2 cups (250 to 500 mL) fifteen minutes before the activity.

While You Are Active

Unless your workout lasts more than one hour, you probably do not need to eat during the activity. If you do, eat carbohydrate-rich foods that are easy to digest, such as a banana or a rice cake.

If you do not replace fluids lost through sweating, you may suffer from dehydration. **Dehydration** is a significant loss of body fluids. Symptoms start with thirst and fatigue, and can progress to weakness, confusion, muscle cramps, and heat exhaustion. In severe cases, dehydration can cause death.

During vigorous activity, drink ½ to 2 cups (125 to 500 mL) of water. The amount depends on how much you sweat. Do not drinks excessively. During vigorous activity your kidneys cannot eliminate extra water fast enough. In extreme cases, this can even be fatal.

Math in Action

Daily Allowance of Water

Sara decides to drink 3 cups (750 mL) of water before a soccer game. She measured her drinking glasses, and found that they hold 12 oz each. How many times should she refill a 12-oz glass to get that amount of water?

Math Concept **Multiply/Divide**
Rational Numbers When a word problem requires organizing things into different-size groups, use multiplication and division to solve it.

Starting Hint First, determine the number of ounces in 3 cups of water. Then, divide by the size of the glass. If necessary, round up to the next whole number.

NCTM Number and Operations Understand the meanings of operations and how they relate to one another.

Math For more math help, go to the Math Appendix.

Chapter 11 Fuel Up for Sports 163

To the Student

Study with Features

Skills You Can Really Use at School and in Life!

As you read, look for feature boxes throughout each chapter. These features build skills that relate to other academic subjects and prepare you for life on your own.

Math in Action

The Right Pan for the Job

James is making drop cookies with his family. Each is 2 inches in diameter. He must leave at least 2 inches between each cookie and 2 inches around the outside edge. Which size cookie sheet will allow him to bake the most number of cookies on one sheet?

- 17" × 12"
- 15" × 10"
- 16" × 14"
- 12" × 9"

Math Concept Determine the area of a figure given its dimensions.

Starting Hint The easiest way to find the answer is to compare the surface areas of each pan, which is really the area (length × width). You may also wish to sketch a pan to verify your answer.

NCTM Geometry Use visualization, spatial reasoning, and geometric modeling to solve problems.

Math For more math help, go to the Math Appendix.

Make Math Simple You use math every day—even if it is just counting money to buy a drink at your campus store. See how to use starting hints to break down math problems and solve them step by step.

Math Concept The math concept helps you understand what you are solving in the math activity.

Starting Hint The Starting Hint helps you figure out how to solve the math problem.

NCTM Correlation Each math activity is correlated to the National Council of Teachers of Mathematics standards.

Learn the Secrets of Science The secret is that it can be easy! You can use scientific principles and concepts in your everyday activities. Investigate and analyze the world around you with these basic skills.

Science in Action

Beating Egg Whites

Beat egg whites for a light and fluffy omelet or soufflé. Beating egg whites forms air bubbles, creating foam that has up to eight times the volume than before beating. Once you combine and cook the beaten egg whites with other ingredients, the extra volume will be baked in!

Procedure Try beating egg whites at home. Are small bubbles stronger or weaker than bigger bubbles? Do you want strong or weak bubbles when cooking? Compare bubbles to balloons—when are balloons stronger?

Analysis Create a one-page written report about your observations. Conduct research on the structure of bubbles, and add your findings to your report.

NSES Content Standard B Develop an understanding of the structure and properties of matter.

Procedure and Analysis Every Science in Action activity reflects the stages of scientific inquiry to help you plan your work.

To the Student

Features (continued)

Explore Careers in the fields of food, nutrition, and wellness. You can use the skills you develop in school to find career possibilities. You can also find more information about careers at this book's Online Learning Center at **glencoe.com**.

HOT JOBS!

Dietitian
Registered dietitians use up-to-date scientific information to help promote healthful eating habits and healthy living. They also suggest ways for people to improve their health.

Careers Find out more about careers. Go to this book's Online Learning Center through **glencoe.com**.

Nutrition & Wellness Tips

Save Time and Calories

✓ Plan one dish to serve twice: a bowl of chili today and leftover chili over a baked potato tomorrow, for example.

✓ Eat a baked potato with salsa instead of French fries as a side dish.

Useful Tips These tips can help you balance your nutrition, plan activities with your family and friends, and make food more flavorful.

Learn New Kitchen Skills and prepare new dishes with these easy, step-by-step guides.

Food Prep How To

SEPARATE EGGS

1. Place a clean egg separator across the rim of a small bowl.

2. Crack the egg in the center.

3. Hold the egg over the round part of the egg separator. Gently pull the shell apart. Slip the yolk into the egg separator.

4. Let the white flow through into the bowl. Then, drop the yolk into a different bowl.

STEP 4

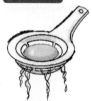

To the Student

Features (continued)

EASY RECIPES — Everyday Favorites

Sunshine Salad

Customary	Ingredients	Metric
4 cups	Spinach leaves, packed	1 L
⅓	Red onion, sliced thin	⅓
⅓	Red bell pepper, sliced	⅓
½	Whole cucumber, sliced	½
2	Oranges, peeled and chopped in bite-sized pieces	2
¼ cup	Bottled low-fat vinaigrette	60

Try This!
Use different greens. Create your own vinaigrette. Top with croutons, toasted nuts, or pumpkin seeds.

Yield: 4 servings, 1 cup (250 mL) each
1. Toss spinach, onion, bell pepper, cucumber, and oranges in a large bowl.
2. Add dressing. Toss lightly.
3. Serve immediately.

Nutritional Information Per Serving: 71 calories, 1 g total fat (0 g saturated fat), 1 mg cholesterol, 150 mg sodium, 14 g total ca... (3 g fiber, 8 g sugars), 2 g protein

Percent Daily Value: vitamin A 25%, vitamin C 80%, calcium 6%...

> **Make Nutrition Count Every Day** Your favorite dishes are easy to prepare with these step-by-step healthful recipes. You can find serving size and nutritional information in each recipe.

Discover International Foods

Vietnam
The food of Vietnam reflects ingredients produced in Southeast Asia, and the Chinese and French who once ruled there. The cuisine uses vegetables, fruits, rice, and noodles. Noodles are made from wheat, rice, and mung beans. They are served in soup, salads, and stir-fries, and mixed with meat, fish, herbs, and vegetables. Nuoc mam (nü-'äk 'mäm), a reddish fish sauce made of fermented anchovies, adds flavor to many Vietnamese dishes. Most dishes are not spicy hot. Fruit is a popular dessert: oranges, bananas, starfruit, rambutans, and loquats are favorite fruits.

Languages Across Cultures
pho *(fō)* noodle dish; as translated "your own bowl." Pho bo is beef-noodle soup seasoned with cinnamon, cloves, and ginger and made with lime, bean sprouts, and onion.

goi cuon *(gòi cuốn)* mixed salad roll with pork, shrimp, herbs, and rice vermicelli wrapped in rice paper.

Recipes Find out more about international recipes on this book's Online Learning Center at glencoe.com.

> **NCTE 9** Develop an understanding of diversity in language use across cultures.

> **International Cuisine** Discover food and cooking trends from around the world. You can also learn more about specific ingredients and dishes from the culture on this book's Online Learning Center at glencoe.com.

EASY RECIPES — International Flavors

Vietnamese Spring Rolls

Customary	Ingredients	Metric
4	Rice paper wrappers	4
½ cup	Rice vinegar	125 mL
½ cup	Sugar	125 mL
1 Tbsp.	Fresh mint	15 mL
½ Tbsp.	Fish sauce	8 mL
1 tsp.	Ginger, minced	5 mL
1 tsp.	Lemon juice	5 mL
2	Carrots, medium size	2
4	Green lettuce leaves	4
8	Cooked shrimp, cold	8

Vietnamese Flavors
Substitute cooked chicken or pork. Try using sprouts or cabbage instead of carrots.

Yield: 4 servings, one roll each.
1. Submerge rice paper wrappers in cold water to rehydrate them.
2. Combine rice vinegar, sugar, mint, fish sauce, ginger and lemon juice in a bowl. Chill for at least one hour.
3. Cut carrots into thin strips about 2 inches long.
4. Dry and spread out one of the rice paper wrappers. Lay down one of the lettuce leaves on top. Near one side, lay down two shrimp. Top with carrot strips and sprinkle with extra mint.
5. Roll up starting from the side with the shrimp. Stop halfway through, tuck in the sides and finish rolling up. Slice the roll diagonally across the middle. Repeat with the other three wrappers.
6. Serve cold with chilled sauce for dipping.

Nutritional Information Per Serving: 150 calories, 1 g total fat, (0 g saturated fat), 22 mg cholesterol, 236 mg sodium, 35 g total carbohydrate (2 g fiber, 28 g sugars), 4 g protein

Percent Daily Value: vitamin A 130%, vitamin C 10%, calcium 4%, iron 8%

> **Recipes Across Cultures** These nutritiousrecipes bring flavors and ingredients from other countries to your table. You can use the tips located in the recipes to substitute ingredients or make recipes more flavorful!

To the Student

Online Learning Center

Use the Internet to Extend Your Learning

Follow these steps to access the textbook resources at the *Food, Nutrition & Wellness* Online Learning Center.

Online Learning Center Icon Look for this icon throughout the text that directs you to this book's Online Learning Center for more activities and information.

Graphic Organizer Go to this book's Online Learning Center at glencoe.com to print out this graphic organizer.

Step 1
Go to glencoe.com.

Step 2
Select **your state** from the pull-down menu.

Step 3
Select **Student/Parent**.

Step 4
Select **Family & Consumer Sciences**.

Step 5
Click **ENTER**.

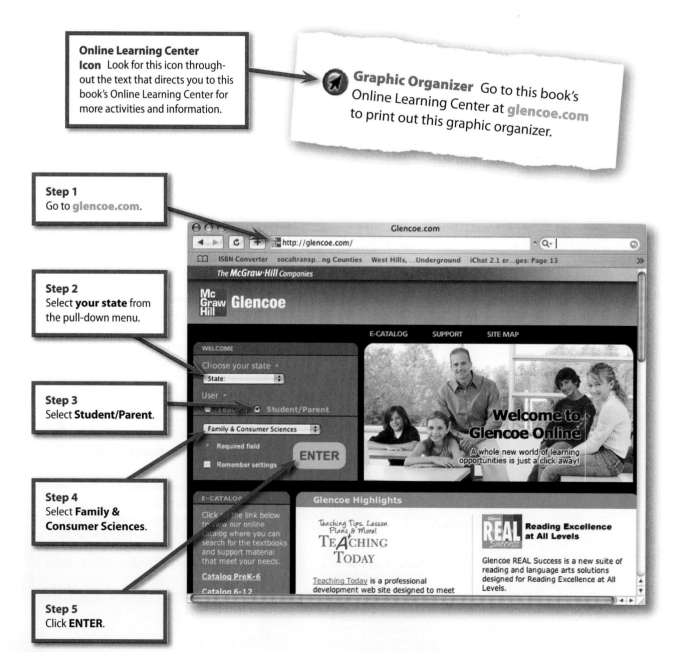

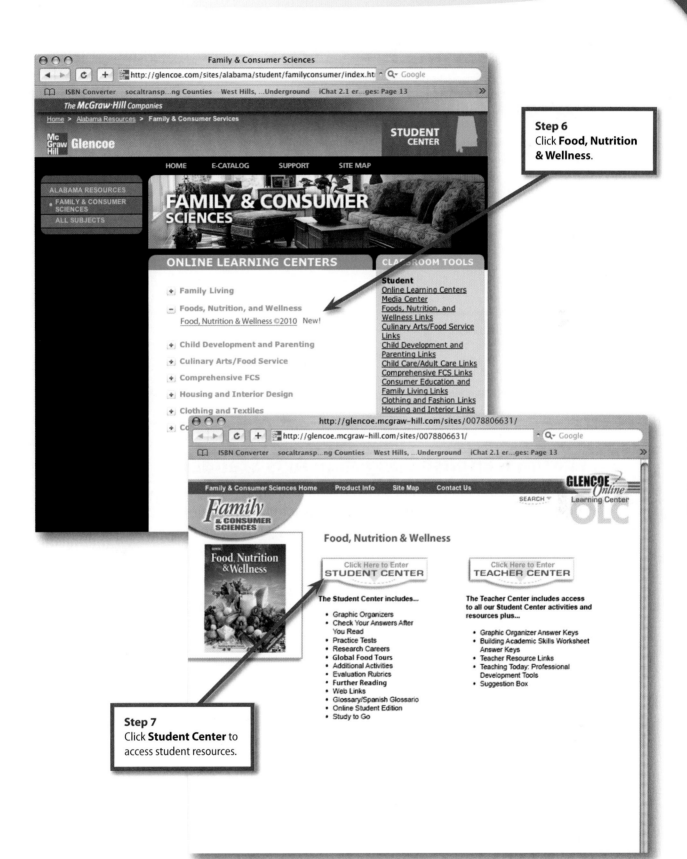

Step 6
Click **Food, Nutrition & Wellness**.

Step 7
Click **Student Center** to access student resources.

Prepare for Academic Success!

By improving your academic skills, you improve your ability to learn and achieve success now and in the future. It also improves your chances of landing a high-skill, high-wage job. The features and assessments in *Food, Nutrition & Wellness* provide many opportunities for you to strengthen your academic skills.

Academic Standards Look for this box throughout the text to know what academic skills you are learning.

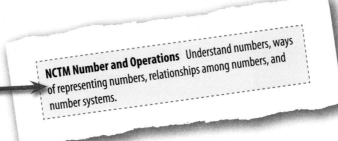

NCTM Number and Operations Understand numbers, ways of representing numbers, relationships among numbers, and number systems.

National English Language Arts Standards

To help incorporate literacy skills (reading, writing, listing, and speaking) into *Food, Nutrition & Wellness,* each section contains a listing of the language arts skills covered. These skills have been developed into standards by the *National Council of Teachers of English and International Reading Association.*

- Read texts to acquire new information.
- Read literature to build an understanding of the human experience.
- Apply strategies to interpret texts.
- Use written language to communicate effectively.
- Use different writing process elements to communicate effectively.
- Conduct research and gather, evaluate, and synthesize data to communicate discoveries.
- Use information resources to gather information and create and communicate knowledge.
- Develop an understanding of diversity in language use across cultures.
- Participate as members of literacy communities.
- Use language to accomplish individual purposes.

National Math Standards

You also have opportunities to practice math skills indicated by standards developed by the *National Council of Teachers of Mathematics*.

- Algebra
- Data Analysis and Probability
- Geometry
- Measurement
- Number and Operations
- Problem Solving

National Science Standards

The *National Science Education Standards* outline these science skills that you can practice in this text.

- Science as Inquiry
- Physical Science
- Life Science
- Earth and Space Science
- Science and Technology
- Science in Personal and Social Perspectives
- History and Nature of Science

National Social Studies Standards

The *National Council for the Social Studies* is another organization that provides standards to help guide your studies. Activities in this text relate to these standards.

- Culture
- Time, Continuity, and Change
- People, Places, and Environments
- Individual Development and Identity
- Individuals, Groups, and Institutions
- Power, Authority, and Governance
- Production, Distribution, and Consumption
- Science, Technology, and Society
- Global Connections
- Civic Ideals and Practices

Reading Skills Handbook

▶ Reading: What's in It for You?

What role does reading play in your life? The possibilities are countless. Are you on a sports team? Perhaps you like to read about the latest news and statistics in sports or find out about new training techniques. Are you looking for a new dish to serve your family? You might be looking for advice about nutrition, cooking techniques, or information about ingredients. Are you enrolled in an English class, an algebra class, or a business class? Then your assignments require a lot of reading.

Improving or Fine-Tuning Your Reading Skills Will:

◆ Improve your grades.
◆ Allow you to read faster and more efficiently.
◆ Improve your study skills.
◆ Help you remember more information accurately.
◆ Improve your writing.

▶ The Reading Process

Good reading skills build on one another, overlap, and spiral around in much the same way that a winding staircase goes around and around while leading you to a higher place. This handbook is designed to help you find and use the tools you will need **before, during,** and **after** reading.

Strategies You Can Use

◆ Identify, understand, and learn new words.
◆ Understand why you read.
◆ Take a quick look at the whole text.
◆ Try to predict what you are about to read.
◆ Take breaks while you read and ask yourself questions about the text.
◆ Take notes.
◆ Keep thinking about what will come next.
◆ Summarize.

▶ Vocabulary Development

Word identification and vocabulary skills are the building blocks of the reading and writing processes. By learning to use a variety of strategies to build your word skills and vocabulary, you will become a stronger reader.

Use Context to Determine Meaning

The best way to expand and extend your vocabulary is to read widely, listen carefully, and participate in a rich variety of discussions. When reading on your own, though, you can often figure out the meanings of new words by looking at their **context,** or the other words and sentences that surround them.

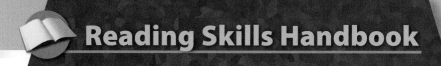

Reading Skills Handbook

Tips for Using Context

Look for clues like these:

◆ A synonym or an explanation of the unknown word in the sentence:
  Elise's shop specialized in millinery, or hats for women.

◆ A reference to what the word is or is not like:
  An archaeologist, like a historian, deals with the past.

◆ A general topic associated with the word:
  The cooking teacher discussed the best way to braise meat.

◆ A description or action associated with the word:
  He used the shovel to dig up the garden.

Predict a Possible Meaning

Another way to determine the meaning of a word is to take the word apart. If you understand the meaning of the **base,** or **root,** part of a word, and also know the meanings of key syllables added either to the beginning or end of the base word, you can usually figure out what the word means.

Word Origins Since Latin, Greek, and Anglo-Saxon roots are the basis for much of our English vocabulary, having some background in languages can be a useful vocabulary tool. For example, *astronomy* comes from the Greek root *astro,* which means relating to the stars. *Stellar* also has a meaning referring to stars, but its origin is Latin. Knowing root words in other languages can help you determine meanings, derivations, and spellings in English.

Prefixes and Suffixes A prefix is a word part that can be added to the beginning of a word. For example, the prefix *semi* means half or partial, so *semicircle* means half a circle. A suffix is a word part that can be added to the end of a word. Adding a suffix often changes a word from one part of speech to another.

Using Dictionaries A dictionary provides the meaning or meanings of a word. Look at the sample dictionary entry on the next page to see what other information it provides.

Thesauruses and Specialized Reference Books A thesaurus provides synonyms and often antonyms. It is a useful tool to expand your vocabulary. Remember to check the exact definition of the listed words in a dictionary before you use a thesaurus. Specialized dictionaries such as *Barron's Dictionary of Business Terms* or *Black's Law Dictionary* list terms and expressions that are not commonly included in a general dictionary. You can also use online dictionaries.

Glossaries Many textbooks and technical works contain condensed dictionaries that provide an alphabetical listing of words used in the text and their specific definitions.

Dictionary Entry

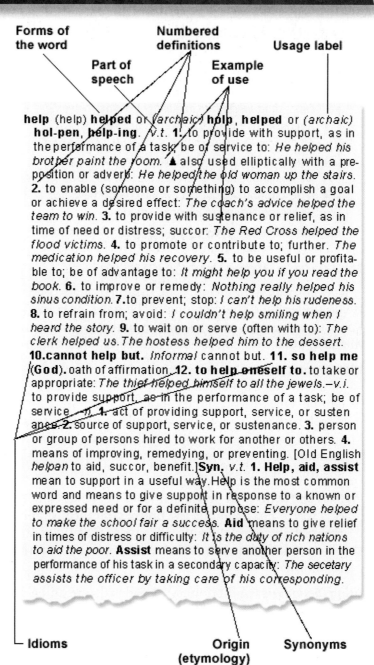

Forms of the word

Numbered definitions

Usage label

Part of speech

Example of use

help (help) helped or (archaic) holp, helped or (archaic) hol-pen, help-ing. v.t. 1. to provide with support, as in the performance of a task; be of service to: *He helped his brother paint the room.* ▲ also used elliptically with a preposition or adverb: *He helped the old woman up the stairs.* 2. to enable (someone or something) to accomplish a goal or achieve a desired effect: *The coach's advice helped the team to win.* 3. to provide with sustenance or relief, as in time of need or distress; succor: *The Red Cross helped the flood victims.* 4. to promote or contribute to; further. *The medication helped his recovery.* 5. to be useful or profitable to; be of advantage to: *It might help you if you read the book.* 6. to improve or remedy: *Nothing really helped his sinus condition.* 7. to prevent; stop: *I can't help his rudeness.* 8. to refrain from; avoid: *I couldn't help smiling when I heard the story.* 9. to wait on or serve (often with to): *The clerk helped us. The hostess helped him to the dessert.* 10. cannot help but. *Informal* cannot but. 11. so help me (God). oath of affirmation. 12. to help oneself to. to take or appropriate: *The thief helped himself to all the jewels.* –v.i. to provide support, as in the performance of a task; be of service. –n. 1. act of providing support, service, or sustenance. 2. source of support, service, or sustenance. 3. person or group of persons hired to work for another or others. 4. means of improving, remedying, or preventing. [Old English *helpan* to aid, succor, benefit.] Syn. v.t. 1. Help, aid, assist mean to support in a useful way. Help is the most common word and means to give support in response to a known or expressed need or for a definite purpose: *Everyone helped to make the school fair a success.* Aid means to give relief in times of distress or difficulty: *It is the duty of rich nations to aid the poor.* Assist means to serve another person in the performance of his task in a secondary capacity: *The secetary assists the officer by taking care of his corresponding.*

Idioms

Origin (etymology)

Synonyms

Recognize Word Meanings Across Subjects Have you learned a new word in one class and then noticed it in your reading for other subjects? The word might not mean exactly the same thing in each class, but you can use the meaning you already know to help you understand what it means in another subject area. For example:

Math Each digit represents a different place **value**.

Health Your **values** can guide you in making healthful decisions.

Economics The **value** of a product is measured in its cost.

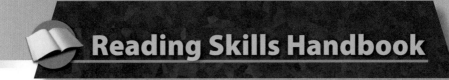

▶ Understanding What You Read

Reading comprehension means understanding—deriving meaning from—what you have read. Using a variety of strategies can help you improve your comprehension and make reading more interesting and more fun.

Read for a Reason

To get the greatest benefit from your reading, **establish a purpose for reading.** In school, you have many reasons for reading, such as:

- to learn and understand new information.
- to find specific information.
- to review before a test.
- to complete an assignment.
- to prepare (research) before you write.

As your reading skills improve, you will notice that you apply different strategies to fit the different purposes for reading. For example, if you are reading for entertainment, you might read quickly, but if you are reading to gather information or follow directions, you might read more slowly, take notes, construct a graphic organizer, or reread sections of text.

Draw on Personal Background

Drawing on personal background may also be called activating prior knowledge. Before you start reading a text, ask yourself questions like these:

- What have I heard or read about this topic?
- Do I have any personal experience relating to this topic?

Using a KWL Chart A KWL chart is a good device for organizing information you gather before, during, and after reading. In the first column, list what you already **know,** then list what you **want** to know in the middle column. Use the third column when you review and assess what you **learned.** You can also add more columns to record places where you found information and places where you can look for more information.

K (What I already know)	W (What I want to know)	L (What I have learned)

Adjust Your Reading Speed Your reading speed is a key factor in how well you understand what you are reading. You will need to adjust your speed depending on your reading purpose.

Scanning means running your eyes quickly over the material to look for words or phrases. Scan when you need a specific piece of information.

Skimming means reading a passage quickly to find its main idea or to get an overview. Skim a text when you preview to determine what the material is about.

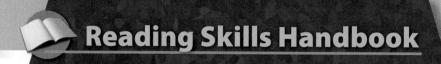

Reading for detail involves careful reading while paying attention to text structure and monitoring your understanding. Read for detail when you are learning concepts, following complicated directions, or preparing to analyze a text.

▶ Techniques to Understand and Remember What You Read

Preview

Before beginning a selection, it is helpful to **preview** what you are about to read.

> **Previewing Strategies**
>
> ◆ Read the title, headings, and subheadings of the selection.
> ◆ Look at the illustrations and notice how the text is organized.
> ◆ Skim the selection: Take a glance at the whole thing.
> ◆ Decide what the main idea might be.
> ◆ Predict what a selection will be about.

Predict

Have you ever read a mystery, decided who committed the crime, and then changed your mind as more clues were revealed? You were adjusting your predictions. Did you smile when you found out that you guessed who committed the crime? You were verifying your predictions.

As you read, make educated guesses about story events and outcomes; that is, **make predictions** before and during reading. This will help you focus your attention on the text and will improve your understanding.

Determine the Main Idea

When you look for the **main idea**, you are looking for the most important statement in a text. Depending on what kind of text you are reading, the main idea can be located at the very beginning (news stories in a newspaper or a magazine) or at the end (scientific research document). Ask yourself the following questions:

• What is each sentence about?
• Is there one sentence that is more important than all the others?
• What idea do details support or point out?

Reading Skills Handbook

Take Notes

Cornell Note-Taking System There are many methods for note taking. The **Cornell Note-Taking System** is a well-known method that can help you organize what you read. To the right is a note-taking activity based on the Cornell Note-Taking System.

Graphic Organizers Using a graphic organizer to retell content in a visual representation will help you remember and retain content. You might make a **chart** or **diagram,** organizing what you have read. Here are some examples of graphic organizers:

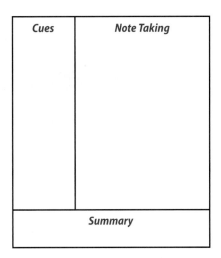

Venn Diagrams When mapping out a compare-and-contrast text structure, you can use a Venn diagram. The outer portions of the circles will show how two characters, ideas, or items contrast, or are different, and the overlapping part will compare two things, or show how they are similar.

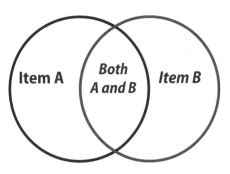

Flow Charts To help you track the sequence of events, or cause and effect, use a flow chart. Arrange ideas or events in their logical, sequential order. Then, draw arrows between your ideas to indicate how one idea or event flows into another.

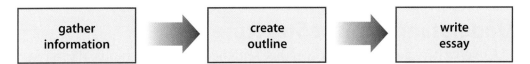

Visualize

Try to form a mental picture of scenes, characters, and events as you read. Use the details and descriptions the author gives you. If you can **visualize** what you read, it will be more interesting and you will remember it better.

Question

Ask yourself questions about the text while you read. Ask yourself about the importance of the sentences, how they relate to one another, if you understand what you just read, and what you think is going to come next.

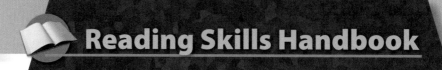
Clarify

If you feel you do not understand meaning (through questioning), try these techniques:

What to Do When You Do Not Understand

◆ Reread confusing parts of the text.
◆ Diagram (chart) relationships between chunks of text, ideas, and sentences.
◆ Look up unfamiliar words.
◆ Talk out the text to yourself.
◆ Read the passage once more.

Review

Take time to stop and review what you have read. Use your note-taking tools (graphic organizers or Cornell notes charts). Also, review and consider your KWL chart.

Monitor Your Comprehension

Continue to check your understanding by using the following two strategies:

Summarize Pause and tell yourself the main ideas of the text and the key supporting details. Try to answer the following questions: Who? What? When? Where? Why? How?

Paraphrase Pause, close the book, and try to retell what you have just read in your own words. It might help to pretend you are explaining the text to someone who has not read it and does not know the material.

▶ Understanding Text Structure

Good writers do not just put together sentences and paragraphs, they organize their writing with a specific purpose in mind. That organization is called text structure. When you understand and follow the structure of a text, it is easier to remember the information you are reading. There are many ways text may be structured. Watch for **signal words**. They will help you follow the text's organization. (Also, remember to use these techniques when you write.)

Compare and Contrast

This structure shows similarities and differences between people, things, and ideas. This is often used to demonstrate that things that seem alike are really different, or vice versa.

Signal words: similarly, more, less, on the one hand/on the other hand, in contrast, but, however

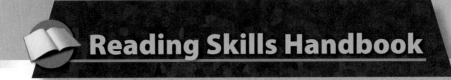

Reading Skills Handbook

Cause and Effect

Writers use the cause-and-effect structure to explore the reasons for something happening and to examine the results or consequences of events.

Signal words: so, because, as a result, therefore, for the following reasons

Problem and Solution

When they organize text around the question *how?*, writers state a problem and suggest solutions.

Signal words: how, help, problem, obstruction, overcome, difficulty, need, attempt, have to, must

Sequence

Sequencing tells you in which order to consider thoughts or facts. Examples of sequencing are:

Chronological order refers to the order in which events take place.

Signal words: first, next, then, finally

Spatial order describes the organization of things in space (to describe a room, for example).

Signal words: above, below, behind, next to

Order of importance lists things or thoughts from the most important to the least important (or the other way around).

Signal words: principal, central, main, important, fundamental

▶ Reading for Meaning

It is important to think about what you are reading to get the most information out of a text, to understand the consequences of what the text says, to remember the content, and to form your own opinion about what the content means.

Interpret

Interpreting is asking yourself, "What is the writer really saying?" and then using what you already know to answer that question.

Infer

Writers do not always state exactly everything they want you to understand. By providing clues and details, they sometimes imply certain information. To **infer** involves using your reason and experience to develop the idea on your own, based on what an author implies, or suggests. What is most important when drawing inferences is to be sure that you have accurately based your guesses on supporting details from the text. If you cannot point to a place in the selection to help back up your inference, you may need to rethink your guess.

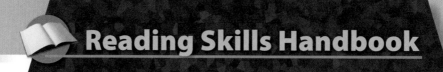

Draw Conclusions

A conclusion is a general statement you can make and explain with reasoning, or with supporting details from a text. If you read a story describing a sport where five players bounce a ball and throw it through a high hoop, you may conclude that the sport is basketball.

Analyze

To understand persuasive nonfiction (a text that discusses facts and opinions to arrive at a conclusion), you need to analyze statements and examples to see if they support the main idea. To understand an informational text (a text, such as a textbook, that gives you information, not opinions), you need to keep track of how the ideas are organized to find the main points.

Hint: Use your graphic organizers and notes charts.

Distinguish Between Facts and Opinions

This is one of the most important reading skills you can learn. A fact is a statement that can be proven. An opinion is what the writer believes. A writer may support opinions with facts, but an opinion cannot be proven. For example:

Fact: California produces fruit and other agricultural products.

Opinion: California produces the best fruit and other agricultural products.

Evaluate

Would you take seriously an article on nuclear fission if you knew it was written by a comedic actor? If you need to rely on accurate information, you need to find out who wrote what you are reading and why. Where did the writer get information? Is the information one-sided? Can you verify the information?

▶ Reading for Research

You will need to **read actively** to research a topic. You might also need to generate an interesting, relevant, and researchable **question** on your own and locate appropriate print and nonprint information from a wide variety of sources. Then, you will need to **categorize** that information, evaluate it, and **organize** it in a new way to produce a research project for a specific audience. Finally, **draw conclusions** about your original research question. These conclusions may lead you to other areas for further inquiry.

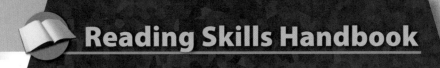
Locate Appropriate Print and Nonprint Information

In your research, try to use a variety of sources. Because different sources present information in different ways, your research project will be more interesting and balanced when you read a variety of sources.

Literature and Textbooks These texts include any book used as a basis for instruction or a source of information.

Book Indices A book index, or a bibliography, is an alphabetical listing of books. Some book indices list books on specific subjects; others are more general. Other indices list a variety of topics or resources.

Periodicals Magazines and journals are issued at regular intervals, such as weekly or monthly. One way to locate information in magazines is to use the *Readers' Guide to Periodical Literature*. This guide is available in print form in most libraries.

Technical Manuals A manual is a guide or handbook intended to give instruction on how to perform a task or operate something. A vehicle owner's manual might give information on how to operate and service a car.

Reference Books Reference books include encyclopedias and almanacs, and are used to locate specific pieces of information.

Electronic Encyclopedias, Databases, and the Internet There are many ways to locate extensive information using your computer. Infotrac, for instance, acts as an online readers' guide. CD encyclopedias can provide easy access to all subjects.

Organize and Convert Information

As you gather information from different sources, taking careful notes, you will need to think about how to **synthesize** the information—that is, convert it into a unified whole, as well as how to change it into a form your audience will easily understand and that will meet your assignment guidelines.

1. First, ask yourself what you want your audience to know.
2. Then, think about a pattern of organization, a structure that will best show your main ideas. You might ask yourself the following questions:

   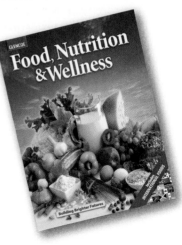

   - When comparing items or ideas, what graphic aids can I use?
   - When showing the reasons something happened and the effects of certain actions, what text structure would be best?
   - How can I briefly and clearly show important information to my audience?
   - Would an illustration or even a cartoon help to make a certain point?

How to Use Technology

Introduction

Technology affects your life in almost every way, both at home and at work. Computers can do wonderful things. They are a path to the libraries of the world. They enhance and enrich your life. You can find the answers to many of your questions on the Internet, often as quickly as the click of your mouse. However, they can also be misused. Knowing some simple guidelines will help you use technology in a safe and secure way.

Practice Safe Surfing!

The Internet can also be a dangerous place. Although there are many Web sites you can freely and safely visit, many others are ones you want to avoid. Before you sign on to any site or visit a chat room, there are several things to consider:

- **Know to whom you are giving the information.** Check that the URL in your browser matches the domain you intended to visit and that you have not been redirected to another site.

- **Never give personal information of any sort** to someone you meet on a Web site or in a chat room, including your name, gender, age, or contact information.

- **Think about why you are giving the information.** For example, if a parent orders something online to be delivered, he or she will need to give an address. But you should never give out your Social Security number, your birth date, or your mother's maiden name without adult consent.

- **Check with a parent or other trusted adult** if you are still unsure whether it is safe to give the information.

Tips for Using the Internet for Research

The Internet is probably the single most important tool for research since the creation of the public library. There is so much information to access on the Internet that it can be difficult to know where to begin.

A good place to start is with a search engine, such as Google. Google is an automated piece of software that searches the Web looking for information. By typing your topic into the search bar, the search engine looks for sites that contain the words you type. You may get many more sites than you expect. Here are some ways to get better results:

> To get the best results when conducting a search online, be sure to spell all your search words correctly.

- ✦ **Place quotes around your topic,** for example, "sports medicine." This will allow you to find the sites where that exact phrase appears.

- ✦ **Use NEAR.** Typing *sports NEAR medicine* will return sites that contain both words and have the two words close to each other.

- ✦ **Exclude unwanted results.** Simply use a minus sign to indicate the words you do not want, for example, "sports medicine" – baseball.

- ✦ **Watch out for advertisements.** If you are using Google, know that the links on the right-hand side of the page, or sometimes at the top in color, are paid links. They may or may not be worth exploring.

- ✦ **Check for relevance.** Google displays a few lines of text from each page and shows your search phrase in bold. Check to see if the site is appropriate for your work.

- ✦ **Look for news.** After you have entered your search phrase and have looked at the results, click on a *News* link on the page. This will show you recent stories about your topic.

- ✦ **Try again!** If you have made an extensive search and not found what you want, start a new search with a different set of words.

- ✦ **Check other sources.** Combine your Internet search with traditional research tools, such as books and magazines.

How to Evaluate Web Sites

Even though there is a ton of information available online, much of this information can be deceptive and misleading, and often incorrect. The books in your library and classroom have been evaluated by scholars and experts. There is no such oversight on the Web. Learning to evaluate Web sites will make you a more savvy surfer and enable you to gather the information you need quickly and easily. When you are trying to decide whether a Web site provides trustworthy information, consider the following:

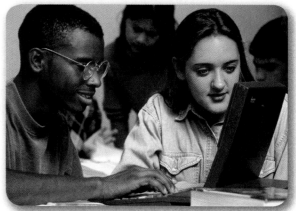

◇ **First, ask, "Who is the author?"** Once you have the name of the author, do a quick Web search to see what else the author has written. Search online for books he or she has written. This information will help you consider whether the person is credible.

◇ **Look at the group offering the information.** Be wary if it is trying to sell a product or service. Look for impartial organizations to provide unbiased information.

◇ **Look for Web sites that provide sources for each of their facts,** just as you do when you write a term paper. Also, look for clues that the information was written by someone knowledgeable. Spelling and grammatical errors are warning signs that the information may not be accurate.

◇ **Check for the date the article was written and when it was last updated.** The more recent the article, the more likely it will be accurate.

◇ **Finally, when using information from a Web site, treat it as you would treat print information.** Anyone can post information on a Web site. Never use information that you cannot verify with another source.

Plagiarism

Using your computer in an ethical manner is simple if you follow certain guidelines. Plagiarism is the act of taking someone else's ideas and passing them off as your own. It does not matter if it is just one or two phrases or an entire paper. Be on guard against falling into the trap of cutting and pasting. This makes plagiarism all too easy.

It is acceptable to quote sources in your work, but you must make sure to identify those sources and give them proper credit. Also, some Web sites do not allow you to quote from them. Be sure to check each site or resource you are quoting to make sure you are allowed to use the material. Remember to cite your sources properly.

Copyright

A copyright protects someone who creates an original work. This can be a single sentence, a book, a play, or a piece of music. If you create it, you are the owner. Copyright protection is provided by the Copyright Act of 1976, a federal statute.

If you want to use a portion of a copyrighted work in your own work, you need to obtain permission from the copyright holder. That might be a publisher of a book, an author, an organization, or an estate. Most publishers are willing to grant permission to individuals for educational purposes. If you want to reproduce information you found on the Web, contact the Webmaster or author of the article to request permission.

Once a work's copyright has expired, anywhere from 28 to 67 years from the date of creation, it is considered to be in the public domain and anyone can reprint it as he or she pleases. Remember the following tips:

◇ **What is copyrighted?** Original work published after March 1989 is copyrighted, whether it says so or not.

◇ **Can I copy from the Internet?** Copying information from the Internet is a serious breach of copyright. Check the site's *Terms of Use* to see what you can and cannot do.

◇ **Can I edit copyrighted work?** You cannot change copyrighted material, that is, make "derivative works" based on existing material.

Student Organizations and FCCLA

What Is a Student Organization?

A student organization is a group or association of students that is formed around activities, such as:

- Family and consumer sciences
- Student government
- Community service
- Social clubs
- Honor societies
- Multicultural alliances
- Technology education
- Artists and performers
- Politics
- Sports teams
- Professional career development

A student organization is usually required to follow a set of rules and regulations that apply equally to all student organizations at a particular school.

Why Should You Get Involved?

Being an active part of a student organization opens a variety of experiences to you. Many student clubs are part of a national network of students and professionals, which provides the chance to connect to a wider variety of students and opportunities.

What's In It for You?

Participation in student organizations can contribute to a more enriching learning experience. Here are some ways you can benefit:

- Gain leadership qualities and skills that make you more marketable to employers and universities.
- Demonstrate the ability to appreciate someone else's point of view.
- Interact with professionals to learn about their different industries.
- Explore your creative interests, share ideas, and collaborate with others.
- Take risks, build confidence, and grow creatively.
- Learn valuable skills while speaking or performing in front of an audience.
- Make a difference in your life and the lives of those around you.
- Learn the importance of civic responsibility and involvement.
- Build relationships with instructors, advisors, students, and other members of the community who share similar backgrounds/world views.

Find and Join a Student Organization!

Take a close look at the organizations offered at your school or within your community. Are there any organizations that interest you? Talk to your teachers, guidance counselors, or a parent or guardian. Usually, posters or flyers for a variety of clubs and groups can be found on your school's Message Board or Web site. Try to locate more information about the organizations that meet your needs. Then, think about how these organizations can help you gain valuable skills you can use at school, at work, and in your community.

Student Organizations and FCCLA

What Is FCCLA?

Family, Career and Community Leaders of America (FCCLA) is a national career and technical student organization for students in Family and Consumer Sciences. Involvement in FCCLA offers members the opportunity to expand their leadership potential and explore careers. FCCLA lets you make a difference in your family, your career, and your community. Involvement offers members the opportunity to expand their leadership potential and develop skills for life—planning, goal setting, problem solving, decision making, character development, interpersonal communication, and career development.

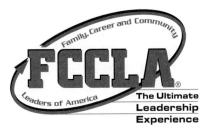

STAR Events Program

STAR Events (Students Taking Action with Recognition) are competitive events in which members are recognized for proficiency and achievement in chapter and individual projects, leadership skills, and occupational preparation. FCCLA provides opportunities for you to participate at local, state, and national levels.

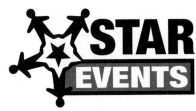

What Are the Purposes of FCCLA?

1. Provide opportunities for personal development and preparation for adult life.
2. Strengthen the function of the family as a basic unit of society.
3. Encourage democracy through cooperative action in the home and community.
4. Encourage individual and group involvement in helping achieve global cooperation and harmony.
5. Promote greater understanding between youth and adults.
6. Provide opportunities for making decisions and for assuming responsibilities.
7. Prepare for the multiple roles of men and women in today's society.
8. Promote family and consumer sciences and related occupations.

Unit 1

Choose Wellness

Chapters in this Unit

Chapter 1   Wellness and Food Choices
Chapter 2   Physical Fitness and Active Living

Unit Thematic Project Preview

Study Physical Activities

While studying this unit, you will learn the importance of following good health practices for a lifetime. You will learn that physical activity and healthful foods are a big part of a healthy lifestyle. In the unit thematic project at the end of this unit, you will find out how different types of physical activity benefit you in different ways. You will also find out about places in your community where you can take part in various types of physical activities.

My Journal

Food choices and physical activity have a huge impact on an individual's overall health and wellness for a lifetime. Write a journal entry that answers these questions:

- What are your favorite foods and why?
- In what physical activities did you participate this week?
- Do your food choices and physical activities have a positive impact on your health? Why or why not?

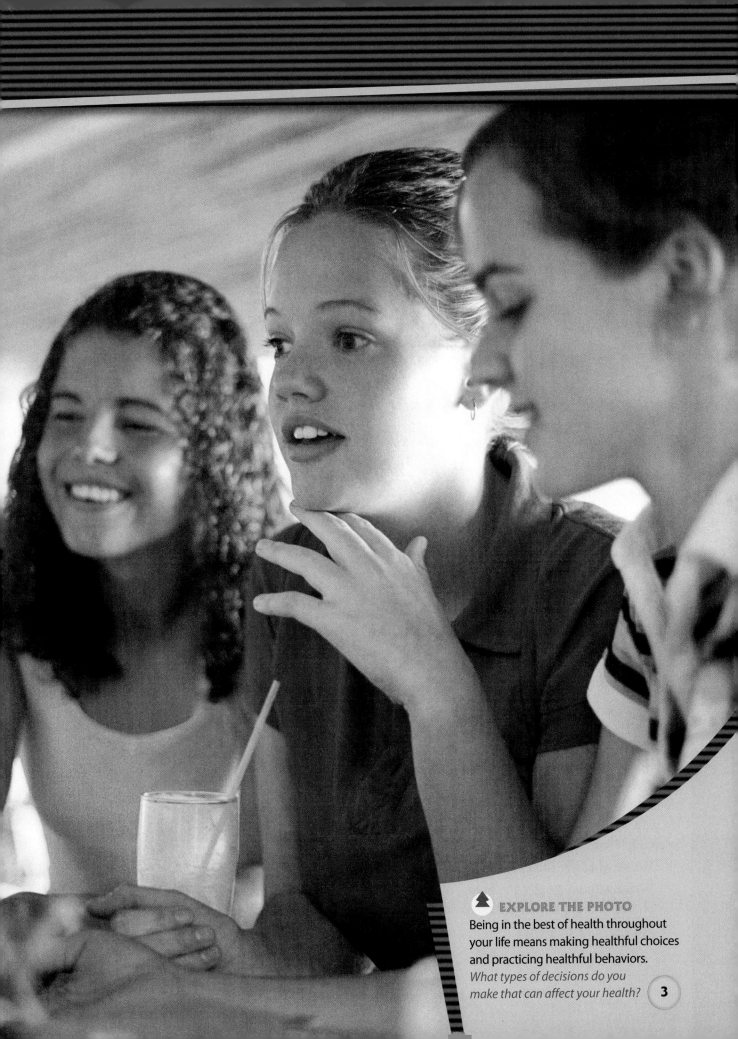

EXPLORE THE PHOTO
Being in the best of health throughout
your life means making healthful choices
and practicing healthful behaviors.
*What types of decisions do you
make that can affect your health?*

3

CHAPTER 1
Wellness and Food Choices

Explore the Photo ▶▶
The key to wellness is making the most of who you are! *How can you take personal responsibility for your health and well-being now?*

Writing Activity
Freewriting

Write About an Event Remember a family get-together, party, or other event where food was served. Freewrite about the event, the food, and the people. Describe how the food tasted, smelled, and looked. Remember the people you ate with and the conversations you had.

Writing Tips

1. **Write** whatever comes to mind.
2. **Write** without stopping to reread, re-phrase, or rethink what you are saying.
3. **Set** a definite time limit.

Reading Guide

Before You Read

Preview Read the Key Concepts below. Write one or two sentences predicting what you think this chapter will be about.

Read to Learn

Key Concepts

- **Identify** four aspects of wellness.
- **Describe** influences on your food choices.
- **Explain** how appetite, hunger, and flavor affect wellness.
- **Demonstrate** how to make decisions and reach goals for wellness.

Main Idea

It is your responsibility to make choices that lead to good health. The key to good health is a healthful lifestyle.

Content Vocabulary

- ◇ wellness
- ◇ lifestyle
- ◇ nutrition
- ◇ stress
- ◇ culture
- ◇ hunger
- ◇ appetite
- ◇ flavor
- ◇ papillae
- ◇ action plan

Academic Vocabulary

You will find these words in your reading and on your tests. Use the glossary to look up their definitions if necessary.

- ■ factor
- ■ resource

Graphic Organizer

Use a graphic organizer like the one below to write notes about the different influences on the foods you eat and enjoy. In each circle, write things that influence your wellness in that area.

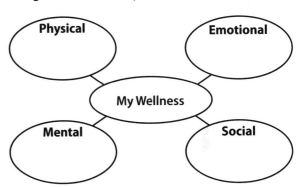

 Graphic Organizer Go to this book's Online Learning Center at **glencoe.com** to print out this graphic organizer.

Academic Standards ●

 English Language Arts
NCTE 12 Use language to accomplish individual purposes.

 Mathematics
NCTM Measurement Apply appropriate techniques, tools, and formulas to determine measurements.

NCTM Number and Operations Understand the meanings of operations and how they relate to one another.

 Science
NSES Content Standard F Develop an understanding of personal and community health.

NCTE National Council of Teachers of English
NCTM National Council of Teachers of Mathematics

NSES National Science Education Standards
NCSS National Council for the Social Studies

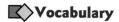
Vocabulary

You can find definitions in the glossary at the back of this book.

Wellness Is Your Choice for Life!

Wellness means reaching for your best level of health. Good health can improve your appearance, self-esteem, ability to handle stress, and physical and mental performance. Healthy people generally live longer and spend less on health care. To achieve wellness, you need to take actions to achieve good physical, mental, emotional, and social health.

Wellness does not mean having a perfect body or never having health problems. Many factors that affect your health are out of your control, such as genetics or a certain life event. A **factor** is an element that contributes to a particular result. When wellness is a lifelong priority, however, you reduce your risk for illness and get well faster when you do get sick.

A Healthful Lifestyle Is the Key to Good Health

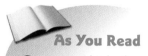
As You Read

Connect Think of some of the things that you do to improve your health.

The key to overall good health is a healthful **lifestyle**, which includes how you live your life and everything you do. For example, if you are always on the go, you may plan quick meals or eat away from home a lot. For a healthful lifestyle, you need:

◆ Regular physical activity.

◆ Effective ways to manage stress.

◆ Good nutrition. **Nutrition** refers to the processes by which your body uses nutrients in food for growth, energy, and maintenance.

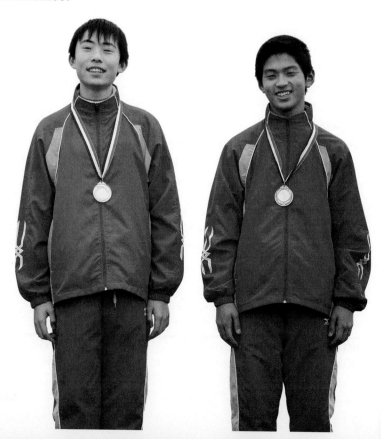

Your Wellness Habits Staying well is its own reward. Making smart choices now can help you live an active, enjoyable life for many years to come. *Name at least four actions that can help you to maintain or improve your physical health.*

Good Physical Health

When your body is working the way it should, you are in good physical health. You have firm skin, clean teeth and healthy gums, good muscle tone, erect posture, healthy weight, and bright, clear eyes. You also have all the energy you need for daily living. You grow at a normal rate, your body resists illness, and you are able to relax and sleep well.

Take Action for Your Physical Health

Follow these guidelines to promote or improve your physical health:

- Eat enough nutritious foods, and do not overeat.
- Eat breakfast daily.
- Choose meals and snacks wisely.
- Maintain a healthy weight.
- Drink enough water or other fluids daily.
- Include physical activity in your life—at least 60 minutes daily.
- Sleep at least eight hours daily. Growing, changing bodies need more sleep than adult bodies do.
- Follow good hygiene habits.
- Wear your seatbelt in the car and safety gear for sports.
- Get regular medical and dental checkups.
- Avoid tobacco, alcoholic beverages, and harmful drugs.
- Stay informed about nutrition and wellness.

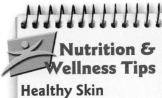

Nutrition & Wellness Tips

Healthy Skin

✓ For acne control, cleanse your skin each morning and night.

✓ Get enough rest.

✓ Eat for good nutrition.

Mental and Emotional Health

How you deal with daily life and how you feel about yourself reflect your mental and emotional health. Feelings affect health more than you might think. For example, overeating or avoiding food when you are unhappy or bored can affect your weight.

People with good mental and emotional health have a positive attitude. They are often in good physical health and enjoy life. They are able to cope with change, face problems, and handle anger and disappointment. Emotionally healthy people are open-minded, confident, sensitive to the needs and feelings of others, and able to work toward goals.

How to Deal with Stress

Most people feel tense or overwhelmed from time to time. These reactions are forms of stress. **Stress** is mental, emotional, or physical strain. Stress is unavoidable, but you can control how you react to it.

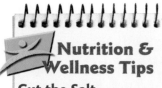

**Nutrition &
Wellness Tips**

Cut the Salt

✓ If you cut back on salt in your food gradually, your desire for salty foods will decrease gradually, too.

Stress is a part of life. It is not always bad. It can give you energy to face challenges and do your best. Uncontrolled stress, however, can have negative effects on you. For example, being upset for too long can disturb your sleep and digestion.

Follow these guidelines to handle stress in positive ways:

◆ Maintain good physical health.

◆ Balance school and work responsibilities with time for family and friends. Do not try to do too much.

◆ Take time every day for rest and fun. Enjoy a hobby.

◆ Accept that you cannot control every situation. Relax and do something constructive to avoid tension.

◆ Admit mistakes and learn from them, but do not dwell on them.

◆ Be an optimist. Find the good in people and situations.

◆ Keep a sense of humor. Laughter relieves tension.

◆ Discuss things that worry you with someone you trust.

◆ Set goals and priorities and make positive decisions. Break large tasks into smaller steps so you can stay on track.

Social Health

Social health involves your relationships. When you are socially healthy, you can:

◆ Praise others, and accept and appreciate their differences.

◆ Enjoy friends of both genders and all ages.

◆ Be helpful and considerate.

◆ Accept rules and be responsible.

◆ Handle conflict in constructive ways.

◆ Communicate well.

◆ Handle peer pressure in ways that respect your values.

✓ **Reading Check** **List** What are some characteristics of physical, mental and emotional, and social health?

Why You Eat What You Eat

People's food choices and eating patterns differ for many reasons. It is important to recognize the factors that influence your food choices. Culture is one important factor. **Culture** is the shared beliefs, values, and behaviors of a group of people. Resources are another factor. A **resource** is something you use to get what you want, meet goals, and complete tasks. Resources include time, money, and personal energy. **Figure 1.1** on page 9 lists and describes many factors that influence what you eat.

Figure 1.1   **Influences on Eating**

Food Choice Factors It is important to recognize the factors that influence your food choices. *Which of these influences do you think has the greatest effect on your personal food choices?*

Influence	Description
Your Family	Many food likes and dislikes, eating habits, and food traditions begin at home. For example, you may like chicken the way your family makes it. Your favorite dish also may be part of your family heritage.
Your Friends	Eating is often part of getting together with friends. People within a group often eat the same kind of food. Does peer pressure affect your food choices? Are you a good influence on your friends' choices?
Culture and Religion	Music, art, and foods are expressions of culture. Cultural influences include your local community, ethnic or religious group, nation, and region. Different cultural and religious groups have different food traditions.
Available Foods	The foods you eat are mostly those sold or grown near where you live. What can you get from grocery stores, farmers' markets, schools, restaurants, vending machines, and perhaps your garden?
Lifestyle, Energy, and Budget	The foods you buy and the ways you prepare them are influenced by your resources, which are the time, money, and personal energy that help you reach goals and complete tasks. When time is short, you might use prepared foods or eat out.
Trends and Technology	New discoveries, lifestyle trends, and health concerns can affect your food choices. For example, the introduction of the microwave oven made it easy to cook food quickly. Because of the obesity trend in the United States today, health agencies are urging people to eat more vegetables, fruits, and whole-grain foods.
The Media	Advertisements can influence you to buy certain foods, whether you need them or not. The media also provides useful information, such as news about fitness and healthful eating.
Knowledge	Knowing the facts about food, nutrition, and wellness can help you buy, prepare, and eat foods that fit your wellness goals.
Emotions	Food is often linked to emotions. You may want comfort foods when you feel negative emotions, such as loneliness, boredom, or sadness. Handling emotions in a positive way can help you eat healthfully.
Priorities	When you make wellness a priority, healthful eating habits follow.

Make Time for Family Meals

For families with busy schedules, eating together is often a special occasion instead of a regular event. Many families make a special effort to eat together at home as often as possible. Dining together helps parents set a good example for their children. It can also promote positive feelings about healthful eating. In some families, all members help cook the meal and clean up afterward.

Studies show that eating together helps family members eat healthier. Research has shown that children who regularly have meals with their parents eat more fruits, vegetables, and calcium-rich foods. They also eat more vitamins and nutrients and more nourishing food. Some research shows that family members who regularly eat together are at lower risk for unhealthy behaviors such as smoking and drug and alcohol use.

Help your family make the most of mealtime with the following tips:

◆ Plan at least one meal a week when your whole family can be together.

◆ Stay at the table until everyone is finished.

◆ Join in on family conversation. Save unpleasant topics for later. Turn off the TV.

◆ Extend your time together by sharing the cooking and cleaning duties.

✓ **Reading Check** **Explain** What factors influence people's food decisions?

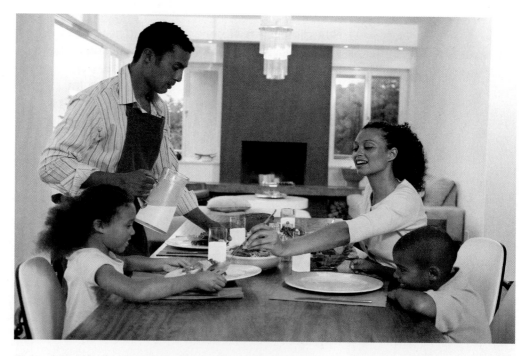

Eat as a Family Family meals offer a chance to share everyday experiences, enjoy being together, and learn from one another. *How can you make family meals at home a fun experience?*

Enjoying Food for Wellness

Think about the last time you walked into your house while someone was cooking, or the last barbeque you went to. Did the smells make you hungry? The taste and the aroma, or smell, of food make eating one of life's great pleasures. When you eat for wellness, you choose from a wide variety of great-tasting foods. Your food choices and eating experiences will add enjoyment to your everyday life.

Hunger or Appetite?

Sometimes, just the sight of tasty food can make your mouth water. If a delicious aroma reaches your nose, you might find it hard to think about anything else! Is this hunger you are experiencing, or is it your appetite?

- ◆ **Hunger** An empty stomach that contracts or growls signals hunger. **Hunger** is a physical need for food. Hunger pangs tell your body that you need a fresh supply of energy and nutrients. Tiredness or a light-headed feeling signals hunger, too. Once you have eaten enough, your hunger disappears after about 20 minutes. That is how long it takes for your stomach to send a full message to your brain. Instead of gulping your food, eat slowly. You will enjoy it more and be less likely to overeat.

- ◆ **Appetite** The sight, aroma, and taste of food can stimulate your appetite. An **appetite** is a psychological desire for food. The sight of appealing food can make you think you are hungry, even when you are not. Even sound, such as popping corn or food sizzling on a grill, can stir up your appetite. A good appetite is a sign of wellness.

How can you tell whether you are hungry, or whether you simply crave a certain appetizing food? Think about whether you would be satisfied by a healthful meal or snack, such as a salad, a sandwich, or a piece of fruit. If not, perhaps you are craving a food simply because it looks appetizing.

You can make nutritious food look appetizing by serving it in an appealing way. How food looks affects your desire to eat in a powerful way.

Math in Action

Increasing Recipes

Recipes indicate the amount they yield, or produce. If you want more or less yield, you will need to adjust the ingredient quantities. Convert the measurements in the Fruit, Granola, and Yogart Parfait recipe on page 14 so that the recipe will yield twice as much. Rewrite the recipe using both customary and metric units.

Math Concept **Convert Measurements**
To convert measurements, you will use multiplication or division. You multiply to increase the value. You divide to reduce it.

Starting Hint To double whole numbers, all you need to do is to multiply by 2. To double fractions, multiply by $\frac{2}{1}$.

NCTM Measurement Apply appropriate techniques, tools, and formulas to determine measurements.

 Math For more math help, go to the Math Appendix

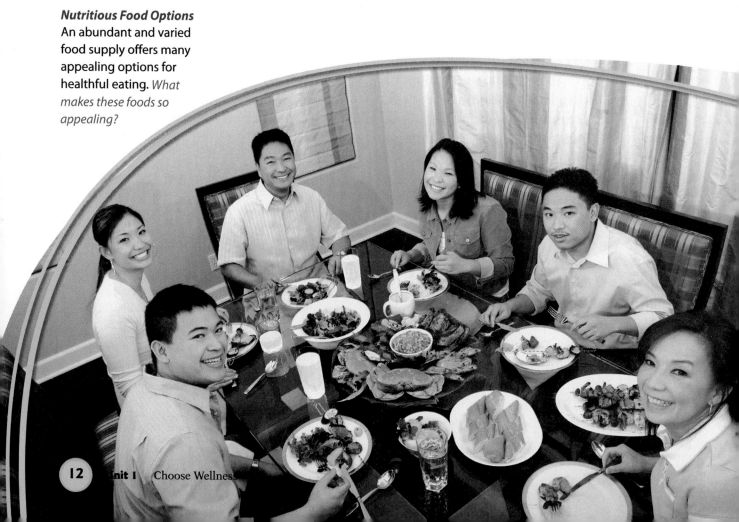

Nutrition & Wellness Tips

Snacks on Hand

✓ Ask your family to keep nutritious snack foods, such as raw vegetables, fruit, cheese and whole-grain crackers, and fat-free milk, on hand to satisfy your hunger.

Sensing Food's Flavor

Your senses help you experience and enjoy food. Chile peppers may feel fiery hot; ice cream feels cold and creamy.

When people talk about taste, they often mean flavor. **Flavor** is the combination of a food's taste, smell, and texture. People experience flavor differently. That is one reason why different people like different foods. Flavors of spinach or salsa may seem stronger to you than to a friend. Children often have a keener flavor sense than adults do—especially older adults.

You taste with your mouth, mostly with your tongue. Your tongue is covered with papillae. **Papillae** (pə-'pi-(ˌ)lē) are tiny bumps that contain taste buds. Each papilla has hundreds of taste buds, which distinguish sweet, sour, salty, bitter, and umami. Umami (ü-'mä-mē) is the brothlike taste in meat, vegetables, and cheese. Other nerve endings in your mouth sense foods' texture and temperature.

Have you noticed that food does not taste the same when you have a cold? The flavor changes because you cannot smell as well. Smell accounts for about 80 percent of flavor. Illness and medication can dull your senses and take away your sense of flavor.

✓ **Reading Check** **Compare** What is the difference between hunger and appetite?

Nutritious Food Options An abundant and varied food supply offers many appealing options for healthful eating. *What makes these foods so appealing?*

Steps to Wellness

When you make decisions for wellness, you make a positive difference in your life both today and in the future. Making responsible decisions and taking positive action are important skills.

Choose Wellness

Every day, you make many decisions. Will you eat breakfast? Will you walk to school? Over time, these decisions add up and affect your health. To reach your wellness goals, follow a decision-making process of seven steps:

1. **Identify the decision to make.** It may be simple or complex.

2. **Collect information and identify your resources.** Get facts from reliable sources. Use critical thinking skills to judge what you see, read, and hear.

3. **Identify possible choices.** You have many different options for food and physical activity. For physical activity. For example, you can jog alone, or join a team.

4. **Consider possible choices.** What are the pros and cons of each option? What are your priorities? When health is a priority, wellness decisions are easier to make.

5. **Choose the best option.** Make choices based on facts, goals, priorities, and values, not peer pressure. An ice cream sundae may not be the best snack if you are watching your weight.

6. **Take action.** Use the action steps for wellness on page 14.

7. **Evaluate your decision.** Did you get the results you expected? How did your decision affect others? What did you learn? Would you make the same choice again?

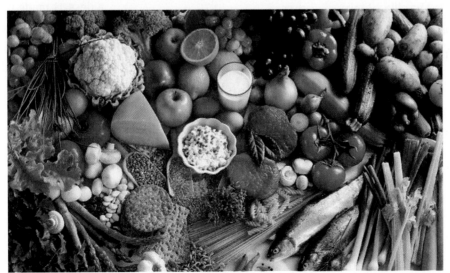

Family and Consumer Sciences Teacher

Family and consumer sciences teachers teach life skills, including wellness skills. They plan and teach lessons and work with students, parents, and school administrators.

Careers Find out more about careers. Go to this book's Online Learning Center at glencoe.com.

Take Action for Wellness

An **action plan** is a step-by-step strategy to identify and achieve your goals. Follow these action steps for wellness. Set goals and track your progress toward meeting them:

1. **Set realistic goals.** Match your goals to your abilities and needs.

2. **Make a plan.** Use the decision-making process to choose the best option for reaching your goal.

3. **Identify small, doable steps.** Each small step builds self-confidence and brings you closer to success.

4. **Take action.** Make your plan a reality.

5. **Stick with it.** Challenges happen. Find ways to get back on track when you are low on energy or time.

6. **Get support.** Ask family, friends, and teachers to support you. Return the favor and support others.

7. **Check your progress and your efforts.** Are your goals realistic? Are you giving your best effort? How close are your goals? Learn from experience. Revise your plan as needed.

8. **Reward yourself.** Reward yourself in a healthful way when you reach a goal. Enjoy taking care of yourself!

EASY RECIPES
Everyday Favorites

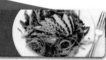

Fruit, Granola, and Yogurt Parfait

Customary	Ingredients	Metric
½ cup	Low-fat granola	125 mL
6 oz.	Low-fat vanilla or lemon yogurt	175 g
½ cup	Sliced strawberries or bananas	125 mL
1 Tbsp.	Chopped nuts	15 mL

Did You Know!
A parfait (pär-fā) is a dessert made of ice cream or yogurt layered with garnishes and served in a tall glass.

Yield: 1 serving, 1¾ cups (425 mL)

❶ Layer ¼ cup (60 mL) granola, 3 oz. (90 g) yogurt, and ¼ cup (60 mL) strawberries or bananas in a clear drinking glass or bowl.
❷ Repeat the layers of granola, yogurt, and strawberries or bananas.
❸ Top with nuts.

Nutritional Information Per Serving: 432 calories, 9 g total fat, (2 g saturated fat), 4 mg cholesterol, 190 mg sodium, 71 g total carbohydrates (6 g fiber, 49 g total sugars), 16 g protein

Percent Daily Value: vitamin A 0%, vitamin C 70%, calcium 30%, iron 4%

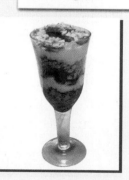

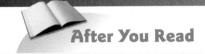

After You Read

CHAPTER SUMMARY
Wellness involves all aspects of your health: physical, emotional, mental, and social. Good nutrition is key to wellness. Factors that influence your food preferences, food choices, and eating habits include culture, resources, food availability, and knowledge. Appetite, hunger, and the sensory qualities of food affect your desire and need to eat. To eat smart and live a healthful lifestyle, set goals, make responsible decisions, and follow a careful action plan that matches your needs and lifestyle.

Vocabulary Review

1. Use each of these vocabulary words in a sentence.

Content Vocabulary
- wellness (p. 6)
- lifestyle (p. 6)
- nutrition (p. 6)
- stress (p. 7)
- culture (p. 8)
- hunger (p. 11)
- appetite (p. 11)
- flavor (p. 12)
- papillae (p. 12)
- action plan (p. 14)

Academic Vocabulary
- factor (p. 6)
- resource (p. 8)

Review Key Concepts

2. Identify four aspects of wellness.

3. Describe influences on your food choices.

4. Explain how appetite, hunger, and flavor affect wellness.

5. Demonstrate how to make decisions and reach goals for wellness.

Critical Thinking

6. Evaluate the following scenario and give suggestions to help Jamie manage her time and energy for wellness. Jamie feels overwhelmed. She plays trumpet in a marching band, works part-time, and serves as Spanish Club treasurer. She eats lunch and dinner but often skips breakfast.

7. Compare and contrast positive stress and negative stress. Write two paragraphs that give at least two examples of stressful situations that many teens face.

8. Design a wellness action plan to achieve a goal that would promote your health, such as fitting more regular physical activity into your daily life.

9. Explain how positive and negative relationships with people may affect wellness.

Real-World Skills and Applications

Decision Making

10. Promote Family Meals Eating as a family is linked to healthful eating and wellness. Family meals can be hard to fit into busy schedules, especially for teens. With your family, set a goal for regular family meals. Write a list of actions your family can take together to meet that goal.

Technology

11. Wellness Technology Many new occupations related to wellness have been created in the past few decades. Locate a wellness, health, or fitness business that uses new technology. Make an oral presentation and explain how the business uses technology to promote wellness.

Interpersonal

12. Leadership Achieving wellness requires taking responsibility for your own health. Write a paragraph that answers these questions: What responsibility, if any, do individuals have for the health of others? How can you take a leadership role in promoting wellness in your community?

Financial Literacy

13. Save Money and Help the Environment Some grocery stores give a small discount when customers bring their own bags. Imagine that you reuse five bags a week for a year. If the store subtracts 5¢ per bag from the bill, how much will you save by reusing bags for a year?

14. Community Wellness Many hospitals and community agencies sponsor wellness programs and events, such as health fairs, fitness events, walk-a-thons, and wellness classes. Find out about a community wellness program or event where you live. Write a paragraph describing it. Explain how people in the community can volunteer to help.

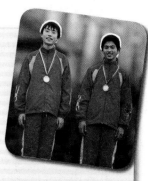

15. School Wellness Policy Schools with government-funded breakfast and lunch programs must have a Local School Wellness Policy. Find out if your school has such a policy. What does it say? Who developed it? How is it carried out? Write an article for your school newspaper that tells how teens can support it.

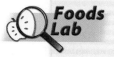

16. Blind Taste Test Conduct a blind taste test of these foods: apple, orange, broccoli, mustard, and onion. While blindfolded, try to identify each food by its taste and smell. Hold your nose and repeat the demonstration. Can you identify the foods now? Write a summary of the experiment and explain your conclusions.

Additional Activities For additional activities go to this book's Online Learning Center at glencoe.com.

Academic Skills

 English Language Arts

17. Identifying Influences Think of a recent meal in which each food you chose was the result of one or more influences. Create a menu for the meal. Annotate the menu with the various influences for each food.

> **NCTE 12** Use language to accomplish individual purposes.

 Science

18. Risks and Benefits An action plan is a step-by-step strategy to identify and achieve your goals. Create an action plan for wellness.

Procedure Conduct research about things that you can do to maintain good health.

Analysis Make a list of three things you can do to maintain good health. Then list the risks and benefits of the three items. Include social, physical, time-related, environmental, and mental factors.

> **NSES Content Standard F** Develop an understanding of personal and community health.

 Mathematics

19. Calculate Cooking Time Darcy and Bennet are cooking a roast for Sunday dinner. It takes approximately 25 minutes of cooking time for every pound of roast beef used. The recipe they are making calls for a 3-pound (1 kg) roast. How long should Darcy and Bennet cook the meat before it is safe to eat? How will they know for certain that the roast is done?

Math Concept **Time** In problems that involve measuring time, it is important to remember conversions. There are 60 seconds in a minute. There are 60 minutes in an hour.

Starting Hint First, find the minutes needed to cook 1 pound of meat:
25 minutes × 3 lbs. = x

 For more math help, go to the Math Appendix

> **NCTM Number and Operations** Understand the meanings of operations and how they relate to one another.

STANDARDIZED TEST PRACTICE

MULTIPLE CHOICE
Read the following paragraph and choose the best answer. Write your answer on a separate piece of paper.

Test-Taking Tip After you have read the paragraph, read the question and the answer choices. Read the paragraph again before choosing the answer. Skim the paragraph once more if you are still unsure.

Everyone needs fiber. Fruits and vegetables contain fiber. Fiber is also found in whole-wheat pasta, oatmeal, brown rice, and whole-grain breads. All of these foods come from plants.

20. Based on the paragraph, which of the following statements is true?
   a. Fiber is only for older people.
   b. One serving of spaghetti is enough fiber for the week.
   c. Fiber comes from plants.
   d. Doctors do not recommend fiber.

CHAPTER 2
Physical Fitness and Active Living

Explore the Photo ▶▶

Daily Activity Moving more and sitting less is a smart habit for teens to follow. *Why do you think living an active lifestyle is a smart decision to make?*

✏ Writing Activity

Write About an Event

Active Living Think about the last time you spent an active day. How did you feel at the end of the day? Write two paragraphs about that day and how you felt when it was over. Were you tired? Were you energized? Think about the rewards that come with active living.

Writing Tips

1. **Describe** what you did that day.
2. **Explain** how you felt before and after.
3. **Use** details that make the day come to life for the reader.

Reading Guide

Before You Read

Preview Look at the photos and figures in this chapter and read their captions. Begin thinking about how physical activity benefits overall health.

Read to Learn
Key Concepts
- **Describe** how physical activity promotes fitness.
- **Identify** the benefits of active living.
- **Discuss** your plan for making physical activity part of your daily life.
- **Identify** safety and health precautions for physical activity.
- **Explain** how to check the progress of your plan for active living.

Main Idea
When you enjoy physical activity and do it regularly, it can become a lifelong habit. Many activities offer fitness benefits.

Content Vocabulary
- physical fitness
- physical activity
- strength
- endurance
- cardiorespiratory endurance
- aerobic activity
- flexibility
- calorie
- sedentary
- intensity
- dehydration

Academic Vocabulary
You will find these words in your reading and on your tests. Use the glossary to look up their definitions if necessary.
- percentage
- potential

Graphic Organizer
As you read, use a pyramid like the one below to list the activities you do every day and plan how often you should do them.

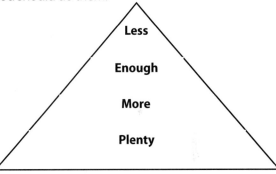

Less

Enough

More

Plenty

 Graphic Organizer Go to this book's Online Learning Center at glencoe.com to print out this graphic organizer.

Academic Standards

 English Language Arts
NCTE 7 Conduct research and gather, evaluate, and synthesize data to communicate discoveries.
NCTE 8 Use information resources to gather information and create and communicate knowledge.
NCTE 9 Develop an understanding of diversity in language use across cultures.

 Mathematics
NCTM Number and Operations Understand the meanings of operations and how they relate to one another.

 Science
NSES Content Standard A Develop understandings about scientific inquiry.

 Social Studies
NCSS IV D Individual Development and Identity Apply concepts, methods, and theories about the study of human growth and development.

NCTE National Council of Teachers of English
NCTM National Council of Teachers of Mathematics
NSES National Science Education Standards
NCSS National Council for the Social Studies

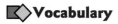
Vocabulary

You can find definitions in the glossary at the back of this book.

What Is Physical Fitness?

Physical fitness means having the energy and ability to do everything you want and need to do in your daily life. You are fit if you can meet the physical demands of an active lifestyle. This includes regular chores as well as exercise.

Along with good nutrition, the way to achieve physical fitness is through exercise, or physical activity. **Physical activity** means using your muscles to move your body. The more physically active you are, the more fit you are likely to be.

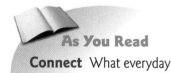

As You Read

Connect What everyday activities do you do that help increase your strength?

Muscular Strength and Endurance

Strength is the power to work your muscles against resistance. When your muscles push and pull, they get stronger. Strong muscles help you lift heavy objects without strain. Common ways to build strength include push-ups, chin-ups, by using resistance bands, or even dancing. **Endurance** is the ability to continue physical activity for a long time without your muscles becoming too tired.

Cardiorespiratory Endurance

Cardiorespiratory endurance is how well your heart and lungs can keep up with your activity. The prefix *cardio* refers to your heart, while *respiratory* refers to your lungs.

To increase their cardiorespiratory endurance, many teens take part in aerobic activities. An **aerobic activity** is an activity that works the heart and lungs. These activities require you to take in and use more oxygen than when you are at rest. The better your body uses oxygen, the longer your muscles can work before you get tired. Some ways to build endurance include brisk walking, climbing stairs, and bicycling for a length of time.

Flexibility

The ability to move your muscles and joints through their full ranges of motion is called **flexibility**. Gentle stretching helps make your muscles and joints more flexible, which in turn makes it easier for you to bend, reach, and stretch. When you stretch your muscles in the correct way, you help prevent injury from other physical activities.

Coordination and Balance

For many actions, such as hitting a tennis ball and riding a bicycle, you need to have good coordination and balance. These abilities help you control your muscles and stay upright as you move.

Body Composition

Body composition is a measure of the different amounts of fat, muscle, bone, and fluid that make up your weight. Physically active people tend to have a higher percentage of muscle in their bodies than inactive people. **Percentage** describes a part of a whole expressed in hundredths. Chapter 10 tells more about body composition. With more muscle, it is easier and more fun to be active!

✓ **Reading Check** **List** What five qualities define physical fitness?

Benefits of Active Living

A physically active lifestyle helps you look and feel your best. When you make physical activity a habit, you enjoy the benefits now—and for a lifetime. This includes maintaining a healthy weight, managing stress, and moving with speed and balance. People who are physically active usually have a positive outlook on life.

Look Your Best and Control Weight

Physical activity helps firm and tone your muscles. Physical activity also helps you manage your weight. During physical activity, your body burns up calories from the food you eat. A **calorie** is a unit of energy. By using calories for energy, your body will not store as many of them as body fat.

Discover International Foods

Spain

Many people in Spain walk to the market daily for produce, meat, fish, bread, and cheese. Tomatoes, onions, garlic, olives, and olive oil are common ingredients in paella, *cocida* (a thick soup), salads, and other mixed dishes. Thanks to a warm climate, many vegetables, fruits, and beans are available year-round. Citrus fruit, apricots, dates, and figs are among the most popular fruits. Spain is also surrounded by water, and many Spaniards enjoy seafood such as bacalao (salted cod), shellfish, and other fish.

Languages Across Cultures

gazpacho *(gə-'spä-chō)* a cold soup of chopped tomatoes and cucumber, softened bread, and garlic

paella *(pä-'ā-yə)* a rice dish, often prepared with chicken, tomatoes, red peppers, shellfish, peas, onions, olives, and garlic; named for the two-handled pan it is cooked in

 Recipes Find out more about International recipes on this book's Online Learning Center at glencoe.com.

NCTE 9 Develop an understanding of diversity in language use across cultures.

Move with Ease, Speed, and Balance

Your muscles help you control your movements and posture. As you work your muscles and joints through regular physical activity, you become stronger, more coordinated, and more flexible. You have better balance.

Stay Healthy

Physical activity benefits your health in many ways. For example, weight-bearing activities such as walking, soccer, and dancing help strengthen your bones. When you also get enough calcium and vitamin D from your food choices, you help build strong, dense bones that are less likely to break. Physical activity also strengthens your heart muscle. Active people have less risk of health problems such as type 2 diabetes, heart disease, osteoporosis, and colon cancer as they get older.

Think Positively and Manage Stress

Physical activity helps you feel good about yourself. Many teens who begin physical activity discover that it improves their mood, energy level, stress level, self-esteem, and sense of well-being. It also helps them cope with unhappy emotions. You also sleep better, so you feel more alert during the day.

If being active feels like a chore instead of a good time, you will be less likely to stick with it. Try different physical activities to find the ones you enjoy. Exercise with friends and family to spend quality time together. Team fitness activities build friendships and communication skills.

✓ **Reading Check** **Identify** What are five benefits of regular physical activity?

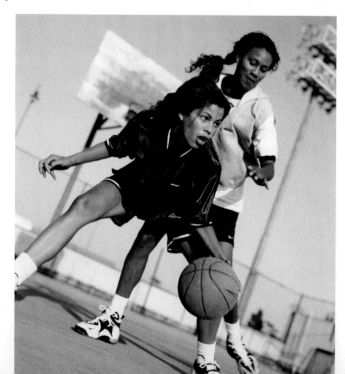

Get Moving You can fill your day with physical activity that is not a sport. *Can you think of ways to keep moving during the day?*

Get Physically Fit

You can be fit regardless of your shape, size, or physical abilities. Everyone has a different fitness potential. **Potential** is the possibility that something can happen. Reaching your fitness potential depends on the activities you do and how often you do them. Even busy teens can find time to add physical activity to their daily routines. To help prevent unexpected injuries or other health problems, get a medical examination before beginning any fitness program.

When you set fitness goals for yourself, know where you are starting from. First consider how physically active you are now. Then set realistic goals and make a plan to reach them. By taking small but steady steps, you can reach your full fitness potential.

What Is Stopping You?

Below are some common excuses people give for being inactive. Fortunately, good solutions exist for each one. Can you think of other solutions besides the ones listed here?

- ◆ **"I don't have time."** Make fitness a top priority, and you will find the time. Try breaking your activity into short segments. For example, walk for 15 minutes as you talk on the phone or dance for a few minutes after school with friends.

- ◆ **"It isn't fun."** Find activities you enjoy. If you are not an athlete, find other fun ways to get moving. Dancing, doing yoga, or taking your dog to the dog park are all fun ways to be active.

- ◆ **"I don't like to sweat."** Sweating is good for you—it cools you off. However, physical activity does not need to be intense. Any kind of movement helps you stay fit.

- ◆ **"My friends don't do it."** You are being active for you—not your friends. You can be a role model. Show how good you feel from being active. Before long, your friends may want to join you!

- ◆ **"I'm too uncoordinated."** Physical activity helps with coordination. Start with activities that match your abilities. As you gain confidence, add others.

Science in Action

Weight Machines

A weight machine is an exercise machine used for strength training. They help people build muscle. Used properly, they reduce the risk of injury because they control the user's range of motion.

Procedure To build muscle, trainers usually suggest using heavy weights and lifting them a few times until your muscles get tired. Ten or twelve repetitions (reps) are usually enough. Then, take a break and do another set. Try to include strength training in your workout three times a week for 10 to 20 minutes. Conduct research to find out how else you could vary your workout to gain strength.

Analysis Write a paragraph explaining other techniques to build strength without a weight machine.

NSES Content Standard A
Develop understandings about scientific inquiry.

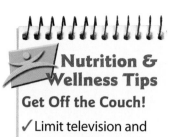

Nutrition & Wellness Tips

Get Off the Couch!

✓ Limit television and computer time to 1 to 2 hours a day.

✓ Move more whenever possible.

How Much Physical Activity Is Enough?

For the best health, most teens need at least 60 minutes of moderately intense physical activity on most days, in addition to their everyday activities. Look for ways to include activity in your life. There are plenty of ways to get moving!

Know your limits, and increase your activity level a little at a time. Too much sudden activity can cause injury. Some women find that being overactive causes problems with their reproductive cycles. A doctor can help you set healthful limits.

Set Your Goals

Decide what you want from physical activity. You may want to feel good, look your best, slim down, build muscle, improve your health, or just have fun outside. The best goals are challenging but realistic.

Choose Your Physical Activities

There are plenty of physical activities for people of all ages. Which activities listed below appeal to you?

- ◆ **Outdoor Recreation** Bicycling, in-line skating, running, walking, hiking, downhill or cross-country skiing, canoeing.

- ◆ **Indoor Recreation** Stationary cycling, dancing, stair climbing, aerobics, jumping rope.

- ◆ **Sports** Basketball, soccer, volleyball, softball, football, track and field, gymnastics, tennis, swimming.

- ◆ **After-school Activities** Marching band, building theater sets, dance class, gardening.

- ◆ **Jobs** Packing groceries, babysitting, mowing lawns.

- ◆ **Lifestyle Activities** Walking to school, washing the car, shoveling snow, vacuuming, raking leaves.

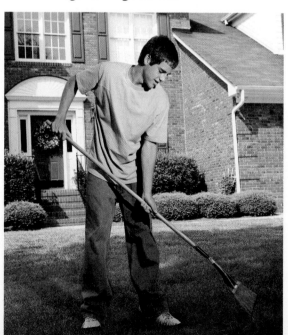

After-School Activities Many after-school activities and everyday chores count toward your 60 minutes of daily physical activity. *What after-school activities in your community can help you be more physically active?*

Look at **Figure 2.1** on the next page. There are plenty of activities in which you can participate. You will need to consider convenience, cost, which activities meet your fitness goals, and whether special equipment or clothes are required.

Ready, Set, Go!

Once you have chosen activities that appeal to you, it is time to put action in your fitness plan. Follow these guidelines to start your fitness plan safely:

- **Start slowly.** This is important, especially if you have been sedentary. **Sedentary** means physically inactive. Make changes to your routine gradually.

- **Split your goals into steps.** If one goal is to build strength, set a mini-goal, such as doing a certain number of push-ups. Do a few more each time you work out.

- **Challenge yourself.** When you achieve a mini-goal, challenge yourself with another doable target.

✓ **Reading Check** **Describe** How much physical activity do teens need?

Play It Safe

Safety is an important part of any physical activity. By making safety a priority, you will help prevent injuries and discomfort.

Warm Up, Know Your Limits, and Cool Down

Warm up before and cool down after more intense activity. Also, know your your limits so that you do not push yourself too hard. These simple actions lower your risk of injury and help reduce soreness.

- **Warm up.** Warming up gets your muscles ready. It causes your heart rate to rise gradually. Do 5 to 10 minutes of a slow, gentler version of your activity. For example, pedal your bicycle slowly before riding fast.

- **Know your limits.** The talk-sing test is a measure of physical activity. If you can talk while working out, your pace is probably right. If you are too breathless to talk, slow down. If you can sing, you may not be working hard enough.

- **Cool down.** Do 5 to 10 minutes of a slow, gentler version of your workout. Gradually decrease the intensity. **Intensity** refers to how hard your body has to work during an activity. Do gentle stretching to prevent stiffness and soreness.

| Figure 2.1 | The Activity Pyramid |

Move It! The Activity Pyramid offers advice about the types, amounts, and benefits of different physical activities. *Why are certain activities shown at the top of the Activity Pyramid, while others appear at the bottom?*

Move It!

Choose your FUN!

Your body counts on you to be active to help strengthen your bones and heart, and build muscles.

How much physical activity do kids need?

• GET AT LEAST 60 minutes a day of moderate activity, most days of the week.

TEAM
NUTRITION·USDA

United States
Department of
Agriculture

Food and
Nutrition
Service

September 2000

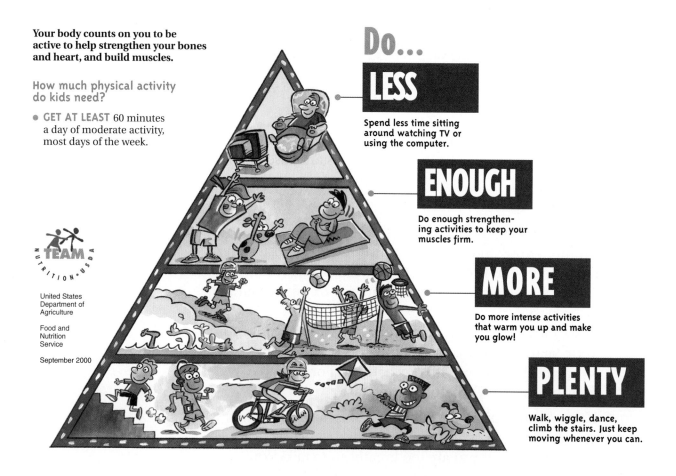

Do...

LESS
Spend less time sitting around watching TV or using the computer.

ENOUGH
Do enough strengthening activities to keep your muscles firm.

MORE
Do more intense activities that warm you up and make you glow!

PLENTY
Walk, wiggle, dance, climb the stairs. Just keep moving whenever you can.

Get in Gear

Safety is an important part of wellness. Always follow safety laws and guidelines where you are. The proper gear also keeps you safe. Wear protective gear, such as a helmet and knee pads, for activities such as in-line skating, bicycling, snowboarding, and skateboarding. Wear reflectors in the dark. Choose appropriate clothing and use sunscreen for outdoor physical activity.

Fuel and Fluids to Go On

Eat nutritious foods—including whole grain foods, fruits, and vegetables—to fuel your active lifestyle. They will give you the energy you need when you are active. Drink plenty of fluids before, during, and after your activity. This will help prevent dehydration. **Dehydration** is a serious health problem caused by a lack of water. Refer to chapter 11 for more information about the importance of water and the danger of dehydration when you are physically active.

✓ **Reading Check** **Explain** When you do intense exercise, why should you warm up first, know your limits, and cool down afterward?

Maintain Physical Fitness

As you work toward your goals, get help from family, friends, and coaches. Their encouragement helps you succeed. If you miss physical activity for a day or more, figure out what caused you to miss it and adjust your plan. For example, if homework keeps you busy at night, be active after school. If you do not enjoy an activity, try a different one! Follow these guidelines to track your progress toward your physical fitness goals:

- ◆ Keep a fitness log of your daily physical activities, including intensity and time spent.

- ◆ Compare your log to your goals and action plan. For example, can you run faster and longer now?

- ◆ If you are not making progress, adjust your strategies. Maybe your goal is too big for now. Maybe you need more time. Remember that slow progress and some setbacks are natural when reaching for a goal.

- ◆ When you reach your goal, set a new, more challenging goal as one more step toward fitness. Reward yourself with something you want that is not food.

✓ **Reading Check** **Predict** What is the benefit of being physically active with friends?

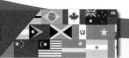

Gazpacho

Customary	Ingredients	Metric	
½ medium	Onion	½	medium
1 small	Cucumber	1	small
1 small	Green pepper	1	small
2 stalks	Celery	2	
4 cups	Tomato juice	1	L
2 Tbsp.	Olive oil	30	mL
1 clove	Garlic	1	clove
½ tsp.	Worcestershire sauce	2	mL
¼ tsp.	Black pepper	1	mL
2 drops	Hot pepper sauce	2	drops
1 large	Tomato, finely chopped	1	large
1	Lemon, cut in 6 wedges	1	

Try This!
Use diced canned tomatoes for better flavor if fresh tomatoes are not in season.

Yield: 6 servings, 1 cup (250 mL) each

❶ Peel onion and cucumber. Remove seeds from cucumber. Remove core and seeds from green bell pepper. Coarsely chop onion, cucumber, green pepper, and celery.

❷ Put 2 cups (500 mL) of tomato juice in blender. Add onion, cucumber, green pepper, celery, olive oil, garlic, Worcestershire sauce, black pepper, and hot pepper sauce. Puree in blender.

❸ Slowly add the remaining 2 cups (500 mL) tomato juice to the pureed mixture.

❹ Mix in chopped tomato. Chill.

❺ Serve gazpacho cold in 6 individual bowls. Garnish with lemon wedges and chopped tomatoes.

Nutritional Information Per Serving:
92 calories, 5 g total fat (1 g saturated fat), 0 mg cholesterol, 458 mg sodium, 13 g carbohydrates (2 g fiber, 9 g total sugars), 4 g protein

Percent Daily Value: vitamin A 20%, vitamin C 100%, calcium 4%, iron 6%

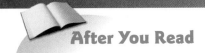

After You Read

CHAPTER SUMMARY

Physical fitness includes muscular strength and endurance, cardio-respiratory endurance, flexibility, coordination and balance, and healthy body composition. Regular physical activity can help you look and feel good. Teens need at least 60 minutes of moderately intense activity daily. You can get physical activity through many physical activities, not just sports. Stay safe and follow an action plan for lifelong physical fitness.

Vocabulary Review

1. Use each of these vocabulary words in a sentence.

Content Vocabulary

◇ physical fitness (p. 20)
◇ physical activity (p. 20)
◇ strength (p. 20)
◇ endurance (p. 20)
◇ cardiorespiratory endurance (p. 20)

◇ aerobic activity (p. 20)
◇ flexibility (p. 20)
◇ calorie (p. 21)
◇ sedentary (p. 25)
◇ intensity (p. 25)
◇ dehydration (p. 27)

Academic Vocabulary

■ percentage (p. 21)
■ potential (p. 23)

Review Key Concepts

2. Describe how physical activity promotes fitness.

3. Identify the benefits of active living.

4. Discuss your plan for making physical activity part of your daily life.

5. Identify safety and health precautions for physical activity.

6. Explain how to check the progress of your plan for active living.

Critical Thinking

7. Evaluate this scenario. Jamal invited Derek for 30-minute morning walks. Derek says getting up early will make him tired. Do you agree? Explain.

8. Analyze how building homes within walking distance of stores, schools, libraries, and other services might impact residents' physical and mental wellness.

9. Assess how teens might encourage parents and other adults in their families to be physically active. How could they help younger relatives play actively?

Real-World Skills and Applications

Make Decisions and Set Goals

10. Count Your Steps Predict how many steps you take in a day. Borrow a pedometer from your school's physical education department to count your steps. Make a plan to reach or maintain 10,000 steps a day. Chart your progress. Did you reach your goal? Why or why not? How can you adjust your plan?

Interpersonal and Collaborative

11. After-School Fun Follow your teacher's instructions to form groups. Work with your group to create a game that gets teens moving. Do the activity together. Draw conclusions about the benefits of physically active games.

Technology

12. Safe Stretches Find recommended stretches to improve flexibility. What muscle(s) does each one stretch? What are correct and incorrect ways to perform the stretches? Should they be done before exercise, after exercise, or both? Prepare a visual report using technology for the class to show safe stretching.

Financial Literacy

13. Calculate Exercise Cost Mi-Young swims three times a week at the recreation center. She pays a monthly fee of $30 to use the pool. If she swims 50 weeks per year, how much is she paying for each swim session?

14. Expert Advice Think of an athlete whom you admire. Conduct research to find out what activities are a part of the athlete's training program during a typical week. Learn what he or she does to stay motivated. How can you apply what you learned?

15. Fitness Survey Ask family members, friends, and classmates to cite reasons people give for not being active. Discuss with them how these obstacles could be overcome. Create a chart showing the results of your survey using percentages. Compare the results to the obstacles and solutions in this chapter.

> **NCTE 7** Conduct research and gather, evaluate, and synthesize data to communicate discoveries.

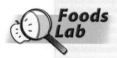
16. Make a Trail Snack Find recipes for snacks you could take on a day trip such as a hike or canoe trip. Prepare one of the snacks. Rate its flavor, texture, appeal, and nutrition. Write a paragraph that explains whether the snack is healthful and easy to prepare and take along.

Additional Activities For additional activities go to this book's Online Learning Center at glencoe.com.

Academic Skills

English Language Arts

17. Protective Gear Helmets can prevent serious injuries. Not all teens use them, however. Find out how many sports-related injuries occur among teens each year. Write an article for the school or community newspaper encouraging teens to use protective gear.

> **NCTE 8** Use information resources to gather information and create and communicate knowledge.

Social Studies

18. Conduct a Survey Write questions for a survey about exercise and fitness attitudes and habits. For example, you might ask people how often and for how long they exercise and what they include or exclude in their diet. Organize a table, chart, or diagram to display your findings.

> **NCSS IV D Individual Development and Identity** Apply concepts, methods, and theories about the study of human growth and development.

Mathematics

19. Steps to a Mile Many high schools have tracks that are open to the public to walk or run laps. Each lap on a track is ¼ mile. The average full-grown man's stride is 2½ feet long. The average full-grown woman's stride is 2¼ feet long. A mile is 5,280 feet long. How many steps will it take the average man to walk a mile on a track? How many steps will it take the average woman to walk a mile on a track?

Math Concept **Fractions and Decimals** Fractions and decimals are similar to each other in that they are used to represent parts of a whole.

Starting Hint Convert 2½ and 2¼ to decimals before solving each of the problems.

 For more math help, go to the Math Appendix

> **NCTM Number and Operations** Understand the meanings of operations and how they relate to one another.

STANDARDIZED TEST PRACTICE

MULTIPLE CHOICE
Read the paragraph and choose the best answer. Write your answer on a separate piece of paper.

Test-Taking Tip When answering multiple-choice questions, predict the correct answer before you look at the options. Then, choose the option that best matches your prediction.

In Australia, more people bought bicycles than cars in 2006. A large percentage of wealthy Australians commute on bicycles. This may be because they are aware of the benefits to the environment as well as the health benefits.

20. Based on the paragraph, which of the following statements is true?
   a. When people ride their bicycles instead of cars, it helps the economy.
   b. Australians do not like cars.
   c. Poor people do not ride bicycles.
   d. Bicycle riding has benefits.

Study Physical Activities

Engaging in physical activity and choosing healthful foods are a big part of a healthy lifestyle. Do you know what physical activities are available at your school and in your community? Understanding the health benefits of different kinds of physical activities can help you make better choices in the future.

My Journal

If you completed the journal entry from page 2, refer to it to see if your food choices and physical activities have a positive impact on your health.

Project Assignment

In this project you will:

- Describe your favorite sports and physical activities.
- Find out about places in your community you can participate in your favorite sports and physical activities.
- Write interview questions.
- Interview someone in a fitness-related profession about the effects of different types of physical activities on health and well-being.
- Make a presentation to your classmates on the findings of your research and interview.

Academic Skills You Will Use . . . .
English Language Arts

NCTE 5 Use different writing process elements to communicate effectively.

NCTE 12 Use language to accomplish individual purposes.

STEP 1 Choose and Research a Topic

Choose your favorite physical activities. Conduct research about the activities and their health benefits. Write a summary of your research that:

- Describes your favorite activities
- Explains how they impact your health and well-being
- Explains where in your community you can participate in your favorite physical activities

STEP 2 Plan Your Interview

Use the information you gathered about your favorite physical activities to formulate questions you will use during an interview you will hold with someone in a fitness-related profession. Ask questions about the impact of various types of physical activities on your physical, mental/emotional, and social health and well-being.

Writing Skills
- Use complete sentences.
- Use correct spelling and grammar.
- Organize your questions in the order you want to ask them.

STEP 3 Connect with Your Community

Using the list of interview questions you wrote in Step 2, interview a physical trainer, coach, gym teacher, or another adult in a physical fitness-related profession. Ask about the effect of different types of physical activities on your health and well-being.

Interviewing Skills
- Record responses and take notes.
- Listen attentively.
- When you transcribe your notes, write in complete sentences and use correcet spelling and grammar.

STEP 4 Create Your Final Report

Use the Unit Thematic Project Checklist to plan a presentation and give an oral report. Use these speaking skills as you present your final report.

Speaking Skills
- Speak clearly and concisely.
- Be sensitive to the needs of your audience.
- Use standard English to communicate.

STEP 5 Evaluate Your Presentation

Your project will be reviewed and evaluated based on:
- Depth of research information
- Content of your presentation
- Mechanics—presentation and neatness

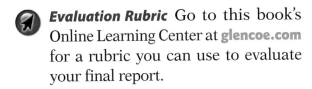 *Evaluation Rubric* Go to this book's Online Learning Center at glencoe.com for a rubric you can use to evaluate your final report.

Project Checklist	
Plan	✓ Conduct research about your favorite physical activities. ✓ Write a summary of your research. ✓ Write interview questions. ✓ Conduct an interview. ✓ Transcribe the notes from your interview. ✓ Plan a five-minute oral presentation.
Present	✓ Make a presentation to your class that explains the results of your research and interview. ✓ Invite classmates to share information about their favorite activities and community facilities where they take part in physical activities. ✓ Invite the students of the class to ask any questions they may have. Answer these questions. ✓ When students ask questions, demonstrate in your answers that you respect their perspectives. ✓ Turn in your research summary, interview questions, and interview notes to your teacher.
Academic Skills	✓ Conduct research to gather information. ✓ Communicate effectively. ✓ Organize your presentation so the audience can follow along easily. ✓ Thoroughly express your ideas.

Unit 2

The World of Food

Chapters in this Unit

Chapter 3   Food and Culture
Chapter 4   Food and the Marketplace

Unit Thematic Project Preview

Explore Ethnic Cuisines

While studying this unit, you will learn about regional and ethnic cooking in the United States. In the unit thematic project at the end of this unit, you will research the ethnic cuisine of your choice. You will interview a community member who is qualified to discuss ingredients and preparation of foods from the cuisine you researched. Then, you will give a presentation on the results of your research.

My Journal

The variety of cuisines available impacts your food choices. If you learn about ingredients and dishes from diverse cultural cuisines, you will be more likely to try interesting and delicious foods from around the world. Write a journal entry that answers these questions:

- What are some unusual foods you have eaten?
- What are some ethnic foods you like to eat?
- What new ethnic foods would you would you like to try?

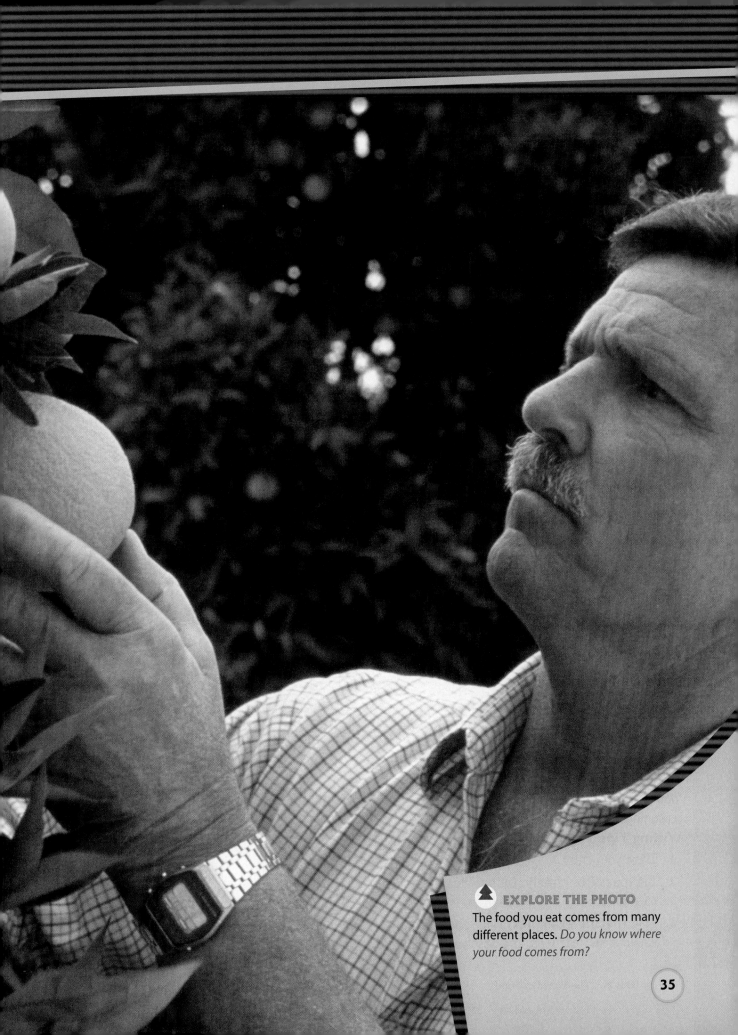

CHAPTER 3
Food and Culture

Explore the Photo ▶▶
Cultural Foods Delicious food is found everywhere. *What are the benefits of enjoying foods from other cultures?*

Writing Activity
Journal Entry

Ethnic Food Every country has its own foods, cuisine, and eating styles. Write a journal entry about the foods you have grown up eating. Think about your family traditions, the way the food is cooked, and the herbs, spices, and other seasonings used to flavor your food.

Writing Tips

1. **Date** your entry.

2. **Let ideas flow freely.** Let one idea lead to another.

3. **Use specific examples.** Write about experiences, reactions, and observations.

Reading Guide

Before You Read

Preview Choose a Content Vocabulary word that is new to you. Find it in the text and write down its definition.

Read to Learn

Key Concepts

- **Explain** the connection between culture and food choices.
- **Describe** influences on the development of the cuisines of the United States and Canada.
- **Identify** ways to learn about healthful foods from other cultures.

Main Idea

Culture and food supply determine the food customs of different regions and groups. Foods of other cultures can offer wellness.

Content Vocabulary

- ◇ diversity
- ◇ cuisine
- ◇ culture
- ◇ custom
- ◇ ethnic food
- ◇ environment
- ◇ regional food

Academic Vocabulary

You will find these words in your reading and on your tests. Use the glossary to look up their definitions if necessary.

- ■ trait
- ■ community

Graphic Organizer

As you read, write notes about the many influences on your food choices.

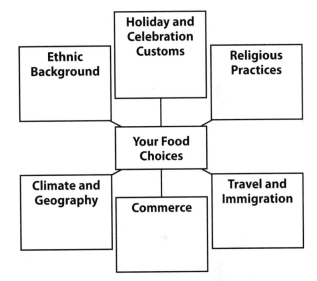

Holiday and Celebration Customs

Ethnic Background

Religious Practices

Your Food Choices

Climate and Geography

Commerce

Travel and Immigration

 Graphic Organizer Go to this book's Online Learning Center at **glencoe.com** to print out this graphic organizer.

Academic Standards ■

 English Language Arts
NCTE 9 Develop an understanding of diversity in language use across cultures.

 Mathematics
NCTM Measurement Apply appropriate techniques, tools, and formulas to determine measurements.
NCTM Algebra Represent and analyze mathematical situations and structures using algebraic symbols.

 Social Studies
NCSS I A Culture Analyze and explain the ways groups, societies, and cultures address human needs and concerns.
NCSS III I People, Places, and Environments
Describe and assess ways that historical events have been influenced by, and have influenced, physical and human geographical factors in local, regional, national, and global settings.

NCTE National Council of Teachers of English	**NSES** National Science Education Standards
NCTM National Council of Teachers of Mathematics	**NCSS** National Council for the Social Studies

Chapter 3 Food and Culture **37**

Different Foods, Different Customs

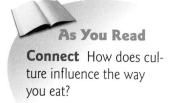

As You Read

Connect How does culture influence the way you eat?

Throughout history, food has connected people from different places. Consider the history of these popular foods:

◆ Yogurt was first produced in ancient times. Food historians think it was probably made by Middle Eastern nomads.

◆ Oranges, which first grew in Asia 20 million years ago, were brought to the Americas by the Spanish.

The flavors of healthful eating today show the rich diversity of global foods and cultures. **Diversity** is the variety of people of different races and cultures. No matter where you go in the world, you will find cuisines with foods that are like and unlike those you grew up with. **Cuisine** is the typical foods and ways of preparing foods associated with a region, country, or cultural group.

Sometimes, the same foods are prepared in different ways in different cultures. For example, salmon is often served raw in Japan, while it is typically smoked or grilled in Alaska and British Columbia. Sometimes, different foods are made in the same ways. For example, skewers of grilled meat are found in many places. Middle Eastern cooks usually make them with lamb, while many American cooks use beef.

People eat differently around the world. Some use only spoons. Others use chopsticks or their fingers. In some places, people pass dishes of food from person to person. Elsewhere, people reach into a large family bowl in the middle of the table. Culture and the food supply influence these differences.

Vocabulary

You can find definitions in the glossary at the back of this book.

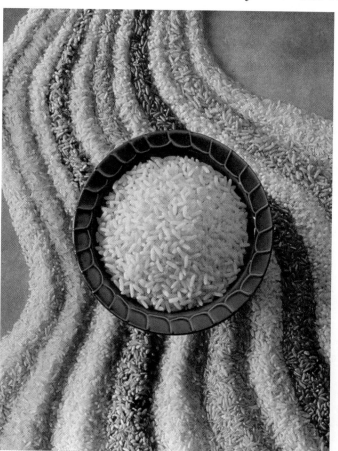

Rice Around the World In Japan, people eat rice plain or with chopped vegetables or fish. Italians enjoy a rice dish called risotto. Rice and beans are popular in parts of Latin America. *How do other cultures use rice in their cooking?*

Food and Culture

Culture is the beliefs, values, attitudes, behaviors, history, and expressions shared by a group of people. Some parts of culture are easy to recognize, such as food, clothing, music, and language. Culture also includes people's thoughts and beliefs.

Culture determines many food customs. A **custom** is the way a group of people traditionally behave. Food customs include how food is prepared as well as when, where, how, and with whom it is eaten. Groups within a culture also have customs. Besides pizza and hamburgers, what foods are associated with American teens? Besides vegetables and whole grains, what foods may be popular among health-focused people?

Some foods are considered special. These foods have a high cultural status. For example, many Americans put a higher status on steak and lobster than on ground beef and canned tuna. The status of foods often varies from one culture to another. In some countries, for example, insects are considered to be special treats.

Ethnic Background

An ethnic group includes people with common cultural **traits**, or characteristics. Nationality, race, and religion affect ethnicity. An **ethnic food** is a food commonly enjoyed by an ethnic group. Ethnic food traditions are passed from parents to children, who learn to enjoy their family's ethnic foods. Food traditions of many ethnic groups shaped today's American cuisine.

Religious Practices

Many religions use foods for symbolic purposes and feasts. Fasting, or not eating, is another religious custom. Some religions forbid certain foods and have strict rules for others. For example, Orthodox Jews do not eat meat and dairy products at the same meal. Many Christians avoid eating meat on Fridays during Lent. Muslims and Orthodox Jews do not eat pork. In strict Hinduism, beef is not allowed. In many religious cultures, sharing food with friends and even strangers is an important part of life.

Holiday and Celebration Customs

In most cultures, certain foods are linked with certain events. For example, many cultures celebrate harvests, national holidays, and religious holidays by having feasts. Families celebrate birthdays, graduations, and weddings with foods from their family and culture. Food traditions are important in life's special moments.

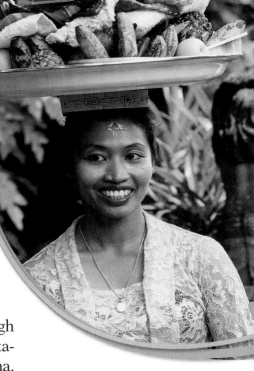

Culture and Food People around the world eat food that is influenced by their culture. *What are some dishes that you know of from another culture?*

Nutrition & Wellness Tips

Eat Japanese Style

✓ Learn to eat with chopsticks to help you eat more slowly and enjoy food more.

✓ Try sushi for a fresh heart-healthy alternative to fried fish.

Local Food Supply

People's food choices are influenced by their environment. **Environment** is the external factors influencing the life and the activities of people. Plentiful and locally available foods are usually more important to a culture's food customs than hard-to-find foods. What foods are plentiful where you live? What makes those foods easy to grow or to buy?

Climate and Geography

A culture's traditional foods depend largely on what grows nearby. For example, cuisines from coastal areas often include a lot of seafood.

Because of modern transportation and food preservation, today's cuisines depend less on locally grown foods. Many people, however, value local foods for their fresh flavor and cultural importance.

Commerce

Throughout history, people have exchanged foods through commerce. That explains why the same foods are grown in different places and why many cuisines include foods grown elsewhere. For example, bananas that first came from Asia now grow in Central America, where they are exported to the United States. Politics, trade policies, and food safety regulations affect commerce and food prices.

Immigration and Travel

Travel has always been an important way to learn about new foods. When people move to a new place, they often want the comfort of familiar foods. In colonial days, European settlers brought chickens, cows, wheat, oats, oranges, and carrots to the Americas. European explorers brought tomatoes, potatoes, and chocolate from the Americas to Europe.

✓ **Reading Check**

Identify What are some factors that affect people's food choices and customs?

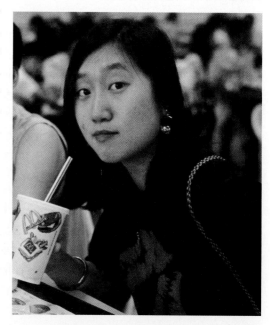

Global Connections
Through international commerce, American fast food is sold around the world.
What foreign foods are sold in the United States?

Foods of the United States and Canada

The United States and Canada have food traditions that range from everyday foods like fried chicken and corn on the cob to holiday favorites like turkey and pumpkin pie. What food traditions does your family observe?

Our Food Heritage

American and Canadian food customs started with foods grown, gathered, and hunted by Native Americans—such as turkey, squash, corn, peppers, and cranberries. Many immigrant groups have influenced American and Canadian cuisine as well. Consider these groups and the dishes they brought:

- Germans: apple strudel
- Scandinavians: meatballs
- British Islanders: fish and chips
- Italians: pasta dishes
- Mexicans: tortillas
- Chinese: stir-fried vegetables

American cuisine continues to change. Immigrants from Latin America, Asia, Eastern Europe, Africa, the Middle East, and elsewhere continue to add new foods and flavors to our food choices.

Foods that the Americas Gave the World

The foods tomatl, mahiz, and papa may sound unfamiliar, but they are eaten every day in America. *Tomatl* is the Aztec (ancient Mexican) name for tomato. *Mahiz* meant corn among the Arawak people of the Caribbean. *Papa* is the word for potato in Quechua, an ancient South American language. Until about five hundred years ago, all these foods grew only in the Americas. Then explorers brought them to the rest of the world. People in other countries embraced the new foods.

Corn, beans, and squash sustained Native Americans before the Europeans arrived. Most corn in the United States grows in the Midwest, while beans and squash are plentiful in many areas, including Northern and Southern regions.

Math in Action

Doubling Twice

To make one banana lassi (yogurt drink) from India, mix these ingredients in a blender: ½ cup (125 mL) sliced bananas, 1 cup (250 mL) plain yogurt, ½ cup (125 mL) water, 2 tsp. (3 mL) sugar, and 1 tsp. (1 mL) cardamom. How much banana and yogurt do you need to make two lassis?

Math Concept **Ratios** You can use ratios to compare two related numbers. The ratio of bananas to yogurt is 1:½, or 2:1. You can also express ratios using fractions with whole numbers as the numerator and denominator: 2/1

Starting Hint Ratios are easy to double because you multiply both numerator and denominator by 2.

NCTM Measurement Apply appropriate techniques, tools, and formulas to determine measurements.

For more math help, go to the Math Appendix.

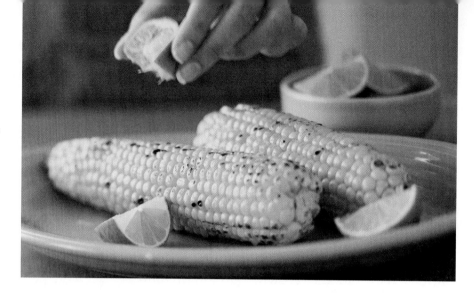

An American Original
Corn is an American original—and one of the most important crops in the United States. *What are three ways that people in the United States eat corn?*

Regional Foods

Have you tasted Florida key lime pie, or fiddlehead soup from New Brunswick? Every region of the world has regional foods. **Regional foods** are foods that are special to one geographic area.

Most regional foods develop because the climate and land are good for producing the ingredients. Many regions in the United States are well known for their popular foods.

◆ The South is known for peach desserts and pecan pies.

◆ Maple syrup flavors many dishes in New England and Southeastern Canada.

◆ Typical Midwestern meals include pork and corn.

◆ The area surrounding the lakes of Minnesota and central Canada are ideal for growing wild rice.

◆ The upper Pacific Coast is famous for salmon and berries.

◆ Alaskan cuisine features game meat such as deer and elk.

◆ Pineapple is used in many Hawaiian dishes.

Regional Foods that Reflect Ethnic Diversity

Some regional foods reflect ethnic diversity. For example, creole cooking in Louisiana combines the cooking styles of French, Spanish, Native American, and African settlers. Southern cooking—with foods such as grits, okra, and catfish—blends the traditions of African slaves, European settlers, and Native Americans. On the West Coast and in Hawaii, foods reflect the influence of Asian immigrants. Southwestern cuisine has strong influences from Mexico, Central America, and South America.

✓ **Reading Check** **Explain** What factors influence an area's regional foods?

Your Passport to Nutrition

Nutritious and tasty foods come from every part of the world. When you enjoy meals and snacks from other cultures, you learn about those cultures and get the benefits of food variety.

Healthful Foods from Many Cultures

Consider the nutritional benefits of including regional and ethnic foods in your meals and snacks. Remember that eating plenty of vegetables, fruits, beans, and whole-grain foods is good nutrition advice no matter where you live in the world.

- In some Asian cuisines, meals often include sliced vegetables and tofu.
- Many Mediterranean cuisines feature fresh salads.
- Fruit soups and yogurt are common in Middle Eastern cultures.
- Hispanic cuisines include combinations of beans and rice seasoned with herbs, spices, and vegetables.

Explore the World of Food

Whether you travel within your local **community**, or area, or visit another country, you can explore regional and ethnic ingredients and dishes. Try these tips:

- Visit local farmers' markets and farms.
- Try foods at regional or ethnic festivals.
- Look for regional or ethnic foods in your supermarket.
- Eat local foods when you travel.
- Find interesting ethnic or regional recipes in cookbooks.
- Watch television shows about regional or ethnic foods.
- Eat at ethnic restaurants. Ask about unfamiliar foods.

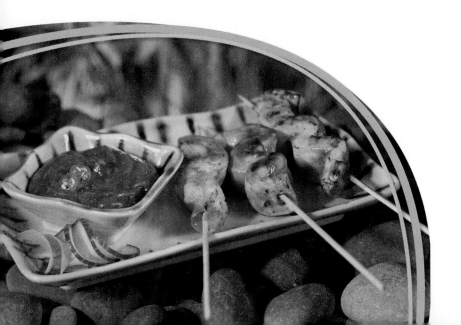

Ethnic Flavors Many ethnic foods are identified by their seasonings. Italian foods often include garlic and olive oil, while foods from India are often seasoned with curry. Many Middle Eastern foods include lemon and parsley. *How would you cook chicken to give it an ethnic flavor?*

Respect Food and Cultural Diversity

Learning about food customs helps you respect the similarities and differences among different peoples. When you watch, listen, and ask questions about other cultures, you can avoid stereotyping other people, their culture, or their foods. A cultural stereotype is a biased or exaggerated belief about the traits of a group of people.

Some foods may seem ethnic that are not. For example, fried tortillas for tacos are an American version of Mexican food. These crisp tacos are popular in Tex-Mex cuisine. Similarly, chop suey is served in many Chinese restaurants, but the dish was created in America.

Remember that cultures change over time, and so do their food customs.

Recognize foods and food customs you have in common with other cultures. Enjoy and learn from the similarities as well as the differences!

✓ **Reading Check** **Identify** What are three ways you could add cultural diversity and ethnic flavors to your food choices?

EASY RECIPES

Everyday Favorites

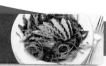

Hummus

Customary	Ingredients	Metric
1 cup	Canned garbanzo beans	250 mL
¼ cup	Tahini (sesame seed paste)	75 mL
2 Tbsp.	Lemon juice	30 mL
1 clove	Garlic, minced	1 clove
dash	Salt	dash
1 Tbsp.	Minced fresh parsley	15 mL

Yield: About 1¼ c (300 mL)

1. Drain and rinse the beans, then puree them in a blender (or mash with a fork).
2. Add tahini, lemon juice, garlic, and salt. Blend until smooth.
3. Place mixture in a serving bowl. Garnish with minced parsley.
4. Serve as a spread or a dip for toasted pita chips or raw vegetables.

Nutritional Information Per Serving: 93 calories, 5 g total fat (1 g saturated fat), 0 mg cholesterol, 161 mg sodium, 8 g carbohydrates (2 g fiber, 1 g total sugars), 4 g protein

Percent Daily Value: vitamin A 2%, calcium 6%, vitamin C 6%, iron 4%

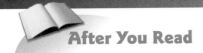

After You Read

CHAPTER SUMMARY

Culture and the food supply influence cuisine and food customs around the world. Cultural influences include ethnic background and religious practices. Foods for holidays and celebrations reflect culture. The food supply is influenced by climate, type of land, commerce, immigration, and travel. Regional foods, including regional American foods, reflect many influences. Learning to enjoy a variety of foods from different cultures and regions can add flavor, pleasure, and nutrition to your meals and snacks.

Vocabulary Review

1. Use each of these vocabulary words in a sentence.

Content Vocabulary
- ◇ diversity (p. 38)
- ◇ cuisine (p. 38)
- ◇ culture (p. 39)
- ◇ custom (p. 39)
- ◇ ethnic food (p. 39)
- ◇ environment (p. 40)
- ◇ regional food (p. 42)

Academic Vocabulary
- ■ trait (p. 39)
- ■ community (p. 43)

Review Key Concepts

2. Explain the connection between culture and food choices.

3. Describe influences on the development of the cuisines of the United States and Canada.

4. Identify ways to learn about healthful foods from other cultures.

Critical Thinking

5. Explore how exposing young children to foods from different cultures might help them to be more open-minded as they get older.

6. Analyze how modern methods of travel and communication affect and will continue to affect cultural and regional food customs.

7. Distinguish how corn, beans, and squash are used in American cuisine. Why have they been important parts of American cuisine?

8. Analyze how a regional Louisiana gumbo reflects the influences of several cultures.

9. Distinguish how regional cuisine develops. Why are some foods popular in different regions of the United States?

Real-World Skills and Applications

Problem Solving

10. Making Decisions You invite a foreign exchange student from Indonesia to your home for dinner. You want to prepare a meal that she can eat and enjoy. Write a paragraph to describe the things you should consider when deciding what foods to serve.

Interpersonal and Collaborative

11. Make Connections Interview a relative to learn about your family history and food customs. Take notes during your interview. Find out about favorite family recipes. Share what you learned with your class. Explain the importance of the recipes in your family's culture.

Financial Literacy

12. Plastic or Ceramic? At a coffee shop you can buy coffee in a paper cup for $1.50 or in a refillable ceramic mug for $6. Refills of the ceramic mug are $1. How many refills do you need to buy to make buying the mug a better value than buying individual paper cups of coffee?

Technology

13. Electronic Recipe File Start a recipe collection in an electronic file. Collect and label at least three recipes for each category: 1) local regional dishes, 2) other regional American dishes, and 3) ethnic or global recipes. Share your recipe collection with your classmates.

14. Learn About Ethnic Cuisine Get a menu from an ethnic restaurant where you live, or, with your teacher's permission, find one online. Identify all the menu terms that are unique to the ethnic cuisine, and define them. Create a poster to display the menu and definitions in class.

15. Potatoes Around the World Trace the geography and history of the potato. Where did potatoes originate? In what countries are they grown and eaten today? How are potatoes prepared in different countries? How did potatoes affect history in Ireland? Make a world map that shows key points in the history of the potato in the form of a timeline.

NCSS III I People, Places, and Environments Describe and assess ways that historical events have been influenced by, and have influenced, physical and human geographical factors in local, regional, national, and global settings.

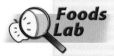

16. Chips and Dip Prepare three styles of chips and dip with foods from different cultures. You might choose Mexican salsa or guacamole with tortilla chips, Indian chutney with chapati, and Middle Eastern baba ghanoush with toasted pita triangles. Compare the textures and flavors.

Additional Activities For additional activities go to this book's Online Learning Center at glencoe.com.

Academic Skills

English Language Arts

17. Foreign Food Glossary Write a glossary of ten food-related terms. Include the spelling, pronunciation, and meaning of the words. Combine your list of words with your classmates' lists of words to make a classroom reference of food terms from around the world. Present your classroom food glossary reference to the school librarian for other students to use.

> **NCTE 9** Develop an understanding of diversity in language use across cultures.

Social Studies

18. Compare/Contrast Many cuisines feature noodles. Choose two noodle dishes from separate countries. Use a chart, paragraph, or Venn diagram to describe how they compare and contrast.

> **NCSS I A Culture** Analyze and explain the ways groups, societies, and cultures address human needs and concerns.

Mathematics

19. Create a Chart Injera is a flat Ethiopian bread resembling a large pancake. One batch of injera makes six pieces. Cait made two batches for a party, then tore each piece into three strips for dipping. Create a chart showing how many pieces and strips of injera you can make from two, three, and four batches.

Math Concept **Variables and Expressions** Use variables, or placeholders, for batches (b), pieces (p), and strips (s) to solve the multiplication problems for the table.

Starting Hint Create a chart with the following column headings: Batches, Pieces, Strips. Complete four rows showing different numbers of batches.

 For more math help, go to the Math Appendix

> **NCTM Algebra** Represent and analyze mathematical situations and structures using algebraic symbols.

STANDARDIZED TEST PRACTICE

MULTIPLE CHOICE
Read the paragraph and choose the best answer. Write your answer on a separate piece of paper.

Pizza is one of the most popular foods in the world, but it comes in different forms. Europe has a strict definiton of traditional Italian pizza. English muffin pizzas would not make the cut. Frozen pizzas prepared in the American way do not. But then, you might not recognize Sicilian pizzas with all the toppings baked right into the crust!

20. Based on the paragraph, which of the following statements is true?
   a. Everyone loves pizza.
   b. All Italians like English muffin pizzas.
   c. Europeans do not freeze pizza.
   d. People often use different ways to make pizza.

> **Test-Taking Tip** Be careful when you see generalizations. Sentences using words such as *all, none, always, never,* or *every* are often stereotypes.

CHAPTER 4
Food and the Marketplace

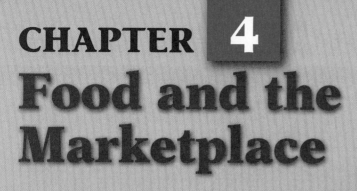

Explore the Photo ▶▶
The foods available in the United States and Canada are varied and abundant. *What are some food plants that grow in your region?*

Writing Activity

Write Using Details

Describe Foods Supermarket trips can be adventures! Write a descriptive paragraph about an unfamiliar food you would like to try. What does it look like? Why does it interest you?

Writing Tips

1. **Decide** what mood you want to create in the paragraph.

2. **Write** a strong topic sentence.

3. **Present Details** to the reader by arranging details in logical order.

4. **Select** precise transition words.

Before You Read

What Do You Want to Know? Write a list of what you need to know about food and the marketplace. Then write the headings in this chapter that provide this information.

Read to Learn

Key Concepts

- **Describe** the steps that bring food from the farm to the consumer.
- **Explain** how technology increases your food choices.
- **Distinguish** government, food industry, and consumer roles in food safety.
- **Identify** factors that may limit the world's food supply.

Main Idea

Bringing food to the table is a complex business. Production, processing, and packaging keep food healthful, safe, and appealing.

Content Vocabulary

- ◇ yield
- ◇ sustainable agriculture
- ◇ organic farming
- ◇ food processing
- ◇ shelf life
- ◇ irradiation
- ◇ additive
- ◇ enrich
- ◇ fortify

Academic Vocabulary

You will find these words in your reading and on your tests. Use the glossary to look up their definitions if necessary.

- ■ require
- ■ exceeds

Graphic Organizer

As you read, write what you know about where food comes from, and what you want to find out. After you read, add what you learned and how you can learn more.

What I Know	What I Want to Find Out	What I Learned	How I Can Learn More

Graphic Organizer Go to this book's Online Learning Center at glencoe.com to print out this graphic organizer.

Academic Standards ■

English Language Arts
NCTE 7 Conduct research and gather, evaluate, and synthesize data to communicate discoveries.
NCTE 9 Develop an understanding of diversity in language use across cultures.

Mathematics
NCTM Number and Operations Compute fluently and make reasonable estimates.

Science
NSES Content Standard A Develop understandings about scientific inquiry.
NSES Content Standard F Develop an understanding of personal and community health.

NCTE National Council of Teachers of English	**NSES** National Science Education Standards
NCTM National Council of Teachers of Mathematics	**NCSS** National Council for the Social Studies

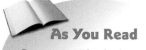

As You Read

Connect Think about the food you eat and where it is grown.

◇**Vocabulary**

You can find definitions in the glossary at the back of this book.

Food Supply Chain

People rely on the food industry for abundant, nutritious, and safe foods. The food business also provides jobs for millions of people. The foods in your kitchen may come from local growers and farms, from other parts of the country, or from another country. **Figure 4.1** shows the roles that people must perform to bring food to you.

Today's Agriculture

Farming can **require**, or need, big investments and risks. To produce a good yield and create profit, farmers must find efficient ways to care for the land and use seed and other resources. **Yield** is how much food a farm produces per acre or area.

Many farmers use methods of sustainable agriculture. **Sustainable agriculture** is the responsible use of resources to produce food without damaging the environment. This includes conserving natural resources such as water and fuel and avoiding poisons. Taking action to care for the environment is sometimes called being green.

For high crop yields, farmers use fertilizers. They must also manage pests such as insects, fungus, mold, and rodents. Pesticides protect crops against pest damage. Farmers must follow government regulations to use only safe amounts of fertilizers and pesticides. Another approach to farming is organic farming. **Organic farming** is growing foods without synthetic fertilizers or pesticides. Organic farmers find other ways to manage pests. Organically grown foods often cost more to produce.

What Affects Food Prices?

One week, a head of lettuce costs $1.49. The next week, it costs $1.99. Why? There are many things that affect food prices. Most of these reasons fit in two categories:

- ◆ **Production and Distribution Costs** Each step in producing food and distributing it to consumers adds cost to food prices. For example, if the cost of fuel or labor rises for businesses in the food supply chain, those increases are passed on to consumers.

- ◆ **Supply and Demand** When the food supply **exceeds**, or is more than, consumer demand, prices go down. When demand exceeds supply, prices go up. This can be caused by an increase in consumer desire, weather, pest damage, or other factors that damage crops or reduce yields.

✓ **Reading Check** **Predict** What are some factors that increase the cost of food you buy?

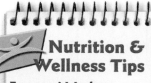

Nutrition & Wellness Tips

Farmers' Market

✓ Visit a farmers' market and talk to the farmers to learn about foods that are locally grown.

Figure 4.1   **From the Field to Your Plate**

How Food Gets to Your Table We often take for granted that we can go to a store and buy any food we want. *Why do you think there are so many stages before food can be brought home to your kitchen?*

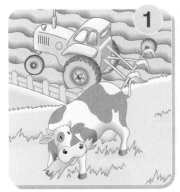

1. **Production Farmers** Producers grow crops and raise livestock and seafood.

2. **Product Research** Product developers work at food and agricultural companies to research and develop farm equipment and new food products.

3. **Processing** Crops, livestock, eggs, and milk are trucked from farms to processing plants. Processing methods include slaughtering, cleaning, sorting, freezing, canning, and packaging.

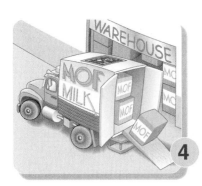

4. **Distribution** Food that is ready to sell is shipped from the processing plant to a distributor. Distributors store food in warehouses. Then they sell and transport the food to retailers.

5. **Marketing** Advertising and marketing agencies help food companies to promote food products to industry buyers and to consumers.

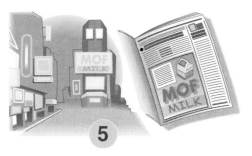

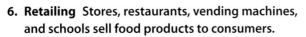

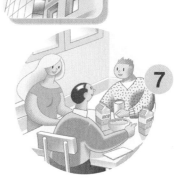

6. **Retailing** Stores, restaurants, vending machines, and schools sell food products to consumers.

7. **Consumption** A consumer like you buys foods to prepare, serve, and enjoy.

Technology and the Food Supply

Two hundred years ago, people relied mostly on foods produced locally. Since then, advances in technology have improved food production, processing, storage, and transportation. Consumers now have access to a wide variety of high-quality foods from other states, provinces, and countries. Consumers also have more choices.

New Methods of Agriculture

Using new technologies, farmers can produce more and different food.

- ◆ **Hydroponics** Vegetables grow indoors in a nutrient-rich solution rather than soil. Light, temperature, and humidity are controlled.

- ◆ **Aquaculture** Fish and shellfish are farmed in enclosed areas of water. Farmers section off areas of the ocean for easy harvest and greater yields of seafood. Fish farms in ponds produce freshwater fish.

- ◆ **Biotechnology** Scientists have learned a lot about genes, the information in living cells that determine specific traits. With this information, scientists have raised plants with certain qualities, such as resistance to disease and tolerance to severe weather. Scientists also have developed fruits that ripen on the tree without quickly spoiling, and crops with extra vitamins or without certain allergens.

- ◆ **Computers** Farmers use computers to predict disease and weather conditions, so they can use fewer pesticides. They also use global positioning systems with satellites to guide farm equipment in the field.

Food Processing

Foods come in many forms. In addition to whole apples, for example, you can buy applesauce, bottled apple juice, frozen apple pie, frozen apple juice concentrate, and dried apple slices. These are all processed foods. **Food processing** is preparing and handling food for safety, nutrition, convenience, and appeal. Even whole apples undergo some processing—they are washed, and often waxed to retain their quality longer.

How Food Is Preserved

Once they are ripe, peaches stay fresh for just a few days. If you put them in cans or freeze them, however, they will keep for weeks and even months. Preserving foods gives them a longer shelf life. **Shelf life** is the length of time foods stay safe, nourishing, and appealing to eat. Thanks to the following preservation methods, you can enjoy your favorite foods year-round:

◆ Freezing uses cold to slow the growth of bacteria.

◆ Canning uses high heat to destroy harmful bacteria. Food is sealed in airtight containers.

◆ Drying removes moisture that bacteria need to survive.

◆ **Irradiation** is passing food through radiant energy. It kills some disease-causing bacteria without nutrient loss. By law, irradiated foods must be labeled as such.

◆ Curing uses ingredients such as salt, sugar, spices, and vinegar for preservation. Ham and bacon are cured.

Foods lose some of their nutrients during harvesting and preservation. Canned and frozen foods have almost as many nutrients as fresh, cooked versions of the same foods. If fresh foods are not handled properly, they may be less nutritious than canned or frozen foods.

Food Additives

An **additive** is a substance added to foods during processing to make them safer, more appealing, or more nutritious. Some additives extend the shelf life of food. Some **enrich** food, or add back nutrients lost in processing. Others **fortify** food, or add nutrients that are not naturally present. Flavorings and colorings make foods more appealing. Additives also can have special functions. One additive helps make ice cream smooth and thick. Another keeps salt from clumping. The Food and Drug Administration makes rules about the safe use of approved additives.

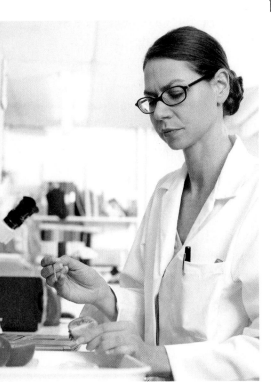

Testing New Products Food technologists work in test kitchens to develop products that meet consumer needs. *What new food products have you seen at your supermarket, and how do you think they meet consumer needs?*

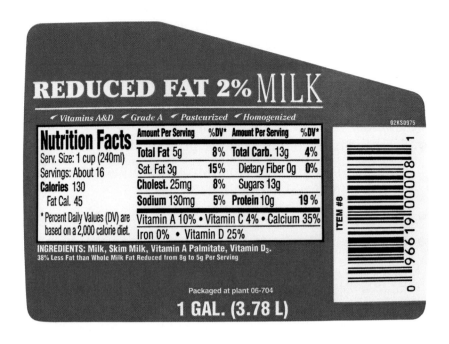

Additives on the Label The label on a food package lists any additives the food contains, as well as their function in some cases. *How can information about additives on food labels be useful to you?*

Food Packaging

Packaging keeps food safe, preserves quality, and provides facts about the food inside. Sometimes, the package serves as a cooking or serving utensil. Newer types of packaging include:

◆ Aseptic packaging, which allows perishable foods to stay fresh at room temperature for several months without preservatives.

◆ Microwave-safe packaging, which can go directly into the microwave oven and sometimes even a conventional oven.

◆ Recyclable packaging, which helps reduce waste.

Convenience Foods

Many packaged foods are partly or fully prepared. They include frozen pizza, canned chili, and dehydrated soups. Most convenience foods cost more than unprepared foods.

✓ **Reading Check** **Explain** Why are foods processed and packaged?

Safe Food Supplies

The government, food industry, and consumers share responsibility for the safety of the food supply in these ways:

◆ Government agencies set food safety rules and standards, including for pesticide and additive use. Agencies make sure the food industry meets or **exceeds** the standards. They also set standards for consumer information, such as food labels.

◆ The food industry must obey government rules. This includes farmers, manufacturers, stores, and restaurants. The industry also provides food safety information. That includes consumer hotlines to report food safety problems.

◆ Consumers must stay informed and handle food safely from the store to the table.

✓ **Reading Check** **Explain** How do the government and the food industry protect the safety of the food you buy?

Nutrition & Wellness Tips

Edible Garden

✓ Grow one or more vegetables or herbs in a backyard or container garden to enjoy the fresh flavor.

World Hunger

In every country, some people go hungry. Hunger exists for many reasons:

◆ Climate, geographical conditions, and poor farming methods.

◆ Lack of modern transportation to deliver food.

◆ Natural disasters, such as drought or floods.

◆ Rapidly growing populations.

◆ Wars and other political conflicts.

Discover International Foods

Peru

Peru has three geographic areas bring a bounty of food: the Amazon rain forest, with its tropical fruits and freshwater fish; the Pacific coastline, with its abundant saltwater fish; and the Andes mountains, where potatoes, beans, quinoa, corn, and other crops grow. Hundreds of different potato, corn, and bean crops grow there in a rainbow of colors! Many foods, from seafood stew to potato salad, are flavored with fiery-tasting yellow chili peppers.

Languages Across Cultures

ceviche (sə-'vē-(,)chā) raw cold seafood marinated in lemon juice, peppers and onions.

quinoa ('kēn-wä) a sweet, nutty grain considered a super grain because it contains more protein than any other grain.

 Recipes Find out more about Latin American recipes on this book's Online Learning Center at glencoe.com.

NCTE 9 Develop an understanding of diversity in language use across cultures.

World Hunger Solutions

The solutions to the problem of world hunger are complex. Many organizations, governments, and volunteers provide immediate aid such as food and water to prevent starvation. Other solutions are long-term, including the following:

◆ Teach people affordable ways to grow more food.

◆ Support efficient farming. This may include inexpensive fertilizers, irrigation systems, and farm equipment.

◆ Develop new crop varieties that grow in harsh conditions.

◆ Build roads, and facilities to transport and store food.

◆ Work to resolve political problems so people can live in a more peaceful world.

✓ Reading Check **Discuss** What are some ways to solve world hunger?

EASY RECIPES 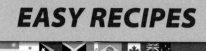 International Flavors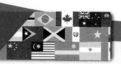

Lime Quinoa with Vegetables

Customary	Ingredients	Metric
1 cup	Water	250 mL
1 cup	Corn	250 mL
¾ cup	Vegetable broth	200 mL
2	Carrots, large, diced	2
½ cup	Quinoa	125 mL
½ cup	Zucchini, diced	125 mL
3	Limes	3
¼ cup	Olive oil	60 mL
3	Green onions, sliced thin	3
1 Tbsp.	Cilantro, chopped	15 mL

Try This!
Try adding chopped tomatoes or other vegetables.

Yield: 6 servings, 1 cup (250 mL) each

❶ Put water, corn, vegetable broth, carrots, quinoa, and zucchini in a large saucepot. Bring to a boil and cook 15 minutes.

❷ Juice limes and pour juice and olive oil into pot. Add green onions and cilantro and mix. Serve in bowls.

Nutritional Information Per Serving: 176 calories, 10 g total fat (1 g saturated fat), 0 mg cholesterol, 416 mg sodium, 20 g carbohydrate (3 g fiber, 3 g total sugars), 4 g protein

Percent Daily Value: vitamin A 80%, vitamin C 20%, calcium 2%, iron 10%

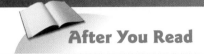

After You Read

CHAPTER SUMMARY

Food goes through many steps before it gets to the table, including production, processing, distribution, marketing, and retailing. Supply and demand, as well as the cost to produce and distribute food, affect food prices. Technological advances in producing, processing, preserving, and packaging food have led to a safer, more appealing, and more healthful food supply. The government, the food industry, and consumers are responsible for keeping the food supply safe. Feeding the world population is a global problem, with complex challenges, and complex solutions.

Vocabulary Review

1. Use each of these vocabulary words in a sentence.

Content Vocabulary
- yield (p. 50)
- sustainable agriculture (p. 50)
- organic farming (p. 50)
- food processing (p. 52)
- shelf life (p. 53)
- irradiation (p. 53)
- additive (p. 53)
- enrich (p. 53)
- fortify (p. 53)

Academic Vocabulary
- require (p. 50)
- exceed (p. 55)

Review Key Concepts

2. Describe the steps that bring food from the farm to the consumer.

3. Explain how technology increases your food choices.

4. Distinguish government, food industry, and consumer roles in food safety.

5. Identify factors that may limit the world's food supply.

Critical Thinking

6. Predict the impact if the wheat yield was unusually high for one or two years. How might that affect farmers, the food industry, and consumers? Explain your reasoning.

7. Analyze the reasons why a U.S. farmer today can feed an average of 128 people, while just 75 years ago a U.S. farmer fed only 20 people.

8. Debate the effect of local and imported foods on global warming. Consider the larger issues of food production, not just transportation of food.

9. Examine why math and science skills are needed to research and to develop new food products.

Real-World Skills and Applications

Set Goals and Make Decisions

10. Weigh Your Options You are shopping with friends to make a homemade pizza. You need to decide whether to buy fresh, sun-dried, or canned diced tomatoes to put on the pizza. How will you decide? What are the pros and cons of each? Write a paragraph to answer.

Interpersonal and Collaborative

11. Food in Many Forms Follow your teacher's instructions to form groups. As a group, choose a food. With your group, brainstorm ways that your food can be processed. Identify as many different processed products as possible that use this food.

Technology

12. Agriculture Time Line Many technological advances have changed agriculture. In food processing, advances include pasteurization, canning, freezing, and microwaveable food products. Create a visual presentation with a time line, showing these and other milestones.

Financial Literacy

13. Packing Lunch vs. Dining Out Erin spends $7 at the deli buying sandwiches for lunch each weekday. She plans to pack herself a more nutritious lunch for $2, and still eat at the deli once every five workdays. How much will Erin save each week?

14. Chefs and Farmers In many places, chefs and farmers work together to serve local foods to their communities. Find out how farms and restaurants, and perhaps your school's food service program, work together. Identify local or regional foods on a restaurant or school menu.

15. The Perfect Vegetable Imagine you are a bioengineer, designing the perfect vegetable. Determine your vegetable's health and/or food production benefits. Describe its color, texture, flavor, and how it would be prepared. Provide a written description and visual sketch of your vegetable.

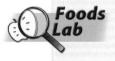

16. Make Raisins Wash white seedless grapes. Remove the stems. Place the grapes in a strainer, then dip them in boiling water to break their skins. Spread them on a tray. Dry them overnight in a 140°F (60°C) oven until they become dry and chewy. Then write a paragraph that answers this question: How does drying preserve grapes?

Additional Activities For additional activities go to this book's Online Learning Center at glencoe.com.

Academic Skills

 English Language Arts

17. Food Relief Choose a country or region where food supplies are limited, and conduct research on causes of the shortage. Find out how the problem is being addressed. Write a report to share in class.

> **NCTE 7** Conduct research and gather, evaluate, and synthesize data to communicate discoveries.

 Science

18. Freezing Produce Some things are preserved better in the freezer than others.

Procedure In separate plastic wrap or sealable plastic bags, freeze a whole tomato, chopped celery and peas. Put the items in the freezer and remove them after two days. Let them thaw and then observe them.

Analysis Write a paragraph that answers these questions: Which of the items look appetizing after freezing? Which do not? Why do you think some items did better than others?

> **NSES Content Standard F** Develop an understanding of personal and community health.

 Mathematics

19. The Cost of a Pineapple A grocery in Arizona sells pineapples at wholesale for $3.99 each. The cost includes the farmer's price plus shipping. The fruit was flown 2,315 miles to San Francisco at $0.0015 per mile per pineapple. Truckers charged $0.0005 per mile per pineapple for trucking it 752 miles to Arizona. How much did the farmer in Hawaii actually get for each pineapple?

Math Concept **Estimation by Rounding** When working with monetary decimals, round your final answer to the nearest cent. Look at the digit in the thousandths place. Round up if it is 5 or greater. Round down if it is 4 or less.

Starting Hint Work backwards to solve this multi-step problem. First, multiply to find the shipping costs.

 For more math help, go to the Math Appendix

> **NCTM Number and Operations** Compute fluently and make reasonable estimates.

STANDARDIZED TEST PRACTICE

MULTIPLE CHOICE
Read the paragraph and choose the best answer. Write your answer on a separate piece of paper.

> **Test-Taking Tip** Look for key words in answer choices that also appeared in the chapter. Ask if an option supports the definition in the chapter. Does it answer the question?

Green grapes can be purchased for $2 per pound in summer months, when they are in season and plentiful. The price of green grapes during winter months, when they are either grown in hothouses or outside the country, can be two or three times as much.

20. Based on the paragraph, which of the following statements is true?
    a. Grapes are very popular in June.
    b. Supply and demand drive prices.
    c. Grapes do not sell well.
    d. Grapes are always expensive.

Explore Ethnic Cuisines

In this unit, you have learned about the diverse cultural influences on American food choices. The United States is a melting pot of people from countless ethnic backgrounds. Your food choices are influenced by the diversity around you, including your family, friends, environment, and family heritage. Learning about ethnic foods and ingredients will broaden your knowledge of our national cultural diversity.

My Journal

If you completed the journal entry from page 34, refer to it to see if you want to add any foods to your list of foods to try.

Project Assignment

In this project you will:

- Select your favorite ethnic cuisine or an ethnic cuisine that interests you.
- Conduct research to gather information about the cuisine you select.
- Write a summary of your research.
- Interview a qualified community member about ingredients and preparation of foods from diverse cultural cuisines.
- While interviewing, take notes, and after interviewing, transcribe your notes.
- Make a presentation to your classmates on the findings of your research and interview.

Academic Skills You Will Use . . . .
English Language Arts

NCTE 4 Use written language to communicate effectively.
NCTE 7 Conduct research and gather, evaluate, and synthesize data to communicate discoveries.

STEP 1 Choose and Research a Topic

Select your favorite ethnic cuisine or one you are interested in. Research recipes and ingredients used in the cuisine you select. While you conduct your research, save electronic files of photos of ingredients and dishes from the cuisine. Write a summary of your research that:

- Describes the cuisine and some of its characteristics, recipes, and ingredients
- Includes one recipe from the cuisine
- Includes a written grocery list of ingredients needed to prepare the recipe

STEP 2 Plan Your Interview

Use the information you gathered in your research to formulate interview questions. You will interview someone in your community who is qualified to discuss ingredients and preparation of foods from the cuisine you researched.

Writing Skills
- Use complete sentences.
- Use correct spelling and grammar.
- Organize your questions in the order you want to ask them.

STEP 3 Connect with Your Community

Using your list of interview questions from Step 2, interview someone in your community who is familiar with the preparation of dishes from the cuisine you researched. Consider interviewing a chef, a culinary professor, or an ethnic foods grocer.

Interviewing Skills
- Record responses and take notes.
- Listen attentively.
- When you transcribe your notes, write in complete sentences and use correct spelling and grammar.

STEP 4 Create Your Final Report

Use the Unit Thematic Project Checklist to plan a presentation and give an oral report. Use these speaking skills as you present your final report.

Speaking Skills
- Speak clearly and concisely.
- Be sensitive to the needs of your audience.
- Use standard English to communicate.

STEP 5 Evaluate Your Presentation

Your project will be reviewed and evaluated based on:
- Depth of research information
- Content of your presentation
- Mechanics—presentation and neatness

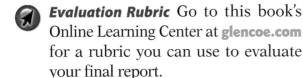 **Evaluation Rubric** Go to this book's Online Learning Center at glencoe.com for a rubric you can use to evaluate your final report.

Project Checklist

Plan **Plan**	✓ Conduct research. ✓ Collect photos of dishes and ingredients. ✓ Write a summary of your research. ✓ Write interview questions. ✓ Conduct an interview. ✓ Transcribe the notes from your interview. ✓ Create a presentation of photos of ingredients and dishes from the cuisine and the recipe you selected. ✓ Plan a five-minute oral presentation that explains the results of your research and interview.
Present	✓ Make a presentation to your class to discuss the findings of your research and interview and to show and describe the photos you collected. ✓ Invite the students of the class to ask any questions they may have. Answer these questions. ✓ When students ask questions, demonstrate in your answers that you respect their perspectives. ✓ Turn in your research summary, recipe, grocery list, interview questions, interview notes, photo presentation, and report outline to your teacher.
Academic Skills	✓ Conduct research to gather information. ✓ Communicate effectively. ✓ Organize your presentation so the audience can follow along easily. ✓ Thoroughly express your ideas.

Unit 3

Food and Kitchen Safety

Chapters in this Unit
Chapter 5   Food Safety and Sanitation
Chapter 6   Kitchen Safety

Unit Thematic Project Preview

Plan a Safe Kitchen

While studying this unit, you will learn about food safety and sanitation, and how they relate to your life. In the unit thematic project at the end of this unit you will interview someone in your community whose place of business is regulated by the health department. Then, you will create a visual of a kitchen that promotes safety and sanitation practices and present it to your class.

My Journal

You probably have already had some experience with food and kitchen safety, either positive or negative. Write a journal entry about one of the topics below.
- Has anyone you know ever suffered from food poisoning?
- Has anyone you know ever had an accident in the kitchen that could have been prevented?
- What food and kitchen safety guidelines do you already follow?

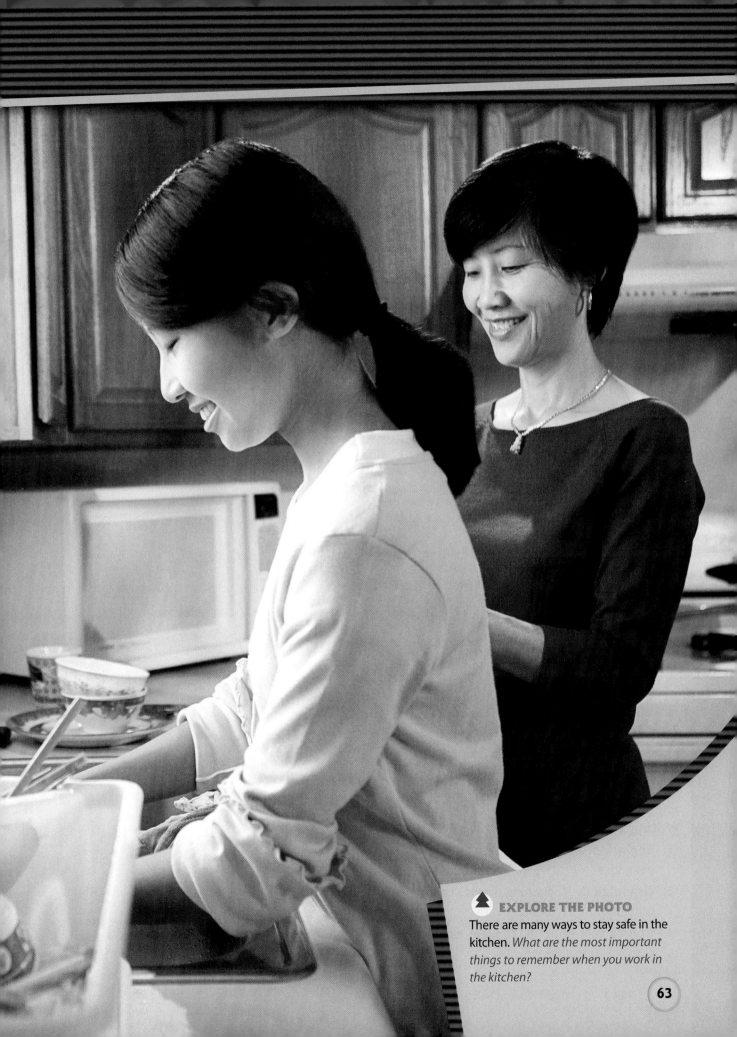

EXPLORE THE PHOTO
There are many ways to stay safe in the kitchen. *What are the most important things to remember when you work in the kitchen?*

63

CHAPTER 5

Food Safety and Sanitation

Explore the Photo ▶▶

Handle with Care Storing and handling food properly helps protect your health. *What do you think are your responsibilities for keeping food safe to eat?*

Writing Activity

Write a Paragraph

Food Safety You will be giving a short presentation about food safety. To prepare, write a paragraph about how you practice safely handling food. Include specific details about what you do, why you do it, and why it is important.

Writing Tips

1. **Begin** with a topic sentence that states the main idea.

2. **Organize** the supporting details in a logical order.

3. **Reread** your paragraph to make sure it is clear for your audience.

Reading Guide

Before You Read

Predict Before reading the chapter, browse the content by reading the headings, bold terms, and photo captions. Then predict what you will learn.

Read to Learn

Key Concepts

- **Describe** the causes, effects, and treatment of foodborne illness.
- **Explain** proper kitchen sanitation.
- **Discuss** how to protect food from cross-contamination.
- **Identify** proper food storage procedures.
- **Explain** how to keep food out of the temperature danger zone.

Main Idea

From farm to table, food requires proper handling. Cleanliness and proper storage are important, as well as keeping food at safe temperatures.

Content Vocabulary

◇ foodborne illness
◇ bacteria
◇ contaminate
◇ sanitation
◇ cross-contamination
◇ freezer burn
◇ perishable
◇ danger zone

Academic Vocabulary

You will find these words in your reading and on your tests. Use the glossary to look up their definitions if necessary.

- signal
- anticipate

Graphic Organizer

As you read, prepare a food-safety checklist. List what to do before, during, and after preparing food.

Before	During	After

 Graphic Organizer Go to this book's Online Learning Center at **glencoe.com** to print out this graphic organizer.

Chapter 5 Food Safety and Sanitation

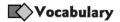
Vocabulary

You can find definitions in the glossary at the back of this book.

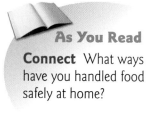

As You Read

Connect What ways have you handled food safely at home?

What Is Foodborne Illness?

Foodborne illness is caused by unsafe food. It is also called food poisoning. Bacteria, parasites, fungi, viruses, and harmful chemicals can make food unsafe. Some symptoms may seem like a mild flu and can last a day or two. Some cases lead to more serious or long-term illnesses, even death. You can avoid most foodborne illness by handling food properly.

Anyone can get sick from unsafe food. Infants, children, pregnant women, older adults, and people with certain health problems, such as cancer, are at greater risk. They often have weaker immune systems that are less able to fight infection.

Bacteria Facts

Bacteria are microscopic living organisms. They are everywhere—on your skin, in the air, and on the things you touch. Many bacteria are harmless. Some foods and medicines are made with helpful or friendly bacteria that help keep you healthy. Most foodborne illnesses occur when harmful bacteria contaminate food. To **contaminate** is to make impure. Food can become contaminated at any step from farm to table.

When Is Bacteria Harmful?

Eating small amounts of bacteria usually will not make you sick. But some bacteria can be toxic even in small amounts.

Bacteria can also multiply to harmful levels wherever there is food (nutrients), moisture, and warmth. Meats, poultry, fish, eggs, and soy and milk products have protein, a nutrient ideal for growing bacteria. **Figure 5.1** shows common illness-causing bacteria. To stop harmful bacteria from multiplying, handle and cook food properly.

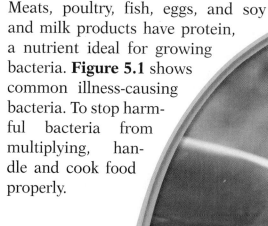

Wash Fresh Fruits and Vegetables Wash all fruits and vegetables under running water to remove residue before you eat, cut, or cook them. *What kinds of residue might be present on fresh fruits and vegetables?*

Figure 5.1 **Bacterial and Viral Illness**

Foodborne Illnesses Harmful bacteria and viruses can cause foodborne illnesses. *What foodborne bacteria live in unpasteurized milk?*

Bacteria	Possible Sources	Symptoms	Timing After Eating Contaminated Food
Campylobacter jejuni	Raw or undercooked poultry and meat, unpasteurized milk, untreated water	Fever, headache, muscle pain followed by diarrhea (sometimes bloody), abdominal pain, nausea	*Start:* 2 to 5 days *Continues:* 7 to 10 days
Clostridium botulinum	Commercial and home-canned foods that are improperly processed or stored, improperly handled home-prepared oils	Double vision; droopy eyelids; difficulty speaking, swallowing, and breathing; paralysis; can be fatal without immediate treatment	*Start:* 4 hours to 8 days (usually 18 to 36 hours) *Fatal:* 3 to 10 days if not treated
Clostridium perfringens	Meat dishes, stews, casseroles, gravies held at low temperatures (often on buffets and steam tables)	Diarrhea, abdominal pain, nausea, vomiting	*Start:* 8 to 24 hours *Continues:* usually 1 day or less, but may persist for 1 to 2 weeks
Escherichia coli (E. coli)	Raw or undercooked ground meat, unpasteurized milk, unwashed produce, unpasteurized apple cider, person-to-person contact	Severe abdominal pain, diarrhea (often bloody), nausea, vomiting; can cause life-threatening problems	*Start:* 2 to 5 days *Continues:* about 8 days
Listeria monocytogenes	Ready-to-eat foods such as hot dogs, luncheon meats, cold cuts, fermented or dry sausage, and other deli-style meat; poultry; soft cheeses; unpasteurized milk	Fever, chills, muscle aches, headache, nausea, diarrhea, vomiting; may be more serious for pregnant women, newborns, older adults, and people with weakened immune systems	*Start:* up to 3 weeks *Continues:* varies
Salmonella	Raw and undercooked eggs, poultry, meat, fish, unpasteurized milk	Nausea, vomiting, abdominal pain, diarrhea, fever, headache	*Start:* 8 to 72 hours *Continues:* 1 to 2 days
Staphylococcus aureus (Staph)	Meat; poultry; egg products; mixtures such as tuna, chicken, potato, or egg salad; cream-filled pastries	Nausea, vomiting, abdominal pain, exhaustion, headache, muscle pain	*Start:* 1 to 6 hours *Continues:* 2 to 3 days; longer if severe dehydration occurs
Viral gastroenteritis (norovirus)	Any food, liquid, or surface that has been contaminated with the norovirus	Nausea, vomiting, diarrhea, stomach cramps, fever, aches, chills, and tiredness	*Start:* 12 to 48 hours *Continues:* 1 to 2 days

Other Contaminants

Food can be contaminated by chemicals or poisons, such as cleaning solutions. Bits of glass or metal can also get into food. Here are some other common food contaminants:

◆ Parasites are organisms that feed on living things. The trichina worm can be transferred to humans through undercooked pork.

◆ Fungi are organisms that spread through invisible spores. Some fungi produce poisons. Mold is a fungus.

◆ Viruses are microorganisms that infect cells. They may come from polluted water or the fish caught there.

When Foodborne Illness Strikes

Foodborne illness can cause flu-like symptoms, including diarrhea, nausea, abdominal pain, headache, muscle pain, and fatigue. Most symptoms appear within four to forty-eight hours after eating contaminated food.

Some symptoms may signal serious illness that requires immediate medical attention. **Signal** means to show signs of something. Symptoms of serious illness include bloody diarrhea, frequent diarrhea or vomiting, a stiff neck, paralysis, severe headache, dizziness, blurred vision, and a high or persistent fever.

If you suspect a foodborne illness, take these steps:

◆ Rest and drink plenty of fluids. If symptoms get worse or last more than a day or two, call a doctor.

◆ Wrap up the bad food as evidence. Label it Danger and refrigerate it. For packaged food, save the can or package.

◆ Report the illness to your local health department. Report the food source and if other people may have eaten it.

✓ Reading Check

Explain How can bacteria cause foodborne illness?

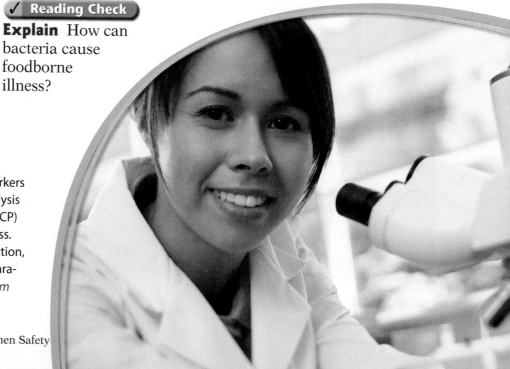

A Team Effort Food service workers use a system called Hazard Analysis and Critical Control Points (HACCP) to help prevent foodborne illness. HACCP steps cover food production, processing, handling, and preparation. *How might the HACCP system affect your life?*

Keep Food Clean

Food safety is supervised by federal government agencies, such as the U.S. Food and Drug Administration and the U.S. Department of Agriculture. However, everyone has a duty to keep the food supply safe and follow sanitation practices. By using proper sanitation, you can help keep harmful bacteria out of food. **Sanitation** is maintaining cleanliness. Everyone should **anticipate**, or expect and prepare for, risks and follow strict sanitation rules.

Wash Hands Properly

Food safety requires good hygiene. Wash your hands with warm, running water and soap for at least 20 seconds. Scrub your hands entirely, between your fingers, and under your fingernails. Use a paper towel to turn off the faucet. Dry your hands well with a clean towel or air dryer. Wash your hands:

◆ Before preparing food or setting the table.

◆ Between handling different kinds of food.

◆ After touching raw food, including meat, fish, or eggs.

◆ After cleaning appliances or dishes.

◆ After handling garbage or dirty laundry.

◆ After using the toilet or changing a diaper.

◆ After using a phone or computer, or touching animals.

◆ After coughing, sneezing, blowing your nose, or touching your face, hair, skin, or a sore.

Avoid Spreading Bacteria

Besides washing your hands, do the following to avoid spreading bacteria:

◆ Do not handle other people's food if you are sick.

◆ Cover an open sore with a clean waterproof bandage. Wear clean rubber or plastic gloves, and use clean utensils.

◆ Cover your nose and mouth with clean tissue when you sneeze or cough.

◆ Tie back long hair before preparing food.

◆ Wear a clean apron and roll up long sleeves.

◆ Use a clean spoon for each tasting. Do not taste foods containing raw or partly cooked meat, poultry, fish, or eggs.

◆ Do not touch surfaces that contact food or drinks. That includes the rims and insides of glasses, forks, and plates.

◆ Never dip more than once into a common dish.

◆ Use paper towels to wipe or dry your hands.

Keep the Kitchen Clean

Food crumbs, spills, and dirty dishes help bacteria multiply. They also attract insects and mice that leave harmful bacteria. To clean your kitchen, use a disinfectant, a mixture of chlorine bleach and water, or hot, soapy water. Rinse and dry the area.

- Wash countertops before and after preparing food.
- Disinfect kitchen surfaces, appliances, and storage areas.
- Keep dirty dishes, pots, and pans away from food preparation areas. Wash dirty dishes right away in hot, soapy water. Rinse washed dishes in hot water.
- Use a stiff nylon brush to wash cutting boards after each use, or wash them in a dishwasher. Replace worn boards.
- Clean the can opener every time. Wipe unopened can lids.
- Wipe up spills right away and sweep the floor when needed.
- Use different towels for drying dishes and your hands.
- Wash cloth towels, dishcloths, and sponges often.
- Keep garbage tightly covered. Empty daily.
- Wash cans and jars before putting them in a recycling bin.
- Keep pets away from food, appliances, and work surfaces.

✓ **Reading Check** **Discuss** If you were making lunch, when would you need to wash your hands?

Avoid Cross-Contamination

Bacteria from raw meat, poultry, fish, and eggs can spread to foods that will not be cooked, such as fruits or vegetables. The spreading of harmful bacteria from one food to another is called **cross-contamination**.

- Keep raw meat, poultry, fish, and their juices away from ready-to-eat foods at all times.
- Keep a separate cutting board just for raw meat, poultry, and fish, and one for fruits, vegetables, and breads.
- Use plastic cutting boards that are free of cracks.
- Clean all cutting boards with hot, soapy water and a brush, or place them in the dishwasher.
- Wash everything that touches raw food before reusing it.
- Use paper towels to wipe up food scraps, spills, or meat juices. Then wash the counter and your hands right away.

✓ **Reading Check** **Describe** How can you avoid cross-contamination when you prepare chicken?

Store Food Safely

Proper food storage ensures safety and preserves food's freshness, flavor, and nutrients. It also protects food from moisture; drying out; and dirt, dust, insects, and other pests.

Food Safety and Shopping

Keep safety in mind as you shop for food. To keep food safe when shopping, make sure to:

◆ Put raw meat, poultry, and fish in plastic bags so they will not drip on other food.

◆ Check package labels for safe-handling instructions and use-by dates.

◆ Pick canned goods without dents, bulges, rust, or leaks. Bulging cans signal botulism. Dents, rust, and leaks are signs that a can's seal has been broken.

◆ Choose high-quality, fresh produce. Refrigerated foods should feel cold and frozen foods should be solid. Avoid discolored or mushy frozen packages. Ice crystals signal food that was thawed and refrozen.

◆ Shop for refrigerated, frozen, and deli foods last. They will have less time to warm up.

◆ Avoid food packages with holes, tears, and broken, or puffy safety seals.

◆ Take groceries home right away. Avoid making additional trips to other stores. If the trip takes more than 30 minutes, bring an insulated cooler for perishable foods.

Labeled for Safety These safe-handling instructions appear on labels for raw and partially cooked meat and poultry products. Eggs also carry safe-handling instructions to control *Salmonella*. *What does an egg carton say about safe handling?*

SAFE HANDLING INSTRUCTIONS

THIS PRODUCT WAS PREPARED FROM INSPECTED AND PASSED MEAT AND/OR POULTRY. SOME FOOD PRODUCTS MAY CONTAIN BACTERIA THAT COULD CAUSE ILLNESS IF THE PRODUCT IS MISHANDLED OR COOKED IMPROPERLY. FOR YOUR PROTECTION. FOLLOW THESE SAFE HANDLING INSTRUCTIONS.

KEEP REFRIGERATED OR FROZEN. THAW IN REFRIGERATOR OR MICROWAVE

KEEP MEAT AND POULTRY SEPARATE FROM OTHER FOODS. WASH WORKING SURFACES (INCLUDING CUTTING BOARDS), UTENSILS, AND HANDS AFTER TOUCHING RAW MEAT OR POULTRY.

COOK THOROUGHLY.

KEEP HOT FOODS HOT. REFRIGERATE LEFTOVERS IMMEDIATELY OR DISCARD.

Store Food Properly

Put food away as soon as you get home. Check package labels for storage instructions. A food's shelf life is how long it can be stored and still be safe to eat. Put away frozen foods first, then refrigerated foods, and then other foods. Put bulk foods in sealed containers. Put new packages behind older ones to help you follow the first in, first out rule, which states that foods should be used in the order they were purchased.

Freezer Storage

You can keep packaged frozen foods, meat, poultry, fish, bread, and home-prepared mixed dishes safe and appealing by properly freezing them. Some foods do not freeze well, such as cooked egg whites, lettuce, and dishes with mayonnaise or salad dressing.

For longer storage, keep your freezer at 0°F (-8°C) or less. If your freezer temperature is 10°F to 15°F (-12°C to -9°C), limit freezing to just a few weeks. Here are some freezer storage guidelines:

◆ Store frozen foods in their original packages.

◆ Wrap foods properly so they do not spoil or get **freezer burn**. Freezer burn is harmless, but it causes unappealing, dried-up white areas on food. To prevent freezer burn, wrap foods airtight in freezer paper, heavy-duty foil, freezer-quality plastic bags, or plastic freezer containers. Light-duty containers, such as margarine tubs, do not protect food in the freezer.

◆ Label foods with names, date frozen, and serving amounts.

Refrigerator Storage

Perishable foods are foods that spoil easily, such as meat, poultry, fish, dairy foods, eggs, fresh fruits and vegetables, and leftovers. A refrigerator helps keep perishable foods fresh.

Keep your refrigerator as cold as possible without freezing foods. Safe temperatures range from 32°F to 40°F (0°C to 4°C). The **danger zone** is the temperature range in which bacteria grow fastest: 40°F to 140°F (4°C to 60°C). Inside shelves and drawers stay colder than door shelves. Here are some refrigerator storage guidelines:

◆ Use foil, plastic wrap, zippered plastic bags, or airtight containers to cover and protect food.

◆ Put meat, poultry, fish, milk, and eggs on inside shelves. Use door shelves for most condiments.

◆ Place raw meat, poultry, and fish on a plate or in a plastic bag, on the bottom shelf so they do not drip onto other foods.

◆ Leave space for cold air to circulate around food.

◆ Wipe spills right away. Sanitize drawers. Throw away spoiled foods.

Dry Storage

Keep nonperishable foods in a cabinet or pantry. This includes grains such as rice, cereal, flour, and crackers. Oils, dry herbs, and unopened cans and jars can also be stored safely in a cabinet or pantry. Dry storage should be clean, dry, dark, and cool (below 85°F or 29°C). Tips for dry storage include:

◆ Do not store foods above the refrigerator or stove, or near a furnace outlet.

◆ Do not keep food under a sink. Openings around pipes cannot be sealed. Pests and moisture from pipes can spoil food.

◆ Do not store cleaning products or trash near food. Cleaners, detergents and other household chemicals can contaminate food.

◆ Store opened packages and bulk food in tightly covered containers to keep out insects and moisture.

◆ Read the labels on food packaging. Some foods need refrigeration after being opened.

What If Food Spoils?

Food spoils when it is stored improperly or for too long. Bacteria and other organisms, such as mold, cause spoilage. Changes in moisture content also make food less appealing.

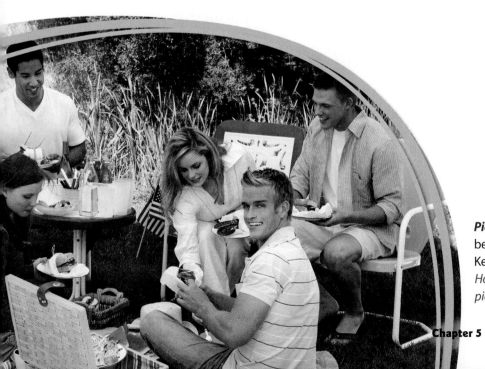

Picnic Safety Perishable foods should be kept at the proper temperature. Keep hot foods hot and cold food cold. *How can you keep foods safe while you picnic?*

Spoiled food may have an unusual color, odor, or texture. Throw away this food. Discard leaky or bulging cans, jars with cracks or loose or bulging lids, and containers that spurt liquid when opened. Wrap moldy food well before throwing it away. Since mold spreads, check nearby foods, and clean the container and the refrigerator.

Some spoiled foods show no signs that they have gone bad. Throw away leftovers more than four days old or that may have been stored improperly. Remember: When in doubt, throw it out!

✓ **Reading Check** **Explain** Why is it a good idea to put new packages of food behind older ones?

Control Food Temperature

Food must be properly thawed, cooked, and served to keep bacteria from growing. When you thaw, cook, and serve food, remember to keep the food out of the danger zone temperatures. Use a NSF International® approved thermometer to ensure accuracy.

Thaw Food Safely

Some frozen foods should be thawed before cooking them. Never thaw food at room temperature. Bacteria can grow on the outside before the inside thaws. Use one of these methods:

♦ **Refrigerator** Place frozen foods on the lowest shelf in a plastic bag so they do not drip. Allow enough time. Frozen turkey, for example, may take several days.

♦ **Cold Water** Place food in a watertight plastic bag, then in cold water. Change the water every 30 minutes to stay cold.

♦ **Microwave Oven** Defrost on the low or defrost setting. Cook microwave-thawed food immediately.

Cook Food Completely

To destroy harmful bacteria, cook food long enough to reach the proper temperature on the inside. (See **Figure 5.2**.) Color and texture changes are not reliable signs of doneness. Follow these guidelines to ensure complete cooking:

♦ Cook food fully. For example, roasting turkey for half the cooking time and then finishing on another day is unsafe.

♦ Check the internal (inside) temperature with a clean meat thermometer. Do not rely on a pop-up thermometer already inserted in poultry.

♦ Avoid raw or partly cooked eggs.

◆ Use proper microwave cooking techniques for even heating. Some microwave and convection ovens have temperature probes. These probes shut off the oven when food reaches the right internal temperature.

Serve Food Safely

Temperatures must be controlled when serving food. If the air is 90°F (32°C) or higher, do not keep food out for longer than one hour. If the air is below 90°F (32°C), do not keep food out for longer than two hours. Follow these three basic rules to serve food safely:

◆ **Keep hot foods hot.** If they will not be eaten immediately, keep foods above 140°F (60°C) in a slow cooker or oven.

◆ **Keep cold foods cold.** Refrigerate cold foods until serving. Put cold buffet platters on ice or use an insulated cooler with ice or freezer packs.

◆ **Limit serving time.** Perishable foods should not be kept out of the refrigerator. This includes meat, poultry, fish, eggs, mayonnaise, and soy and dairy dishes.

Figure 5.2	Food Temperature

Cook to a Safe Temperature Use a meat thermometer to make sure that food is completely cooked. *Why should you use a meat thermometer to check the inside temperature of a hamburger?*

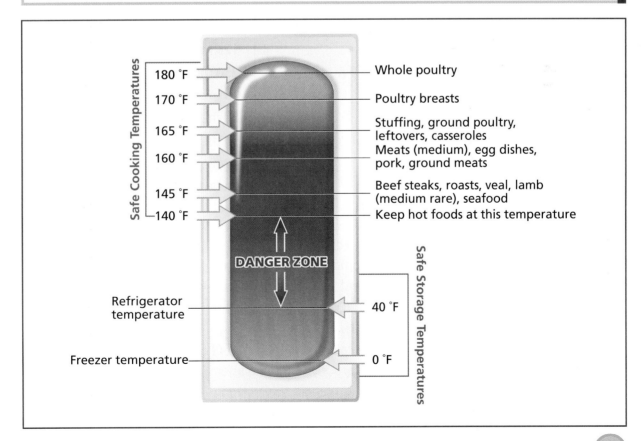

Handle Leftovers Properly

Leftovers must be stored properly to be safe. Follow these rules for keeping leftovers:

◆ Throw away food that is kept too long at room temperature.

◆ Refrigerate or freeze leftovers as soon as the meal is done.

◆ Eat refrigerated leftovers within three to four days.

◆ Reheat leftover solid foods to 165°F (74°C).

◆ Boil leftover soups, sauces, and gravies before eating.

Practice the food safety procedures described in this chapter. You will stay healthier, enjoy food more, and save money, too.

✓ **Reading Check** **Identify** What are three ways to serve food safely?

EASY RECIPES
International Flavors

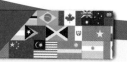

Pasta Salad

Customary	Ingredients	Metric
1 cup	Orzo pasta	250 mL
1 cup	Carrots, chopped	250 mL
1 cup	Green pepper, chopped	250 mL
¼ cup	Red onion, chopped	125 mL
1 cup	Yellow corn, cooked	250 mL
1 Tbsp.	Parsley, chopped	15 mL
¼ cup	Olive oil	60 mL
2 Tbsp.	Red wine vinegar	30 mL
¼ tsp	Salt	1 mL
To taste	Pepper	To taste

Try This!
Try using different vegetables and vinegars.

Yield: 4 servings, 1½ cup (375 mL) each

❶ Cook pasta in boiling water. Drain and chill.

❷ Put the carrots, green pepper, corn, onion, and parsley into a large bowl. Add chilled pasta.

❸ Mix olive oil, red wine vinegar, salt, and pepper in a small bowl and then pour over the pasta salad.

❹ Toss well and serve cold.

Nutritional Information Per Serving: 398 calories, 15 g total fat (2 g saturated fat), 0 mg cholesterol, 174 mg sodium, 58 g total carbohydrates (5 g fiber, 7 g total sugars), 10 g protein

Percent Daily Value: vitamin A 110%, vitamin C 60%, calcium 4%, iron 15%

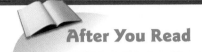

After You Read

CHAPTER SUMMARY

Eating food contaminated with large numbers of bacteria, parasites, viruses, or fungi is the main cause of foodborne illnesses. Poisons and bits of other material can also contaminate food. If warmth, moisture, and food all are present, bacteria can multiply quickly to dangerous levels. Prevent most foodborne illnesses by following good hygiene and sanitation rules. Handle food safely when you shop for, store, prepare, and serve it. Avoid cross-contamination. Keep food out of the temperature danger zone so harmful bacteria cannot thrive. Cook food to a safe internal temperature. Store food properly to avoid contamination.

Vocabulary Review

1. Define each vocabulary term in your own words.

Content Vocabulary
- foodborne illness (p. 66)
- bacteria (p. 66)
- contaminate (p. 66)
- sanitation (p. 69)
- cross-contamination (p. 70)
- freezer burn (p. 72)
- perishable (p. 72)
- danger zone (p. 72)

Academic Vocabulary
- signal (p. 68)
- anticipate (p. 69)

Review Key Concepts

2. Describe the causes, effects, and treatment of foodborne illness.

3. Explain proper kitchen sanitation.

4. Discuss how to protect food from cross-contamination.

5. Identify proper food storage procedures.

6. Explain how to keep food out of the temperature danger zone.

Critical Thinking

7. Analyze your responsibility for keeping food safe for yourself and others. Use what you know about food safety. Explain what you would do if you were at someone else's home and saw food being handled in unsafe ways.

8. Predict what could happen if you used the same platter for raw hamburgers and cooked hamburgers. What might the consequences be? Why?

9. Create a sketch, cartoon, or poster describing a top 10 list of food safety mistakes.

Real-World Skills and Applications

Set Goals and Make Decisions

10. Home Food Safety Do a food safety check at home. Identify what your family does to keep food safe and what you could do better. Write a family food safety plan. Put it in action. Record your successes—and any next steps your family needs to take to make food safety a priority.

Interpersonal and Collaborative

11. Teach Handwashing Volunteer to teach proper handwashing to young children, perhaps in a preschool or elementary school. For fun, sing the "ABC song," which takes about 20 seconds—the time needed for proper handwashing. Share your experience in class.

Financial Literacy

12. Bulk Food A bulk goods store sells ground meat in 3-pound (1½ kg) packages and grapefruit by the dozen. Alli paid one-third less for these items at the bulk goods store than at her regular market. But she ended up discarding half of each because of spoilage. Write a paragraph that explains whether these purchases were a good deal for Alli.

Technology

13. Emergency Preparedness Create a visual presentation, such as a poster, computer presentation, or video, on preparing for emergencies such as hurricanes and power outages. Include an emergency food checklist. Explain how to keep food safe for and during emergencies. Show your presentation in class.

 14. Antibacterial Soap Learn about antibacterial soap and detergent. Are they more effective than plain soap? Are they better at removing bacteria from hands than other soaps? What are some possible disadvantages of these soaps? Present your findings to the class.

 15. Food Safety Game Create a crossword puzzle about food safety, including bacteria and other causes of foodborne illness. Include at least 20 terms in your puzzle. Make up an answer sheet. Swap with a classmate, and solve each other's puzzle.

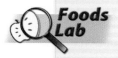 **16. Bacterial Spread** Observe how easily foods can cross-contaminate. Coat a small cheese slice with cinnamon. Put it on a cutting board and cut it in half. Cut another slice of cheese in half using the same cutting board and knife. Compare the two pieces of cheese. Draw conclusions.

 Additional Activities For additional activities go to this book's Online Learning Center through glencoe.com.

Academic Skills

 English Language Arts

17. Investigate a Local Story Write a summary of a recent incident of local foodborne illness. Identify the cause of the illness, learn where the incident occurred, and determine how it could have been avoided. List your resources.

> **NCTE 7** Conduct research and gather, evaluate, and synthesize data to communicate discoveries.

 Science

18. Fresh Eggs How recently an egg was laid is only one factor that affects its freshness.

Procedure Research other factors that affect egg freshness. Take notes on your discoveries.

Analysis Analyze each of the factors you found. Create a chart showing why each is important.

> **NSES Content Standard B:** Develop an understanding of the structure and properties of matter.

 Mathematics

19. Conversions You arrive home to find your power is out. Your brother says the freezer still feels cold, so it is okay to cook a frozen steak. You measure the temperature with a freezer thermometer. It reads 3°C. Dad says that the steak is okay to cook today. Mom says to throw it out. What temperature is the freezer using customary measurement (the Fahrenheit scale)? What should you do with the steak?

 Customary System Celsius is a metric scale with 100° separating freezing and boiling. Fahrenheit is the customary scale with 180° separating freezing and boiling.

Starting Hint To convert from Celsius to Fahrenheit, multiply by $\frac{9}{5}$, then add 32. Remember that your freezer works best at temperatures 0°F to 10°F.

For more math help, go to the Math Appendix

> **NCTM Measurement** Apply appropriate techniques, tools, and formulas to determine measurements.

STANDARDIZED TEST PRACTICE

ESSAY
Read the paragraph, then read the writing prompt and write an essay on a separate piece of paper.

Test-Taking Tip When answering essay questions, make sure that you support generalizations with evidence. Answer even short essay questions with accurate explanations backed up by facts.

All restaurants are inspected by the health department to be sure they are safe and clean. Local news stations often report these findings. Restaurants follow strict rules to maintain food safety. For example, employees who handle food must wash their hands and arms in a certain way.

20. How would your kitchen rate if it were inspected by the health department? Write a short essay about how you, as a good cook, keep food safe.

CHAPTER 6
Kitchen Safety

Explore the Photo ▶▶

Accidents in the Kitchen The most common kitchen accidents are cuts, falls, electrical shock, burns, and poisoning. *What can you do to reduce the chance of accidents in your kitchen?*

Writing Activity

Autobiographical Paragraph

Kitchen Memories People have many memories of time spent in the kitchen. Think of a time when something went wrong in the kitchen. What could have been done differently to prevent the accident? Write an autobiographical paragraph about your memory.

Writing Tips

1. **Tell** what happened.

2. **Explain** how you felt before and after the accident.

3. **Use** details to make the incident come to life for the reader.

Reading Guide

Before You Read

Vocabulary Divide a piece of paper into two columns. Label the left column *Vocabulary* and the right column *What Is It?* Skim the chapter. Write each vocabulary word in the left column and a brief definition in the right column.

Read to Learn

Key Concepts
- **Identify** common kitchen hazards.
- **Explain** how to handle kitchen emergencies.

Main Idea

Kitchen safety means preventing burns, cuts, falls, electrical shocks, choking, and poisoning. If accidents happen, you need to be prepared to take fast action.

Content Vocabulary

◇ flammable
◇ pesticide
◇ poison control center
◇ antidote
◇ first aid
◇ Heimlich maneuver
◇ cardiopulmonary resuscitation (CPR)

Academic Vocabulary

You will find these words in your reading and on your tests. Use the glossary to look up their definitions if necessary.

▪ appropriate
▪ crucial

Graphic Organizer

As you read, write five steps you can take to be prepared for kitchen emergencies.

Prepare for Kitchen Emergencies
1.
2.
3.
4.
5.

 Graphic Organizer Go to this book's Online Learning Center at glencoe.com to print out this graphic organizer.

Academic Standards ▪ ▪ ▪ ▪ ▪ ▪ ▪ ▪ ▪ ▪ ▪ ▪ ▪ ▪ ▪ ▪ ▪ ▪ ▪

 English Language Arts

NCTE 4 Use written language to communicate effectively.

NCTE 8 Use information resources to gather information and create and communicate knowledge.

NCTE 9 Develop an understanding of diversity in language use across cultures.

 Mathematics

NCTM Number and Operations Understand numbers, ways of representing numbers, relationships among numbers, and number systems.

 Science

NSES Content Standard B Develop an understanding of the structure and properties of matter.

NSES Content Standard B Develop an understanding of motions and forces.

NCTE National Council of Teachers of English
NCTM National Council of Teachers of Mathematics

NSES National Science Education Standards
NCSS National Council for the Social Studies

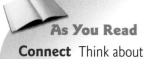

As You Read

Connect Think about how you can be safer in the kitchen.

How to Prevent Accidents

You can prevent most kitchen accidents. The most common cause of accidents is simply being careless. Start with these basic safety rules to avoid injuring yourself and others:

◆ Keep hair, loose clothing, jewelry, or apron strings from dangling. They could catch fire or get tangled in appliances.

◆ Pay attention to your tasks.

◆ Use the right tool for each job.

How to Prevent Cuts

Vocabulary

You can find definitions in the glossary at the back of this book.

Knife safety can help you prevent cuts. Keep knives sharp. Dull knives are more dangerous than sharp ones because you have to push harder on the blade to make it cut. This may cause the knife to slip. Always cut away from yourself. Never cut toward others or point sharp objects at anyone. Other tips for preventing cuts include:

◆ Use a cutting board. Do not hold food in your hand to cut.

◆ Do not try to catch a falling knife.

◆ Use knives only to cut food. They are not **appropriate**, or proper, tools for opening cans or tightening screws.

◆ Do not swing your arms when walking with a knife. Keep the knife loosely pressed against your thigh.

◆ Wash knives separately from other dishes.

◆ Store knives in a knife block, rack, or drawer divider.

◆ Use a can opener that makes a smooth edge. Throw away the lid immediately.

◆ Throw away chipped or cracked plates and glasses.

◆ Never pick up broken glass with bare fingers. Use a broom to pick up large pieces and a wet paper towel to grab tiny pieces.

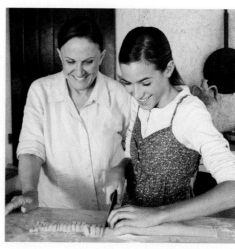

Knife Safety To cut safely, use the right knife for the job. Hold your hand so that your fingertips are under your knuckles, and be careful of the thumb holding the food! Never push with your hand on the end of the knife blade. *What other advice would you give for using a knife safely?*

How to Prevent Falls, Bruises, and Back Injuries

Falls, bruises, and back injuries are common kitchen accidents. Prevent them by following a few simple rules:

◆ Clean up spills immediately.

◆ Never walk on a wet floor. Clear away floor clutter.

◆ Use a sturdy ladder or step stool to reach high shelves. Chairs tip over easily.

◆ Choose kitchen rugs with nonskid backing.

◆ Store heavy items within easy reach. Lift them with care.

◆ Close drawers and cabinet doors after you open them.

How to Prevent Electrical Shocks and Burns

Electricity can give a shock or burn, or even kill you. Follow these safety rules to prevent shocks and burns:

◆ Keep electrical appliances and cords away from water, the sink, the stove, and other heat sources.

◆ Never use electrical appliances when your hands are wet or when you are standing on a wet floor.

◆ Unplug appliances before cleaning them. Do not put electrical appliances in water unless the label reads immersible.

◆ Keep appliances and their cords in good condition.

◆ Hold the plug, not the cord, when you unplug an appliance. Tugging on the cord may damage it.

◆ Do not run electrical cords under a rug.

◆ If food gets stuck in an appliance, disconnect it first. For a toaster, turn it upside down. If the food does not easily shake loose, take the appliance to a repair person.

◆ Never insert a fork or other object into an appliance. You could get a shock. The appliance also could be damaged.

◆ Do not plug too many appliances into one outlet.

◆ If someone around you gets shocked, do not touch them until it is safe! Turn off and disconnect any appliance. You may need to turn off the electricity at the main switch. This will protect you from getting shocked, too.

Science in Action

Kitchen Fires

Fire requires three ingredients: heat, fuel, and oxygen. When you add some type of ignition source, you have a fire! The ignition is the mechanism that ignites the fuel. To ignite is to cause to start burning.

Procedure Choose one type of kitchen fire to analyze. Conduct research to identify what might cause this type of fire. Also, find out about safe ways to put out this type of fire.

Analysis Write a report on your findings. In your report, describe the type of fire, typical causes, and safe ways to put out that type of fire.

NSES Content Standard B Develop an understanding of the structure and properties of matter.

Cafeteria Cook

Most schools have cafeterias. Kitchen safety is essential for cafeteria cooks, who prepare large quantities of nutritious meals for students.

Careers Find out more about careers. Go to this book's Online Learning Center at **glencoe.com**.

How to Prevent Burns and Fires

Several kitchen hazards can burn you or cause fires. Follow these guidelines to prevent burns and fires:

◆ Wear close-fitting clothes. Roll up sleeves. Tie back hair.

◆ Keep flammable materials at least 3 feet (1 meter) away from the range. **Flammable** means easy to catch on fire.

◆ Keep equipment clean. Grease buildup is very flammable.

◆ Use dry potholders and oven mitts to handle hot items. Damp ones can cause steam burns.

◆ Turn pot and pan handles toward the center of the range. This keeps someone from bumping a hot pan off the range.

◆ Watch foods carefully while they cook on the range.

◆ Tilt the cover of a hot pan so steam flows away from you.

◆ Wait until appliances cool before cleaning them.

◆ Stand to one side as you open a hot oven.

◆ Keep aerosol cans away from heat. They can explode if heated. Their spray may also be flammable.

◆ Keep a fire extinguisher nearby and learn how to use it.

How to Prevent Poisoning

Many cleaning and pest control products are poisonous. This makes it **crucial**, or important, to follow label directions exactly.

◆ Keep food away from pesticides. A **pesticide** is a poison that kills insects or other pests.

◆ Point spray containers away from people.

◆ Keep household chemicals in their original containers.

◆ Never mix chemicals or store them near food.

Kitchen Safety and Physical Challenges Safe kitchens can be designed for people with physical challenges such as impaired vision, limited hand strength, and difficulty standing or walking. *What simple changes can make a kitchen safer for someone who uses a wheelchair?*

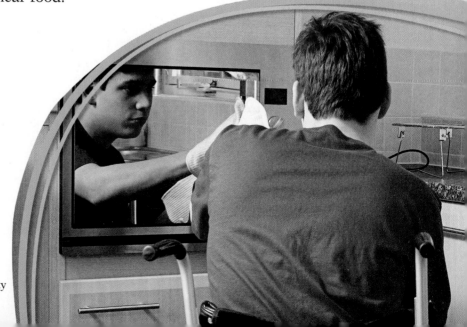

If someone is poisoned, call the poison control center. A **poison control center** is a medical facility that gives free advice about handling poison emergencies. Tell the kind of poison, how much and when it was swallowed, and any symptoms. Look on the container to find out if there is an antidote. An **antidote** is a substance that works against a poison.

✓ **Reading Check** **Explain** Why is it important to be careful when using electricity?

How to Handle Kitchen Emergencies

It is important to be prepared in case an accident happens. (See the First Aid Appendix at the back of this book for more information.) Follow these five steps to be prepared to handle accidents:

1. Keep emergency telephone numbers by the telephone.

2. Keep a first-aid kit nearby. **First aid** is immediate care that prevents more injury and relieves pain. Call for help immediately for a serious injury.

3. Have an action plan in case of a fire.

4. Learn the Heimlich maneuver. The **Heimlich maneuver** is a life-saving technique to help someone who is choking.

5. Learn **cardiopulmonary resuscitation** (CPR), a life-saving technique to restart someone's breathing and heartbeat.

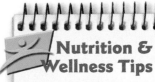

Nutrition & Wellness Tips

Poison Control

✓ Handle kitchen chemicals safely by keeping them tightly closed in their original containers, with the labels intact.

Discover International Foods

China

Chinese cuisine features a nutritious combination of vegetables, rice, and noodles; small amounts of meat, poultry, fish, and tofu; and seasonings such as soy sauce. Ingredients are often cut in small pieces and cooked in a wok. Regional dishes reflect different cooking styles. Meals are served family-style with spoons and chopsticks.

Languages Across Cultures

dim sum *('dim-'səm)* light meal with many small dishes, such as *shaomai* (small dumplings), *bau* (stuffed buns), or spring rolls, served in a steamer basket or on a small plate

tofu *('tō-(,)fü)* cheese-like food, high in protein, and made from soybeans

 Recipes Find out more about international recipes on this book's Online Learning Center at glencoe.com.

NCTE 9 Develop an understanding of diversity in language use across cultures.

How to Put Out a Kitchen Fire

◆ Use the right fire extinguisher to put out a small fire.

◆ Use baking soda, salt, or a fire extinguisher to put out a grease fire. Water may cause grease to spatter and burn you.

◆ Put the cover on a pan or close an appliance door if food is burning inside. This will smother the fire.

◆ Leave a burning pan on the range. You could spill burning grease or spread the fire if you try to move it.

◆ Turn off the heat source or disconnect the appliance.

◆ If your clothing is on fire, stop what you are doing, drop to the ground, and roll back and forth to put out any flames.

◆ Leave if the fire seems out of your control. Alert others in the building. Call 911 once you are clear of the building.

✓ Reading Check **Describe** How should you put out a grease fire?

EASY RECIPES International Flavors

Asian Stir-Fried Vegetables

Customary	Ingredients	Metric
1 cup	White onion	250 mL
1 cup	Carrots	250 mL
1 cup	Zucchini	250 mL
1 cup	Green bell pepper	250 mL
1 ½ tsp.	Vegetable oil	7 mL
1 cup	Bean sprouts	250 mL
2 tsp.	Low-sodium soy sauce	10 mL
¼ tsp.	Ground ginger	1 mL

Try This!

For more protein, stir-fry thin strips of beef or chicken first. Remove the cooked meat from the wok, then stir-fry the vegetables. Return the meat and mix all in the wok. Serve with cooked rice.

Yield: 4 servings, ½ cup (125 mL) each

❶ Cut the vegetables into thin strips about two inches long. Heat a wok or heavy skillet over high heat. Add oil, then the onion and carrots. Stir-fry for 2 minutes.

❷ Add the zucchini and bell pepper. Continue stir-frying for 1 minute.

❸ Add the bean sprouts. Stir-fry for 45 to 60 seconds or until hot. Turn off the heat, add the soy sauce and ginger and mix gently. Serve immediately.

Nutritional Information Per Serving: 74 calories, 2 g total fat (0 g saturated fat), 0 mg cholesterol, 117 mg sodium, 12 g carbohydrate (3 g fiber, 6 g total sugars), 4 g protein

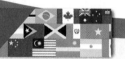

Percent Daily Value: vitamin A 100%, vitamin C 100%, calcium 4%, iron 6%

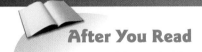

After You Read

CHAPTER SUMMARY

You can prevent most kitchen accidents by following the rules of kitchen safety. Cuts, falls, electrical shocks, burns and fires, and poisoning are common kitchen accidents. Being prepared for accidents makes them easier to handle. This includes reacting quickly, knowing how to handle fires, giving first aid, calling for help in emergencies, and following instructions until help arrives.

Vocabulary Review

1. Use each of these vocabulary words in a sentence.

Content Vocabulary
◇ flammable (p. 84)
◇ pesticide (p. 84)
◇ poison control center (p. 85)
◇ antidote (p. 85)
◇ first aid (p. 85)
◇ Heimlich maneuver (p. 85)
◇ cardiopulmonary resuscitation (CPR) (p. 85)

Academic Vocabulary
■ appropriate (p. 82)
■ crucial (p. 84)

Review Key Concepts

2. Identify common kitchen hazards.

3. Explain how to handle kitchen emergencies.

Critical Thinking

4. Describe what you would do if you were frying chicken in oil and a fire started in the pan. Also, explain how you could have prevented it.

5. Analyze the following situation: Tanika has two knives: one is dull, and the other is sharp. She uses the dull knife to avoid cutting herself. Is she correct? Explain.

6. Examine the proper and safe procedure for using an oven cleaner.

7. Analyze how you would teach young children about poison safety. What safety rules would you share? How would you get children to remember and understand them?

8. Describe similarities in the five steps for handling kitchen emergencies.

9. Evaluate an action plan for home fire emergency. Find and critique an action plan. Is it complete and easy to understand?

Real-World Skills and Applications

Set Goals and Make Decisions

10. Accident-Free Kitchens The Occupational Safety and Health Administration (OSHA) requires food service kitchens to follow safety rules to prevent accidents. Interview your school's food service director to learn about OSHA rules. Find out how the school reaches its kitchen safety goals. Report your findings in class.

Collaborative and Interpersonal

11. Household Safety Follow your teacher's directions to break into small groups. Choose a common kitchen injury. Discuss the injury and how you would help a victim, provide first aid, and avoid further injury. Summarize your discussion for the class.

Technology

12. Kitchen Safety Training Create a script for a training video to show the safe operation of a gas range. The script should describe how a gas range and its burners operate. Also, describe how to prevent a grease fire from occurring, and from spreading if it happens. Include visual directions in your script.

Financial Literacy

13. Need Sharp Knives? You could have your kitchen knives sharpened professionally at FoodMart for $5 each. Or, you can buy a good knife sharpener for $40 and sharpen them yourself. If you have 7 kitchen knives, which option would cost more? Why?

14. Disposal of Chemicals Contact a local or state agency or waste treatment company to learn the safe, legal way to dispose of dangerous kitchen chemicals. Learn why proper disposal is important. Write two paragraphs describing wrong and right ways. Share your findings with the class and your family.

> **NCTE 8** Use information resources to gather information and create and communicate knowledge.

15. Develop a First-Aid Kit Develop a complete supply list of what is needed to make a home first-aid kit. Identify the supplies you would need to help victims of the many different accidents that can occur in a kitchen.

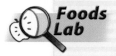

16. Chemicals in the Kitchen Create a table of the types of household chemicals that are in the foods lab at school or in your kitchen at home. Indicate if the products are stored correctly. Note whether any warnings or special instructions are given on the labels. Write a paragraph to summarize the safe storage of each chemical.

Additional Activities For additional activities, go to this book's Online Learning Center at glencoe.com.

Academic Skills

 English Language Arts

17. Kitchen Safety Poster Create a poster about kitchen safety for your school foods lab. Decide on one main message about preventing accidents in the kitchen. Consider your audience and message, and the best way to deliver that message. As a class, decide which posters to hang.

> **NCTE 4** Use written language to communicate effectively.

 Science

18. Step Stool Safety If you must use a step stool to reach something, it is important to use it in the safest way possible.

Procedure Position a step stool near something out of reach. What might happen if you used the step stool sideways? What is the safest way to use a step stool?

Analysis Write a paragraph to explain which position is safest and why.

> **NSES Content Standard B** Develop an understanding of motions and forces.

 Mathematics

19. Unintentional Poisoning According to the Home Safety Council, about 20,000 people die each year from unintentional home injuries. Of that number, 4,833 deaths were from unintentional poisoning. What percentage of the total deaths were from unintentional poisoning?

Math Concept **Percents** Percent means "for each hundredth." So 10% = 0.10, or 10 hundredths. 4% = 0.04, or 4 hundredths.

Starting Hint Divide the number of unintentional poisoning deaths (4,833) by the total number of deaths (20,000). Then, convert the decimal to a percentage by moving the decimal two places to the right.

 For more math help, go to the Math Appendix

> **NCTM Number and Operations** Understand numbers, ways of representing numbers, relationships among numbers, and number systems.

STANDARDIZED TEST PRACTICE

ESSAY
Read the paragraph, then read the writing prompt. Write your essay on a separate piece of paper.

Test-Taking Tip When answering an essay question, focus on one main idea. Do not write long introductions and conclusions; spend most of your time answering the question.

The kitchen can be a dangerous place. About 30% of all U.S. fires start there. A stove can tip over while you clean it. Also, many people have been burned by boiling water or by steam. One moment of inattention can cause a serious burn.

20. Think of what you learned in this chapter. Then, write a short essay about how your kitchen can be made safer for the people who work in it.

Unit 3 Thematic Project

Plan a Safe Kitchen

Not only is it important for your health to eat well, you must also ensure that your food is properly handled and prepared. In addition, you must follow kitchen safety guidelines because even the most routine tasks can be dangerous if not done properly. Think about the kitchen safety and sanitation regulations required by the health department. Why do you think these rules were developed?

My Journal

If you completed the journal entry from page 62, refer to it to see if you were aware of important kitchen sanitation requirements.

Project Assignment

In this project you will:
- Research kitchen safety and sanitation regulations.
- Write a summary of your research.
- Write a list of interview questions.
- Interview someone in the community whose place of business is regulated by the health department.
- While interviewing, take notes, and after interviewing, transcribe your notes.
- Plan a kitchen that promotes safety and sanitation practices.
- Create a graphic that includes callouts that explain the parts of the kitchen and how they promote food and kitchen safety.
- Make a presentation to your classmates.

Academic Skills You Will Use ∙ ∙ ∙ ∙
English Language Arts

NCTE 7 Conduct research and gather, evaluate, and synthesize data to communicate discoveries.

NCTE 8 Use information resources to gather information and create and communicate knowledge.

STEP ① Research Safety and Sanitation Regulations

Conduct research about kitchen safety and sanitation regulations required by your local health department. Write a summary of your research that:
- Describes safety and sanitation regulations
- Explains why it is important to have uniform sanitation regulations for all kitchens
- Lists ways safety and sanitation regulations affect your life

STEP ② Plan Your Interview

Use the results of your research to develop a list of interview questions. Keep these writing skills in mind as you form your questions.

Writing Skills
- Use complete sentences.
- Use correct spelling and grammar.
- Organize your questions in the order you want to ask them.

STEP 3 Connect with Your Community

Interview someone in your community whose place of business is regulated by the health department. For example, you might interview a local restaurant owner or the manager of a school or hospital cafeteria. Use the questions you formed in Step 2 to interview him or her.

Listening Skills
- Make eye contact with your subject when he or she answers questions.
- Ask additional questions to ensure your understanding.
- Show your interest by responding appropriately.

STEP 4 Create Your Final Presentation

Use the Unit Thematic Project Checklist to plan and give an oral report. Use these speaking skills as you present your final report.

Speaking Skills
- Speak clearly and concisely.
- Be sensitive to the needs of your audience.
- Use standard English to communicate.

STEP 5 Evaluate Your Presentation

Your project will be reviewed and evaluated based on:
- Depth of interview and questions
- Content of your presentation
- Mechanics—presentation and neatness

Evaluation Rubric Go to this book's Online Learning Center at glencoe.com for a rubric you can use to evaluate your final report.

Project Checklist	
Plan	✓ Conduct research on safety and sanitation regulations. ✓ Write a summary of your research. ✓ Write interview questions. ✓ Conduct an interview. ✓ Transcribe the notes from your interview. ✓ Create a graphic of a kitchen with callouts that indicate the ways the kitchen complies with safety and sanitation regulations. ✓ Create a five-minute oral presentation.
Present	✓ Make a presentation to your class to explain the results of your research and interview. ✓ Display and describe the various aspects of safety and sanitation represented in your kitchen graphic. ✓ Speak slowly and clearly. ✓ Invite the students of the class to ask any questions they may have. Answer these questions. ✓ When students ask questions, demonstrate in your answers that you respect their perspectives. ✓ Turn in your research summary, interview questions, interview notes, and your kitchen graphic to your teacher.
Academic Skills	✓ Conduct research to gather information. ✓ Communicate effectively. ✓ Organize your presentation so the audience can follow along easily. ✓ Thoroughly express your ideas.

Unit 4

Food and Your Body

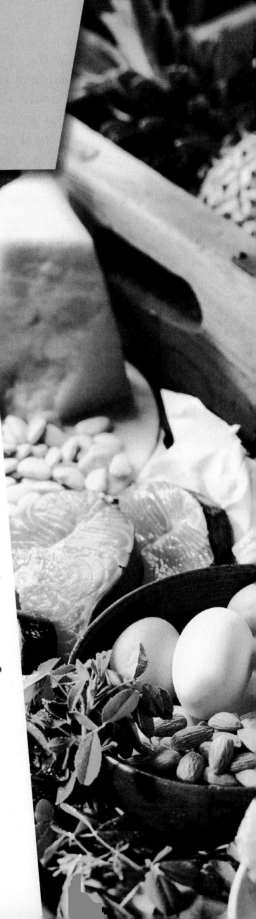

Chapters in this Unit

Chapter 7   Nutrients: From Food to You
Chapter 8   Dietary Guidelines
Chapter 9   MyPyramid and You

Unit Thematic Project Preview

Investigate Food Trends

In the unit thematic project at the end of this unit, you will research a current food trend. You will then interview someone in your community about the trend. You will examine the health effects of the trend and record your findings. Then, you will prepare a presentation to share what you have learned.

My Journal

Food trends may influence the food choices you make. You can make better food choices now if you remember the food choices you have made in the past.

Write a journal entry that answers these questions:
- What did you eat today?
- What did you eat yesterday?
- How might your food choices have been improved?

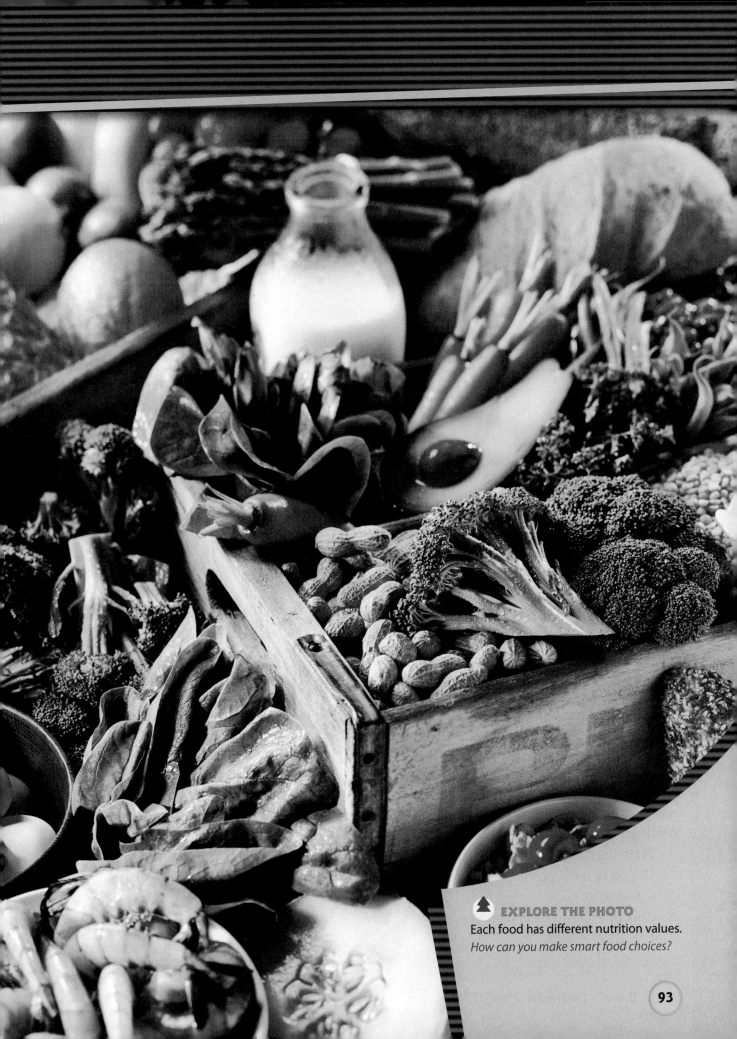

CHAPTER 7
Nutrients: From Food to You

Explore the Photo ▶▶

Food tastes good. It also provides substances that your body needs to be healthy. *What nourishing foods have you eaten today?*

Writing Activity

Write a Paragraph

Eat Nourishing Meals for Good Health Food provides nutrients. These are substances that your body needs to work properly. Write a paragraph that describes a healthful meal that you like to eat and explains why you think it is healthful.

Writing Tips

1. **State** the main idea with a topic sentence.
2. **Organize** the supporting details in a logical order.
3. **Reread** your paragraph to make sure it is clear for your audience.

Reading Guide

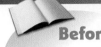

Before You Read

Understanding It is normal to have questions when you read. Write any questions you have about nutrients on a separate sheet of paper. Cross off the questions that you answer as you read. Ask your teacher any questions that are still on your list when you finish reading.

Read to Learn

Key Concepts

- **List** the three main nutrient functions.
- **List** the six categories of nutrients.
- **Explain** energy balance.
- **Describe** the possible effects of getting too few or too many nutrients.
- **Describe** the safe use of dietary supplements.

Main Idea

Nutrients provide energy, build and repair body cells, and keep your body working.

Content Vocabulary

- ◇ nutrient
- ◇ carbohydrate
- ◇ sugar
- ◇ starch
- ◇ fiber
- ◇ proteins
- ◇ vitamins
- ◇ minerals
- ◇ Recommended Dietary Allowances
- ◇ malnutrition
- ◇ supplement

Academic Vocabulary

You will find these words in your reading and on your tests. Use the glossary to look up their definitions if necessary.

- ▪ process
- ▪ appropriate

Graphic Organizer

Use a graphic organizer like the one below to list the six categories of nutrients.

Nutrients
1.
2.
3.
4.
5.
6.

 Graphic Organizer Go to this book's Online Learning Center at **glencoe.com** to print out this graphic organizer.

Academic Standards · · · · · · · · · · · · · · · ·

 English Language Arts
NCTE 2 Read literature to build an understanding of the human experience.

 Social Studies
NCSS III J People, Places, and Environments
Analyze and evaluate social and economic effects of environmental changes and crises resulting from phenomena such as floods, storms, and drought.

 Mathematics
NCTM Numbers and Operations Understand numbers, ways of representing numbers, relationships among numbers, and number systems.

NCTM Geometry Analyze characteristics and properties of two- and three-dimensional geometric shapes and develop mathematical arguments about geometric relationships.

NCTE National Council of Teachers of English
NCTM National Council of Teachers of Mathematics

NSES National Science Education Standards
NCSS National Council for the Social Studies

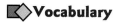
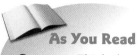

As You Read

Connect Think about how the nutrients in your lunch will be used by your body.

Nutrients for Wellness

A **nutrient** is a substance that performs a job in your body. More than 40 nutrients belong in six groups: carbohydrates, fats, proteins, vitamins, minerals, and water. You need larger amounts of macronutrients: carbohydrates, proteins, and fats. You need small amounts of micronutrients: vitamins and minerals. Eat a variety of foods to get a variety of nutrients. The "Nutritive Value of Foods" Appendix shows nutrient amounts in specific foods.

What Nutrients Do for You

When you are well nourished, you feel good, grow properly, and perform your best. Nutrients work in three main ways:

♦ **Nutrients give you energy.** Your body uses energy, even as you sleep. Carbohydrates, fats, and proteins supply energy.

♦ **Nutrients build and repair body cells.** A healthy body constantly replaces worn-out or damaged cells. Proteins help build and repair your cells and help you grow.

♦ **Nutrients regulate body processes.** Body **processes**, or functions, include breathing, digesting food, and building red blood cells, and all your body functions.

How Digestion and Absorption Work

To use nutrients, your body must digest the food you eat. Digestion is the breaking down of food in the body. After your body digests food, nutrients are absorbed into your bloodstream so they can be used by your body.

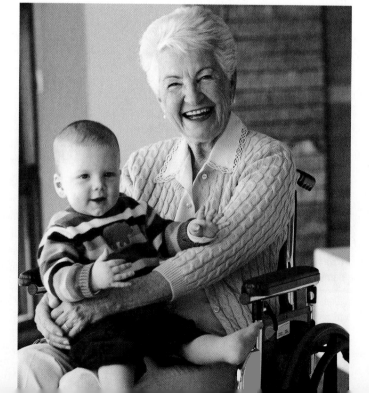

Choose Nutritious Foods
People of all ages need to eat foods with enough nutrients. Think of the foods you eat. *Do you get the nutrients you need?*

Digestion and absorption occurs in many parts of the body:

◆ **Mouth** Saliva in the mouth starts to break down food chemically. Chewing breaks down food physically.

◆ **Esophagus** Your esophagus carries food to the stomach.

◆ **Stomach** Gastric juices break down food chemically.

◆ **Small Intestine** Digestive juices produced in the liver, pancreas, and small intestine fully break down food. Nutrients are absorbed into the bloodstream.

◆ **Liver** Nutrients are taken to the liver, where they are made ready for use. They are then transported in the bloodstream to cells throughout the body.

◆ **Large Intestine** Waste material, such as fiber, moves into the large intestine, or colon. Water, potassium, and sodium are removed and the rest is eliminated from the body.

✓ **Reading Check**) **List** What are the three main jobs of nutrients?

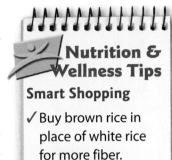

Meet the Nutrients

Each nutrient category, and each specific nutrient, has unique functions. Different foods supply different nutrients. The six categories of nutrients—carbohydrates, fats, proteins, vitamins, minerals, and water—work together to perform their functions.

Carbohydrates: Your Main Energy Source

A **carbohydrate** is a nutrient that serves as the body's main energy source. If you do not eat enough carbohydrates, your body uses proteins and fats for energy. Without carbohydrates, proteins and fats cannot do their regular jobs. Extra calories from any source, including carbohydrates, may lead to weight gain.

There are two types of carbohydrates: simple and complex. Simple carbohydrates are sugars. Complex carbohydrates are starches and fiber.

◆ **Sugar** is a simple carbohydrate that is digested quickly. It is simple because sugars are made of one or two sugar units.

◆ **Starch** is made of many sugar units attached together. During digestion, your body breaks down starches into single sugars, which are used to make energy.

◆ **Fiber** comes from plant material that cannot be digested. Fiber helps your digestive system work properly. It may also help protect your body from heart disease and cancer.

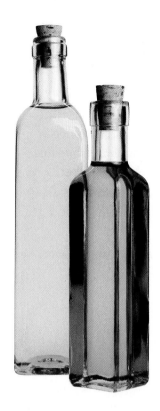

Saturated or Unsaturated?
Unsaturated fats are better for your health than saturated fats. *What are 3 sources of unsaturated fats?*

Foods With Carbohydrates

Sugars occur naturally in some foods. Fruit and milk contain natural sugars, along with other nutrients. Sugars can be added to sweeten foods. Be careful not to eat too many foods with added sugars. Complex carbohydrates come from plant sources of food. Some of these foods, including whole grains, legumes, and many vegetables, are good fiber sources.

◆ Grain products, such as bread, cereal, rice, grits, and pasta

◆ Starchy vegetables, such as squash, potatoes, and corn

◆ Legumes such as beans, peas, and lentils

Fats: Nutrients Essential to Your Health

Fat is a food and a nutrient that provides energy. It gives food flavor and texture. Your fingers may feel slippery after eating chips or fried foods because you feel the fat in these foods. You need some fat for healthy skin and normal growth. Fats transport some vitamins. They also slow digestion in your stomach so you feel full longer.

Your body makes fat from the excess fats, carbohydrates, and proteins that you eat, body fat is a reserve energy supply. It also insulates you from heat and cold, and cushions vital organs.

Types of Fats

Fats are a mixture of saturated or unsaturated fatty acids. Fatty acids occur naturally in solid fats and oils. The level of cholesterol in your blood can be affected by the amount and type of fat you eat.

◆ **Saturated Fats** Saturated fats are solid at room temperature. They come mostly from animal sources and tropical oils: coconut, palm, and palm kernel. Fish usually has less saturated fat than meat or poultry. Saturated fats tend to *raise* the cholesterol level in blood.

◆ **Unsaturated Fats** Unsaturated fats are usually liquid at room temperature. Vegetable oils, except tropical oils, are mostly unsaturated. Nuts, olives, and avocados also have unsaturated fat. Unsaturated fats help *lower* the cholesterol level in blood. One type, omega-3 fatty acid from salmon, other fatty fish, canola oil, and walnuts may be good for your heart.

◆ **Trans Fats** Oils can be hydrogenated, or processed to be firm. For example, stick margarine is made from hydrogenated oil. Hydrogenation forms trans fats. Some processed foods, such as some cookies often have trans fats. Trans fats tend to *raise* blood cholesterol levels.

Foods With Fats

Fats are naturally present in meat, poultry, fish, dairy foods, and nuts. Vegetable oil is liquid fat. Butter, margarine, cream, and mayonnaise are almost entirely fat. They are often used in foods such as salad dressings, gravy, and cookies. Fried foods are high in fat because they are fried in fat. Eating too much fat, especially saturated and trans fats, increases your risk for heart disease. A high-fat diet can also contribute to health problems.

What Is Cholesterol?

Cholesterol is a fat-like substance found in body cells. It helps carry out many body processes. Your body makes all the cholesterol it needs. Cholesterol also comes from meat, poultry, fish, egg yolks, and dairy foods. Foods from plant sources have none. High levels of cholesterol in the bloodstream are linked to heart disease.

Proteins: Your Body's Building Blocks

Proteins are substances that the body uses to build new cells and repair injured ones. They are needed for growth and fighting disease. Protein can help give you energy if you do not take in enough carbohydrates and fat.

Proteins are made of many small units called amino acids. Of the 22 amino acids, nine are essential, meaning they must come from food. Your body can make the other 13. Your body arranges them in different ways to make many different proteins for muscles, blood, bones, and more.

Most people get enough protein from their daily food choices. Extra protein will not build bigger muscles. Only physical activity can build more muscle. If you consume enough calories, any excess protein breaks down and is stored by your body as fat.

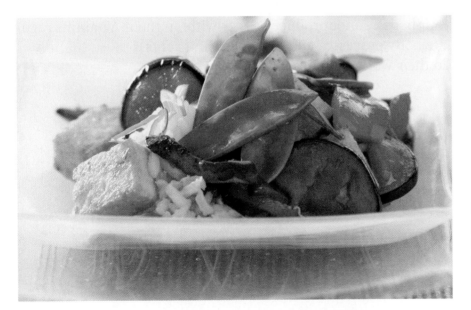

Meatless Dishes Many people are choosing to eat meatless meals, such as this one. *What are some high-protein, meatless dishes you would like to try?*

Types and Sources of Protein

Proteins are either complete or incomplete, depending on the kinds of amino acids they contain.

◆ **Complete proteins** have all nine essential amino acids in the right amounts. Foods from soybeans and from animal sources, such as meat, poultry, fish, eggs, and dairy products, provide complete proteins.

◆ **Incomplete proteins** lack one or more essential amino acids. Except for soy protein, the protein in plant sources is incomplete. Eating a variety of foods from plant sources daily can provide all the essential amino acids you need. Beans and peas, grains, and nuts have more protein than vegetables and fruits, but it is not complete protein.

Water Is a Nutrient!

Every body cell contains water. Water carries nutrients, helps regulate body temperature, and helps perform life-supporting functions. It also helps the digestive process by eliminating wastes.

Your body loses water every day through breathing, sweat, and body waste. To replace your body's fluids, you need to drink water and eat food every day. Moisture from food can provide 20 percent of your water intake. When you perspire a lot, you need to drink more water. If you drink more fluids than you need, the excess fluids pass through your body in urine. Get most of your water from plain water, juice, milk, and soups. Teenage girls need about 78 ounces (2.3L) of water per day. Teenage boys need about 112 ounces (3.3L) a day.

Vital Vitamins

Vitamins are nutrients. They are needed in small amounts. Vitamins do not provide energy or build body tissue. However, your body cannot produce energy without them. Vitamins regulate body processes and help other nutrients do their work.

Drink Enough Water Thirst signals a need for water. Make an effort to drink water and other liquids throughout the day so you get enough fluids.
What are the best sources of fluids?

Water-Soluble Vitamins

Water-soluble vitamins dissolve in water. Most cannot be stored by the body. Your body gets rid of excess amounts of water-soluble vitamins in urine. **Figure 7.1** below shows seven key water-soluble vitamins.

| Figure 7.1 | Functions and Sources of Water-Soluble Vitamins |

Getting Your Vitamins Eating a variety of foods provides the many different vitamins your body needs. *What water-soluble vitamins did your breakfast foods provide today?*

Water-Soluble Vitamins	Where You Can Find Them
Thiamin (Vitamin B$_1$) • Helps in energy production • Maintains healthy nerves	• Enriched and whole-grain breads and cereals • Lean pork • Dry beans and peas
Riboflavin (Vitamin B$_2$) • Helps in energy production • Helps the body resist infections	• Enriched and whole-grain breads and cereals • Milk products • Dry beans and peas • Meat, poultry, fish
Niacin (a B-vitamin) • Helps in energy production • Needed for a healthy nervous system	• Meat, poultry, fish • Liver • Enriched and whole-grain breads and cereals • Dry beans and peas, peanuts
Vitamin B6 • Helps in energy production • Needed for a healthy nervous system • Helps protect against infection	• Poultry, fish, meat • Dry beans and peas • Whole-wheat products • Some fruits and vegetables • Liver
Vitamin B12 • Helps build red blood cells • Needed for a healthy nervous system • Helps in energy production	• Meat, poultry, fish • Eggs • Dairy products • Some foods, such as breakfast cereals, that are fortified with vitamin B12
Folate (Folic Acid) (a B-vitamin) • Helps build red blood cells • May help protect against heart disease • In pregnant women, helps to prevent birth defects	• Bread, cereal, rice, pasta, flour, and other grain products that are fortified with folic acid • Dark green, leafy vegetables • Dry beans and peas • Fruits
Vitamin C (Ascorbic Acid) • Increases resistance to infection • Maintains healthy teeth and gums • Helps wounds heal • Helps keep blood vessels healthy	• Citrus fruit • Other fruits (such as cantaloupe, berries, mango, kiwifruit) • Some vegetables (such as tomatoes, green peppers, potatoes, broccoli, cabbage)

Fat-Soluble Vitamins

Fat-soluble vitamins dissolve in fat—both in foods and in your body. Your body stores extra fat-soluble vitamins in body fat and in your liver. When you need them, your body pulls some out of storage. Excess amounts of fat-soluble vitamins can build up to harmful levels in your body. Fat-soluble vitamins are A, D, E, and K, as shown in **Figure 7.2**.

Mighty Minerals

Your body uses **minerals** for many processes. Some minerals regulate body processes. Some minerals become a part of your body in the form of cells, fluids, muscles, teeth, and bones. Minerals also work together. For example, calcium and phosphorus work together, along with vitamins D and A, to help build strong bones and teeth. **Figure 7.3** shows the functions and food sources of some important minerals.

Figure 7.2	Functions and Sources of Fat-Soluble Vitamins

Building a Strong Body Eggs, fish, and dark green vegetables are good sources of some fat-soluble vitamins. *Why do you think milk is fortified with vitamin D?*

Fat-Soluble Vitamins	Where You Can Find Them
Vitamin A • Helps bones, teeth, skin, and hair stay healthy • Helps eyes adjust to darkness • Helps body resist infections	• Dairy products • Egg yolk • Liver • Dark green vegetables (such as spinach) and deep yellow-orange fruits and vegetables (such as carrots, pumpkin, winter squash, cantaloupe, peaches, apricots) These contain beta carotene, which the body turns into vitamin A.
Vitamin D • Helps build strong bones and teeth • Helps the body absorb and use calcium	• Fortified milk • Fatty fish (such as salmon, mackerel) • Egg yolk • The body can also produce vitamin D from exposure to sunlight
Vitamin E • Helps form red blood cells and muscles • Helps protect cells from damage by oxygen	• Vegetable oils • Whole-grain breads and cereals • Dark green, leafy vegetables • Dry beans and peas • Nuts and seeds
Vitamin K • Needed for normal blood clotting	• Dark green, leafy vegetables • Wheat bran and wheat germ • Some fruits • Egg yolk • Liver

Build Strong Bones for Life

Bones grow with the help of calcium, phosphorus, and magnesium. Your body constantly removes and replaces the calcium stored in your bones. Before age 30 to 35, more calcium is added than removed. This makes bones stronger and heavier. After age 30 to 35, more calcium is taken away than put back. Then bones gradually lose strength. Losing too much calcium can lead to osteoporosis, a condition that causes bones to weaken and break easily.

Your need for calcium is highest during your teen years. Eat plenty of calcium-rich foods, such as milk and yogurt. Eat foods with other bone-building nutrients, including vitamin D, phosphorus, and magnesium. (See **Figure 7.3** on page 104.) This can help build strong bones and prevent osteoporosis. Be physically active. Activities that carry your body weight, such as walking, help strengthen your bones.

Eat Right for Healthy Blood

Iron helps red blood cells carry oxygen to all your cells. If you do not eat enough foods with iron, you may develop anemia. Anemia is a condition in which the blood does not have enough red blood cells to carry oxygen to body cells where energy is made. Anemia makes you feel tired and weak. Teenage girls and younger women are more likely than men to get anemia because the female reproductive system requires more iron.

✓ **Reading Check** **Explain** Why do you need to consume enough calcium during your teen years?

Nutrients and Energy

Your body uses energy for everything you do. That includes walking or running, recovering from illness, growing, solving math problems, and even staying alive. What you eat and drink affects your long-term health.

What Are Calories?

Calories are not a food ingredient or a nutrient. Instead, a calorie is a unit that measures energy from food and energy used by the body. One calorie is the same amount of energy, whether it comes from hamburger, cake, broccoli, or candy. Calories are not good or bad. Everyone needs them to live. Be sure to get the right number of calories from foods that have the right nutrients for your health. You can use extra calories you eat or drink through more physical activity.

Nutrition & Wellness Tips

Drink Nutrients

✓ Drink 100-percent fruit juice for breakfast as a source of vitamin C and other nutrients.

✓ Choose low- or non-fat milk or soy milk, with calcium and vitamin D added to get bone-building nutrients.

Figure 7.3   **Functions and Sources of Minerals**

Understanding Minerals Calcium and iron are just two of the minerals that teens need to build strong bodies. *What foods can help you build strong bones?*

Calcium • Helps build and renew bones and teeth • Helps your heart, muscles, and nerves work properly	• Milk, yogurt, cheese • Dark green, leafy vegetables • Canned fish with edible bones • Dry beans • Calcium-fortified juices, soy foods, and cereals
Phosphorus • Helps build and renew bones and teeth • Helps your body produce energy	• Milk, yogurt, cheese • Meat, poultry, fish • Egg yolks • Whole-grain breads and cereals
Magnesium • Helps build and renew bones • Helps nerves and muscles work properly	• Whole-grain products • Dark-green, leafy vegetables • Dry beans and peas • Nuts and seeds
Sodium, Chloride, and Potassium • Help maintain the water balance in your body • Help with muscle and nerve actions • For potassium, needed for normal heartbeat	• Sodium and chloride: Salt and foods that contain salt; many ingredients also contain sodium. • Potassium: Fruits (such as bananas and oranges), vegetables, meat, poultry, fish, dry beans and peas, dairy products
Iron • Helps red blood cells carry oxygen	• Meat, poultry, fish • Egg yolks • Dark-green, leafy vegetables • Dry beans and peas • Enriched grain products • Dried fruits
Zinc • Helps heal wounds and form blood • Helps the body make proteins	• Meat, liver, poultry, fish • Dairy products • Dry beans and peas • Whole-grain breads and cereals • Eggs
Fluoride • Helps prevent tooth decay by strengthening teeth	• Small amounts are added to the water supply in many communities. • Toothpaste also has fluoride, which can be absorbed by brushing teeth.

Some other minerals you need:
• Copper
• Iodine
• Manganese
• Selenium
• Chromium

Energy in Food

Three nutrients provide energy: carbohydrates, proteins, and fats. Other nutrients (water, vitamins, and minerals) do not. Different foods supply different amounts of energy. Fatty foods tend to be high in calories. One gram of carbohydrate or protein has 4 calories; one gram of fat has 9 calories.

The sources of your calories are just as important as the number of calories supplied by your food. Teens should get 45 to 65 percent of their calories from carbohydrates and 10 to 35 percent of their calories from proteins. For teens, fats should comprise 25 to 35 percent, with no more than 10 percent of those fats coming from saturated fats. The advice for trans fats is to eat as little as possible. The energy, or calories, in your food choices depends on the foods themselves, how they were prepared and the amount you eat.

Energy Your Body Uses

Food provides energy so your body can do its work. How much energy do you need? That depends on how much energy you use. **Figure 7.4** shows the daily recommended energy needs for teens who are active, moderately active, and sedentary. People who are sedentary get very little exercise.

Energy for Body Processes

Even when you sleep, your body works. You need energy for breathing, circulating blood, building cells, and other basic processes. These processes make up your metabolism.

Figure 7.4	Daily Recommended Energy Needs for Teens

Calorie Needs Look at the chart to find the approximate number of calories you may need every day. *How many calories do you need today?*

Age	Boys			Girls		
	Sedentary	Moderately Active	Active	Sedentary	Moderately Active	Active
13	2,000	2,200	2,600	1,600	2,000	2,200
14	2,000	2,400	2,800	1,800	2,000	2,400
15	2,200	2,600	3,000	1,800	2,000	2,400
16–18	2,400	2,800	3,200	1,800	2,000	2,400

*Sedentary = less than 30 minutes a day of moderate physical activity in addition to daily activities. **Moderately Active** = at least 30 minutes and up to 60 minutes a day of moderate physical activity in addition to daily activities. **Active** = 60 or more minutes a day of moderate physical activity in addition to daily activities*

The speed at which your body uses energy for body processes is called your basal metabolic rate (BMR). A person with a high BMR uses more calories when resting than someone with a low BMR. BMR differs from person to person depending on body build and size, age, gender, and genetic make-up. Muscle uses more energy than body fat. On average, adults use about 1,200 calories daily for body processes. Teens use more energy because they are growing.

Energy for Physical Activity

Every movement you make, such as getting dressed, playing sports, and raking leaves, uses energy. The amount you use depends on how active you are. Longer, more strenuous exercise uses more energy. For example, walking briskly for 15 minutes uses more energy than walking slowly for 15 minutes.

Energy in Balance

Consuming the same amount of energy, or calories, as your body uses is called energy balance. When you balance the energy from your food and drinks with the amount your body uses, you maintain your weight. If you eat more calories than the amount your body uses, you gain weight. If you eat fewer calories than the amount your body uses, you lose weight.

✓ **Reading Check** **Explain** What does energy balance mean? How does it affect body weight?

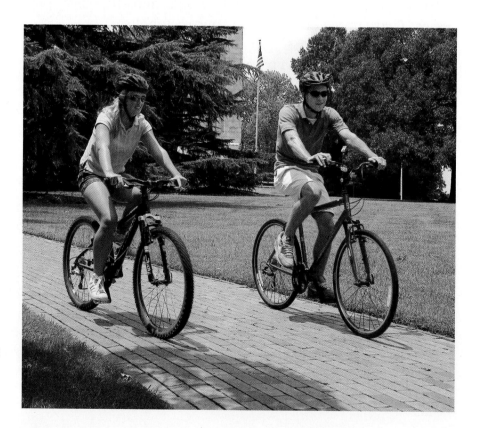

Enjoy Exercise Activities that you enjoy can help you burn calories in food. *What are some activities that you enjoy?*

Nutrient Advice

The **Recommended Dietary Allowances** (RDAs) give advice about daily nutrient needs for most healthy people. They are part of the Dietary Reference Intakes (DRIs) from the Institute of Medicine, a nonprofit, nongovernmental organization established by the U.S. National Academy of Sciences. The DRIs also give an upper level for many nutrients. That is the maximum amount that probably will not be harmful. DRIs are used mainly by health professionals.

Discoveries About Nutrition

One new frontier in nutrition science is the study of *phytonutrients,* or natural chemicals found in plants. (*Phyto* means plant.) Plants use phytonutrients as a natural protection from bacteria, fungi, and viruses. The phytonutrients in grain products, vegetables, fruits, and beans and peas have benefits for humans, too. They may help protect you from health problems such as heart disease and cancer.

Getting Too Few Nutrients

A nutrient deficiency, or shortage, over time may result in poor health or a lack of energy. The effects of some nutrient deficiencies may take a long time to become visible. For example, if you do not get enough calcium now, your bones may break easily when you get older.

A nutrient deficiency is one form of **malnutrition**, or poor nutrition. It can be caused by health problems that keep the body from using nutrients. Malnutrition can also result from food shortages or poverty. Even people who have enough to eat can develop malnutrition if they make poor food choices.

Getting Too Many Nutrients

Too much of some nutrients over time can be harmful. Exra energy from carbohydrates, proteins, or fats turn to body fat. Too much fat increases heart disease risk later in life. Excess amounts of fat-soluble vitamins can build up in the body. Excess water-soluble vitamins pass out of your body as waste, however too much Vitamin C can cause diarrhea. Excess vitamins usually come from supplements, not from food.

✓ **Reading Check** **Define** What are the RDAs?

Dietary Supplements

A dietary **supplement** contains nutrients or other food substances that add to your diet. They may be sold as pills, capsules, liquids, or powders. With wise food choices, you probably do not need a supplement.

Be Smart with Supplements

Food contains all the nutrients people need. Supplements do not contain only known nutrients. Ask your doctor before taking any supplement. If your doctor advises a supplement, follow the recommended dose. High doses can be harmful. Store them away from children.

✓ **Reading Check** **Explain** In what circumstances might a doctor advise dietary supplements?

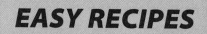

EASY RECIPES   Everyday Favorites

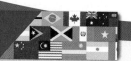

Italian-Style Chicken Strips

Customary	Ingredients	Metric
¼ cup	Italian-style dry bread crumbs	60 mL
½ tsp.	Italian seasoning (low-sodium)	2 mL
½ tsp.	Garlic powder	2 mL
¼ tsp.	Ground black pepper	1 mL
1 lb.	Boneless chicken breasts	500 g
1 tsp.	Olive oil	5 mL
½ cup	Prepared spaghetti sauce, heated	125 mL

Yield: 4 servings (4 ounces or 120 g chicken each)

1. Preheat oven to 425°F (220°C).
2. Combine bread crumbs, Italian seasoning, garlic powder, and pepper in a medium bowl.
3. Cut chicken in ½-inch (1.25-cm) strips. Put in bowl with bread crumbs and stir to coat.
4. Place chicken in a single layer on a nonstick baking sheet. Drizzle oil over chicken.
5. Bake 9 minutes. Turn pieces. Bake 7 to 11 more minutes or until thoroughly cooked. Serve with sauce.

Nutritional Information Per Serving: 90 calories, 2 g total fat (0 g saturated fat), 0 g trans fat, 16 mg cholesterol, 281 mg sodium, 9 g total carbohydrate (1 g fiber, 3 g sugars), 8 g protein

Percent Daily Value: vitamin A 4%, vitamin C 4%, calcium 2%, iron 4%

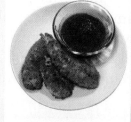

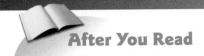

After You Read

CHAPTER SUMMARY

Carbohydrates, fats, proteins, vitamins, minerals, and water are nutrients. They work together to give you energy, build and repair your body, and keep your body processes running smoothly. Some foods are especially good sources of certain nutrients. Carbohydrates, fats, and proteins provide the energy needed for body processes and physical activity. Your body needs enough of each nutrient for health and growth. Supplements used appropriately can provide needed nutrients for people in special circumstances.

Vocabulary Review

1. Use each of these vocabulary words in a sentence.

Content Vocabulary
- ◇ nutrient (p. 96)
- ◇ carbohydrate (p. 97)
- ◇ sugar (p. 97)
- ◇ starch (p. 97)
- ◇ fiber (p. 97)
- ◇ proteins (p. 99)
- ◇ vitamins (p. 100)
- ◇ minerals (p. 102)
- ◇ Recommended Dietary Allowances (p. 107)
- ◇ malnutrition (p. 107)
- ◇ supplement (p. 108)

Academic Vocabulary
- ▪ processes (p. 96)
- ▪ appropriate (p. 108)

Review Key Concepts

2. List the three main nutrient functions.

3. List food sources of carbohydrates, fats, proteins, vitamins, minerals, and water.

4. Explain energy balance.

5. Describe the possible effects of getting too few or too many nutrients.

6. Describe the safe use of dietary supplements.

Critical Thinking

7. Critique this statement: "The best way to lose weight is to cut fat completely out of your diet." Is this statement true? Explain why or why not.

8. Deconstruct a food you enjoy. What nutrients does the food contain? Check the charts in the appendix to find out. Write a summary explaining your answers.

9. Explain why supplements cannot replace food. Write a paragraph that explains your answers.

Real-World Skills and Applications

Decision-Making

10. Decisions for Bone Health Learn more about osteoporosis. Besides not getting enough of certain minerals, what are some other risk factors for osteoporosis? What decisions can you make now to prevent it later? Write a brief report on your findings.

Interpersonal and Collaborative

11. Interpersonal Skills A friend takes large doses of a multivitamin supplement. You think he might not know about the dangers of large doses of some vitamins and minerals. What would you tell your friend? Write him a letter of advice.

Technology

12. Research Careers Online Conduct research on a food or nutrition career path that interests you. Use a word processing application to describe the career, the skills needed to succeed in that career, and the education and training needed for the career.

Financial Literacy

13. Food Costs Choose three food items with similar nutritive value. Research the price of each item at a store in your area. What do they cost in two other locations, one in your state and another across the country. Create a table summarizing the results of your research.

14. Get Enough Fluids Track the amount and type of liquids you drink for three days. How much was plain water, fruit juice, or milk? How much was coffee, tea, or soda? Create a chart or graph of your records. Include information about the nutrients in your drinks. Draw conclusions.

15. Taste-Test Experiment During digestion, saliva breaks down one type of carbohydrate, starch, into another, sugar. Test this by placing a little cornstarch on the tip of your tongue. Mix it with saliva and let it remain there. What change in taste do you notice? How do you explain this change?

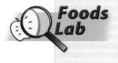

16. Test for Hidden Fats Rub a very small amount of margarine on brown paper. Label the spot. Repeat with foods like these: apple, carrot, avocado, cheese, bread, cracker, nuts. Label each spot; let it dry. Which foods left a permanent spot? Which left an oily spot? What can you conclude?

Additional Activities For additional activities go to this book's Online Learning Center through **glencoe.com**.

Academic Skills

English Language Arts

17. Research Scurvy For centuries, sailors on long voyages became ill with scurvy, caused by a nutrient deficiency. Conduct research to learn more about the history of scurvy or another deficiency disease and its cure. Write a one-page report. Include your sources.

> **NCTE 2** Read literature to build an understanding of the human experience.

Social Studies

18. Malnutrition The serious lack of adequate nutrition for individuals and whole populations is a problem throughout the world. Poverty, famine, floods and overpopulation are causes in some countries. Research a country where many people suffer from malnutrition. Write a paragraph about the causes of malnutrition in that country and possible solutions.

> **NCSS III People, Places, and Environments** TK

Mathematics

19. Pizza Party Romi and Keisha invited friends over to celebrate winning the big game. They ordered six vegetable pizzas for a party. Each circular pizza came in a square box. The top of each pizza box had a surface area of 169 in². If each pizza was as wide as the box, what was the total surface area of all of the pizzas?

Math Concept **Surface Area** The surface area of geometric objects can be found using simple equations. The equation for rectangular objects is area = length × width. For circular objects, the equation is area = π × radius².

Starting Hint If a circle is drawn inside of a square, the width of the square equals the diameter of the circle.

 For more math help, go to the Math Appendix.

> **NCTM Geometry** Analyze characteristics and properties of two- and three-dimensional geometric shapes and develop mathematical arguments about geometric relationships.

STANDARDIZED TEST PRACTICE

Test-Taking Tip When answering true/false questions, pay close attention to the wording as you read the questions. Look for words such as *not, nor, any,* or *all.* These words are important in determining the correct answer.

TRUE/FALSE QUESTIONS

Review the chapter and answer the following questions with a T for *True* or F for *False.*

20. Starches are simple carbohydrates.

21. The body cannot store water-soluble vitamins.

CHAPTER 8
Dietary Guidelines

Explore the Photo ▶▶
Following the Dietary Guidelines provides benefits now—and lowers your chances for developing health problems later. *What does this meal suggest about healthful eating?*

Writing Activity

Write a Letter

Choose Food for Health Write a letter to your teacher about how healthful foods available can improve the health of your community. Suggest a community project for improving health through good nutrition.

Writing Tips

1. **Write** concise sentences that clearly state your thoughts to the person receiving the letter.

2. **Link** your sentences together clearly and logically.

Reading Guide

Before You Read

Create an Outline Use this chapter's headings to create an outline. Make the headings into Level 1 main ideas. Add supporting information to create Level 2, 3, and 4 details. Use the outline to predict what you are about to learn.

Read to Learn

Key Concepts

- **Describe** the purpose of the Dietary Guidelines for Americans.
- **List** the nine Dietary Guidelines topics.
- **Identify** five tips for making the Dietary Guidelines help you live more healthfully.

Main Idea

The Dietary Guidelines provide advice about healthful eating and active living.

Content Vocabulary

- ◇ Dietary Guidelines for Americans
- ◇ health risk
- ◇ diet
- ◇ nutrient-dense food
- ◇ risk factor

Academic Vocabulary

You will find these words in your reading and on your tests. Use the glossary to look up their definitions if necessary.

- ■ minimize
- ■ affect

Graphic Organizer

As you read, use a graphic organizer like the one below to write the nine topics of the Dietary Guidelines for Americans.

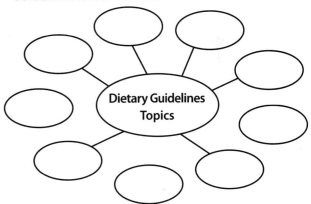

Dietary Guidelines Topics

 Graphic Organizer Go to this book's Online Learning Center at glencoe.com to print out this graphic organizer.

Academic Standards ●

English Language Arts
NCTE 4 Use written language to communicate effectively.
NCTE 9 Develop an understanding of diversity in language across cultures.

Mathematics
NCTM Number and Operations Compute fluently and make reasonable estimates.

Science
NSES Content Standard A Develop understandings about scientific inquiry.

Social Studies
NCSS II F Time, Continuity, and Change Apply ideas, theories, and modes of historical inquiry to analyze historical and contemporary developments, and to inform and evaluate actions concerning public policy issues.
NCSS IV E Individual Development and Identity Examine the interaction of ethnic, national, or cultural influences in specific situations or events.

NCTE National Council of Teachers of English
NCTM National Council of Teachers of Mathematics

NSES National Science Education Standards
NCSS National Council for the Social Studies

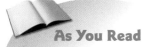

Vocabulary

You can find definitions in the glossary at the back of this book.

As You Read

Connect Think about ways you can improve your health through the Dietary Guidelines.

Good Health Making food choices for good health can benefit you now and when you are older. *What healthful food choices have you made recently?*

What Are the Dietary Guidelines?

The **Dietary Guidelines for Americans** provide advice to help people live longer, healthier lives. These science-based guidelines about nutrition and physical activity are meant for healthy Americans two years and older. They are published by the U.S. Department of Agriculture (USDA) and the U.S. Department of Health and Human Services (HHS). The guidelines are revised every five years to keep them current. Many nutrition programs, such as school meals and food stamps, reflect the Dietary Guidelines. The Dietary Guidelines reflect what is known about:

◆ What nutrients and other food substances do.

◆ Where nutrients are found.

◆ How much nutrients people need for a healthful, active life.

◆ How healthy weight, physical activity, and food safety help reduce health risks. A **health risk** is the likelihood of developing health problems, such as heart disease, diabetes, and some cancers.

✓ **Reading Check** **Explain** What do the Dietary Guidelines for Americans provide?

Advice from the Dietary Guidelines

When you think of the word *diet,* do you think of losing weight or a special medical diet? A **diet** is an eating plan. Diet refers to everything you eat and drink. The Dietary Guidelines have 41 different recommendations, grouped into nine topics. Following these guidelines can help you feel good and stay healthy.

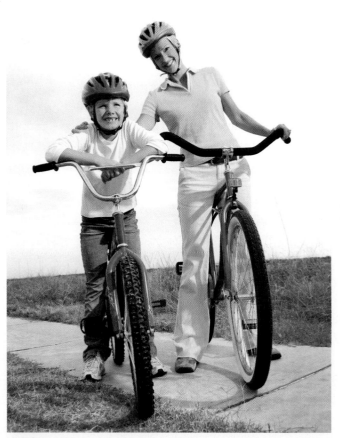

Get Enough Nutrients Within Your Calorie Needs

You need a certain amount of calories in a day. The amount depends on your age, activity level, and whether you are trying to gain, maintain, or lose weight. You will learn more about your daily calorie budget in Chapter 9. If you use your daily calorie budget on only a few high-calorie foods, then you will not get some of the important nutrients you need.

- Many teens do not get enough calcium, potassium, magnesium, vitamin E, and fiber.

- Teens tend to eat too much saturated and *trans* fats, cholesterol, added sugars, and sodium.

To get enough nutrients, eat a variety of nutrient-dense foods: whole grains, vegetables, fruits, low-fat and fat-free milk and milk products, and lean meats and beans. A **nutrient-dense food** is a food that provides high amounts of vitamins and minerals for relatively few calories. Stay within your calorie limits. Limit foods with saturated and *trans* fats, cholesterol, added sugars, and salt.

Maintain a Healthy Weight

Keep your body weight in a healthy range. It helps you look and feel better throughout your life. Having too much extra body fat increases the workload on your heart, lungs, and body frame. Being overweight is a risk factor for many health problems. A **risk factor** is a condition that increases your chances of developing a problem. Health problems that can be caused by having too much body fat include:

- Diabetes
- Heart disease
- High blood pressure
- Some types of cancer
- Arthritis

The key to weight management is energy balance. The energy you consume should equal the energy you use. To maintain a healthy weight, find a balance between food and physical activity. Calories in should equal calories out. As you set your weight goals, remember: your body is changing. You are no longer a child, but not yet an adult. Your growth and physical development are factors in weight gain.

Being underweight also has health risks. An underweight person does not have much body fat as an energy reserve. Underweight people can also suffer from health problems. Underweight people may need to increase their weight.

People at a healthy weight should strive to stay that way. Increasing physical activity and small decreases in food and beverage calories are important.

Keep Moving! Physical activity means more than just exercise or sports. *How can you be physically active and help your family or community at the same time?*

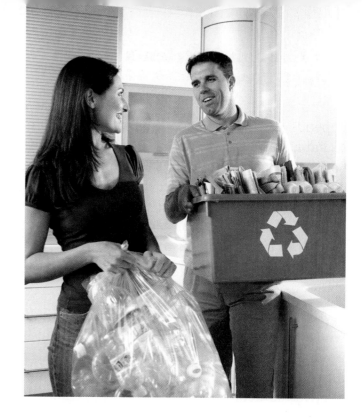

Be Physically Active Every Day

Physical fitness is about physical activity *and* healthful eating. Physical activity includes any activity that gets your body moving. Active living helps you:

◆ Control your weight.

◆ Strengthen your heart and lungs.

◆ Increase your endurance and flexibility.

◆ Reduce your risk for future health problems.

Teens should build 60 minutes or more of moderate to vigorous physical activity into their daily routine. Longer and more strenuous activity gives more benefits. Follow these guidelines to build physical activity into your daily routine:

◆ Get involved in a team or individual sport.

◆ Walk briskly or ride a bike rather than ride in a car or bus.

◆ Spend less time watching television and more time doing fun activities, such as bowling or skating.

◆ Use the stairs instead of the elevator.

◆ Help with chores such as mowing the lawn or raking leaves.

Choose Whole Grains, Fruits, Vegetables, and Milk

Whole-grain products, vegetables, and fruits should be a main part of your meal and provide most of your calories. Mix up your choices. These foods are nutrient rich, cholesterol free, and naturally low in fats and calories. They also help protect against heart disease, cancer, and other health problems.

- Make whole-grain products the star of your meals.
- Enjoy fruit or vegetables with meals and as snacks.
- Eat fruit instead of sugary dessert.
- Eat meals featuring cooked dry beans or peas.
- Drink fruit or vegetable juice with your meals or as a snack.
- Eat a variety of yellow, deep-green, orange, and red fruits and vegetables for their different nutrients.
- Drink yogurt smoothies for snacks. Add low-fat cheese to sandwiches.

Limit Fats and Cholesterol

You need to eat fat but only in small amounts. It is an essential nutrient. If you eat too much fat—especially saturated fats and trans fats—and too much cholesterol, you raise your risk of developing heart disease. You will also consume more calories than you need. Remember, fat provides more calories per gram than carbohydrates or protein.

Most Americans consume too much fat. For most children and teens, 25 to 35 percent of the calories consumed over several days should come from fat. See **Figure 8.1** on the next page. Cutting back on fat usually lowers cholesterol intake. Read food labels to compare the amount of total fat, saturated fat, trans fat, and cholesterol in foods.

What Is on Your Plate?
Here is a quick hint for healthful eating: Three-quarters of your meal should be grain products, vegetables, and fruit. The small area remaining is just the right amount for lean meat, poultry, or fish. *What healthful beverages could you enjoy with a meal like this?*

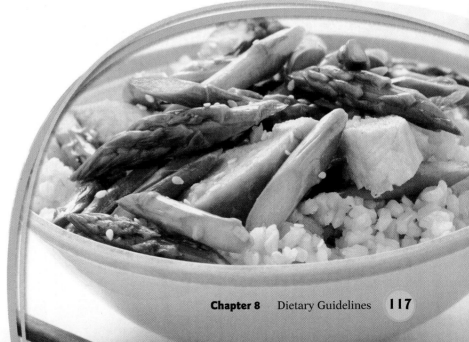

Figure 8.1   **Amounts of Fat in a Day**

How Much Fat Is Enough? Your upper limit for fat intake depends on how many calories you need. *If you consume 2,000 calories a day, what is the maximum number of grams of fat you should consume each day?*

Calories Consumed per Day	1,800 calories	2,000 calories	2,600 calories
Total Fat Consumed per Day in Grams	50–70 grams	56–78 grams	72–101 grams
Total Fat Consumed per Day in Calories	450–630	504–702	648–909

Follow these guidelines to stick to an eating plan that is moderate in total fat and low in saturated fats, *trans* fats, and cholesterol:

◆ Keep saturated fats to less than 10 percent of your calories.

◆ Eat as few foods containing trans fats as possible.

◆ Limit cholesterol to less than 300 milligrams per day.

◆ Choose mostly foods prepared with little or no fat.

◆ Eat dairy foods that are mostly reduced-fat, low-fat, and fat-free.

◆ Get most of your fat from fish, nuts, and healthy oils.

◆ Buy lean meat and poultry. Remove skin from chicken and turkey. Trim excess fat from meat.

◆ Eat egg yolks and whole eggs in moderation. Use egg substitutes sometimes.

◆ Choose fewer solid fats, such as butter and stick margarine.

✓ Reading Check **Explain** How can you cut down on fats and reduce your risk of heart disease?

Be Choosy About Carbohydrate Foods

Foods have sugars and starches, two types of carbohydrate. Some sugars are naturally present in nutrient-rich fruit and milk. Foods with added sugars, such as candy and soft drinks, are high in calories but often low in vitamins, minerals, complex carbohydrates, and protein. Sugars, along with starches, also promote tooth decay. Limit your intake of sugary foods. Corn sweetener, fructose, honey, maltose, molasses, and syrup are all sugars. Any ingredient that ends with *ose* is a sugar. Eat fiber-rich vegetables, fruits, and whole grains often for nutrients without added sugar.

Reduce Sodium and Increase Potassium

Sodium helps control body fluids. However, too much sodium is linked to high blood pressure, heart attack, and stroke. As people get older, they may become more sensitive to sodium without knowing it. Some foods contain sodium naturally. However, processed foods usually have large amounts of added sodium.

Potassium helps counteract sodium's effects on blood pressure. Many fruits and vegetables are good sources of potassium. To **minimize**, or lower, the amount of sodium you eat, flavor your food with herbs and spices instead of salt. Avoid eating salty snacks. Choose processed foods wth less salt or sodium.

Avoid Alcoholic Beverages

Teens should avoid alcoholic beverages, including beer and wine. Drinking them can **affect**, or influence, your judgment, and that can lead to accidents and injuries. Heavy drinking also increases the chance of accidents and injuries, violence, emotional problems, dependency, and other problems. Alcohol has calories but almost no nutrients. Drinking also puts others at risk.

Keep Food Safe

Safe food is healthful food that is free from harmful bacteria and other contaminants. When food is not properly handled, stored, and prepared, it can cause foodborne illness.

✓ **Reading Check** **Discuss** Why is food safety an important Dietary Guideline?

Discover International Foods

British Isles

One of Ireland's dietary guidelines is: Enjoy foods! People in the British Isles greet their day with a hearty breakfast, which may include cereal, fruit, eggs, meat, mushrooms, tomatoes, toast, and jam. Lunch may include a meat stew, often served with potatoes and vegetables. Late afternoon is tea time with sandwiches, tea cakes, or cookies, and hot tea. Dinner is often a light meal, followed by cheese and crackers.

Languages Across Cultures

kipper ('ki-pər) herring, a type of fish, that is salted, dried, and smoked, and eaten at any meal including breakfast

scone ('skōn) small, dense breads in a variety of shapes that are often served with tea

 Recipes Find out more about international recipes on this book's Online Learning Center at glencoe.com.

NCTE 9 Develop an understanding of diversity in language use across cultures.

Five Tips to Make the Dietary Guidelines Work for You

The following five tips from the Dietary Guidelines Alliance can help you achieve and maintain wellness. Making good food and lifestyle choices will give you the best chance to do all the things in life you want to do.

1. **Be realistic!** Make small changes over time in what you eat and your level of activity. Small steps work better than giant leaps.

2. **Be adventurous!** Enjoy a variety of foods.

3. **Be flexible!** Balance what you eat and the physical activity you do over several days.

4. **Be sensible!** Enjoy all foods, just do not overdo it.

5. **Be active!** Walk the dog. Do not just watch the dog walk.

EASY RECIPES

International Flavors

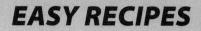 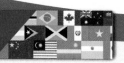

Beans and Chopped Vegetables on Toast

Customary	Ingredients	Metric
⅛ cup	Diced red peppers	30 mL
⅛ cup	Diced onions	30 mL
1 Tbsp.	Olive oil	5 mL
15 oz. can	Baked beans	454 g
¼ cup	Diced tomatoes	60 mL
8 slices	Bread	8 slices

Try This!
Use whole-grain bread for a healthful spin on this British favorite.

Yield: 8 servings, ½ cup (125 mL) each

1. Sautee the diced red pepper and onion in olive oil in a pan.
2. After 2 minutes, add the chopped tomatoes and the beans to the pan.
3. Add pepper to taste.
4. Toast the bread.
5. When the toast is crisp and hot, pour the beans and vegetables onto the toast.

Nutritional Information Per Serving: 331 calories, 5 g total fat (1 g saturated fat), 79 mg cholesterol, 764 mg sodium, 62 g total carbohydrate (5 g fiber, 5 g total sugars), 11 g protein

Percent Daily Value: vitamin A 4%, vitamin C 8%, calcium 10%, iron 15%

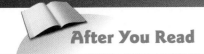

After You Read

CHAPTER SUMMARY

The Dietary Guidelines for Americans provide advice about healthful eating and active living. Get the most nutrition for your calories by eating a variety of nutrient-dense foods. Focus on whole grains, fruits, vegetables, low-fat or fat-free dairy foods, and lean protein. Keep active. Achieve or maintain your appropriate weight and stay healthy. Know the limits on fats, especially saturated fat and *trans* fats and cholesterol. Limit your consumption of foods high in added sugars and sodium. Avoid alcoholic beverages. Keep food safe to eat.

Vocabulary Review

1. Use each of these vocabulary words in a sentence.

Content Vocabulary
- ◇ Dietary Guidelines for Americans (p. 114)
- ◇ health risk (p. 114)
- ◇ diet (p. 114)
- ◇ nutrient-dense foods (p. 115)
- ◇ risk factor (p. 115)

Academic Vocabulary
- ■ minimize (p. 119)
- ■ affect (p. 119)

Review Key Concepts

2. Describe the purpose of the Dietary Guidelines for Americans.

3. List the nine Dietary Guidelines topics.

4. Identify five tips for making the Dietary Guidelines help you live more healthfully.

Critical Thinking

5. Compare and contrast the nutrient density of chocolate cake and whole-grain wheat bread. Which has more fat? Which has more sugar? Which one has the higher nutrient density?

6. Outline what you could do on a daily basis to stay healthy and active.

7. Predict how ignoring the advice of the Dietary Guidelines could impact your daily life and affect your lifestyle and future health.

8. Analyze some obstacles that may make the Dietary Guidelines difficult to follow. Then determine some ways to overcome those obstacles.

9. Extend your knowledge of the Dietary Guidelines. Your community wants to host an event that promotes the Dietary Guidelines and healthful living every day. Create a plan for the event. Include activities for each Dietary Guideline.

Real-World Skills and Applications

Goal Setting

10. Wellness Challenge You want to help your classmates do well on physical fitness tests. Design a fitness poster to promote goals for being physically active. In your poster, suggest ways that your audience can stay motivated and reach their fitness goals.

Interpersonal and Collaborative

11. Dietary Guidelines Around the World Follow your teacher's instructions to form into small groups. With your group, research the dietary guidelines in Canada or in one other country. Make a classroom display to compare and contrast U.S. Guidelines with the other country's guidelines.

Technology

12. Food Substitutes Research one substitute for sugar or fat. How is it used in food and beverages? What are its pros and cons? Are all food items with the substitute low in calories? Summarize your research in a one-page document using a word-processing program.

Financial Literacy

13. Compare Values You can buy 48 ounces (1.5 L) of juice with water added for $3. You can buy 48 ounces (1.5 L) of 100% juice for $4. You buy the 100% juice and add water. How much water must you add for the price per ounce to be the same for both?

14. Sugars in Sodas A 12-ounce (375 g) can of soda may contain 9 to 12 teaspoons (45 to 60 mL) of added sugar. Estimate how much sugar you get from sodas in a week if you drink one can each day.

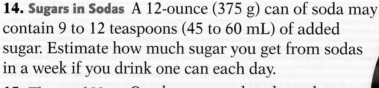

15. Then and Now Conduct research to learn how and why the Dietary Guidelines have changed every five years since they were written in 1980. Find out when they will be updated again. Create a time line to illustrate your findings. Share the results of your research with your class.

NCSS II F: Time, Continuity, and Change Apply ideas, theories, and modes of historical inquiry to analyze historical and contemporary developments, and to inform and evaluate actions concerning public policy issues.

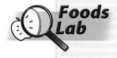

16. Too Much Sodium? Shake salt onto a paper plate as if you were salting food. Measure how much you shook onto the plate. One-quarter teaspoon of salt has 500 milligrams of sodium. Check your answer to see how that amount compares to the amount of sodium in the *Daily Values and DRIs for Teens* appendix at the back of this book.

Additional Activities For additional activities go to this book's Online Learning Center at glencoe.com.

Academic Skills

English Language Arts

17. Write a News Story Write an article for your school newspaper about one recommendation of the Dietary Guidelines for Americans. In the article, explain why that advice helps promote health. Offer tips to follow that advice. Tell how to learn more.

> **NCTE 4** Use written language to communicate effectively.

Social Studies

18. How Much Sodium? The RDA (recommended daily allowance) for sodium (salt) in the United States is less than 2,400 milligrams for adults. In England, the RNI (recommended nutritional intake) for sodium is 1,600 mg. Find what is recommended in a third country. Why do you think the recommendations vary?

> **NCSS IV E Individual Development and Identity** Examine the interaction of ethnic, national, or cultural influences in specific situations or events.

Mathematics

19. Adding Large Numbers Knowing that you should have less than 2,400 milligrams of sodium each day, keep track of your sodium intake for one day. Remember to look at labels of drinks as well as everything you eat. If you eat in a restaurant, you may find nutrition facts about the menu on the Internet.

Math Concept **Add Large Numbers** To add large numbers, line up numbers starting in the ones place. You may wish to add groups of numbers, or use a calculator.

Starting Hint To be sure your total is correct, predict what the total will be using estimation. Then, compare the total with your estimate to check whether it was reasonable.

 For more math help, go to the Math Appendix

> **NCTM Number and Operations** Compute fluently and make reasonable estimates.

STANDARDIZED TEST PRACTICE

MULTIPLE CHOICE

Read the paragraph and choose the best answer. Write your answer on a separate piece of paper.

Food labels can be confusing. MSG (monosodium glutamate) makes people crave more food. MSG gives some people headaches and contains no healthful nutrients. However, the government allows food manufacturers to list MSG on labels as a spice.

20. Based on the paragraph, which of the following statements is true?
   a. Unknown ingredients get into food.
   b. Knowledge about nutrition helps to understand food labels.
   c. All food labels hide the truth.
   d. Reading labels is too difficult.

> **Test-Taking Tip** When answering multiple-choice questions, ask yourself if each option is true or false. This may help you find the best answer.

CHAPTER 9
MyPyramid and You

Explore the Photo ▶▶
Think of the foods you enjoy. Categorize some of them in lists. *In what food group does each of your favorite foods belong?*

Writing Activity

Prewriting

Wellness Check-Up Playing sports, walking the mall, riding a bike, or washing the car are all active physical activities. Think about your activities. Are they a part of a healthful lifestyle? How do the foods you eat fit into a healthful lifestyle? How nutritious are your food choices?

1. **Identify** two smart food choices you usually make.

2. **List** two ways you could improve your food choices.

3. **Write** two questions about your own eating decisions.

Reading Guide

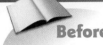

Before You Read

Preview Look at the photos and figures and read their captions. Then think about how the foods you eat fit into the MyPyramid food guide.

Read to Learn

Key Concepts
- **Identify** the key ideas in MyPyramid.
- **Summarize** how to use MyPyramid.
- **Describe** the five food groups and oils.
- **Name** nutrient dense foods.
- **Explain** the importance of portion sizes.

Main Idea

MyPyramid is your daily guide for healthful eating and active living. Eating a variety of foods in the right amounts provides the nutrients and energy you need.

Content Vocabulary

◇ MyPyramid
◇ combination foods
◇ empty-calorie foods
◇ discretionary calories

Academic Vocabulary

You will find these words in your reading and on your tests. Use the glossary to look up their definitions if necessary.
- estimate
- influence

Graphic Organizer

Use a graphic organizer like the one below to list your favorite foods according to their food group.

Food Group	Favorite Foods
Grain Group	
Vegetable Group	
Fruit Group	
Milk Group	
Meat & Beans Group	
Oils	

Graphic Organizer Go to this book's Online Learning Center at **glencoe.com** to print out this graphic organizer.

Academic Standards ■

English Language Arts
NCTE 4 Use written language to communicate effectively.

Mathematics
NCTM Measurement Understand measurable attributes of objects and the units, systems, and processes of measurement.

Science
NSES Content Standard A Develop understandings about scientific inquiry.

Social Studies
NCSS II C Understand time, continuity, and change to develop a historical perspective.

NCTE National Council of Teachers of English
NCTM National Council of Teachers of Mathematics

NSES National Science Education Standards
NCSS National Council for the Social Studies

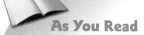

Vocabulary

You can find definitions in the glossary at the back of this book.

As You Read

Connect Think of some healthful food choices you have made recently.

All About MyPyramid

MyPyramid is a food guidance system from the U.S. Department of Agriculture (USDA). It was developed as a guide for healthful eating and active living for healthy people ages two and over. MyPyramid shows how much and what kinds of foods you need daily for your nutrient and food energy needs. It also gives physical activity advice. (See **Figure 9.1**)

How to Interpret MyPyramid

♦ Choose a variety of foods, as represented by the six colored stripes. Each stripe stands for a food group or oils. The yellow stripe represents oils, which are not one of the basic food groups.

♦ Eat more of some foods and less of others. Each stripe is a different width. That suggests the proportion of foods you need from each group. Stripes for grains, vegetables, fruits, and milk are wider than those for meat and beans and for oils. The different widths are **estimates**, not exact amounts.

♦ Make smart choices from every group. In each group some foods are more healthful than others. The wider base of MyPyramid stands for foods with little or no solid fats or added sugars. Eat these foods more often. For example, low-fat milk is a smarter choice than fried cheese sticks. Some foods have a lot of added sugars or fats. Eat them less often.

Stay Active Staying phyically active does not mean you have to spend money. *What activities do you participate in that are free?*

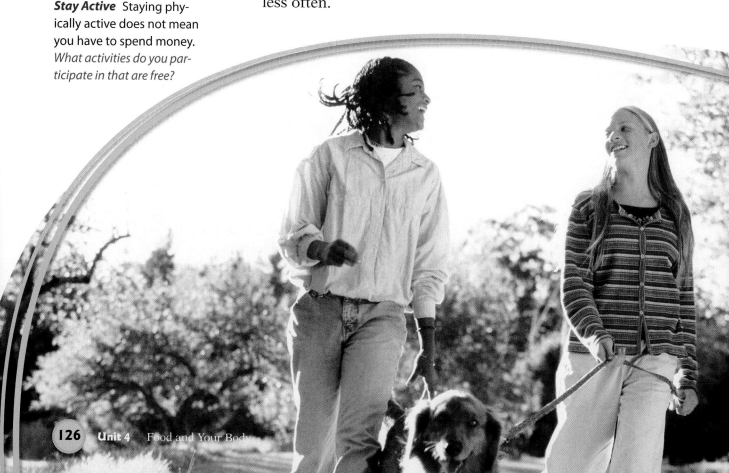

◆ Be physically active every day. The person climbing up the stairs on the left side of MyPyramid reminds you to exercise. Most teens need 60 minutes of physical activity daily. You might want to join a sports team or take daily walks.

◆ Match MyPyramid's advice to you. Each person has different physical needs, food preferences, and family and cultural traditions that **influence** food choices. Influence means that traditions can affect food choices.

◆ Take small steps to healthier eating and living. Make changes gradually.

Check **www.MyPyramid.gov** to learn more.

✓ **Reading Check** **Identify** What do the stripes represent on MyPyramid?

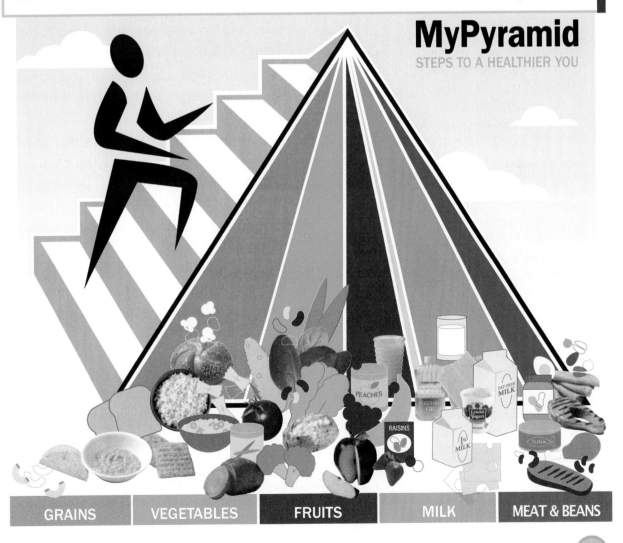

Figure 9.1 **MyPyramid**

Stay Active Make small changes to eat healthier and be more active. Start with one little step. Add others as often as possible. Small steps add up to better health. *What steps can you take to eat healthier and to move more?*

MyPyramid
STEPS TO A HEALTHIER YOU

GRAINS VEGETABLES FRUITS MILK MEAT & BEANS

Build Your Pyramid

Follow these guidelines to use MyPyramid as your personal action plan for your whole day's meals and snacks.

◆ Choose the right foods in the right amounts daily to get the nutrients you need for growth, energy, and wellness.

◆ Get the most nutrition from your calories to stay within your daily calorie needs.

◆ Balance your food intake and your physical activity to maintain a healthy weight.

◆ Make smart choices from every food group. Go easy on fat and added sugars.

MyPyramid is a flexible guide for a lifetime of healthful eating and active living. Adjust it as your life and your activity level change.

Math in Action

Conversions

Some recipes use the metric system, even though most people in the United States use customary measurements. Convert the following customary measures to metric.

  2 tablespoons olive oil

  6½ fluid ounces tomato juice

  ⅓ cup raisins

Math Concept Customary measures usually are written with fractions or mixed fractions. Metric measures are written as decimals or mixed decimals because they show part of a whole.

Starting Hint Use these equivalents to convert these measurements: 14.7 milliliters equals 1 tablespoon or 0.5 fluid ounces, and 1 cup equals 250 mL.

> **NCTM Measurement** Understand measurable attributes of objects and the units, systems, and processes of measurement.

 For more math help, go to the Math Appendix.

How MyPyramid Works

Follow these steps to put MyPyramid in action:

1. Go and visit the MyPyramid Web site at **www.MyPyramid.gov** to calculate how many calories you need on most days.

2. Determine the amounts of foods from the food groups you need based on your overall calorie level.

3. Get familiar with each food group. Choose the foods you want to eat from each food group. Pick foods you like. Try some new ones. Choose nutrient-dense foods.

4. Estimate the amounts of foods you need to eat daily.

5. Put together a daily eating plan that includes amounts of foods that match your calorie level. Include discretionary calories if you have extra calories to spend.

6. Stay physically active to balance your weight!

7. Follow your daily eating and physical activity plan, one step at a time.

✓ **Reading Check** **Discuss** How can you use MyPyramid to choose the kinds and the amounts of foods you need?

Five Food Groups Plus Oils

Foods in MyPyramid fit into five food groups, plus the oils category. Each group is important.

Why Foods Belong Together

Foods are grouped in food groups because their nutrient content is similar. For example, Milk Group foods provide calcium for healthy bones and protein for building body cells. Meat and Beans group foods can be great sources of protein, and some B vitamins, iron, and zinc.

Within each food group, different foods contain different nutrient amounts. In general, the Vegetable and Fruit Groups are good sources of vitamins A and C, folate, potassium, carbohydrates, and fiber. Carrots and apricots are excellent sources of vitamin A, while oranges and broccoli are excellent sources or vitamin C. Because their nutrients differ, vary your fruits and vegetables. For vegetables you might choose carrots, broccoli, and potatoes one day, and spinach, tomatoes, and corn the next.

Grain Group foods provide starches (complex carbohydrates), several B vitamins, and iron. Whole grain foods, such as brown rice and whole-wheat bread, are good sources of fiber. Refined grain products, such as white rice and most white bread, are not. For more fiber make at least half of your Grain Group choices whole grain.

Why Variety Is Important

No single food or food group supplies all the nutrients your body needs. Eat a variety of foods among and within the food groups for different nutrients, great flavors, and fun. To learn more about the five food groups and oils, see **Figure 9.2** on page 130.

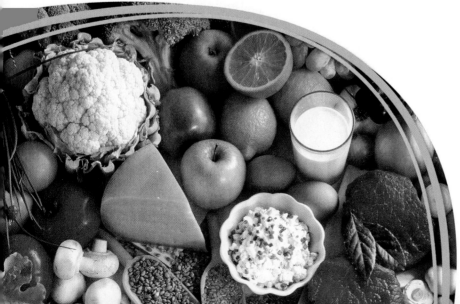
The Five Food Groups Each food group provides you with different nutrients. *What are some nutrients in these foods?*

Figure 9.2   **MyPyramid's Five Food Groups Plus Oils**

The Five Food Groups Food is grouped into food groups because their nutrient content is similar.
How can you be sure that you are getting all of the nutrients your body needs?

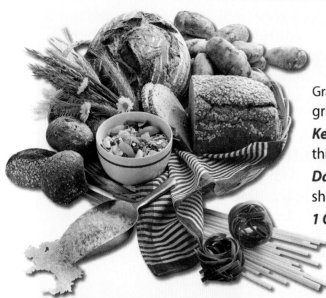

Grain Group

Grain Group includes cereal, rice, pasta, breads, and grits.

Key Nutrients: carbohydrates, B vitamins, especially thiamin, niacin, folate; minerals, including iron; fiber

Daily Amount: 6-ounce equivalents, at least half should be whole grain*

1 Ounce Is: 1 slice of bread; 1 cup (250 mL) ready-to-eat cereal; ½ cup (125 mL) cooked cereal, rice, pasta, or grits; 1 small muffin; 1 small tortilla

Vegetable Group

Vegetable Group includes broccoli, carrots, spinach, lettuce, asparagus, and beans.

Key Nutrients: Carbohydrates; vitamins, especially vitamins A and C and folate; minerals, including potassium; fiber

Daily Amount: 2½ cups*

1 Cup Is: 2 cups (500 mL) raw leafy vegetables; 1 cup (250 mL) cooked or chopped raw vegetables; 1 cup (250 mL) vegetable juice

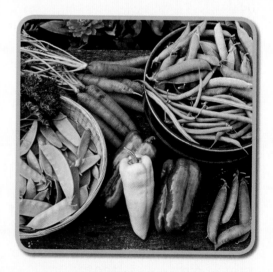

Fruit Group

Fruit Group includes apples, oranges, tomatoes, avocados, blueberries, plums, and grapes.

Key Nutrients: Carbohydrates; vitamins, especially vitamins A and C and folate; minerals, especially potassium; fiber

Daily Amount: 2 cups*

1 Cup Is: 1 cup (250mL) cut up cooked or raw fruit; 1 cup (250mL) fruit juice; 1 large banana or orange; 1 small apple; ½ cup (125mL) dried fruit

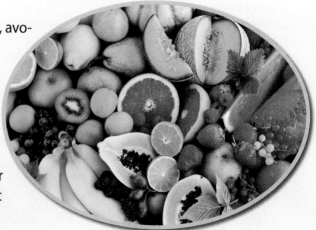

*Amount for a 2,000-calorie daily eating plan.

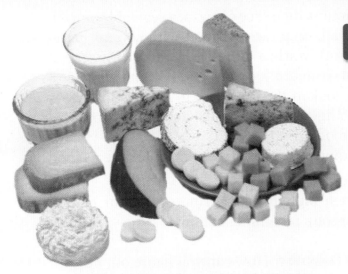

Milk Group

Milk Group includes milk, yogurt, and cheese.

Key Nutrients: protein, calcium, and other minerals, B vitamin (riboflavin), Vitamin D

Daily Amount: 3 cups*

1 Cup Is: 1 cup (250 mL) milk or yogurt; 1½ ounces (42 g) natural cheese; 2 ounces (56 g) processed cheese

Meat and Beans Group

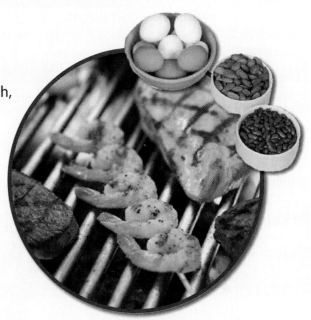

Meat Group includes all meats, poultry, fish, legumes, eggs, nuts, and seeds.

Key Nutrients: protein, B vitamins (thiamin and niacin), iron, zinc

Daily Amount: 5½-ounce equivalents*

1 Ounce Is: 1 ounce (28 g) cooked lean meat, poultry, or fish; ¼ cup (50 mL) cooked dry beans (legumes); 1 egg; 1 tablespoon (15 mL) peanut butter; ½ ounce (14 g) nuts or seeds

Oils

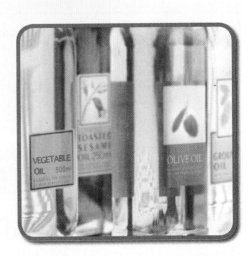

Healthful oils are not considered a food group. Many different foods from the five food groups contain healthful oils. Healthful oils include fish oil, vegetable and olive oils; liquid, at room temperature.

Key Nutrients: Fats (unsaturated)

Daily Amount: 6 teaspoons (from fish, nuts, and some vegetable oils)*

*Amount for a 2,000-calorie daily eating plan.

What About Mixed Foods?

Where do mixed foods fit in MyPyramid? How do you estimate food-group amounts for a slice of pizza, a vegetable omelet, a chicken Caesar salad, or a taco? A food with several ingredients is called a **combination food**, or a food with several ingredients from two or more food groups. For an example of a combination food, look at the sandwich in **Figure 9.3** below. Follow these steps to figure out how much a combination food provides from each food group:

◆ Estimate the amount of each ingredient and name its food group.

◆ Decide how each ingredient contributes to your calorie level and food-group recommendations.

✓ **Reading Check**) **Describe** How can you figure out how a combination food fits into MyPyramid?

Figure 9.3	Food Groups in a Pita Sandwich

Mixed Foods A pita sandwich includes foods from several food groups. *What are some other combination foods you like?*

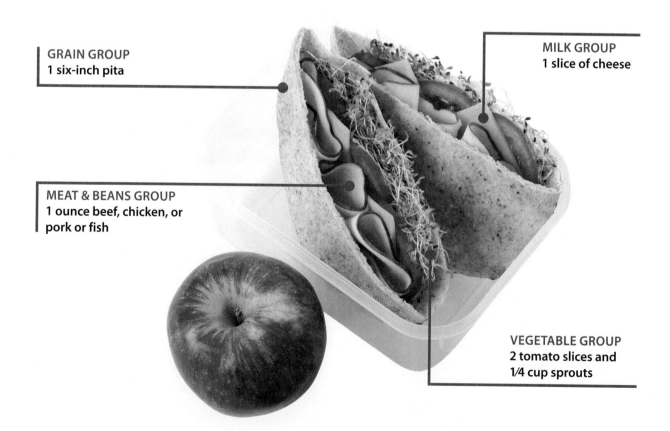

GRAIN GROUP
1 six-inch pita

MILK GROUP
1 slice of cheese

MEAT & BEANS GROUP
1 ounce beef, chicken, or pork or fish

VEGETABLE GROUP
2 tomato slices and
1/4 cup sprouts

Make Wise Choices

In each food group some foods contain more nutrients. Nutrient-dense foods provide high amounts of vitamins and minerals and fewer calories than others in the same food group. The more nutrients a food has in relation to its calories, the higher its nutrient density. Sweet potatoes are nutrient dense; potato chips are not.

Added sugars and fats add calories. Smart food choices have low amounts of solid fats or added sugars: choose mostly fat-free or low-fat milk instead of whole milk, and unsweetened rather than sweetened applesauce. Food preparation also can add sugars and fats. Skinless baked chicken has less fat than fried chicken. Fruit pie has added sugars; fresh fruit does not.

Regular soft drinks and candy are **empty-calorie foods**. Their calories come from added sugars, fat, or both. These foods supply few nutrients and do not count as food-group foods.

Get the Most Nutrition for Your Calories

Follow these guidelines to select nutrient-dense foods that are smart food-group choices:

◆ Make at least half of your grain foods whole grains for more fiber. Grain foods are valuable energy sources.

◆ Vary your veggies. Choose different colors. Many teens do not to eat enough dark-green or orange vegetables and beans (legumes). These foods deliver nutrients such as vitamin A and fiber.

◆ Focus on fruit. Many teens need to eat more fruit. Choose mostly whole or cut-up fruit. Go easy on fruit juice. It has less fiber than whole fruit.

◆ Eat calcium-rich foods. Choose mostly low-fat and fat-free milk, yogurt, and similar dairy foods for calcium. Teens need calcium for growing bones. If you cannot or do not drink milk, eat other calcium-rich foods.

◆ Go lean with protein. Eat enough lean meat, poultry, fish, eggs, nuts, or beans for iron and protein. Teens need iron and protein from food for new blood cells.

Foods with solid fats tend to increase the level of cholestorol in your body. Eating these foods raises your risk of heart disease. Eating some healthy oils, but not solid fats, is important. Since they provide calories, you do not need much. Some healthy oils also come from olives, avocados, seeds, and nuts.

✓ **Reading Check** **Explain** What is the difference between a nutrient-dense and an empty-calorie food?

The Right Amount for You

Before you can track your food amounts, you need to know how much food you need. Use *MyPyramid Tracker* on the www.MyPyramid.gov Web site to find out.

MyPyramid offers food plans at 12 calorie levels. A teenage athlete may need 2,600 calories daily, while a less-active teen may need only 2,000 calories. Your energy needs also depend on your age and gender. Each food plan gives specific amounts for each food group. See **Figure 9.4**.

Watch Your Portion Sizes!

Knowing portion sizes helps you stay within your energy needs. A portion, or helping, is the specific amount of a food or drink eaten in a meal or snack. It may differ from the serving size, a fixed amount, on a food label. See how your portions contribute to the daily amounts recommended for each food group in **Figure 9.4**.

Your portions may be bigger or smaller than you think. A typical portion could be enough for a day. For example, one bagel may weigh 5 ounces! Big portions can lead to overeating and too many calories, fat, and added sugars.

You do not need to measure every time. You just need to know how to estimate. Two slices of bread are worth about 2 ounces from the Grain Group. To check your typical portions, you can:

◆ Measure the bowls, cups, and plates you usually use.

◆ Compare your portion sizes to common objects shown in **Figure 9.5**.

How much you eat in a whole day is what counts. The total of your portions should match your daily food-group targets.

Figure 9.4	MyPyramid Advice

A Plan for Healthy Eating These three plans show how much to eat for three different calorie (food-energy) levels if most choices are lean, low-fat, fat-free and without added sugars. *Which calorie level is right for you?*

Food Groups	About 1,800 Calories	About 2,000 Calories	About 2,600 Calories
Fruit Group	1½ cups	2 cups	2 cups
Vegetable Group	2½ cups	2½ cups	3½ cups
Grain Group	6-ounce equivalents	6-ounce equivalents	9-ounce equivalents
Meat and Beans Group	5-ounce equivalents	5½-ounce equivalents	6½-ounce equivalents
Milk Group	3 cups	3 cups	3 cups
Oils	5 teaspoons*	6 teaspoons*	8 teaspoons*

Healthy oils come from some vegetable oils, as well as nuts, seeds, and some fish, such as salmon.

Figure 9.5 **How Much Do You Eat?**

Know Your Portions These common objects can help you get to know the size of common measures, such as ½ cup, or 1 cup, or 1 ounce. The column on the right shows the amount of food needed for a 2,000 calorie eating plan. *How do these common objects compare to your usual portion sizes?*

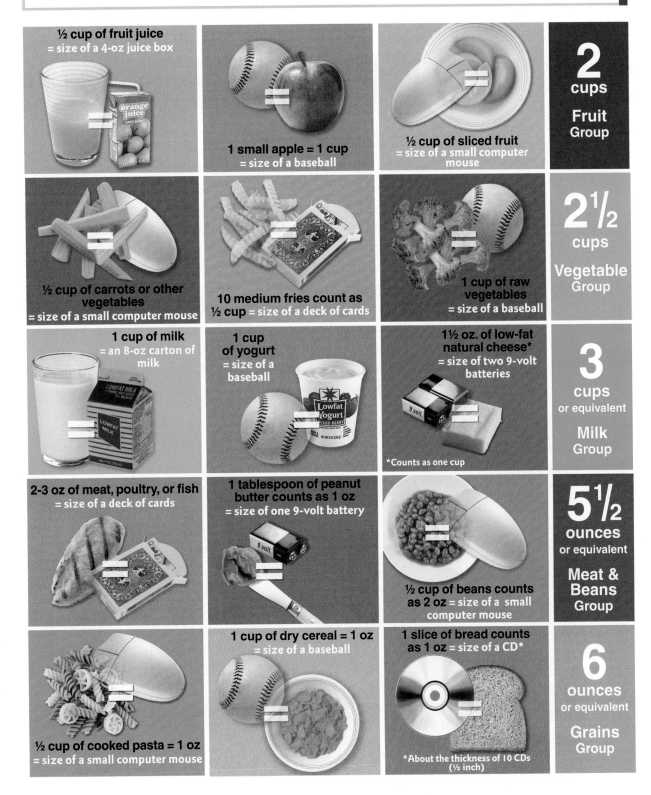

½ cup of fruit juice
= size of a 4-oz juice box

1 small apple = 1 cup
= size of a baseball

½ cup of sliced fruit
= size of a small computer mouse

2 cups Fruit Group

½ cup of carrots or other vegetables
= size of a small computer mouse

10 medium fries count as
½ cup = size of a deck of cards

1 cup of raw vegetables
= size of a baseball

2½ cups Vegetable Group

1 cup of milk
= an 8-oz carton of milk

1 cup of yogurt
= size of a baseball

1½ oz. of low-fat natural cheese*
= size of two 9-volt batteries

*Counts as one cup

3 cups or equivalent Milk Group

2-3 oz of meat, poultry, or fish
= size of a deck of cards

1 tablespoon of peanut butter counts as 1 oz
= size of one 9-volt battery

½ cup of beans counts as 2 oz = size of a small computer mouse

5½ ounces or equivalent Meat & Beans Group

½ cup of cooked pasta = 1 oz
= size of a small computer mouse

1 cup of dry cereal = 1 oz
= size of a baseball

1 slice of bread counts as 1 oz = size of a CD*

*About the thickness of 10 CDs (½ inch)

6 ounces or equivalent Grains Group

Plan Your Daily Menu

You can make good food choices if you know what and how much you should eat. Think about the day's meals in advance to make sure you eat as healthfully as possible. **Figure 9.6** shows the amounts and types of foods you might eat in a day based in a total of 2,000 calories. **Figure 9.7** shows a daily meal plan that includes the amounts and types of foods shown in Figure 9.6. Young children and inactive women need less food than what is shown in the two figures. Teen boys and grown men need more food than what is shown in the two figures.

Your Calorie Extras

Your food-group choices provide calories as well as nutrients. Depending on the foods and your portion sizes, they may contribute all the calories, or food energy, you need. If not, you have extra calories to spend. That may happen if most of your food-group choices have little or no fat and added sugars, if you eat the right amount without overeating, and if you are more physically active.

These extra calories are **discretionary calories**. They are the extras you can have if you eat enough from all food groups, and if you stay within your total calorie budget. Be careful. Even with smart food choices, you may have only 200 to 300 calories to spare.

Figure 9.6	Food for a Day

Food Group Choices This shows specific amounts and kinds of foods for each of the food groups, for a total of 2,000 calories a day. *Who might need smaller or larger portions?*

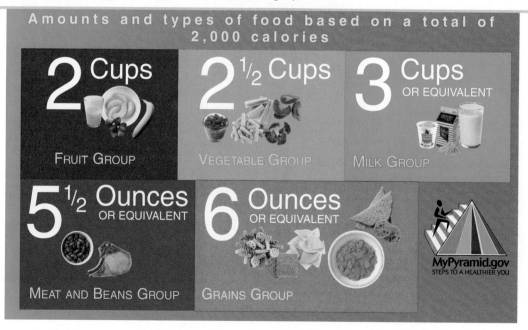

Figure 9.7   **Putting It All Together**

A Daily Meal Plan It is important to enjoy different foods in your meals and snacks. This daily meal plan includes the amounts and types of foods based on a total of 2,000 calories as shown in Figure 9.6. *What are the discretionary calorie foods in this chart?*

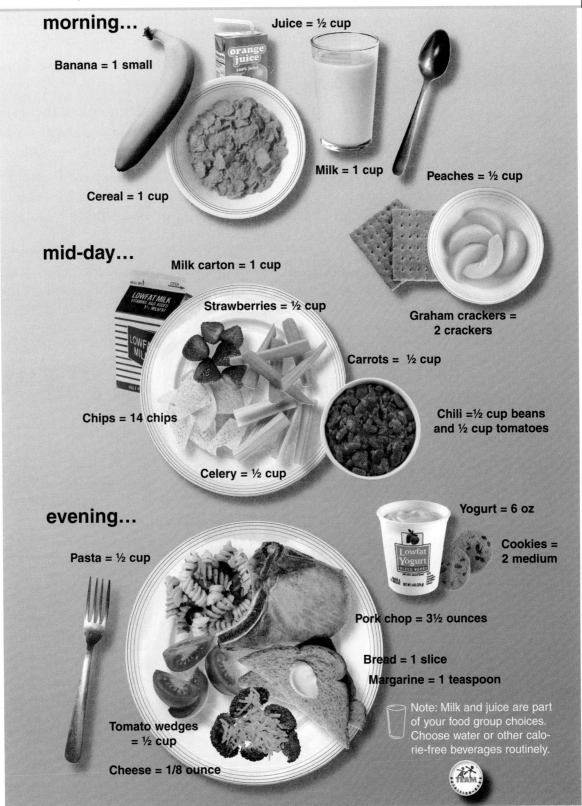

morning...

Banana = 1 small

Juice = ½ cup

orange juice 100% Juice

Cereal = 1 cup

Milk = 1 cup

Peaches = ½ cup

mid-day...

Milk carton = 1 cup

LOWFAT MILK

Strawberries = ½ cup

Graham crackers = 2 crackers

Carrots = ½ cup

Chips = 14 chips

Chili = ½ cup beans and ½ cup tomatoes

Celery = ½ cup

evening...

Yogurt = 6 oz

Lowfat Yogurt

Cookies = 2 medium

Pasta = ½ cup

Pork chop = 3½ ounces

Bread = 1 slice

Margarine = 1 teaspoon

Tomato wedges = ½ cup

Note: Milk and juice are part of your food group choices. Choose water or other calorie-free beverages routinely.

Cheese = 1/8 ounce

How to Spend Your Discretionary Calories

There are four ways to spend you discretionary calories:

◆ Eat foods that are nutrient dense.

◆ Eat small amounts of food-group foods that have more calories from fat or added sugars. Cheese, sweetened cereal, sausage, or biscuits are examples foods with more fat or added sugars than other foods in their food groups.

◆ Add just a little fat or sugars to foods, for example, butter, salad dressing, or jelly.

◆ Enjoy some empty-calorie foods every now and then, such as a soft drink or piece of candy. When you eat empty-calorie foods, remember to keep your portions small!

How can you earn more discretionary calories? Remember to choose food-group foods with fewer calories, and less fat and added sugars. Participate in sports or move more to increase your need for food energy.

✓ **Reading Check** **Describe** What are some foods that have more fats or added sugars than other foods in their food groups?

EASY RECIPES

Everyday Favorites

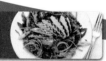

Balsamic Vinaigrette

Customary	Ingredients	Metric
1 cup	Olive oil	250 mL
½ cup	Balsamic vinegar	125 mL
1 Tbsp.	Dijon mustard	15 mL
1 tsp.	Dried oregano	5 mL
½ tsp.	Dried thyme	2 mL
½ tsp.	Dried basil	2 mL
½ tsp.	Salt	2 mL
½ tsp.	Pepper	2 mL

Try This!
Fresh herbs add flavor to this lively dressing.

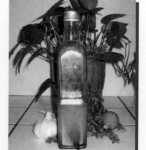

Yield: 18 servings, ¾ fluid ounce (25 mL) each

❶ Combine all ingredients in a mixing bowl and whisk until vinaigrette is mixed well.

❷ Pour into a carafe or jar and store. Serve cold and toss with salad.

Nutritional Information Per Serving: 118 calories, 13 g total fat (2 g saturated fat), 0 mg cholesterol, 87 mg sodium, 1 g total carbohydrate (0 g fiber, 1 g sugars), 0 g protein

Percent Daily Value: Vitamin A 0%, vitamin C 0%, calcium 0%, iron 2%

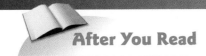

After You Read

CHAPTER SUMMARY

MyPyramid was developed by the USDA to help people make healthful food choices and stay physically active. MyPyramid places foods into five food groups and the oils category based on nutrient content. You need to eat a variety of nutrient-dense foods in the right amounts from these groups for energy, growth, and wellness. The right amount is based on calorie level for your age, gender, and physical activity level. MyPyramid is your personal action plan for your whole day's meals and snacks and for active living.

Vocabulary Review

1. Use each of these vocabulary words in a sentence.

Content Vocabulary
- MyPyramid (p. 126)
- combination foods (p. 132)
- empty-calorie foods (p. 133)
- discretionary calories (p. 136)

Academic Vocabulary
- estimate (p. 126)
- influence (p. 127)

Review Key Concepts

2. Identify the key ideas in MyPyramid.

3. Summarize how to use MyPyramid.

4. Describe the five food groups and oils.

5. Name five nutrient-dense foods.

6. Explain the importance of portion sizes.

Critical Thinking

7. Evaluate why nutrition experts advise teens to choose whole-grain foods, fruit, dark-green or orange vegetables, dried beans, low-fat or fat-free milk, and lean and low-fat protein foods.

8. Design a meal that includes foods from all five food groups.

9. Analyze why eating a variety of foods is more healthful than eating from one or two food groups.

Real-World Skills and Applications

Problem-Solving

10. Making Decisions Make MyPyramid a roadmap to a healthier you. For each food group, write three simple, specific steps you can take for a healthier you. Make a plan to follow through. Track your progress, then add more steps.

Interpersonal and Collaborative

11. Work in Teams Follow your teacher's instructions to form teams. Work in teams to research and compile a menu for a restaurant that promotes its healthful choices. As a team, share your menu with the class.

Technology

12. Create a Spreadsheet Keep track of your food and drink choices for a day. Create a spreadsheet to show how the foods you eat for a day fill up your MyPyramid goals.

Financial Literacy

13. Food Shopping on a Budget Imagine that you have $50 a week to spend on food for yourself. Plan a week's worth of menus based on MyPyramid, and calculate the cost. Did you come in under or over budget? Share your findings with the class.

14. Estimate Portions Pour a typical amount of cereal in a bowl. Spoon a helping of cooked pasta or rice on a plate. Pour a glass of milk. Estimate the amount, then measure. How close was your estimate to the measured amount? How could common objects be used as clues to help estimate postion sizes?

15. Research Nutrition History Find out about different food guides that have been used to promote healthful eating in the United States over the past 70 years. What nutrition advice does each one provide? How and why did they change? Share your findings as an oral report in class.

> **NCSS II c: Time, Continuity and Change** Understand time, continuity and change to develop a historical perspective

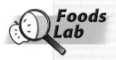

16. Make a Smoothie. Create a recipe for a 12-ounce smoothie. Use whole or cut-up fruit, yogurt, and juice. Determine how each ingredient contributes to its food group and the day's nutrient recommendation for you. Prepare your smoothie. Rate it for flavor and nutrition.

 Additional Activities For additional activities go to this book's Online Learning Center at glencoe.com.

Academic Skills

 English Language Arts

17. Advertise Write a commercial jingle about how to use MyPyramid to make snack choices. In your song, describe the ways that snacks can fit into a healthful eating plan and contribute to your food group needs.

> **NCTE 4** Use written language to communicate effectively.

 Science

18. Form a Hypothesis The scientific method is a way to answer questions. You must collect information, form a hypothesis, study the results, and draw conclusions that can be tested by others. One hypothesis might read: *Obesity is an increasing concern in the United States because people are less active, and eat more than they used to.* Write a list of facts that supports this hypothesis.

> **NSES Content Standard A** Develop understandings about scientific inquiry.

 Mathematics

19. Calculate Average Amounts A local restaurant has installed a salad bar. On a busy night, workers fill a large bowl 3 times, each time with 16 cups of salad greens. This serves 48 guests who order from the salad bar. What is the average portion size of greens for each guest?

Math Concept **Use Variables and Operations** Translating words into algebraic expressions requires knowledge of the meaning of the verbal descriptions. In algebra, a variable is a symbol used to represent a number. Arithmetic operations include addition, subtraction, multiplication, and division.

Starting Hint If x = the average number of salad greens each guest takes at the salad bar, the algebraic expression for the problem is x = (3 × 16) divided by 48. Solve for x.

> **NCTM Measurement** Understand measurable attributes of objects and the units, systems, and processes of measurement.

STANDARDIZED TEST PRACTICE

MULTIPLE CHOICE
Read the paragraph and choose the best answer. Write your answer on a separate piece of paper.

Test-Taking Tip Read the paragraph carefully to make sure you understand what it is about. Read the answer choices. Then read the paragraph again before choosing the answer.

Healthful eating means choosing enough nutrient-dense foods from each food group. The right amount for a day depends on a person's age, gender, and physical activity.

20. Based on the paragraph, which of the following statements is true?
   a. Eating a healthful diet is easy.
   b. Age helps determine a person's daily food needs.
   c. Teens do not need to eat healthfully.
   d. Eating nutrient-dense foods is not important.

Unit 4 Thematic Project

Investigate Food Trends

Understanding good food choices may help you make better choices in the future. Popular food trends can influence your food choices. Research a current food trend. What are some favorite foods and ways of eating? Are they healthful choices? How might food trends affect your own personal food choices?

My Journal

If you completed the journal entry from page 92, refer to it to see if your food choices reflect current trends.

Project Assignment

In this project you will:

- Choose and research a popular food trend that interests you.
- Examine how the food trend you selected reflects or does not reflect the messages of the Dietary Guidelines and MyPyramid.
- Write a list of interview questions about the food trend you selected and its effect on nutrition.
- Interview someone in the community who is qualified to discuss the food trend.
- Take notes during the interview, and type the results of the interview.
- Use what you learned in your research to create an oral presentation.

Academic Skills You Will Use . . . .
English Language Arts

NCTE 4 Use written language to communicate effectively.
NCTE 7 Conduct research and gather, evaluate, and synthesize data to communicate discoveries.

STEP 1 Choose and Research a Topic

Choose a topic or select your own topic and research its effect on health. Possible topics include obesity, fast food, artificial sweeteners, vegetarianism, convenience foods, sustainable eating, organic foods, or trans fats. Write a summary of your research that:

- Describes the food trend
- Explains health effects of the trend
- Relates your topic to the messages of MyPyramid and the Dietary Guidelines
- Includes relevant statistics

STEP 2 Plan Your Interview

Use the results of your research to develop a list of interview questions. Keep these writing skills in mind as you form your questions.

Writing Skills
- Use complete sentences.
- Use correct spelling and grammar.
- Organize your questions in the order you want to ask them.

STEP 3 Connect with Your Community

Interview someone in your community who is qualified to discuss the food trend you chose. For example, you might interview a local farmer or grocer about organic foods; a pastry chef about trans fats; or a doctor, nurse, or dietitian about obesity. Use the questions you formed in Step 2 to interview him or her.

Interviewing Skills
- Record responses and take notes.
- Listen attentively.
- When you transcribe your notes, write in complete sentences and use correcet spelling and grammar.

STEP 4 Create Your Final Report

Use the Unit Thematic Project Checklist to plan and give an oral report. Use these speaking skills as you present your final report.

Speaking Skills
- Speak clearly and concisely.
- Be sensitive to the needs of your audience.
- Use standard English to communicate

STEP 5 Evaluate Your Presentation

Your project will be reviewed and evaluated based on:
- Depth of interview and questions
- Content of your presentation
- Mechanics—presentation and neatness

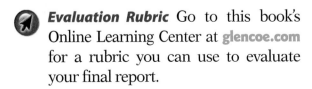 **Evaluation Rubric** Go to this book's Online Learning Center at glencoe.com for a rubric you can use to evaluate your final report.

Project Checklist	
Plan	✓ Research your topic to prepare you for your interview. ✓ Write a summary of your research. ✓ Write your interview questions. ✓ Interview a professional with relevant experience. ✓ Write out the results of your interview. ✓ Create a presentation that illustrates your findings.
Present	✓ Make a presentation to your class to discuss the results of your research about the food trend you selected. ✓ Explain how popular food trends can affect health. ✓ Relate your topic to MyPyramid and the Dietary Guidelines. ✓ Invite the students of the class to ask any questions they may have. Answer these questions. ✓ When students ask questions, demonstrate in your answers that you respect their perspectives. ✓ Turn in the notes from your interview and your research summary to your teacher.
Academic Skills	✓ Conduct research to gather information. ✓ Communicate effectively. ✓ Organize your presentation so the audience can follow along easily. ✓ Thoroughly express your ideas.

Unit 5

Nutrition for Life

Chapters in this Unit

Chapter 10 Choices for Your Healthy Weight

Chapter 11 Fuel Up for Sports

Chapter 12 Nutrition Throughout the Life Cycle

Chapter 13 Vegetarian Choices

Chapter 14 Special Health Concerns

Unit Thematic Project Preview

Plan a Healthy Lifestyle

In the unit thematic project at the end of this unit, you will choose and research a healthy lifestyle that appeals to you. You will plan an entire day's menu with foods from that lifestyle. Then, you will interview someone in your community who is qualified to discuss your choices. Last, you will make a presentation to your class to share what you have learned.

My Journal

Choosing a sensible diet and being physically active are important parts of becoming a healthy adult. There are many lifestyle options to choose from. Some are healthier than others. Write a journal entry that answers these questions:

- What healthy lifestyles appeal to you?
- How close or far are you from currently practicing your preferred lifestyle?
- How can you make better food choices?

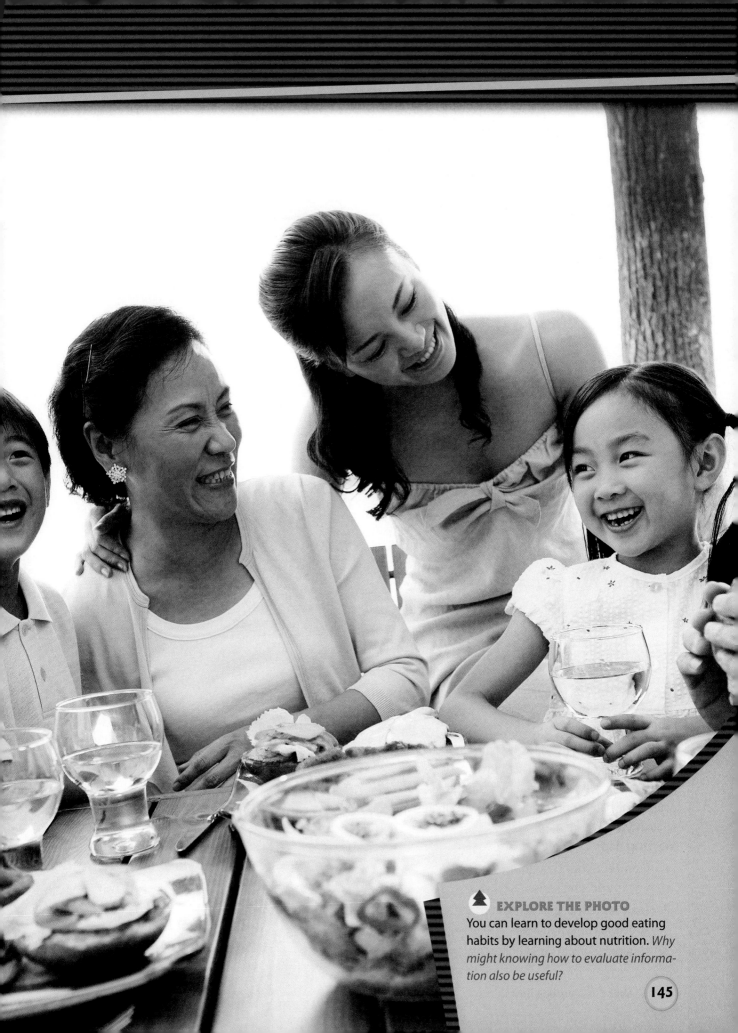

EXPLORE THE PHOTO
You can learn to develop good eating habits by learning about nutrition. *Why might knowing how to evaluate information also be useful?*

145

CHAPTER 10
Choices for Your Healthy Weight

Explore the Photo ▶▶
People come in many sizes and shapes. Your body structure is a trait that helps make you unique. Being different is absolutely normal. *What other qualities make you unique and special?*

Writing Activity

Coherent Paragraph

Healthy Weight for Life! Your teen years are the right time to start a lifelong pattern of smart eating and regular physical activity to achieve a healthy weight. Write a clear paragraph to explain what habits you can adopt now to maintain a healthy weight for life.

Writing Tips

1. **Connect** your thoughts with transition words and phrases.
2. **Link** sentences and paragraphs with parallel structures or synonyms.
3. **Use** pronouns to avoid unnecessary repetition.

Reading Guide

Before You Read

Prior Knowledge Read the Key Concepts below. Write down what you know about each concept and what you want to learn about each concept.

Read to Learn

Key Concepts
- **Explain** the factors that determine your healthy weight.
- **Discuss** the reasons to maintain a healthy weight.
- **Describe** ways to achieve and maintain your healthy weight.
- **Explain** why fad diets do not promote healthful patterns of eating.

Main Idea
A healthy lifelong weight promotes overall wellness. Eat smart and be physically active to reach and maintain your healthy weight.

Content Vocabulary
- healthy weight
- body composition
- Body Mass Index
- underweight
- overweight
- obesity
- body image
- energy balance
- fad diet

Academic Vocabulary
You will find these words in your reading and on your tests. Use the glossary to look up their definitions if necessary.

- determine
- significant

Graphic Organizer
As you read, write the consequences of underweight, overweight, and obesity.

Weight Issue	Consequences
Underweight	
Overweight	
Obesity	

 Graphic Organizer Go to this book's Online Learning Center at **glencoe.com** to print out this graphic organizer.

Academic Standards

 English Language Arts
NCTE 9 Develop an understanding of diversity in language use across cultures.
NCTE 11 Participate as members of literacy communities.

 Mathematics
NCTM Measurement Understand measurable attributes of objects and the units, systems, and processes of measurement.

NCTM Number and Operations Compute fluently and make reasonable estimates.

 Science
NSES Content Standard F Develop an understanding of personal and community health.

 Social Studies
NCSS IV D Individual Development and Identity Apply concepts, methods, and theories about the study of human growth and development.

NCTE	National Council of Teachers of English	NSES	National Science Education Standards
NCTM	National Council of Teachers of Mathematics	NCSS	National Council for the Social Studies

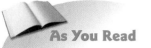
As You Read

Connect Think about the models you see in magazines. How might seeing such images affect a person's body image?

Every Body Is Different

People come in all shapes and sizes. Some have narrow shoulders and big hips. Others have a large waistline and narrow hips. Some are muscular or have bigger bones. Others are lanky. People of all shapes and sizes can be happy and healthy.

Advertisements, movies, and fashions often express the idea that a tall, slim body is the ideal. There is no ideal body shape or size. Very few people will ever look like a fashion model or a superstar athlete.

You Are Still Growing

Your clothes from last year probably do not fit well now. When your teen growth spurt ends, you will probably be 20 percent taller and 50 percent heavier than before. You are experiencing the fastest growth rate since you were an infant.

Gaining weight as you grow is natural. Growth during your teen years often comes in uneven spurts. As your body shape changes, you may get heavier without growing taller. This does not mean you are getting fat, however. Males develop broader shoulders. Females get wider hips and more body fat as their adult shape develops.

Everyone grows at different rates. Females usually start their teen growth spurt before males do. Some teens put on extra body fat before they grow taller. Others grow tall first and put on weight later. Teens who are physically active and eat smart usually grow into a healthy body weight.

Many teens keep growing until their early 20s. Your body will continue to change throughout your life.

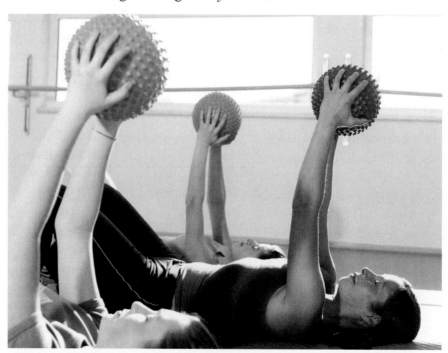

Movement Promotes a Healthy Weight
Physically active teens build muscles, improve their body composition, and control their weight.
Why does body composition make a difference?

Your Healthy Weight

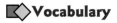

Vocabulary
You can find definitions in the glossary at the back of this book.

Healthy weight varies from one person to the next—for teens as well as adults. Many factors determine your **healthy weight**, or appropriate weight, including your age, height, growth pattern, gender, and body type.

Teens with large body frames have bigger bones and sometimes more muscle than teens with small body frames. Bigger bones and muscles weigh more than body fat. Your **body composition** is the measure of how much bone, muscle, fluids, and body fat you have. Because body types are so different, body composition is a better measure of how fit you are than your body weight alone.

Human bodies need to have some fat. Body fat acts as insulation to protect you from cold and heat. It cushions your bones as well as your heart, lungs, and other organs. Your body also keeps some fat available as a backup source of energy.

Two charts can help you understand your height and weight patterns. The height chart in **Figure 10.1** below shows height in relation to age. The chart of **Body Mass Index (BMI)** shows weight in relation to height. See **Figure 10.2** on page 150. Find your BMI on the charts to determine a range that is right for you. **Determine** means to decide by looking at choices. Remember: Only use these charts to give you a general idea about your healthy weight as your body grows and changes.

Figure 10.1   Height Charts

Height Averages The percentile shows how you compare with an average group of males or females your age. *What percentile is closest to your height and age?*

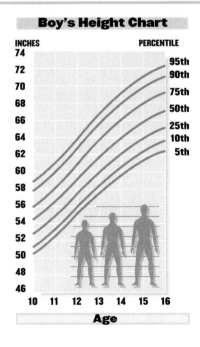

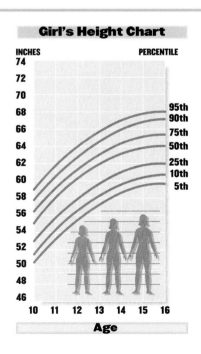

Track Your Height

Follow these steps while you look at **Figure 10.1** on page 149 to see how your height compares to an average group of others your age:

1. Measure your height in inches.
2. Find your height along the left side of the chart.
3. Find your age along the bottom of the chart.
4. Note where your age and height cross on the chart. These charts are just estimates and are one way to judge growth.

What Is Your BMI?

Follow these steps while you look at **Figure 10.2** below to find your BMI.

1. Divide your weight in pounds by your height in inches.

    weight ÷ height = χ

2. Divide this number by your height in inches.

    χ ÷ height = γ

3. Multiply the result by 703.

    $\gamma \times 703 = \text{BMI}$

✓ **Reading Check** **Identify** What are the two charts that can help you understand your height and weight patterns?

Figure 10.2	BMI Charts

Your BMI Your BMI can help you look at your weight and height realistically. Find your age along the bottom of the chart, then find your BMI along the left side of the chart. *Where does your BMI fit on the chart?*

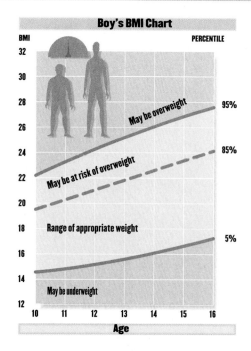

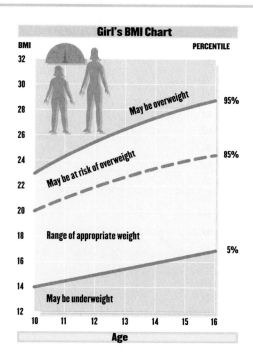

Weight Issues

How much you weigh influences your physical and mental health. You will move more easily and confidently and have a better chance of good overall health if you maintain a healthy weight. You will also have a lower risk of health problems later in life.

Being underweight can be harmful. Being **underweight** means having too little body fat. Being underweight can result from physical or emotional illness, or from a lack of food. It can lead to poor growth, depression, infections, and other diseases. Severe underweight may even lead to death.

Remember that it is natural for some teens to be thin while they are growing quickly. They usually gain some body fat when their growth spurt slows down.

Overweight means having too much body fat. It is also harmful to be overweight. Sometimes, however, very muscular people may weigh more, but not have too much fat. **Obesity** means having a **significant**, or measurably large, amount of excess body fat. Obesity is a growing health problem around the world. People who are obese later in life have a higher risk of diabetes, heart disease, and some types of cancer. Even young people may develop diabetes if they are obese. Not all people who are overweight are obese. However, having too much body fat can also affect a person's mental and social health. It can lead to low self-esteem or avoiding friends. Teens who maintain a healthy weight feel better and move with more ease and confidence.

Accept Your Body Type

Do you see yourself as overweight? Underweight? Just right? Your **body image** is how you view your body. This may differ from the way others see you. Healthy teens do not try to achieve someone else's idea of a perfect body.

Your body type and growth pattern may be like those of a parent or relative. You may lose or gain weight, or gain muscle, but changing your body type is impossible. Teens who try to do so often end up with poor eating and activity habits that harm their health. Remember to get the energy and nutrients you need from the right foods. You also need to stay active to stay healthy.

It is important to accept the body you have. Work to keep it healthy and fit. Base your weight goals on what is right for you. Remember that overall health and the total person are what really count.

✓ Reading Check **Explain** Why is there no ideal body shape and size?

Smart Choices for Your Healthy Weight

If your bathroom scale shows added pounds or your clothes feel tight, does that mean you need to lose weight? In most cases, the answer is no. The extra pounds probably just mean that you are growing. Extra pounds may mean your body is growing.

Teens who diet to lose weight may be taking a big risk. Cutting back on food could rob you of important nutrients, such as calcium and iron, and interfere with your natural growth. If you are concerned about your weight, get advice from a physician or registered dietitian.

Balance the Energy Equation

Calories measure the energy in food. Your body burns calories for physical activities and for body processes, including growth. The rate that energy is used for body processes varies from person to person. For calories in food, check the Nutrition Facts on a food label. You could also check a chart that lists foods with their calories.

You do not need to count calories to control your weight. Instead, to achieve a healthy weight you need to maintain an energy balance. **Energy balance** is when what you eat and how much energy you expend equals the same amount. This means you burn as many calories as you eat.

Stay Balanced

One pound (0.5 kg) of body fat equals about 3,500 calories. To gain 1 pound (0.5 kg) per week, a person would need to eat 500 more calories daily of mostly nutrient-dense foods. To lose one pound (0.5 kg) in a week you would need to eat 500 calories less a day than your body uses, but still follow MyPyramid. You could also eat 250 calories less and burn 250 calories more in physical activity in a day. Remember these points if you want to maintain, lose, or gain weight:

◆ You maintain weight when the calories you eat and drink equal the calories you burn.

◆ You lose weight when the calories you eat and drink are less than the calories you burn.

◆ You gain weight when the calories you eat and drink are greater than the calories you burn.

Keep Your Healthy Weight

Your teen years are the right time to develop habits to keep your healthy weight for the rest of your life. To maintain your healthy weight within an appropriate range for your age and height:

◆ Learn how much you need to eat from each food group in MyPyramid. Choose the right amount of Nutrient-dense foods from each group to provide enough food energy for growth and health. Remember that teens need the equivalent of 3 cups of milk daily from the Milk Group.

◆ Know how many discretionary calories you have to spend. Choose them wisely. (You can find more information on discretionary calories in Chapter 9.)

◆ Stay physically active. Besides receiving other health benefits, you will burn more calories. This will give you more freedom to enjoy a variety of foods.

◆ As you get older, continue to exercise and eat smart to keep the weight that is right for your growing body.

◆ Forget about dieting. Following unhealthy diets or skipping meals is not a smart way to keep your weight on track. Dieting could interfere with your health and growth. When you eat nutrient dense foods regularly, you can manage your weight healthfully.

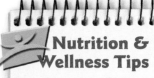

Nutrition & Wellness Tips

Use Common Sense

✓ Talk to a trusted adult if you are concerned about your weight or your BMI.

✓ Never tease or bully someone about body type or size. Instead, recognize the value of the person.

Discover International Foods

France

France is famous for its cuisine, and for having citizens who are often slender. The French enjoy regional favorites prepared mostly with local foods. Small portions are well-prepared, and people enjoy their meals at a relaxed pace. Salads, cheese, and crusty bread are part of everyday meals. Along the Mediterranean, dishes feature seafood, fresh vegetables, and olive oil. Areas bordering Germany enjoy pork and *choucroute*, French for "sauerkraut." Burgundy, in central France, is famous for its cattle industry and its beef dishes.

Languages Across Cultures

baguette *(ba-'get)* a long, crusty white bread, often called French bread

hors d'oeuvre *(òr-'dərv)* first course or appetizer

mirepoix *(mir-'pwä)* a mixture of sautéed diced carrots, onions, celery; used to season stocks, soups, and stews

Recipes Find out more about international recipes on this book's Online Learning Center at **glencoe.com**.

NCTE 9 Develop an understanding of diversity in language use across cultures.

A Slow, Sensible Path to Reach Weight Goals

You may need to lose or gain weight someday. First, talk to your doctor. Then set smart goals that are right for your body size, shape, and age. A realistic and healthful goal may be to gain or lose ½ to 1 pound (0.25 to 0.5 kg) a week.

To help you reach your weight goal, track your food intake and physical activity. Weigh yourself just once a week. It is normal if your weight stays the same for a while as you work toward your goal. See **Figure 10.3** for an estimate of how many calories you burn during daily activities.

Strategies to Lose Weight

If you need to lose weight, many strategies can help you do so safely. The most important strategies include being physically active every day and making healthful food choices.

◆ Eat at least the minimum amounts from MyPyramid's food groups. This adds up to about 1,800 calories from mostly low-fat and fat-free foods.

◆ Choose nutrient-dense foods and snacks.

◆ Do not skip meals. You might overeat later.

◆ Use food labels to find foods with fewer calories.

◆ When you enjoy a high-calorie food, eat a small amount.

◆ Pay attention to portion sizes. Eat from a plate, instead of the package, to know how much you eat.

Figure 10.3	Burn Calories

Energy for Physical Activities Every movement of your body uses energy. The longer and more strenuous an activity, the more energy you use. *For each of these activities, how long would it take you to burn the calories in a 20 oz. (600 mL) bottle of regular cola?*

Activity Level	Approximate Amount of Energy Used*
Little Activity sitting, standing quietly	1 to 2 calories per minute
Light Activity cleaning house, walking	4 calories per minute
Moderate Activity brisk walking, cycling, dancing, playing basketball	6 calories per minute
Strenuous Activity jogging, playing football, swimming	9 to 10 calories per minute
Very Strenuous Activity fast running, playing racquetball, skiing	12 calories per minute

* These figures are for someone who weighs 140 pounds (64 kg). Someone who weighs more would burn slightly more calories. Someone who weighs less would burn slightly fewer calories.

Strategies to Gain Weight

These strategies can help you safely gain weight:

◆ Stay physically active. The weight you gain will be muscle.

◆ Eat a moderate amount of foods with some fat and sugar. Go easy on foods high in fat and added sugars.

◆ Eat nutrient-dense snacks often. Eat your snacks two to three hours before meals so you are hungry at mealtime.

◆ Eat bigger portions or second helpings of nutrient-dense foods.

◆ Use food labels to find nutrient-dense foods with more calories.

◆ Eat several small meals if your appetite is small. Avoid skipping meals.

◆ Do not try to gain weight too fast, or you may add fat instead of muscle. Building muscle takes time.

Why Fad Diets Are Not the Best Choice

Have you heard about "magical" or effortless ways to melt away body fat? A **fad diet** is a weight-loss plan often based on misinformation. Fad diets are usually popular for a short time. Fad diets do not help people develop healthful patterns of eating and physical activity for the long run.

Some fad diets over-restrict the amount and type of foods. They do not provide the nutrients and food energy needed for growth and health. When people follow one fad diet after another, the weight they lose may be muscle. Without exercise, muscle may be replaced with fat. People on fad diets usually do not keep lost weight off.

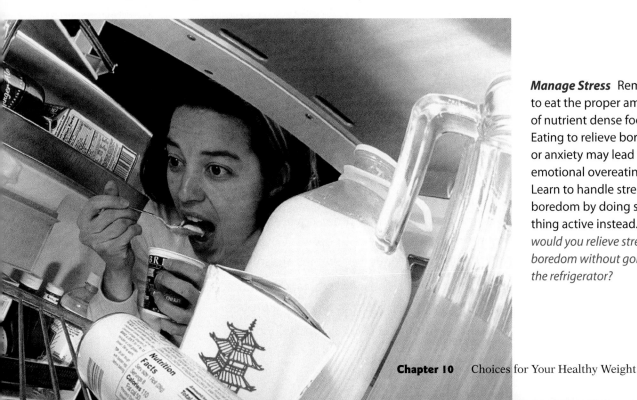

Manage Stress Remember to eat the proper amounts of nutrient dense foods. Eating to relieve boredom or anxiety may lead to emotional overeating. Learn to handle stress and boredom by doing something active instead. *How would you relieve stress or boredom without going to the refrigerator?*

Avoid these risky fad diets, which can damage your health:

◆ **All-Liquid Diets** A low-calorie, all-liquid diet will not provide enough food energy, nutrients, and fiber so you may feel tired. It can have other harmful effects, too.

◆ **Fasting** Denying your body food and fluids, even for a short period of time, can mean your body will not get the nutrients and energy needed to function properly. Your body will use up some protein, which is stored in muscle, for fuel. You also may become dehydrated.

◆ **Diet Pills** Diet pills can work to suppress your appetite, but they also can have harmful side effects such as drowsiness, anxiety, rapid heart rate, and addiction.

✓ **Reading Check** **Explain** Why are fad diets often unhealthy?

EASY RECIPES

International Favorites

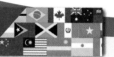

Ratatouille (Vegetable Stew of France)

Customary	Ingredients	Metric
1½ cup	Red onion	375 mL
2 cloves	Minced garlic	2 cloves
1½ cup	Green bell pepper	375 mL
1½ cup	Eggplant	375 mL
1½ cup	Zucchini	375 mL
1½ cup	Peeled tomato	375 mL
3 Tbsp.	Olive oil	45 mL
1 tsp.	Dried basil	5 mL
½ tsp.	Dried oregano	2 mL
⅛ tsp.	Salt	0.5 mL
⅛ tsp.	Pepper	0.5 mL

Try This!
Use fresh basil and oregano. One Tbsp. (15 mL) of chopped fresh herbs equals 1 Tbsp. (15 mL) of dried herbs.

Yield: 6 servings, ¾ cup (185 mL) each

❶ Chop all vegetables into ½-inch cubes. Heat oil in a skillet. Simmer onion and garlic in oil for about 3 minutes.

❷ Add green pepper, eggplant, and zucchini. Simmer, covered, for about 20 minutes.

❸ Add tomato, basil, oregano, salt, and pepper. Stir gently. Cover and continue simmering about 15 minutes, until mixture is thick and vegetables are soft.

Nutritional Information per Serving: 107 calories, 7 g total fat (1 g saturated fat), 0 mg cholesterol, 61 mg sodium, 11 g carbohydrate (3 g fiber, 5 g total sugars, 2 g protein)

Percent Daily Value: vitamin A 10%, vitamin C 80%, calcium 4%, iron 4%

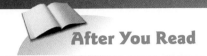

After You Read

CHAPTER SUMMARY
A healthy weight throughout life promotes overall wellness. There is no ideal weight for everyone. Your best weight depends on your body type, gender, and growth stage. Eating smart and being physically active will help you reach and maintain your healthy weight. Follow a healthful action plan to lose or gain weight. Fad diets may not follow guidelines of healthful eating and can harm your health.

Vocabulary Review

1. Use each of these vocabulary words in a sentence.

Content Vocabulary
◇ healthy weight (p. 149)
◇ body composition (p. 149)
◇ Body Mass Index (BMI) (p. 149)
◇ underweight (p. 151)
◇ overweight (p. 151)
◇ obesity (p. 151)
◇ body image (p. 151)
◇ energy balance (p. 152)
◇ fad diet (p. 155)

Academic Vocabulary
■ determine (p. 149)
■ significant (p. 151)

Review Key Concepts

2. Explain the factors that determine your healthy weight.

3. Discuss the reasons to maintain a healthy weight.

4. Describe ways to achieve and maintain your healthy weight.

5. Explain why fad diets do not promote healthful patterns of eating.

Critical Thinking

6. Recommend nutrient-dense foods from the five food groups for a friend who needs to gain weight. He needs more calories because he is growing very fast and he is an athlete.

7. Evaluate the effect of skipping breakfast on healthy weight. Plan a breakfast for a teen that would be part of a smart plan to manage weight.

8. Analyze how society communicates a "thin is in" message to young people today. What are the effects of this message on teens? Suggest how to counter this message with more healthful, positive messages.

9. Evaluate a current fad diet described in a magazine. What clues could help you judge its safety, nutrition, and effectiveness?

Real-World Skills and Applications

Set Goals and Make Decisions

10. Teen Challenges Making choices for a healthy weight is not always easy. List five common excuses that teens give as reasons for quitting a healthy weight plan. For each excuse, list three solutions. Decide which solutions would work for you. Write a paragraph that explains why.

Collaborative and Interpersonal

11. Obesity Weight gain comes from eating more calories than you burn. Brainstorm with two other students about why obesity is a growing problem. Choose one factor and propose a solution. Present your factor and solution in class.

Financial Literacy

12. Vending Machines Candy costs more than fruit and it has more calories. Instead of a 65¢ candy bar, you could have a 20¢ piece of fruit. How much could you save in a week if you ate a candy bar for a snack on two days and a piece of fruit the other five days?

Technology

13. Healthy Body Image Design a Web page or poster that promotes the beauty of the individual, no matter what shape or size. Include positive messages to boost teens' body image and show respect for others' bodies and feelings.

14. Burden of Overweight Explore the burden of excess body fat on your body and health. Carry a 10-pound (5 kg) bag of flour around for an hour, perhaps in a backpack. Record how that extra weight feels. Write a paragraph describing your conclusions about how excess body fat affects you.

> **NCTM Measurement** Understand measurable attributes of objects and the units, systems, and processes of measurement.

15. Snack Survey Do a survey of the after-school snacks and drinks available to you in school vending machines, concession stands, nearby stores, and at home. Create a table to rate the choices for healthfulness and for how well they fit with your weight-management goals.

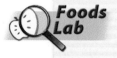

16. Snack Makeover Find a recipe for a nutritious snack. Adapt the recipe to meet the needs of two people: an active teen wanting to gain weight and an adult wanting to lose weight. Work as a class to prepare both versions. Rate them for flavor and nutrition.

Additional Activities For additional activities, go to this book's Online Learning Center at glencoe.com.

Academic Skills

 English Language Arts

17. Different Growth Rates Write a short story in which a fictitious teen is growing and developing at a different rate from that of friends and classmates. Tell how the teen overcomes feelings of being different and learns to appreciate his or her uniqueness.

> **NCTE 11** Participate as members of literacy communities.

 Social Studies

18. Obesity Crisis Obesity is a national and global health crisis. The Centers for Disease Control and Prevention describe it as the most common nutrition problem among Americans today. With your teacher's permission, go online to find statistics on obesity in the United States. Write a two-paragraph summary.

> **NCSS IV D Individual Development and Identity** Apply concepts, methods, and theories about the study of human growth and development.

 Mathematics

19. How Many Laps? Swimming is a great way to get in shape because your whole body is working. Swimming joined the Olympics in 1896. An Olympic-size pool is 50 meters long. Each length of the pool is called a lap. A mile is 1,609.344 meters. Estimate how many laps you would have to swim to travel a mile in the pool.

Math Concept **Estimation by Rounding**
The answer will contain a decimal. First, look at the first digit to the right of the decimal point. If it is 5 or greater, round up. If it is 4 or less, round down.

Starting Hint A good strategy to help you solve word problems is to ask the question another way. For example, "How many lengths are there per mile?" The word *per* suggests division.

 For more math help, go to the Math Appendix

> **NCTM Number and Operations** Compute fluently and make reasonable estimates.

STANDARDIZED TEST PRACTICE

MULTIPLE CHOICE
Read the paragraph and question, and choose the best answer.

Test-Taking Tip If you find an unfamiliar word, read other words and phrases around the word to help you figure out its meaning. The way a word is used will often give you clues to the meaning.

Humans need enzymes to aid in processes such as digestion. Saliva contains enzymes, but not enough to do the job. Uncooked fruits and vegetables provide enzymes, along with other nutrients.

20. Based on the paragraph, which of the following statements is true?
  a. Raw fruit is the best source of healthy enzymes.
  b. The human body needs enzymes only for digestion.
  c. Fresh vegetables can contribute healthy enzymes to your diet.
  d. Enzymes are only found in foods.

CHAPTER 11
Fuel Up for Sports

Explore the Photo ▶▶
Whether you are preparing for tryouts, competing in a sports event, or being active for fun and fitness, smart eating can help you do your very best. *Why is a smart eating plan important for peak performance in sports?*

Writing Activity

Business Letter

Sports are a fun way to stay active and relax. What sports are available near you? Write a business letter to your local chamber of commerce or department of parks and recreation. Request information about sports programs near you. Also, suggest ideas for programs that interest you.

Writing Tips

1. **Be** clear, brief, and considerate.
2. **Use** correct form.
3. **Proofread** to correct errors in grammar, usage, spelling, and punctuation.

Reading Guide

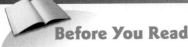

Before You Read

Look It Up Scan the vocabulary words in the chapter. If you see a word that you do not know, look it up in the glossary or the dictionary.

Read to Learn

Key Concepts

- **Describe** how physical activity affects your nutrient needs.
- **Discuss** smart food and fluid choices for before, during, and after physical activity.
- **Analyze** common myths about sports nutrition.

Main Idea

Rigorous physical activity requires smart food choices and more fluids—before, during, and after a workout or competition.

Content Vocabulary

◇ dehydration
◇ electrolyte
◇ steroid
◇ carbohydrate loading

Academic Vocabulary

You will find these words in your reading and on your tests. Use the glossary to look up their definitions if necessary.

■ develop
■ strategy

Graphic Organizer

As you read, write the main messages about eating for peak performance, supported by strategies for before, during, and after strenuous activity.

Eating for Peak Performance		
Before	**During**	**After**

 Graphic Organizer Go to this book's Online Learning Center at **glencoe.com** to print out this graphic organizer.

Academic Standards ▪

 English Language Arts
NCTE 8 Use information resources to gather information and create and communicate knowledge.

 Mathematics
NCTM Number and Operations Understand the meanings of operations and how they relate to one another.

NCTM Data Analysis and Probability Develop and evaluate inferences and predictions that are based on data.

 Science
NSES Content Standard F Develop an understanding of personal and community health.

NCTE National Council of Teachers of English
NCTM National Council of Teachers of Mathematics

NSES National Science Education Standards
NCSS National Council for the Social Studies

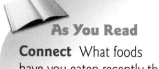

As You Read

Connect What foods have you eaten recently that helped you to feel energetic?

Vocabulary

You can find definitions in the glossary at the back of this book.

Nutrients for Active Living

All teens should follow MyPyramid when planning their meals and snacks. Eating the right amounts of foods from the five food groups will supply all the nutrients you need.

◆ **Carbohydrates** People who are very physically active need extra calories. Most of these calories should come from nutrient-dense foods high in starches, or complex carbohydrates. These include bread, cereal, rice, pasta, dry beans and peas, and starchy vegetables.

◆ **Protein** Eat 5 to 7 ounces daily from the Meat and Beans Group. Extra protein will not help you build bigger muscles. To build muscle, you need muscle-building physical activity, not more protein from food.

◆ **Vitamins and Minerals** Eat a variety of foods to get the vitamins and minerals you need. Iron-rich foods are good for your blood. Calcium-rich foods help **develop**, or promote the growth of, healthy bones. As an athlete, you do not need extra vitamins and minerals.

◆ **Water** During intense activity, your body heats up. To cool down, your body sweats. When you sweat, you must drink fluids to replace lost fluids.

✓ **Reading Check** **Discuss** How does physical activity affect your nutrient needs?

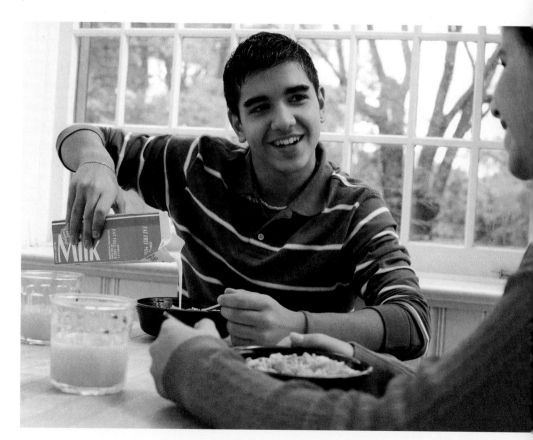

Eat to Succeed Smart eating throughout the year should be part of your body's ongoing training program for sports or any physical activity. *What are some of the nutrients that these breakfast choices supply?*

Choices for Peak Performance

Plan ahead to do your personal best at strenuous physical activity. During your workout, warm-up and cool-down properly. Performance also depends on what you eat and how much you drink before, during, and after activity.

Before You Are Active

About three to four hours before vigorous activity, enjoy a meal that is high in carbohydrates and low in fat and protein. This combination is easy to digest. Carbohydrates also provide energy for the activity. Carbohydrates also provide fuel for your working muscles. Eat until you are satisfied but not too full. These meals are great choices a few hours before physical activity:

◆ Orange juice, bagel, peanut butter, apple slices

◆ Apple juice, pancakes and syrup, low-fat yogurt, strawberries

◆ Tomato soup, grilled cheese sandwich, low-fat milk

Eat a light snack, such as some fruit, about a half hour before an activity if you are hungry. Sugary foods like candy may leave you feeling shaky or cause you to get tired quickly.

Drink at least 2 cups (500 mL) of water about two hours before the activity. Drink another 1 to 2 cups (250 to 500 mL) fifteen minutes before the activity.

While You Are Active

Unless your workout lasts more than one hour, you probably do not need to eat during the activity. If you do, eat carbohydrate-rich foods that are easy to digest, such as a banana or a rice cake.

If you do not replace fluids lost through sweating, you may suffer from dehydration. **Dehydration** is a significant loss of body fluids. Symptoms start with thirst and fatigue, and can progress to weakness, confusion, muscle cramps, and heat exhaustion. In severe cases, dehydration can cause death.

During vigorous activity, drink ½ to 2 cups (125 to 500 mL) of water. The amount depends on how much you sweat. Do not drinks excessively. During vigorous activity your kidneys cannot eliminate extra water fast enough. In extreme cases, this can even be fatal.

Math in Action

Daily Allowance of Water

Sara decides to drink 3 cups (750 mL) of water before a soccer game. She measured her drinking glasses, and found that they hold 12 oz each. How many times should she refill a 12-oz glass to get that amount of water?

Math Concept **Multiply/Divide Rational Numbers** When a word problem requires organizing things into different-size groups, use multiplication and division to solve it.

Starting Hint First, determine the number of ounces in 3 cups of water. Then, divide by the size of the glass. If necessary, round up to the next whole number.

NCTM Number and Operations Understand the meanings of operations and how they relate to one another.

 For more math help, go to the Math Appendix

Fluid Choices

Plain water is the best choice for replacing fluids. Before or after a workout, you might also drink juice or milk. The carbohydrates in these drinks fuel your muscles. Diluted juice is better during a workout because your body absorbs it faster.

For activities lasting over one hour, you could drink sports drinks with easily absorbed glucose, or simple sugar. Sports drinks also supply electrolytes. An **electrolyte** is a mineral such as sodium, chloride, and potassium that helps maintain your body's fluid balance. Your body loses some electrolytes through sweat.

Some choices are not as good. Caffeinated drinks such as cola and energy drinks may increase anxiety. Sugary drinks take longer to absorb. Carbonated drinks may upset your stomach.

After You Are Active

Immediately after an intense workout, drink fluids to replace those you have lost—3 cups (750 mL) of water for each pound of weight lost. Within one to four hours, eat plenty of foods with carbohydrates and some protein and fat.

Athletes who play seasonal sports may not need as much food energy during their off-season. To maintain a healthy weight, the best **strategy**, or plan of action, is to cut down on high-calorie foods or stay as active as you were in season.

✓ **Reading Check** **Recall** How can you avoid dehydration?

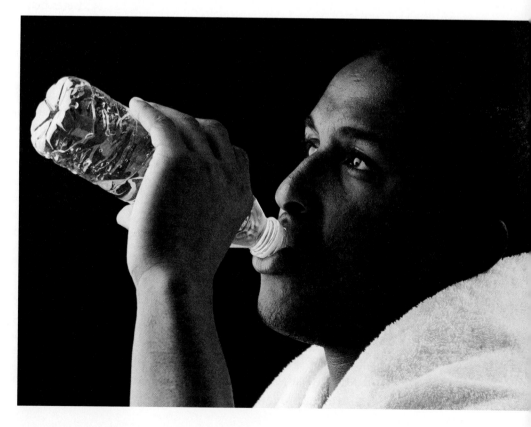

Rehydrate! During physical activity, drink fluids to replace water lost by sweating. Do not wait until you feel thirsty, because you may already be dehydrated. *Why is eating an ice cube not an effective way to replace fluids?*

Sports Facts and Myths

Some athletes believe that special products—such as protein powders, vitamin supplements, and energy bars—will help them win. Be cautious of products that promise to boost your performance. Healthful food choices provide all the nutrients you need.

Get Fit with F.I.T.

You can improve your fitness level with F.I.T. This stands for Frequency, Intensity, and Time. For the best results, gradually increase each part of the F.I.T. formula:

◆ **Frequency**—how often you work out. Start with two workouts a week, then do more as you become stronger.

◆ **Intensity**—the speed and power of your movements. This could mean how much you hustle on the basketball court or how high you step in aerobics class. As you build strength and endurance over time, you can increase the intensity of your workouts.

◆ **Time (duration)**—how long you work out each time. How much time you spend moving is what counts.

Making Weight

To compete in certain sports, like wrestling, athletes need to weigh a specific amount. In other sports, such as gymnastics, athletes may think they need to compete at a low weight, but this is not always true. Teen athletes must remember that their bodies are still growing and compete in the right weight class.

Manage your weight for competition every day you train—not just the days before an event. Fasting, crash diets, or trying to sweat off weight will keep you from doing your best.

Bulk Up Muscles

Adding muscle may improve performance for some athletes. Trying to build muscle too fast and without physical activity, however, may build fat instead. Slow, steady weight gain is best. Do not gain more than 2 pounds (.9 kg) per week.

Lifting heavy weights can damage growing bones. Use your body's own weight to build muscle strength and endurance instead. Try pull-ups, push-ups, and leg lifts.

Stay away from any performance-enhancing steroid. A **steroid** is a drug that acts like male hormones. Teens who use steroids to build muscle often suffer permanent health problems. For example, steroids can damage the reproductive system.

High-Protein Diets

Some athletes think they need to eat a high-protein, low-carbohydrate diet to build muscle and improve physical performance. Instead, eating a variety of foods for well-balanced nutrition is best, both for athletic performance and for overall health. Extra protein from food, protein powders, or supplements will not build muscle. Any extra protein turns into energy or gets stored as fat.

Some athletes use carbohydrates to prepare for competitive events through a practice called carbohydrate loading. **Carbohydrate loading** is strategy to increase the store of energy in the muscles. Several days before an event, athletes gradually decrease training and gradually increase the carbohydrates they eat. For trained endurance athletes, this helps the body store extra carbohydrates. Most people do not benefit from carbohydrate loading. Using this practice repeatedly could interfere with growth. It is not advised for teens.

✓ **Reading Check** **Explain** What is the danger of trying to lose weight for sports such as wrestling a day or two before a competition?

EASY RECIPES

Everyday Favorites

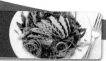

Trail Mix

Customary	Ingredients	Metric
1 cup	Any whole-grain cereal	250 mL
¾ cup	Raisins	180 mL
½ cup	Roasted peanuts	120 mL
¼ cup	Sunflower seeds	60 mL
¼ cup	Dried cranberries	60 mL
¼ cup	Chocolate chips	60 mL

Try This!

Mix and Match
For variety, use a different cereal or add a different dried fruit.

Yield: 4 servings, ¾ cup (250 mL) each

❶ Combine all ingredients and mix in a large bowl.

❷ Store in an airtight container.

Nutritional Information Per Serving: 356 calories, 18 g total fat, (4 g saturated fat), 0 mg cholesterol, 60 mg sodium, 49 g total carbohydrate (6 g fiber, 31 g total sugars), 9 g protein.

Percent Daily Value: vitamin A 2%, vitamin C 4%, calcium 8%, iron 25%

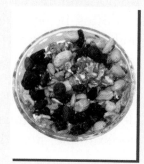

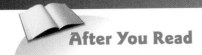

After You Read

CHAPTER SUMMARY

Follow MyPyramid to get enough food energy and nutrients for your peak physical performance. Get most of your food energy from complex carbohydrates, not from extra protein. Carefully plan and choose what you eat and drink before, during, and after physical activity. Focus on frequency, intensity, and time in your workouts. Make nutrition an ongoing training strategy, even in the off-season. Drink enough fluids to avoid dehydration. Plain water is the best choice. Be cautious of eating plans or nutrition supplements that promise top performance or more muscle.

Vocabulary Review

1. Use each of these vocabulary words in a sentence.

Content Vocabulary
- dehydration (p. 163)
- electrolyte (p. 164)
- steroid (p. 165)
- carbohydrate loading (p. 166)

Academic Vocabulary
- develop (p. 162)
- strategy (p. 164)

Review Key Concepts

2. Describe how physical activity affects your nutrient needs.

3. Discuss smart food and fluid choices for before, during, and after physical activity.

4. Analyze common myths about sports nutrition.

Critical Thinking

5. Analyze Which would be a better lunch on the day of a late-afternoon gymnastics meet: a steak sandwich or spaghetti? Explain why. Add foods to your choice to make a balanced pre-competition meal.

6. Analyze this scenario. You are a long-distance runner on your school's track team. How could you use your management skills to make sure you get enough fluids?

7. Design a training regimen for a hockey player. What training activities and eating plan would you recommend? How could he or she stay motivated?

8. Analyze this situation. Your friend Julianna is planning to run a 5K race. She plans to eat only high-protein foods to prepare. Is this a good plan? Explain.

9. Examine the snack choices on your midday school lunch menu. Imagine you will be choosing. You and your classmates will have physical education 30 minutes after this snack. What foods would you choose, and why?

Real-World Skills and Applications

Set Goals and Make Decisions

10. Fueling Exercise Lauren is joining an all-night jump-rope-a-thon to raise funds for the Special Olympics. She wonders what to eat before and during the event to have enough energy to last all night. Write a paragraph to describe solutions that could help her reach her goal.

Collaborative and Interpersonal

11. Think Like a Coach Imagine that you are on the wrestling team. You notice that some team members are crash dieting to try to compete in a weight class lower than their appropriate weight. Write a paragraph to explain how you could help them understand the potential dangers.

Technology

12. Design a Brochure Use publishing software to create a brochure for teen athletes about eating smart for sports. Include information about sports nutrition myths. Share your brochure with a school coach. Offer to share it with a team.

Financial Literacy

13. By the Bar or Box? You visit a local grocery store where granola bars are sold. Granola bars are available individually for $1.19 or in a box of 6 for $6.50. You want to purchase 6 granola bars. Write a paragraph to explain which is a better deal and why.

14. Training Table Menus Create five original menus featuring high-carbohydrate foods that you like and that would help fuel your body before a big sports competition. Trade your recipe list with a classmate and evaluate each other's plans.

15. Energy Bars Compare the calories and nutrients in several energy bars. Use information on food labels. Consider the cost and convenience of each. How would you rate these snacks? What other foods can provide portable nutrition for before or after physical activity?

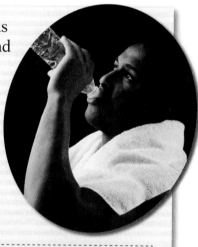

NCTM Data Analysis and Probability Develop and evaluate inferences and predictions that are based on data.

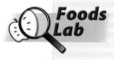

16. Your Sports Drink Create a juice beverage to enjoy after a workout. You might blend more than one juice or other beverage. Write the recipe with its name, ingredients, and directions, and describe why it makes a great drink for after a workout.

Additional Activities For additional activities go to this book's Online Learning Center at **glencoe.com**.

Academic Skills

 English Language Arts

17. Dangers of Steroids Steroids often have dangerous, permanent side effects. Research the damage steroids can do. Write a script for a 60-second public service announcement about steroids.

> **NCTE 8** Use information resources to gather information and create and communicate knowledge.

 Science

18. Sports Drinks Just for Sports Because they contain more sugar and acid than regular soda, sports drinks should be reserved for sports that require endurance. Which types of athletes need sports drinks?

Procedure Research the ingredients and effects of several sports drinks.

Analysis Write a paragraph to explain your findings.

> **NSES Content Standard F** Develop an understanding of personal and community health.

 Mathematics

19. Comparing Bottled Water Zack needs to drink enough water when running long distance. He likes the convenience of pre-bottled water he can buy at the store. He can buy three packs of six ½-liter bottles for $6.99, or he can buy one pack of twelve 1-liter bottles for $9.49. Show how Jack can compare the two packages to find the better deal.

Math Concept **Divide Integers** An integer is a whole number. Finding the better deal requires comparing the costs per unit of measure.

Starting Hint Find the total number of liters for each option, then divide to find the cost per liter. Round up to the nearest hundredth for cost.

 For more math help, go to the Math Appendix

> **NCTM Number and Operations** Understand the meanings of operations and how they relate to one another.

STANDARDIZED TEST PRACTICE

MULTIPLE CHOICE
Read the paragraph and choose the best answer. Write your answer on a separate piece of paper.

Test-Taking Tip When taking a test, if you have time at the end, check your answers and solutions. Did you answer each part of every question? Did you answer the questions asked? Do your answers look reasonable? Do your calculations check out?

The minerals that charge your body are called electrolytes. If you lose too many electrolytes while exercising, cramps, weakness, or nausea can result. Sports drinks contain electrolytes, but so do many foods.

20. Based on the paragraph, which of the following statements is true?
  a. Sports drinks are the only source of electrolytes.
  b. Too many electrolytes will cause cramps.
  c. A healthful eating plan provides plenty of electrolytes.
  d. Your body needs extra electrolytes.

CHAPTER 12

Nutrition Throughout the Life Cycle

Explore the Photo ▶▶

Your meals and snacks have changed since you were a baby. You still need the same nutrients, but in different amounts. As a teen, you can enjoy a variety of foods. *How have your food choices changed since your childhood?*

Writing Activity

Dialogue

Family Memories Nearly everyone has a childhood or family story about food. Write a dialogue in which two people share a childhood or family food experience. Think about funny family stories or warm memories.

Writing Tips

1. **Give** each person their own voice.

2. **Use** dialogue for a purpose.

3. **Choose** language that sounds real and appropriate to the people talking.

4. **Use** quotation marks appropriately.

Reading Guide

Before You Read
Check for Understanding If you have questions as you are reading, that means you are checking your understanding of the material. To get the most out of the text, try to answer those questions.

Read to Learn
Key Concepts
- **Summarize** how nutrition needs change throughout the life cycle.
- **Explain** the importance of good nutrition for pregnancy.
- **Compare** how infant feeding changes in the first year of life.
- **Create** a healthful eating plan for children.
- **Explain** why good nutrition and active living are important for teens.
- **Discuss** how food and nutrition needs change during adulthood.
- **Identify** sources of food assistance.

Main Idea
Throughout the life cycle, people need the same nutrients, but in different amounts. At each life stage, people eat and enjoy different kinds of food.

Content Vocabulary
◇ life cycle
◇ prenatal
◇ fetus
◇ low birth weight
◇ lactate
◇ food jag

Academic Vocabulary
You will find these words in your reading and on your tests. Use the glossary to look up their definitions if necessary.
■ specific
■ environment

Graphic Organizer
As you read, list five ways to make the most of family meals. Use a graphic organizer like the one below to organize your answers.

Family Meals
1.
2.
3.
4.
5.

 Graphic Organizer Go to this book's Online Learning Center at **glencoe.com** to print out this graphic organizer.

Academic Standards ■

 English Language Arts
NCTE 4 Use written language to communicate effectively.
NCTE 5 Use different writing process elements to communicate effectively.
NCTE 9 Develop an understanding of diversity in language use across cultures.

 Science
NSES Content Standard C Develop an understanding of matter, energy, and organization in living systems.

 Mathematics
NCTM Number and Operations Compute fluently and make reasonable estimates.

NCTE National Council of Teachers of English
NCTM National Council of Teachers of Mathematics

NSES National Science Education Standards
NCSS National Council for the Social Studies

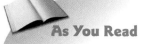

As You Read

Connect Think about how what you eat now differs from what you ate as a young child.

◆ **Vocabulary**

You can find definitions in the glossary at the back of this book.

Nutrition Is Important at Every Age

Good nutrition throughout your life cycle is essential for your growth, energy, and wellness. The **life cycle** is the entire time from before birth through adulthood. The best advice for healthful eating and active living for anyone who is two years of age and older comes from the Dietary Guidelines for Americans and MyPyramid. The Recommended Dietary Allowances give **specific**, or particular, nutrient recommendations for both genders and all ages.

✓ **Reading Check** **Recall** MyPyramid advice is meant for people of what age?

Eat for a Healthy Pregnancy

The **prenatal** period is the time between conception and birth. During the prenatal period, a single cell develops into a baby. The unborn baby is called the **fetus**. The fetus depends on the mother for its nourishment. Maintaining good nutrition and health habits, along with getting proper medical care, are a pregnant woman's most important responsibilities.

Before and During Pregnancy

Good nutrition helps prepare a woman for a healthy pregnancy. Women who are pregnant or may become pregnant need to pay careful attention to several nutrients. Folate, a B vitamin that is also called folic acid, helps the body make new cells. If a pregnant woman does not get enough folate, her baby may have a set of birth defects in the spine called spina bifida. Grain products are required by law to be fortified with folic acid. As the amount of blood increases in both mother and fetus, they both need more iron. Calcium builds the baby's bones and teeth and helps renew the mother's bones.

Foods from the Milk Group provide calcium and protein. Foods from the Meat and Beans Group provide iron as well as protein. Fruits, vegetables, dry beans, and fortified grain products are essential for folate and other nutrients.

Gaining 25 to 35 pounds (11 to 16 kg) during pregnancy is normal. Poor nutrition can lead to low birth weight. **Low birth weight** is a birth weight less than 5½ pounds (2.5 kg). Babies with low birth weight may develop health problems. A pregnant woman should add 300 calories a day from nutrient-dense foods to her diet.

✓ **Reading Check** **Recall** What three nutrients may need special attention among pregnant women?

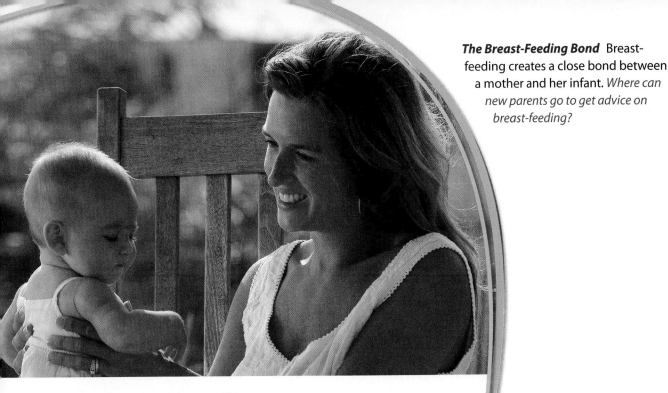

The Breast-Feeding Bond Breast-feeding creates a close bond between a mother and her infant. *Where can new parents go to get advice on breast-feeding?*

Infant Feeding

Infants change quickly during the first year! A baby may grow 50 percent longer and triple in weight. The brain and other organs also continue to develop. A baby needs the right nourishment. At first, mother's milk or infant formula is the only food a baby needs.

Mother's Milk or Formula?

Breast-feeding is an economical, natural way to feed babies. New mothers lactate. To **lactate** is to produce milk. This milk contains important nutrients, as well as antibodies that build immunity to infection. Mother's milk is easily digested, pre-warmed, and germ-free. Breast-feeding mothers should follow MyPyramid and drink enough fluids. This helps to ensure enough milk for their babies and enough nutrients for their own health. Mothers who face difficulty breast-feeding can get advice from a pediatrician, a lactation counselor, the public health department, and the La Leche League, a nonprofit organization that offers information and support to breast-feeding mothers.

Infant formula, prepared correctly, has nutrition similar to mother's milk. Most formulas contain modified, enriched non-fat cow's milk. Babies who cannot tolerate cow's milk can drink soy-based formulas.

Plain cow's milk cannot substitute for mother's milk or formula. It lacks some nutrients babies need. In their first year, babies cannot digest cow's milk properly. After the first year, many children can drink whole milk. It contains fats and proteins essential for growth.

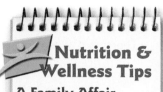
Bottle-Feeding Basics

Prepare bottles carefully to ensure food safety and prevent injury. Always wash your hands before feeding a baby. Bottles and bottle nipples must be clean. The bottle should be warmed (not hot), but should *never* be warmed in a microwave oven! During bottle-feeding, babies must:

◆ Be held in a calm, clean **environment**, or conditions.

◆ Have their head and back securely supported.

◆ Surround the nipple with their lips.

◆ Be burped to release swallowed air.

Babies should rest after eating. It is okay if a baby does not finish a bottle. This usually means the baby is full. Discard any milk left in the bottle. Never put a baby to bed with a bottle. Sipping a bottle in bed can lead to tooth decay.

Solid Foods for Babies

Babies need their food served warm or at room temperature, not hot. They also need calm surroundings and time to chew and swallow. Someone should always be with the baby while he or she eats. Infant feeding progresses in the following stages:

◆ **Usually no sooner than six months:** Babies are physically ready to eat iron-enriched infant cereal.

◆ **By about seven to nine months:** Babies are ready for strained, single-ingredient foods like fruits, vegetables, and poultry. Offer unsweetened juice from a cup. Introduce new foods one at a time to easily identify food allergies.

◆ **By about 10 to 12 months:** Most babies can eat chopped soft foods, unsweetened dry cereals, plain soft bread, and pasta.

◆ **After one year:** Toddlers start to eat many foods that others in their family enjoy.

✓ **Reading Check** **Compare** What can babies eat at eight months compared with what they eat at two months?

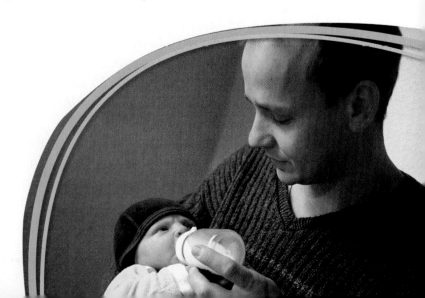

Bottle-Feeding Skills Breast milk can be stored and given to the baby in a bottle. This allows the father to feed the baby. *What bottle-feeding techniques is the father using to properly feed his baby?*

Healthful Eating for Children

For children ages two and older, MyPyramid is the best guide for making healthful choices. Children need the same food variety and nutrients as adults and teens do, but in different amounts. **Figure 12.1** shows how many calories most children need.

Meals and Snacks for Kids

Active, growing children need a regular meal schedule. They also need nourishing snacks because their stomachs are small, but their energy levels are high. They may not be able to eat enough at mealtime to satisfy their food needs.

Some foods are a choking hazard for children under three or four years of age. Avoid small, hard foods such as nuts, popcorn, raw carrot pieces, raisins, and seeds. Avoid hard candy and cough drops. Cut meat and poultry into small pieces, and slice grapes in half.

Safe, Easy, Kid-Friendly Snacks

After school, kids are often hungry. When the kitchen contains nourishing foods, smart snacking is easy and enjoyable. Older children can make these nutritious snacks by themselves:

◆ Tortilla chips or baby carrots and salsa

◆ Apple and cheese slices between crackers

◆ Fruit with milk or yogurt

◆ Peanut butter and banana slices on bread

| Figure 12.1 | Calories for Kids |

How Much for Kids? These recommendations show the average daily calorie needs for a moderately active child. Moderately active means 30 to 60 minutes a day of moderate physical activity in addition to daily activities. *What are the MyPyramid guidelines for calorie needs for a child age 7 to 8 years old?*

Average Daily Calorie Needs for a Moderately Active Child		
Age (years)	Boys	Girls
2	1,000	1,000
3	1,400	1,200
4 to 5	1,400	1,400
6	1,600	1,400
7 to 8	1,600	1,600
9	1,800	1,600
10	1,800	1,800
11	2,000	1,800
12	2,200	2,000

Learning Good Eating Habits

If you have younger brothers or sisters, set a good example by eating healthful foods with them. Find recipes for snacks they will enjoy. With your help, younger children can have positive experiences with food. This will encourage them to become good eaters. It is not wise to reward good behavior with food or to discipline a child by withholding a favorite food. Using food in these ways teaches negative attitudes about eating.

Sometimes a young child goes on a food jag. A **food jag** is wanting just one food for a while. This is a step toward independence and not a cause for worry. Food jags usually do not last long. If a child is hard to please, do not give up. Continue introducing new foods in small amounts as you teach children to eat a variety of foods. Also, remember that:

♦ Children need mealtimes that are pleasant, not pressured.

♦ Children like colorful foods and interesting shapes.

♦ Small servings are best—children can always ask for more.

♦ Children like to participate in preparing meals, serving food, or setting the table.

♦ Children can decide how much they need to eat, and like to feed themselves.

✓ Reading Check **Analyze** Why are snacks important for young children?

Nutrition for Your Teen Years

Healthful eating and active living are two of the smartest ways to be your personal best. The choices you make during your teen years will keep you fit in the years to come.

Eat to Be Your Best

You grow faster during your teen years than at any time since infancy. Like most teens, you probably need more of some food-group foods for a healthful, physically active lifestyle. Eat a small amount of high-fat foods. For energy, choose plenty of nutrient-dense foods that are high in complex carbohydrates.

Pay attention to certain vitamins and minerals during special teen years. Zinc is essential for growth. Iron supports increasing muscle mass. Females also need enough iron to avoid anemia. Calcium helps you grow strong bones. You can get all those nutrients by eating enough of the food-group foods!

Food for a Teen Lifestyle

You can fit healthful eating into your busy schedule with some planning and creativity.

◆ If you have a big after-school appetite, put portable snacks (fruit, crackers and cheese, raisins) in your school bag.

◆ If your after-school schedule interferes with family meals, make a plan with your family. Ask someone to set aside a plate of food for you to eat later. Make time for family meals as often as possible.

◆ If you are still hungry after eating quickly, slow down. Remember that it takes time to feel full.

◆ If you do not have time for breakfast or lunch, make time! You will feel better and perform better at school and at after-school activities.

◆ If you spend time with friends at fast-food places, be a role model. Order juice or milk. Try a salad.

Discover International Foods

Greece

For Greeks, dinner is a family event, often served late in the evening. Greek cuisine is often seasoned with oregano, mint, and garlic, and uses foods that thrive along the Mediterranean. These foods include olives and olive oil, eggplant, zucchini, tomato, green beans, okra, onions, artichokes, and citrus fruits. Lamb, seafood, chicken, feta cheese, yogurt, and honey are typical ingredients, too. The origins of many dishes go back to the ancient Greeks. Many, such as avgolemono (lemon-egg) soup, have Middle Eastern influences.

Languages Across Cultures

moussaka *(mü-'sä-kə)* a dish of layered eggplant with ground lamb or beef, often made with other vegetables and topped with a white sauce

souvlaki *(süv-'lä-kē)* skewered, grilled chicken, pork, swordfish, or shrimp

Recipes Find out more about international recipes on this book's Online Learning Center at glencoe.com.

NCTE 9 Develop an understanding of diversity in language use across cultures.

Eating with Your Friends

Food is part of many teen activities, such as parties, school games, and going to the mall. Plan to eat foods for flavor, nutrition, and fun. Here are some examples:

- ◆ **Party Foods** Vegetable-topped pizza, potato wedges and salsa, sparkling water mixed with juice.
- ◆ **Field Trip Snacks** Apples, granola bars, string cheese and crackers, canned fruit juice.
- ◆ **Mall Foods** Yogurt-fruit smoothie, bagel with hummus, oatmeal cookie.

✓ Reading Check **Discuss** What kinds of nutrient-rich snacks could you choose to satisfy after-school hunger?

Smart Eating During Adulthood

Good nutrition and physical activity are important during every stage of adulthood. Nutrient and energy needs change with adulthood stage: 19 to 30 years, 31 to 50 years, 51 to 70 years, and over 70 years.

Because adults' bodies have stopped growing, their energy needs are typically lower. They may become more sedentary. Adults need less energy for basal metabolism as they get older. Nutrient recommendations also change. Adults must balance calories eaten with calories used. Adults should also choose nutrient-dense foods from different food groups.

Stay Active, Keep Fit Staying physically active throughout life helps people maintain a healthy weight and reduce health risks. *Why do calorie needs decrease as adults get older?*

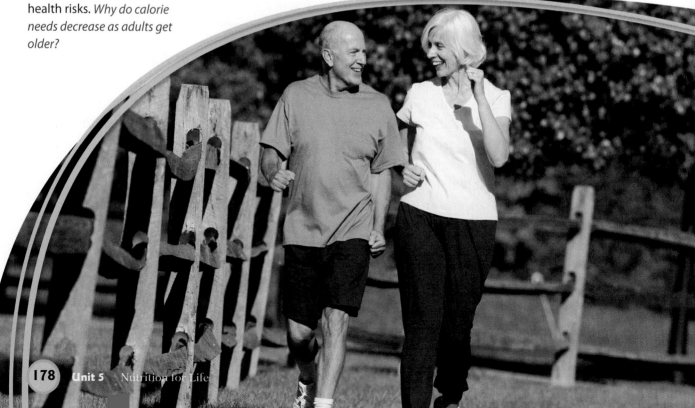

Food for a Changing Life

Different adults have different food needs. Adults who eat well and stay active earlier in life are more likely to be healthy and active later. Other adults may have health problems that require a special diet and limit the foods they can eat.

Lifestyle changes also affect food choices. People who live alone may lose interest in preparing food. An older person who cannot drive or who lives on a limited or fixed income may find it difficult to buy healthful food.

Independence for Older Adults

Most older adults want to stay independent for as long as possible. To do this, they can use the same strategies used by busy families, such as buying convenience foods, cooking ahead, and freezing meals. Community services may provide shopping and meal assistance. Health care aides can teach new cooking skills to people with physical limitations.

Think about older people you know who live alone or have health problems. Could you offer your help with food shopping or meal preparation? Could you bring a meal you prepared or invite the person to your home?

✓ **Reading Check** **Express** What challenges do some older adults face in getting the foods they need?

Healthy Families, Healthy Communities

To eat in a healthful way throughout the life cycle, people need family and community support.

Family Meals

Family meals bring people together and promote healthier eating. How can you make the most of family meals?

◆ Set a regular family mealtime so everyone can be there.

◆ Make family meals simple, quick, and healthful.

◆ Turn off the television. Postpone phone calls.

◆ Eat around a table, so you can talk and listen easily.

◆ Make table talk pleasant.

Healthful Food in Your Community

In almost every community, there are some people who cannot afford to meet the nutritional needs of their families. Fortunately, there are government, community, religious, and private programs that provide help with food and nutrition.

- **Food Stamp Program** This government program helps people with limited incomes buy food at grocery stores and farmers' markets. Food stamps work like cash.

- **Women, Infants, and Children (WIC) Program** This government program gives food assistance and nutrition education to pregnant and nursing women, infants, and preschool children.

- **Home-Delivered Meals** Hot or cold meals are delivered to disabled or frail people who cannot easily leave home.

- **Food Banks** These banks distribute food to people in need. Contributions come from food companies, individuals, community groups, supermarkets, and restaurants.

- **Community Kitchens** Low-cost or free meals may be served in schools, religious institutions, and other centers where older adults gather to eat and be with others.

✓ **Reading Check** **Discuss** How can you make the most of meals with your family?

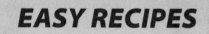

EASY RECIPES — International Flavors

Tzatziki

Customary	Ingredients	Metric
1	Cucumber	1
1 clove	Garlic	1
1 cup	Plain, low-fat yogurt	250 mL
1 Tbsp.	Lemon juice	15 mL
1½ tsp.	Olive oil	7 mL
½ tsp.	Dried mint	2 mL
¼ tsp.	Salt	1 mL

Try This!
Try using fresh mint or dill instead of dried mint. Use vinegar instead of lemon juice.

Yield: 4 servings, 6 oz (155 g) each

1. Peel and remove seeds from cucumber. Coarsely chop cucumber and finely chop garlic.
2. Combine all ingredients and mix well. Refrigerate.
3. Serve cold.

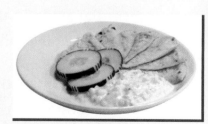

Nutritional Information Per Serving: 77 calories, 3 g total fat (1 g saturated fat), 5 g cholesterol, 201 mg sodium, 9 total carbohydrate (1 g fiber, 7 g total sugars), 4.6 g protein

Percent Daily Value: vitamin A 2%, vitamin C 8%, calcium 15%, iron 4%

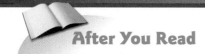

After You Read

CHAPTER SUMMARY

The Dietary Guidelines and MyPyramid offer nutrition advice throughout the life cycle. Healthful eating before and during pregnancy helps ensure that mother and baby get the nutrients they need. Infant feeding progresses from mother's milk or formula to various soft then chopped foods. Children need the same food variety from MyPyramid as adults, but in different amounts. Growing teens need more nutrient-dense foods, especially if they are active. Adult food needs depend on physical activity level, health, and lifestyle. Community programs can support good nutrition for people of all ages.

Vocabulary Review

1. Use each of these vocabulary words in a sentence.

Content Vocabulary
◇ life cycle (p. 172)
◇ prenatal (p. 172)
◇ fetus (p. 172)
◇ low birth weight (p. 172)
◇ lactate (p. 173)
◇ food jag (p. 176)

Academic Vocabulary
■ specific (p. 172)
■ environment (p. 174)

Review Key Concepts

2. Summarize how nutrition needs change throughout the life cycle.

3. Explain the importance of good nutrition for pregnancy.

4. Compare how infant feeding changes in the first year of life.

5. Create a healthful eating plan for children.

6. Explain why good nutrition and active living are important for teens.

7. Discuss how food and nutrition needs change during adulthood.

8. Identify sources of food assistance.

Critical Thinking

9. Compare the calorie and nutrient recommendations for teen girls and boys. Use the Recommended Dietary Allowances in the Appendix. Explain the differences. Predict how these differences might affect food choices.

Real-World Skills and Applications

Set Goals and Make Decisions

10. Malnutrition Among the Elderly Your friends worry about their grandfather. Since their grandmother died recently, he has eaten poorly and lost weight. He does not like to cook or eat alone. How could they help him? What challenges might they face?

Interpersonal and Collaborative

11. When I Was Your Age Interview your grandparents or older family friends. Find out what practices they followed for feeding their children. Ask your family how these practices are different from the way you were raised. How are they similar? Draw conclusions.

Financial Literacy

12. WIC The groceries in Julia's cart at the market cost $65.37. However, some items, such as infant formula, are eligible for rebates under the Women, Infants, and Children (WIC) program. If the value of WIC-eligible groceries is $14.88, how much will Julia's groceries cost?

Technology

13. Health Greeting Card Use a computer to create one health greeting card each for a child, a teen, and an adult. Include wellness messages and healthful eating tips for their age. You can design your own cards or use an online template. Hand out copies of your cards.

14. Babysitter's Handbook Create a handbook of information for babysitters. Research and include information on bottle-feeding a baby. This should include how to safely warm formula, how to clean bottles and bottle nipples after feeding, and how to hold a baby while feeding. Include other babysitting advice.

> **NCTE 4** Use written language to communicate effectively.

15. Community Food Assistance Research food assistance programs in your area. Learn how teens can help. For example, teens can hold a canned food drive, volunteer at a food bank, or help an older adult with grocery shopping. As a group or by yourself, get involved with a program. Report on your volunteering.

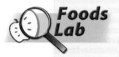

16. Cooking with Kids Find a cookbook for kids. Choose a healthful snack recipe from the book. Prepare it yourself. Then, make a plan to prepare the food with a child. Identify safety precautions and food preparation steps that a child can safely do.

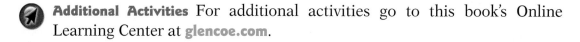

Additional Activities For additional activities go to this book's Online Learning Center at glencoe.com.

Academic Skills

English Language Arts

17. Sing About Good Nutrition Create a call-and-response song to help children learn about healthful fruits and vegetables. Teach the song to your classmates.

> **NCTE 5** Use different writing process elements to communicate effectively.

Science

18. Folic Acid Fortification By law, many grain products must be fortified with folic acid.

Procedure Research to find out the benefits of folic acid.

Analysis Write a paragraph to explain how this law protects the health of developing babies.

> **NSES Content Standard C** Develop an understanding of matter, energy, and organization in living systems.

Mathematics

19. Healthier Baby Food on a Budget Instead of buying 4-ounce jars of baby food for 50¢ each, Kim buys frozen peas for 99¢. Observing all safety rules, Kim makes baby food by putting the peas in a blender. Each bag makes 31 ounces. About how much money is she saving?

Math Concept **Estimation by Rounding** When rounding numbers, look at the digit to the right of the place to which you are rounding. It the digit is 5 or greater, round up. If it is 4 or less, round down.

Starting Hint First, find out how many jars Kim would have to buy to equal the amount of homemade blended peas. Then, subtract the costs to show savings.

 For more math help, go to the Math Appendix

> **NCTM Number and Operations** Compute fluently and make reasonable estimates.

STANDARDIZED TEST PRACTICE

MULTIPLE CHOICE
Read the paragraph and choose the best answer. Write your answer on a separate piece of paper.

Fruit juice can provide part of the day's Fruit Group total. Drinking too much fruit juice, however, can provide too many calories, and can crowd out milk and other nourishing foods. Children ages 1 to years should drink no more than ¾ cup (180 mL) of juice per day; 1½ cups (375 mL) is the maximum amount recommended for youth ages 7 to 18 years.

20. Based on the paragraph, which of the following statements is not true?
   a. Drinking juice can help children and teens follow My Pyramid's Fruit Group recommendations.
   b. Juice provides the same nutrients as milk.
   c. The upper limit for juice is higher for teens than for young children.
   d. Fruit juice is a nourishing beverage—in sensible amounts.

> **Test-Taking Tip** When taking a test, always read the directions before you work on a section. Circle key words such as *not, contrast, similar,* and *different.* Failing to read directions can cause you to misunderstand what the test is asking.

CHAPTER 13
Vegetarian Choices

Explore the Photo ▶▶
Vegetarian eating plans may have no food at all from animal sources. *What vegetarian dishes have you eaten?*

Writing Activity
Descriptive Paragraph

Vegetarian Sensation Do you like the texture of rice or the smell of fresh lemon? Write a descriptive paragraph about a non-meat food or dish that you enjoy. Use your five senses, and use plenty of adjectives in your sentences.

Writing Tips

1. **Include** a strong topic sentence.

2. **Present details** in a logical order for your reader.

3. **Select** precise transition words.

Reading Guide

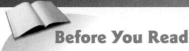

Before You Read

Predict Read the Content Vocabulary words below. Write one or two sentences predicting what this chapter will be about.

Read to Learn

Key Concepts
- **Distinguish** between the different types of vegetarian eating styles.
- **Identify** the nutritional benefits and challenges of vegetarian eating plans.
- **Explain** how to use MyPyramid to make healthful vegetarian food choices.

Main Idea

Vegetarian foods can be healthful and delicious. Like everyone else, vegetarians need to make wise food choices, using MyPyramid as a guide.

Content Vocabulary

◇ vegetarian
◇ lacto-ovo-vegetarian
◇ lacto-vegetarian
◇ ovo-vegetarian
◇ vegan

Academic Vocabulary

You will find these words in your reading and on your tests. Use the glossary to look up their definitions if necessary.

■ examine   ■ obtain

Graphic Organizer

As you read, use this challenge-solution chart to show the seven nutritional challenges that vegetarians face, and their solutions.

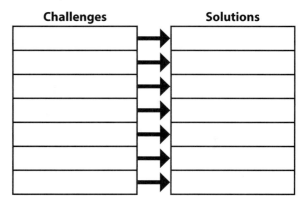

Challenges	Solutions

 Graphic Organizer Go to this book's Online Learning Center at **glencoe.com** to print out this graphic organizer.

Academic Standards •

 English Language Arts
NCTE 5 Use different writing process elements to communicate effectively.

 Mathematics
NCTM Number and Operations Understand numbers, ways of representing numbers, relationships among numbers, and number systems.

 Social Studies
NCSS I E Culture Demonstrate the value of cultural diversity, as well as cohesion, within and across groups.
NCSS IX H Global Connections Illustrate how individual behaviors and decisions connect with global systems.

NCTE National Council of Teachers of English
NCTM National Council of Teachers of Mathematics

NSES National Science Education Standards
NCSS National Council for the Social Studies

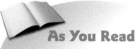

Vocabulary

You can find definitions in the glossary at the back of this book.

As You Read

Connect Think how you would get the nutrients you might miss if you avoided meat or dairy foods.

The Vegetarian Way

A **vegetarian** is a person who avoids eating meat, poultry, and fish, and perhaps eggs and dairy foods. Instead, vegetarians eat foods from plant sources, such as vegetables, fruits, grains and grain products, dry beans and peas, nuts, and seeds. Many vegetarians also eat eggs and dairy products.

Some people are vegetarians for religious or cultural reasons. Others are concerned about the treatment of animals or the sustainability of the world's food supply. Many people are vegetarians for health reasons. A well-planned vegetarian diet is often low in fat and cholesterol and high in fiber, which offers health benefits.

Vegetarians are described by the foods they eat:

- A **lacto-ovo-vegetarian** eats dairy foods and eggs in addition to foods from plant sources. This is the most common vegetarian eating style.

- A **lacto-vegetarian** eats dairy foods and foods from plant sources, but not eggs.

- An **ovo-vegetarian** eats eggs and foods from plant sources, but not dairy foods.

- A **vegan** *('vē-gǝn)* eats only foods from plant sources.

Anyone can enjoy vegetarian meals. Some people might eat vegetarian meals several times each week, but not every day. They might eat poultry and fish, but little or no red meat.

✓ **Reading Check** **Explain** How do the four vegetarian eating plans differ?

Nutrients for Vegetarians

Healthy vegetarians know that food choices matter. The keys to a nutritious, healthful vegetarian eating plan are to follow MyPyramid guidelines, to **examine**, or study, food labels for information, and to eat enough variety every day.

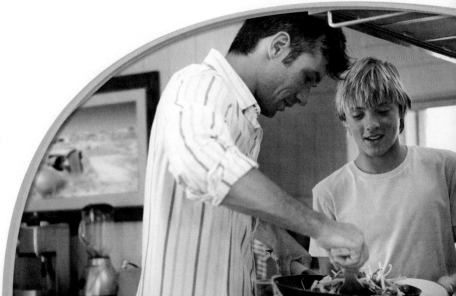

Teen Vegetarians If you decide to become a vegetarian, get family support. Make a shopping list together with plenty of healthful vegetarian food choices.
What vegetarian main dishes could you prepare for a family dinner?

Nutrition Challenges for Vegetarians

Vegetarian diets are not always healthful diets. Some vegetarians eat too many calories, high-fat foods, and sugary foods. Other vegetarians do not eat enough fruits, vegetables, and whole-grain foods. To **obtain**, or receive, enough nutrients, vegetarians must eat enough of a variety of foods. Many vegetarians face these challenges:

- **Energy** High-fiber meals may make people feel full before they get enough calories. Some higher-calorie foods like dried fruits and nuts can help provide enough food energy.

- **Protein** Vegetarians should eat a variety of plant-based foods to get all the essential amino acids. Soybeans are a complete protein. Dry beans and peas, nuts, and seeds are nearly complete. Dairy foods and eggs also provide complete protein.

- **Calcium** Lacto-vegetarians can get calcium from dairy foods. Vegans can get enough calcium from foods such as dry beans, broccoli, calcium-processed tofu, and calcium-fortified orange juice.

- **Vitamin D** Lacto-vegetarians can drink fortified milk for vitamin D. Vegans can get vitamin D from fortified cereals and some soy beverages.

- **Vitamin B_{12}** Vitamin B_{12} is a vitamin that only comes from animal products. This vitamin is often added to foods eaten by vegetarians. It is easy for lacto-ovo-vegetarians to get enough vitamin B_{12}. Fortified foods such as cereal and soy milk can provide B_{12} for vegans.

- **Iron** Enriched, fortified, and whole-grain cereals and breads have iron. Other sources include dry beans, and some dark-green, leafy vegetables.

- **Zinc** Whole-grain products, dry beans, wheat germ, dairy products, and tofu provide zinc.

Children, teens, and pregnant women can be healthy vegetarians if they get enough food variety, nutrients, and food energy.

✓ Reading Check) Recall What nutritional challenges do many vegans face?

Math in Action

Healthy Amounts of Soy

Soy protein may help keep you healthy. Eating 25 grams of soy protein daily—in an eating plan that is low in saturated fat and cholesterol—promotes heart health. If you consume 12 ounces of soy milk, 2 ounces of tofu, and 2 tablespoons of soy nuts in a day, do you get more or less than 25 grams of soy protein? The amount of soy protein is:

- Soy milk: 10 grams in 1 cup
- Firm tofu: 13 grams in 4 ounces
- Roasted soy nuts: 19 grams in ¼ cup

Math Concept **Order of Operations** Equations are solved by first performing any operations within parentheses, then exponents, multiplication and division from left to right, and finally addition and subtraction from left to right.

Starting Hint Multiply the amounts of each food with the grams contained in them, then add the total.

NCTM Number and Operations Understand numbers, ways of representing numbers, relationships among numbers, and number systems.

 For more math help, go to the Math Appendix

Pair Vitamin C and Iron
To help your body absorb iron from rice, pasta, other grain products, beans, and peanut butter, pair them with foods rich in vitamin C, such as tomatoes and orange juice. *What iron-vitamin partnerships might you enjoy in a vegetarian meal?*

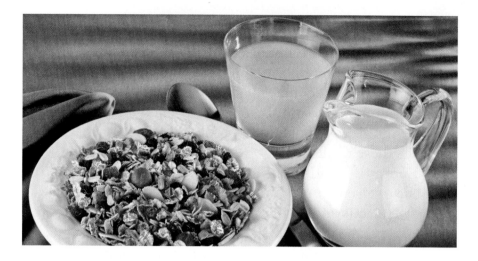

MyPyramid for Vegetarians

MyPyramid is flexible. It is a useful guide for both vegetarians and non-vegetarians. A smart vegetarian eating plan provides enough nutrients. Vegetarians need to choose plenty of fruits, vegetables, and whole-grain products. In addition, they need enough of these food-group foods:

◆ **Meat and Beans Group** Dry beans and peas, soy burgers, tofu, peanut butter, eggs, and sunflower seeds are protein-rich alternatives to meat, poultry, and fish.

◆ **Milk Group** Lacto-vegetarians can enjoy dairy foods. For calcium, vegans can choose fortified soy milk, soy cheese, and soy yogurt. Soy foods fortified with calcium and vitamin D are smart choices.

Vegetarian Meals

Vegetarian meals can be a feast of colors, flavors, and aromas. Planning and preparing vegetarian meals can be easy. Vegetarian meals are often inexpensive as well.

Plan for a variety of food. You can use familiar ingredients, and you can also try new ones. **Figure 13.1** shows sample vegetarian menus for a day.

Adapt Traditional Recipes

It is easy to modify favorite family recipes to make them vegetarian. You can substitute beans, lentils, soy products, and other protein-rich foods in many recipes with meat, poultry, and fish. The following tips can help you to get started thinking about adapting traditional recipes:

◆ Use extra beans in place of meat in chili.

◆ Substitute cooked beans or lentils for meat-based ingredients in a casserole. Top with toasted nuts or seeds for added flavor and crunch.

HOT JOBS!

Food Technologist

Food technologists apply food science to produce and distribute safe, nourishing, and wholesome food. Some specialize in certain products, such as soy.

Careers Find out more about careers. Go to this book's Online Learning Center at **glencoe.com**.

- Add different chopped vegetables and beans to meatless spaghetti sauce.
- Top pizza with extra vegetables and crumbled soy burgers. Use soy cheese in place of mozzarella on pizza.
- Enjoy a bean burrito instead of one made with beef.
- Try crumbled firm tofu in place of ricotta cheese for lasagna.
- Make a stir-fry with soy burgers, firm tofu, or tempeh instead of meat or chicken.
- Use soy milk, soy yogurt, or soy margarine in place of dairy products in baked goods.
- Create a fruit smoothie with silken tofu or soy milk in place of cow's milk.

Figure 13.1 **Vegetarian Menus—Simple and Delicious**

Vegetarian Meals Every style of vegetarian eating is full of variety and flavor! *Which of these three menu plans would a vegan choose? Which menu plan is right for a lacto-vegetarian?*

	MENU 1	MENU 2	MENU 3
Breakfast	Scrambled egg Whole-wheat toast Orange juice Hot cocoa made with milk	Flavored yogurt Raisin bran muffin Cranberry juice	Whole-grain waffles topped with pecans Soy breakfast sausage Calcium-fortified orange juice Calcium-fortified soy milk
Lunch	Three-bean chili Cornbread Raw vegetables Banana Milk	Soy burger with cheese, lettuce, and tomato Broccoli slaw Peach halves Chocolate milk	Vegetable-barley soup Spinach salad with orange slices, almonds, and chickpeas Whole-grain breadsticks Calcium-fortified soy milk
Dinner	Cheese-spinach manicotti with tomato sauce Garden salad French bread slices Frozen yogurt topped with berries Water	Stir-fry with tofu cubes, vegetables, and cashews Brown rice Dinner roll Watermelon slices Milk	Bean and vegetable burrito with salsa Mango slices Spanish rice Baked apple topped with soy cheese Oatmeal cookies Iced tea
Snacks	Crackers with peanut butter Raisins Lemonade	Raw baby carrots Peanuts Apple juice	Pita triangles and hummus Fruit smoothie

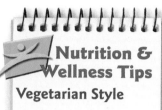
Explore Vegetarian Foods

Vegetarian dishes are enjoyed in everyday meals in many parts of the world. Mexico has soft tacos with beans. In Asia, stir-fried vegetables and rice is a popular dish. Spicy vegetable stews are common in the Middle East.

Try some plant-based dishes from around the world that may be new to you. For example, you could try *mujudarah*, a Saudi Arabian dish. It is made from rice and lentils and flavored with lemon, onion, and cumin. Or try curry dishes from India—cooked vegetables, lentils, and curry seasoning over basmati rice. Peru combines a high-protein grain called *quinoa* with corn, beans, tomatoes, and other vegetables. Look in ethnic and vegetarian cookbooks for recipes. Explore vegetarian dishes at ethnic restaurants, too.

✓ **Reading Check** **Reflect** What are two strategies for fitting vegetarian meals into your day?

EASY RECIPES

Everyday Favorites

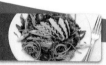

Southwest Salad

Customary	Ingredients	Metric
1 can (15 oz.)	Black beans, drained and rinsed	1 can (420 g)
1 can (11 oz.)	Sweet corn, drained	1 can (300 g)
1	Roma tomato, chopped	1
2 Tbsp.	Green onion, chopped	30 mL
2 Tbsp.	Fresh cilantro, chopped	30 mL
½ tsp.	Chili powder	2 mL
¼ tsp.	Ground cumin	1 mL
¼ cup	Low-fat vinaigrette salad dressing	50 mL

Try This!

Use red, navy, or soybeans instead of black beans. All make complete protein when combined with corn!

Yield: 4 servings, 8 oz. (200 g) each

❶ In a large bowl, stir together all ingredients except salad dressing until well combined.

❷ Divide mixture evenly among four salad plates.

❸ Drizzle 1 Tbsp. (15 mL) dressing over each salad. Serve immediately.

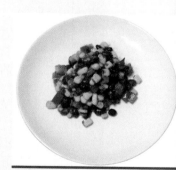

Nutritional Information Per Serving: 173 calories, 3 g total fat, (0 g saturated fat), 0 mg cholesterol, 711 mg sodium, 30 g total carbohydrate (8 g fiber, 3 g total sugars), 8 g protein

Percent Daily Value: vitamin A 4%, vitamin C 15%, calcium 4%, iron 15%

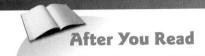

After You Read

CHAPTER SUMMARY
Vegetarians eat foods from plant sources. Many also eat eggs and dairy products. People choose to be vegetarians for various reasons, including religious, cultural, health, and concern for animals. Several nutrients need special attention from vegetarians: protein, calcium, vitamin D, vitamin B$_{12}$, iron, and zinc. MyPyramid can guide vegetarians as they make their own healthful eating plans. Vegetarian meals may include familiar foods or introduce you to new plant-based dishes.

Vocabulary Review

1. Use each of these vocabulary words in a sentence.

Content Vocabulary
◇ vegetarian (p. 186)
◇ lacto-ovo-vegetarian (p. 186)
◇ lacto-vegetarian (p. 186)
◇ ovo-vegetarian (p. 186)
◇ vegan (p. 186)

Academic Vocabulary
■ examine (p. 186)
■ obtain (p. 187)

Review Key Concepts

2. Distinguish between the different types of vegetarian eating styles.

3. Identify the nutritional benefits and challenges of vegetarian eating plans.

4. Explain how to use MyPyramid to make healthful vegetarian food choices.

Critical Thinking

5. Plan a day of healthful meals and snacks for a vegan. Identify the food groups represented. Explain how your menu addresses nutrition challenges vegans may face.

6. Analyze a friend's comment. She said that any eating plan is healthful as long as it contains no meat. Is she right? Explain.

7. Design a vegetarian version of MyPyramid, using the shape and its food groups. Include food choices for all vegetarians, including vegans.

8. Explain how to find vegetarian foods in the supermarket with enough nutrients that vegetarian eating plans often lack.

9. Modify a meat-based recipe. Explain how to change the recipe to make a meal appropriate for a lacto-vegetarian or a vegan.

Real-World Skills and Applications

Set Goals and Make Decisions

10. Order Pizza Write a script for this situation: Four teens are at a pizza place. One is not a vegetarian. The second is a vegan. The third is a lacto-ovo-vegetarian, and the fourth is a lacto-vegetarian. Write a script of the conversation as each describes what to order and why.

Collaborative and Interpersonal

11. Dinner Guests A vegetarian has been invited to a non-vegetarian's home for dinner. Write two or more paragraphs to explain how the vegetarian can use good communication and interpersonal skills to explain his or her dietary needs. The explanation should show respect for the food choices of others.

Technology

12. Vegetarians at School With your teacher's permission, break into groups. Plan a video with two or three other students about healthful vegetarian meals at school. Consider vegetarian foods sold at school and brought from home. Create a storyboard and share it in class.

Financial Literacy

13. Compare Costs A grocery store sells a frozen vegetarian lasagna that serves two people for $7.50. It also has a frozen family-size vegetarian lasagna that serves four people for $12.95. Determine the individual serving cost to find which is the better value.

14. International Vegetarian Dishes People enjoy vegetarian dishes around the world. Collect six main-dish recipes from different countries. List each recipe and the non-meat protein sources in each recipe. Add these recipes to your recipe file with a brief description of the dish and its cultural connection.

> **NCSS I E Culture** Demonstrate the value of cultural diversity, as well as cohesion, within and across groups.

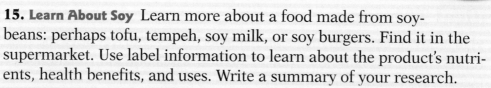

15. Learn About Soy Learn more about a food made from soybeans: perhaps tofu, tempeh, soy milk, or soy burgers. Find it in the supermarket. Use label information to learn about the product's nutrients, health benefits, and uses. Write a summary of your research.

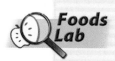

16. Taste Test for Soy Burgers Cook and taste a soy burger. Write a paragraph to answer these questions: What does it taste like? What is its texture and color? How does it compare for nutrition and cost with a cooked beef patty of the same size? How might you use a soy burger in different types of recipes?

Additional Activities For additional activities go to this book's Online Learning Center at glencoe.com.

Academic Skills

 English Language Arts

17. Write a Culinary Article Imagine that you write for a food and travel magazine. Research and write a 500-word article about rice and beans around the world. Organize your information logically in paragraphs with a main theme.

> **NCTE 5** Use different writing process elements to communicate effectively.

 Social Studies

18. All About Soy Soybeans are used in many ways: as human food (tofu, tempeh, soy milk, soy burgers, other soy foods), for vegetable oil, for oil, as livestock feed, and for biofuel. Go online to learn more about soybeans. Write a paragraph to describe different uses and the possible impact of selling soybean crops for different uses.

> **NCSS IX H Global Connections** Illustrate how individual behaviors and decisions connect with global systems.

 Mathematics

19. Percents Meat, poultry, and fish are popular ingredients in many American meals. In the United States in 1980, people ate an average of 180 pounds of meat per year. By 2006, each American ate an average of 220 pounds of meat per year. By what percentage did meat consumption rise?

Math Concept **Fraction, Decimal, and Percent** A percent is a ratio that compares a number to 100. A percent can be converted to a decimal by dividing the percent number by 100.

Starting Hint Start by finding the difference in amounts people ate each year. Divide the recent total into the difference. Then, multiply by 100 to find the percentage.

 For more math help, go to the Math Appendix

> **NCTM Number and Operations** Understand numbers, ways of representing numbers, relationships among numbers, and number systems.

STANDARDIZED TEST PRACTICE

ESSAY
Read the paragraph. Write your answer on a separate piece of paper.

> **Test-Taking Tip** Highlight the content vocabulary terms in your notes to find them easily. Consider taking a section of notes about only vocabulary. One way to write definitions is in this format: <u>vegan</u>—someone who eats no meat or other animal products.

Vegetarian or not, almost everyone can benefit from adding more fruits and vegetables to their meals and snacks. It is easy to add a pear to a salad or fresh spinach to mashed potatoes. Consider adding a dessert of fruit. Eating more fruits and vegetables take a little planning.

20. Think about what you learned in this chapter. Write an essay about how you would plan a vegetarian meal or day's menu for yourself or your family. Include the vegetarian dishes you would choose and the ingredients included in each dish.

CHAPTER 14
Special Health Concerns

Explore the Photo ▶▶
A lifetime of wellness depends on your food choices and active-living habits now. *How could you improve your overall food choices and lifestyle today?*

Writing Activity

Write an Explanation

Your everyday food choices affect your health and wellness. Write a letter to the editor of your local newspaper explaining the importance of making healthy food choices. Discuss which food-related health problems can be prevented and which cannot.

Writing Tips

1. **State** the purpose of your letter.

2. **Explain** clearly how wellness is affected by food choices.

3. **Organize** supporting details in a logical way, and write clearly.

Reading Guide

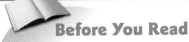

Before You Read

Adjust Reading Speed Adjust your reading speed to match the difficulty of the text. Reread when needed. You will understand and remember more.

Read to Learn
Key Concepts

- **Identify** food and lifestyle recommendations that lower health risks.
- **Describe** eating disorders and their warning signs.
- **Identify** food sensitivities and how to handle them.
- **Discuss** special eating plans used for certain health problems.
- **Propose** meal and snack basics to help someone recovering from an illness or injury.
- **Explain** how food and medications may affect each other.

Main Idea

Smart food choices help prevent, treat, and manage many health problems.

Academic Vocabulary

You will find these words in your reading and on your tests. Use the glossary to look up their definitions if necessary.

- perceive
- minimize

Content Vocabulary

- eating disorder
- lactose intolerance
- gluten intolerance
- food allergy
- allergen
- diabetes
- coronary heart disease
- atherosclerosis
- high blood pressure
- lipid
- high-density lipoprotein
- low-density lipoprotein

Graphic Organizer

As you read, use a table like the one below to show common eating disorders and their characteristics.

Eating Disorder	Characteristics

 Graphic Organizer Go to this book's Online Learning Center at **glencoe.com** to print out this graphic organizer.

Academic Standards ■ ■ ■ ■ ■ ■ ■ ■ ■ ■ ■ ■ ■ ■ ■

 Social Studies
NCSS I A Culture Analyze and explain the ways groups, societies, and cultures address human needs and concerns.

 English Language Arts
NCTE 4 Use written language to communicate effectively.
NCTE 9 Develop an understanding of diversity in language use across cultures.

 Science
NSES Content Standard A Develop abilities necessary to do scientific inquiry.

 Mathematics
NCTM Data Analysis and Probability Formulate questions that can be addressed with data and collect, organize, and display relevant data to answer them.

NCTE National Council of Teachers of English
NCTM National Council of Teachers of Mathematics

NSES National Science Education Standards
NCSS National Council for the Social Studies

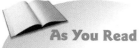
As You Read

Connect Think about how your food choices contribute to your wellness.

Nutrition for Prevention

You can reduce health risks at any age by making good food choices. The Dietary Guidelines for Americans give advice for lowering your risk of health problems such as diabetes, heart disease, high blood pressure, and some forms of cancer. MyPyramid helps you balance your diet and prevent nutrient deficiencies. Your choices can also help prevent problems such as osteoporosis, anemia, obesity, underweight, and injury.

✓ **Reading Check** **Review** Where would you go for advice about lowering health risks?

Eating Disorders

An **eating disorder** is a complex illness that involves harmful attitudes about the body, self, and food. People of all ages and both genders can develop eating disorders. They are most common among teens and young adults, especially females. Common eating disorders are:

◆ **Anorexia Nervosa** People see themselves as fat even if they are dangerously thin, and starve themselves. They often set strict rules for themselves about what, when, and how much they can eat. They also set rules about how much they must exercise.

◆ **Bulimia Nervosa** People binge, or eat too much food. They also purge, or get rid of extra calories, to avoid gaining weight. Bulimics may take laxatives, vomit, exercise very hard, or go on strict diets between binges. Many bulimics have normal weights.

◆ **Binge-Eating Disorder** People binge regularly but do not purge or exercise. They may binge when they are emotionally upset. They may also be overweight, or may lose and gain weight often.

Vocabulary

You can find definitions in the glossary at the back of this book.

Helping People People with some physical impairments—such as arthritis, paralysis, and limited hand strength—may need to modify their food choices to stay properly nourished. *How might you help someone who has difficulty using a fork and knife?*

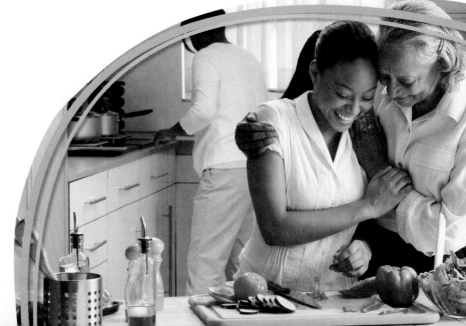

Dangers of Eating Disorders

Eating disorders are emotional illnesses that are dangerous to a person's health. Anorexia can lead to serious illness, even death. Binge eating can cause the stomach or esophagus to burst. Purging can damage teeth and cause heart failure. Other long-term medical problems can result from eating disorders, including heart and kidney problems, breathing difficulties, and digestive troubles.

Warning Signs of Eating Disorders

If you or someone you know shows any of these warning signs, get help:

◆ Refusing to eat, eating tiny amounts, or regularly eating very large amounts of food

◆ Extreme weight loss or weight that seems to go up and down

◆ More frequent and more intense exercise than normal

◆ Eating secretly or disappearing after eating, often to the bathroom

◆ Unhealthy teeth and gums

◆ Loss of menstrual cycle

◆ Use of diet pills or laxatives

How to Get Help

Eating disorders are serious and dangerous. People with these disorders need help to overcome them. To help a person with an eating disorder, you must **perceive**, or see, the problem. People with eating disorders try to keep their habits secret, or deny a problem. Eating disorders are symptoms of emotional problems. As the person learns to recognize and heal from the underlying cause, he or she can begin to eat in a more healthful way.

If you know someone with an eating disorder, talk to a trusted adult, like a parent, teacher, or doctor. The sooner treatment starts, the better. Some people may need long-term care. Treatment often includes medical or dental care, and nutritional and psychological counseling. If you know someone who may have an eating disorder, get help from a trusted adult including a parent, teacher, counselor, or nurse. Family and friends can help:

◆ Be alert to the warning signs.

◆ Encourage the person to seek professional help.

◆ Be supportive and patient.

✓ **Reading Check** **Name** What are some warning signs for bulimia nervosa?

Food Sensitivities

Some people are sensitive to foods or substances in food. This may be a lifelong issue. People with food sensitivities can avoid potential health risks by making careful food choices. Symptoms of food sensitivities may have many causes and it is important to get a medical diagnosis. Always check with your doctor if you think you may be sensitive to a certain food.

Lactose Intolerance

Lactose intolerance is the inability to adequately digest lactose, the sugar found in milk products. Nausea, stomach pain, gas, and diarrhea are some symptoms. Lactose intolerance may be mistaken for an allergy. Lactose-intolerant people can still enjoy milk products, however, by using these strategies:

- Drink small amounts of milk, perhaps one cup or less at a time, and only with other foods.

- Look for lactose-reduced or lactose-free milk products. Buy tablets and drops that reduce lactose when added to milk.

- Ask a doctor about supplements that help digest lactose.

Gluten Intolerance

Gluten intolerance is the inability to digest gluten, a protein found in wheat, rye, barley, and perhaps oats. This is also called celiac ('sē- lē- ˌak) disease. The protein damages the lining of the small intestine of people with this intolerance, so the body cannot properly absorb nutrients. People with a gluten intolerance must avoid foods with gluten, so the small intestine can heal.

The symptoms of gluten intolerance can resemble those of other health problems, such as the flu, and it is often misdiagnosed. People with gluten intolerance should ask a health professional or registered dietitian to help them make gluten-free choices. Gluten intolerance is not a wheat allergy.

People who have a gluten intolerance may have other health problems. This includes malnutrition, arthritis, colon cancer and diabetes. Some foods that can help keep a person with gluten intolerance well-fed are corn, beans, and quinoa ('kēn-ˌwä). Some grocery stores also sell gluten-free flour for baking.

Food Allergies

A **food allergy** is an allergic reaction to a substance in food. When an allergic reaction happens, the body's immune system reacts as if it were fighting an illness. An allergic food reaction can cause a rash, swelling of the eyes, lips or throat, itching, stomach cramps, a runny nose, a headache, nausea, vomiting, diarrhea, or difficulty breathing. Even small amounts of a food can cause symptoms of an allergic reaction. Food allergies may be life-threatening.

Food allergies are not common. Foods that cause most allergic reactions include peanuts, shellfish, tree nuts, fish, and eggs. Some people are allergic to soybeans, wheat, or milk. The only solution is to avoid the food and substitute others.

Consult a qualified health professional to diagnose and treat an allergy if you think you have one. Tests can determine which foods may cause allergic reactions.

Ways to Manage Food Allergies

To manage a food allergy, avoid the **allergen** that causes the reaction. An allergen is a protein substance in food that triggers an allergic reaction. If you have a food allergy:

- Talk to your school nurse or personal physician.

- Eat foods only if you know what the ingredients are and how the food is prepared. Only eat foods prepared especially for you.

- Read food labels. Ask questions when away from home.

- Be prepared for emergencies. Learn how to quickly signal for help.

✓ **Reading Check** **Compare** What is the difference between lactose intolerance and a milk allergy?

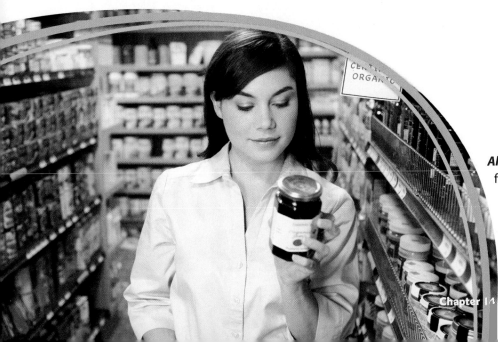

Allergen Labeling on Foods By law, food labels must list potential allergens in food. If you have a food allergy, use the label to identify foods that may cause a reaction. *Why is it important to identify allergens in food?*

Be Aware

✓ Ask friends if they
have special food
needs so you can
provide foods they
can enjoy.

✓ Tell restaurant serv-
ers about any spe-
cial food needs you
have, such as a food
allergy.

Special Eating Plans

Some health conditions require special eating plans as part of medical treatment. These plans can be temporary or last a lifetime. People with high blood pressure, for example, may need to follow a diet low in sodium. Only doctors and other qualified health professionals should prescribe a special eating plan.

Eating plans may be hard to follow at first. Family members can give encouragement. They can help by planning and preparing flavorful meals that fit both the special plan and the food preferences of the whole family. If you are preparing food for someone with special food needs, ask what he or she can eat. Respect those needs to make mealtime enjoyable. Learn to adapt favorite recipes by substituting new ingredients, experimenting with different preparation methods, and eliminating foods that may cause problems.

Diabetes

Diabetes is a condition in which the body cannot control blood sugar properly. The body does not make enough insulin, a chemical that helps blood sugar move into body cells. Without insulin, body cells cannot use blood sugar normally to provide energy. People with pre-diabetes have higher-than-normal blood sugar levels, and may develop diabetes.

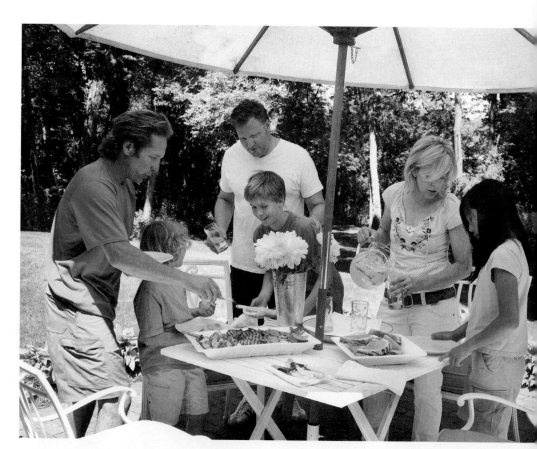

Healthy for All If a family member must follow a special eating plan, there are many ways to support his or her needs. *How could you adapt a main-dish recipe for a family member who follows a low-sodium diet?*

Two types of diabetes are:

- ◆ **Type 1 Diabetes** The pancreas cannot make enough insulin. Heredity or a virus may be the cause.

- ◆ **Type 2 Diabetes** The body does not make enough insulin or the cells do not respond to insulin normally. This is the most common form of diabetes. Overweight and aging contribute to this type. You can develop type 2 diabetes if you have poor eating habits.

Diabetes can damage many parts of the body. With physical activity and the right eating plan, people with diabetes can **minimize**, or lessen, the damage from diabetes. Medication can also help.

Eating Plans for Diabetics

People with diabetes need eating plans with carefully choosen foods. Healthful eating plans can help people with diabetes control their blood sugar levels. People with diabetes generally need a varied diet rich in vegetables, fruits, and whole grains. They also need regular meal and snack times. Eating about the same amount of food at about the same time every day helps control blood sugar levels. Some people with diabetes may need to limit the amounts they eat from each food group each day.

Doctors often recommend managing diabetes by balancing food and energy nutrients. Diabetes management includes physical activity, maintaining a healthy weight, and checking blood sugar levels. Oral medicine or insulin injections may be necessary.

Discover International Foods

Italy

Olive oil, tomato sauces, and vegetables make many Mediterranean foods heart-healthy, especially those from southern Italy. Dishes such as pizza and spaghetti are familiar in the United States, but Italians make them in a simpler style. Pasta is usually the first dish in a meal, followed by meat, fish, or a vegetable dish. Traditional foods in northern Italy use more butter and creamy sauces. Polenta, risotto, and hearty bean soups are popular there.

Languages Across Cultures

polenta (pō-ˈlen-tə) a cornmeal dish from northern Italy, that can be eaten as a mush or cooled, sliced, and fried

risotto (ri-ˈsȯ-tō) a rice dish with a creamy texture, often flavored with chicken, fish, sausage, vegetables, or cheese. It is usually made with a special short-grain rice called Arborio rice.

Recipes Find out more about international recipes on this book's Online Learning Center at glencoe.com.

NCTE 9 Develop an understanding of diversity in language use across cultures.

Coronary Heart Disease

Coronary heart disease is a cardiovascular disease—a disease of the heart and blood vessels. The prefix *cardio* refers to the heart. The adjective *vascular* refers to the arteries, veins, and blood vessels. Before getting a heart attack or stroke, other cardiovascular conditions may affect your circulatory system, including atherosclerosis. **Atherosclerosis**, which is the hardening of the arteries, develops as fatty substances build up in the arteries. **High blood pressure** is too much pressure on the heart and arteries as the heart beats.

Why Arteries Get Blocked

A **lipid** is a fat that circulates in your bloodstream. One type of lipid is blood cholesterol. Your liver makes most of the cholesterol in your body. Some comes from food. Too much blood cholesterol can build up and block arteries.

Cholesterol travels in your bloodstream with proteins. Together, they form two types of lipoproteins. **High-density lipoprotein** (HDL) is often called "good cholesterol." It removes cholesterol from your blood and artery walls to your liver. **Low-density lipoprotein** (LDL) is often called "bad cholesterol." It deposits blood cholesterol on your artery walls, causing atherosclerosis.

Keep your LDL cholesterol low and HDL cholesterol high to maintain good heart health. High LDL is linked to heredity, aging, excess body fat, sedentary living, and poor food choices.

Eating Plans to Prevent Heart Disease

Healthful living and eating can help to prevent heart disease:

- Eat plenty of vegetables, fruits, whole grains, and lean, low-fat, and fat-free foods.
- Limit foods with cholesterol, trans fats, and saturated fats.
- Get at least 60 minutes of physical activity as a teen.
- Avoid smoking and drinking alcoholic beverages.
- Maintain a healthy weight.

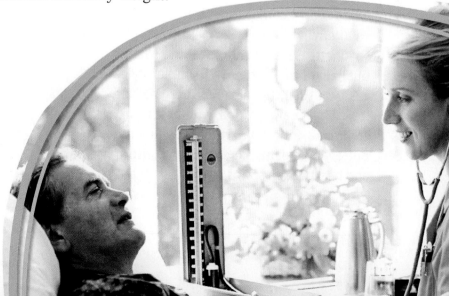

Heart-Conscious Heart conditions sometimes stem from unhealthful food choices. *What is one example of a food pattern that might damage your heart?*

Eating Plans for Other Health Problems

Special eating plans help manage many medical conditions. Eating plans are part of medical nutrition therapy. A registered dietitian evaluates a patient's nutrition, then helps the patient design and follow an eating plan. Conditions that often require special eating plans include:

◆ **Chewing Problems** Oral surgery and certain health problems can lead to difficulty chewing. People can choose soft foods, such as smoothies, soup, or cooked cereal.

◆ **Cancer** Cancer patients often experience loss of taste, loss of appetite, difficulty swallowing, weight loss, and other problems that require special eating plans.

◆ **HIV/AIDS** This disease lowers one's immunity. People with AIDS must protect against weight loss and food-borne illness. Certain foods must be avoided, such as raw sprouts, unpasteurized juice or milk, and soft cheeses.

✓ **Reading Check** **Recall** What kind of eating plan may help lower high blood cholesterol levels?

Nutrition and Illness

Sick or injured people may not be able to eat normally. Illness or medication may decrease their appetite. Good nutrition helps the body to fight illness, repair itself, and return to health. As health improves, appetite and the ability to eat also improve. Follow these guidelines to help someone follow a doctor's instructions for eating:

◆ Help the person sit comfortably before bringing food.

◆ Encourage the person to drink fluids if the doctor advises. Soup and juice, as well as water, are usually appealing choices during illness.

◆ Make meals and snacks appealing. For a sick person with a poor appetite, small, frequent meals may be easier to handle than large ones.

◆ Be calm and patient with the person when he or she is eating.

◆ Ask the doctor about the timing of meals and when to take medicine.

◆ Follow all food safety guidelines. Disposable dishes, cups, napkins, and utensils prevent the spread of illness and infection.

✓ **Reading Check** **Reflect** How can you make a meal more appealing to someone who is sick?

Food and Medications

Some medicine can interfere with the way the body uses nutrients. Some foods keep medicines from working properly.

Always read and follow directions for taking medicines. Know how much medicine to take and when. Some medicines should be taken with food. For example, if you take aspirin, take it with food to keep your stomach from getting upset. Other medicines should be taken on an empty stomach because food may slow the medicine's absorption by the body or its action within the body. It may be necessary to avoid some foods while taking certain medications. If you have questions, ask your doctor or pharmacist.

✓ **Reading Check** **Explain** What might you ask a pharmacist or doctor about medicine and food?

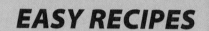

EASY RECIPES

International Flavors
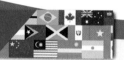

Quick Marinara Sauce

Customary	Ingredients	Metric
¼ cup	Olive oil	50 mL
2 cup	Onions, finely chopped	400 mL
1 cup	Carrots, finely chopped	200 mL
1 cup	Celery, finely chopped	200 mL
3 cloves	Garlic, minced	3 cloves
2 cups	Chicken stock	400 mL
3½ cups	Crushed tomatoes, canned	900 mL
1 tsp.	Ground basil	5 mL
1 tsp.	Ground oregano	5 mL

Try This!

Use additional spices like parsley, crushed red pepper, and bay leaves. Use only half of the chicken stock and cook the mixture longer to make a flavorful pizza sauce.

Yield: 6 servings, ¾ cup (150 mL) each

1. Heat oil in a large saucepan, simmer the chopped onions, carrots, and celery until tender, about 10 minutes. Add garlic and simmer two more minutes.
2. Add chicken stock, crushed tomatoes, and spices, return to simmer and let cook at least 20 minutes. Stir frequently.
3. Serve over your choice of cooked pasta.

Nutritional Information Per Serving: 195 calories, 11 g total fat (1.7 g saturated fat), 2.4 g cholesterol, 335 mg sodium, 21.9 total carbohydrate (4.5 g fiber, 4.8 g total sugars), 5.3 g protein

Percent Daily Value: vitamin A 90%, vitamin C 30%, calcium 8%, iron 15%

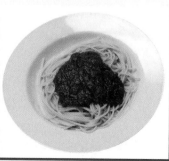

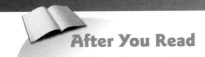

After You Read

CHAPTER SUMMARY
Good nutrition helps lower many health risks. Eating disorders are emotional illnesses that result in extreme, unhealthy ways of eating or exercising. People with food sensitivities—lactose intolerance, gluten intolerance, and food allergies—have unpleasant and even harmful reactions to food. Some health problems, including diabetes, heart disease, and high blood pressure, require special eating plans. Good nutrition helps speed recovery from illness and injury. Food and medication can interact positively and negatively.

Vocabulary Review

1. Use each of these vocabulary words in a sentence.

Content Vocabulary
◇ eating disorder (p. 196)
◇ lactose intolerance (p. 198)
◇ gluten intolerance (p. 198)
◇ food allergy (p. 199)
◇ allergen (p. 199)
◇ diabetes (p. 200)
◇ coronary heart disease (p. 202)
◇ atherosclerosis (p. 202)
◇ high blood pressure (p. 202)
◇ lipid (p. 202)
◇ high-density lipoprotein (p. 202)
◇ low-density lipoprotein (p. 202)

Academic Vocabulary
■ perceive (p. 197)
■ minimize (p. 201)

Review Key Concepts

2. Identify food and lifestyle recommendations that lower health risks.

3. Describe eating disorders and their warning signs.

4. Identify food sensitivities and how to handle them.

5. Discuss special eating plans used for certain health problems.

6. Propose meal and snack basics to help someone recover from an illness or injury.

7. Explain how food and medications may affect each other.

Critical Thinking

8. Analyze whether teens should be concerned about health problems that may not appear until later in life. Support your answer with research.

9. Plan a menu for a friend who will have her wisdom teeth removed.

Real-World Skills and Applications

Set Goals and Make Decisions

10. Getting Help for Eating Disorders Imagine that you suspect a friend has an eating disorder. What signs would you look for? Who would you go to for advice about what to do to help your friend? Write one or more paragraphs to explain your answer.

Collaborative and Interpersonal

11. Diabetes Ask your school nurse to explain the challenges of diabetes, and how teens with diabetes manage their disease. With the nurse, role-play with another student how to be sensitive to a friend with diabetes and how to help if the friend has a diabetic reaction.

Technology

12. Heart Health Create a PowerPoint presentation with 10 slides. Explain what heart disease is, how it develops, and how teens can protect their heart health starting today. Use the American Heart Association Web site as a source for information.

Financial Literacy

13. Best Buy Doug's family drinks soymilk, which costs $3.89 per half-gallon. Sometimes the grocery offers a special two-pack for $6. How much can Doug save if he buys a two-pack containing two half-gallons instead of two separate half-gallons?

14. Community Health Event Identify community events that raise funds and awareness for health issues. Possible events include health fairs, fitness walks, and bicycle tours. Health issues may include heart health, cancer, and diabetes prevention. Create a brochure describing the events. Share the brochure with your classmates.

NCSS I A Culture Analyze and explain the ways groups, societies, and cultures address human needs and concerns.

15. Food Allergies A peanut allergy can pose serious health risks. Some candy bars, cereals, baked goods, and sauces contain peanuts. Some restaurants cook foods in peanut oil. Visit a grocery store. Read product labels to identify at least ten foods with peanuts. Make a list of the foods that people with a peanut allergy must avoid.

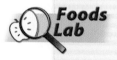

16. Taste Test With classmates, conduct a blind taste test of canned chicken broth—regular, no salt added, and low-sodium. Write one or more paragraphs to describe the flavor of each type and explain how you would enhance the taste and appeal of the various kinds of broth without using salt.

Additional Activities For additional activities go to this book's Online Learning Center at glencoe.com.

Academic Skills

English Language Arts

17. Create a Health Alert Research and report on type 2 diabetes. Find out what causes it, why more children and teens are developing it, and how it is managed and treated. Write a health alert for parents and teens.

> **NCTE 4** Use written language to communicate effectively.

Science

18. Sugar Substitutes Artificial sweeteners are chemical substitutes for sugar. They are often used in soda, snacks, and many other foods. These products may help people with diabetes or those wanting to lose weight. Find a food containing an artificial sweetener. Research this ingredient, its calories and sweetness, and its uses. Write one or more paragraphs to summarize the results of your research.

> **NSES Content Standard A** Develop abilities necessary to do scientific inquiry.

Mathematics

19. Every Little Bit Ana made small changes in her diet to avoid obesity, such as drinking only one soda daily instead of three. She has also gradually increased her activity level. Ana's weight began dropping an average of 2 pounds weekly. Ana started at 170 pounds, and her target weight is 140 pounds. Chart her weekly progress using a line graph.

Math Concept **Line Graphs** A line graph is useful in displaying information about quantities that change over time. In this case, there are two variables to analyze: time and weight lost.

Starting Hint Begin the line with Ana's current weight, then chart her average weight loss down to her goal weight.

 For more math help, go to the Math Appendix

> **NCTM Data Analysis and Probability** Formulate questions that can be addressed with data and collect, organize, and display relevant data to answer them.

STANDARDIZED TEST PRACTICE

MULTIPLE CHOICE
Read the paragraph and write an answer on a separate piece of paper.

Test-Taking Tip To help remember new vocabulary, create a mental picture to go along with the meaning of the word. For example, cholesterol comes from the word parts *chol-* meaning solid and the Greek *stereos,* meaning oil. Do you have a mental picture of solidified oil in your veins?

The *type* of fat you eat is as important as the *amount* you eat. Unsaturated fats may lower LDL and raise HDL. They can be found in fish, olive oil, nuts, and some other plant-based foods.

20. Based on the paragraph, which of the following statements is true?
  a. Unsaturated fats raise HDL.
  b. Olive oil is not a source of unsaturated fats.
  c. Unsaturated fats are only from plants.
  d. A high-fat diet is a healthful diet.

Unit 5 Thematic Project

Plan a Healthy Lifestyle

With so many healthful diets to choose from, it is important to find one that suits you best. Following sensible food choice guidelines can keep you from being tempted by fad diets. Think about some of the fad diets you have heard of. Why are these diets unhealthy?

My Journal

If you completed the journal entry from page 144 refer to it to see if the lifestyle you chose follows the recommendations made by MyPyramid and the Dietary Guidelines for Americans.

Project Assignment

In this project you will:
- Choose and research a healthy lifestyle.
- Create a full day's menu that meets all your nutritional needs.
- Write a summary of your research.
- Write a list of interview questions.
- Interview someone in the community who is qualified to discuss the lifestyle you have chosen.
- While interviewing, take notes, and after interviewing, transcribe your notes.
- Make a presentation to your classmates on the findings of your research and interview.

Academic Skills You Will Use . . . .
English Language Arts

NCTE 5 Use different writing process elements to communicate effectively.

NCTE 9 Develop an understanding of diversity in language use across cultures.

STEP 1 Choose and Research a Healthy Lifestyle

Choose and conduct research on a healthy lifestyle approved by your teacher such as sugar-free, low-fat, vegetarian, or any other healthy lifestyle. You can also design your own lifestyle, such as supporting local fresh food sources. Write a summary of your research that
- Describes your chosen healthy lifestyle
- Includes a day's menu for breakfast, lunch, dinner, and a snack, with drinks and side dishes for each meal
- Explain how your menu provides a full day's nutrition, according to the MyPyramid and Dietary Guidelines recommendations.

STEP 2 Plan Your Interview

Use the results of your research and the menu you have planned to develop a list of interview questions. Keep these writing skills in mind as you form your questions.

Writing Skills
- Use complete sentences.
- Use correct spelling and grammar.
- Organize your questions in the order you want to ask them.

STEP 3 Connect with Your Community

Interview someone in your community who is qualified to discuss your healthy lifestyle. This person can be a dietition, nutrition professor, health care professional, family and consumer sciences teacher, or chef of a restaurant that specializes in healthy cuisine.

Interviewing Skills
- Record responses and take notes.
- Listen attentively.
- When you transcribe your notes, write in complete sentences and use correct spelling and grammar.

STEP 4 Create Your Presentation

Use the Unit Thematic Project Checklist to plan and give an oral report. Use these speaking skills as you present your final report.

Speaking Skills
- Speak clearly and concisely.
- Be sensitive to the needs of your audience.
- Use standard English to communicate.

STEP 5 Evaluate Your Presentation

Your project will be reviewed and evaluated based on:
- Depth of interview and questions
- Content of your presentation
- Mechanics—presentation and neatness

Evaluation Rubric Go to this book's Online Learning Center at glencoe.com for a rubric you can use to evaluate your final report.

Project Checklist

Plan	✓ Research a healthy lifestyle. ✓ Write a summary of your research. ✓ Write interview questions. ✓ Conduct an interview. ✓ Transcribe the notes from your interview. ✓ Plan a five-minute oral presentation.
Present	✓ Make a presentation to your class to discuss the results of your research and interview. ✓ Describe the menu you have created. ✓ Explain how your menu provides a full day's nutrition following MyPyramid and Dietary Guidelines. ✓ Invite the students of the class to ask any questions they may have. Answer these questions. ✓ When students ask questions, demonstrate in your answers that you respect their perspectives. ✓ Turn in your research summary, interview questions, interview notes, and menu to your teacher.
Academic Skills	✓ Conduct research to gather information. ✓ Communicate effectively. ✓ Organize your presentation so the audience can follow along easily. ✓ Thoroughly express your ideas.

Unit 6

Smart Food Choices

Chapters in this Unit

Chapter 15 Consumer Issues:
            Fact vs. Fiction
Chapter 16 Planning Nutritious Meals
            and Snacks
Chapter 17 Shopping for Food
Chapter 18 Eating Well When Away
            from Home

Unit Thematic Project Preview

Consider Nutritional Information

While studying this unit, you will learn about being a smart consumer and choosing nutritious foods. In the unit thematic project at the end of this unit, you will conduct research and create a poster comparing factual nutritional information with the information presented in advertisements for food.

My Journal

To learn how to make good food choices, it helps to think about your past food choices. Write a journal entry about the topics below.

- What did you eat yesterday?
- Did you consider the nutritional value of your food choices?
- How could you have improved your food choices?

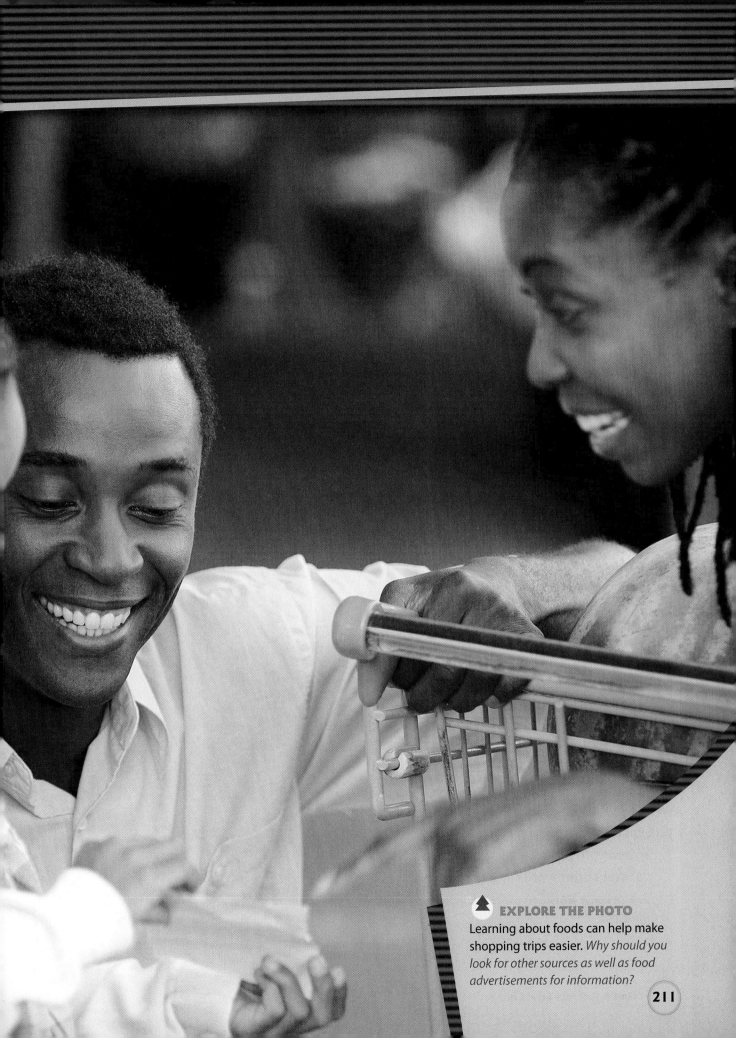

EXPLORE THE PHOTO
Learning about foods can help make
shopping trips easier. *Why should you
look for other sources as well as food
advertisements for information?*

211

CHAPTER 15
Consumer Issues: Fact vs. Fiction

Explore the Photo ▶▶
Smart choices for wellness are based on scientific facts. *Where do you find facts about food and nutrition?*

Writing Activity
Step-by-Step Guide

Expert Advice Get the facts before making food choices. Write a step-by-step guide to finding sound food advice. Include the materials you need to create it and the steps to assemble it.

Writing Tips

1. **Explain** terms the reader may not know.
2. **Write** the steps in chronological order.
3. **Use transition words** in your sentences.
4. **Use precise verbs** to make your explanation clear.

Reading Guide

Before You Read

Prepare with a Partner Before you read, work with a partner. Read the headings and ask each other questions about the topics that will be discussed. Write down the questions you both have about each section. As you read, answer the questions you have identified.

Read to Learn

Key Concepts
- **Identify** sources of reliable food and nutrition information.
- **Evaluate** food advertisements.
- **Recognize** false health claims.
- **Interpret** food and nutrition news.

Main Idea
You can use food and nutrition knowledge, critical-thinking skills, and decision-making abilities to make smart decisions for wellness.

Content Vocabulary
◇ media literacy
◇ health fraud
◇ herbal supplement

Academic Vocabulary
You will find these words in your reading and on your tests. Use the glossary to look up their definitions if necessary.
▪ accurate   ▪ conflict

Graphic Organizer
As you read, use a graphic organizer like the one below to list four generally reliable sources of health information.

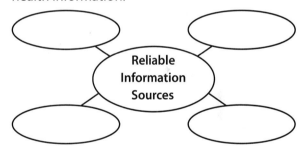

 Graphic Organizer Go to this book's Online Learning Center at **glencoe.com** to print out this graphic organizer.

Academic Standards ▪

 English Language Arts
NCTE 6 Apply knowledge of language structure and conventions to discuss texts.

 Mathematics
NCTM Number and Operations Compute fluently and make reasonable estimates.
NCTM Number and Operations Understand numbers, ways of representing numbers, relationships among numbers, and number systems.

 Social Studies
NCSS VI A Power, Authority, and Governance Examine persistent issues involving the rights, roles, and status of the individual in relation to the general welfare.
NCSS VII H Production, Distribution, and Consumption Apply economic concepts and reasoning when evaluating historical and contemporary social developments and issues.

NCTE National Council of Teachers of English
NCTM National Council of Teachers of Mathematics

NSES National Science Education Standards
NCSS National Council for the Social Studies

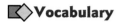

**Nutrition &
Wellness Tips**

Reliable Web Sites

✓ Look for Web sites with URLs that end with .gov (government) or .edu (education). These usually indicate reliable sources of online information.

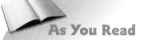**Vocabulary**

You can find definitions in the glossary at the back of this book.

As You Read

Connect Think of some of the sources where you have found nutrition information recently.

Find the Facts on Food and Nutrition

Have you done a report on food or nutrition? If so, you know that nutrition information is everywhere. There are news, talk, and cooking shows on television and radio. Magazines, newspapers, books, pamphlets, and brochures have advice. Many Web sites have cooking, nutrition, and wellness information. Even your family and friends may have advice. With so much information, many people become confused about nutrition and health.

You need to be a good consumer of information to make food choices for wellness. You must have media literacy. **Media literacy** is knowing how to find reliable information sources, evaluate how **accurate**, or factual, the information is, and apply what you learn.

Who Are the Experts?

No matter where the information comes from, make sure the source is reliable, or trustworthy. To be reliable, a writer must either be an expert or present facts from expert sources.

Many food and nutrition experts have degrees in food science or nutrition from colleges and universities. These experts usually offer reliable information. Physicians and nurses also receive nutrition training. Students at culinary schools prepare for careers as chefs and learn cooking techniques for good nutrition.

Most nutrition experts show their science-based education credentials with letters after their names. The letters CFCS mean that a person is certified in family and consumer sciences. The letters RD mean that a person is a registered dietitian.

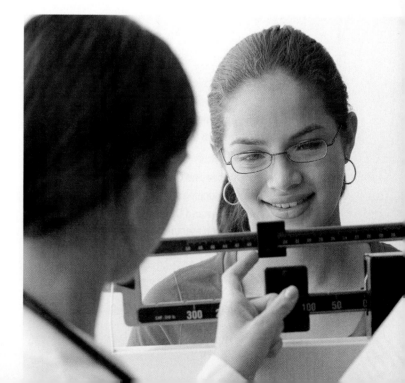

Talk to an Expert Registered dietitians have special training that qualifies them to provide expert advice on nutrition. *What is the advantage of talking with a registered dietitian when you need nutrition advice?*

When You Have Questions

Use reliable sources of information when you have questions about food, nutrition, and wellness. Here are some reliable sources of information:

- **At School** Your school nurse, food and nutrition teachers, health teachers, and family and consumer sciences teachers.

- **In Your Community** Registered dietitians, doctors, city or county nutritionists, specialists from a state university, consumer groups, and the local office of the U.S. Food and Drug Administration (FDA).

- **National Organizations** The American Dietetic Association, American Heart Association, and the American Association of Family and Consumer Sciences.

- **Government Web Sites** National Institutes of Health (NIH), Centers for Disease Control and Prevention (CDC), FDA, and the Food and Nutrition Information Center of the United States Department of Agriculture (USDA).

✓ **Reading Check** **Discuss** Why is media literacy important for wellness?

Math in Action

Vitamin C from Food

Food, not supplements, is the best source of vitamins. Teen boys should get at least 75 mg of vitamin C daily; girls need 65 mg. Use addition to plan a combination of foods from the list below that provides you with the right amount of vitamin C.

- 1 (7.5-in, or 19 cm) carrot — 4 mg
- 1 medium apple — 8 mg
- 1 large tangerine — 26 mg
- 2 cups fresh spinach — 16 mg
- 1 medium tomato — 16 mg

Math Concept **Front-End Estimation**
Front-end estimation can be used to quickly estimate sums and differences before adding or subtracting.

Starting Hint Use addition to find combinations of foods that will total at least 75 mg for boys, or at least 65 mg for girls. While you can have more than one serving of any food, try to use as many different items from the list as possible.

NCTM Number and Operations Compute fluently and make reasonable estimates.

 For more math help, go to the Math Appendix

Advertising

Food companies spend billions of dollars every year on advertising for radio, television, magazines, and newspapers. Putting a food or beverage brand in a movie or TV show is another example of advertising. Advertisements often include information that is biased in favor of the advertiser.

Almost every advertisement has one purpose: to persuade you to buy. Ads may not provide all the facts or options you need to make the best decisions for your health.

Some ads may tempt you to believe that a product or service will make you more popular or attractive. They may use celebrities and athletes, music, and graphics to make the product seem irresistible. Sometimes ads even look like news stories.

✓ **Reading Check** **Recall** How do advertisers try to influence you?

True or False?

Have you ever heard a food or supplement promoted as a cure, secret, breakthrough, guarantee, or miracle food? Words like these are usually hype! There are also many myths about nutrition and supplements. (See **Figure 15.1**.)

The way to stay healthy is with a sensible lifestyle and smart eating. However, many people spend money on products that promise quick and easy health fixes. These products are usually a waste of money and can create a false sense of hope for a cure. Some people who sell these products claim to have qualifications that they do not have. This is why it is important to learn to recognize health fraud. **Health fraud** is false and possibly harmful approaches to health care. The Federal Trade Commission and the FDA help protect Americans from health fraud.

Using a food or supplement as an easy health fix may have serious consequences. For example, very high doses of some vitamins can have harmful side effects. These products are never a good substitute for healthful lifestyle choices and proper medical care.

Figure 15.1 **Nutrition Myths and Truths**

How Food Myths Spread Some beliefs about food are based on myths, not facts. Even so, these myths spread from person to person. *What other food and nutrition myths, besides the ones listed on the chart, have you heard?*

Myth	Fact
"Chocolate and greasy foods cause pimples."	Hormone changes cause acne, not chocolate or greasy foods.
"Sugar makes you hyper."	Hyperactivity is not related to eating candy or sweet drinks. Scientists do not yet know all the reasons for hyperactivity.
"Carbohydrates like bread and pasta make you fat."	Carbohydrates are the body's best energy source. A slice of bread has only about 70 calories. Half a cup of pasta has about 100 calories. Excessive calories come from big portions or high-fat spreads or sauces.
"Nutrient supplements can make up for poor eating."	No single supplement provides all the nutrients and other substances that food supplies. Supplements also do not supply enough food energy to meet your body's needs.
"You can build muscle by eating more protein."	Only physical activity builds muscles. Without physical activity, extra protein from food can become body fat.

Herbal Supplements

An **herbal supplement** is a substance that comes from plants. Herbal supplements are often promoted with health claims. However, scientists do not know everything about what they do, how they interact with medicine, or how safe they are. Some herbal supplements can be dangerous. Always talk to your doctor before taking any herbal supplement. When you are unsure whether advice about food and nutrition is reliable, ask yourself:

◆ Does the advice identify good foods and bad foods? No food is good or bad. Your overall food choices are what count.

◆ Does the advice use emotional appeals and personal stories to prove a claim? Only good research can prove a claim.

◆ Does the advice fit with what you already know?

✓ **Reading Check** **Predict** What might happen if you used an herbal supplement to treat an illness instead of seeking medical care?

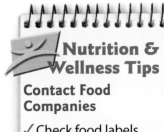

Nutrition & Wellness Tips

Contact Food Companies

✓ Check food labels for the Web site addresses and toll-free phone numbers of food companies for answers to your consumer questions.

Food and Nutrition in the News

You have probably seen news reports about scientific studies on food and nutrition. Do not change your food choices based on a single report. The results of one study are just one piece of a large puzzle. Sometimes, the results of a study **conflict**, or disagree, with the results of other studies. This is a natural part of the scientific process. Scientists must do many studies before they can agree on what the results mean. Research needs to be repeated before it can be considered reliable.

It is important to pay careful attention when you hear news about nutrition studies. Some news reports may exaggerate or not fully explain the results of the research.

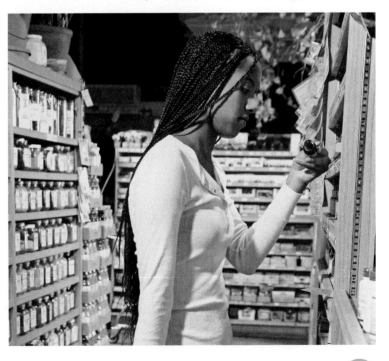

Beware of Claims Supplements such as bee pollen, shark cartilage, and spirulina are often promoted with misleading claims. *What would you say to a friend who thinks you should try the latest herbal supplement?*

Think Critically About News

It is important to use critical thinking skills when reading about health news. If you do not understand something you read, ask a doctor, nurse, registered dietitian, or teacher questions such as:

◆ Who did the research? Are the researchers qualified?

◆ Who paid for the study? This may influence the results.

◆ Was the study performed on animals or humans? Animal studies might not apply to humans.

◆ How large was the study? Small studies may not draw the right conclusions.

◆ What do other experts on the topic or studies about the topic say? Other studies may have reached different conclusions.

◆ Were study participants like you? Even good scientific studies may not apply to you.

✓ **Reading Check** **Explain** Why should you pay careful attention to news reports about nutrition research?

EASY RECIPES — Everyday Favorites

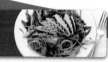

Cinnamon Baked Apples

Customary	Ingredients	Metric	
5	Apples	5	**Try This!** Serve this over waffles or with ice cream.
½ cup	Packed brown sugar	125 mL	
1 tsp.	Cinnamon	1 mL	
1 tsp.	Lemon juice	1 mL	

Yield: 6 servings, ½ cup (125 mL) each

❶ Preheat oven to 350 degrees. Peel, core and slice apples into quarters, then cut each quarter into three pieces. Put into a large bowl and mix with other ingredients.

❷ Pour into a baking dish and put in oven.

❸ Stir occasionally. Serve when apples are tender, about 30 minutes.

Nutritional Information Per Serving: 122 calories, 0 g total fat, (0 g saturated fat), 0 mg cholesterol, 9 mg sodium, 33 g total carbohydrate, (3 g fiber, 30 g total sugars), 1 g protein

Percent Daily Value: vitamin A 0%, vitamin C 10%, calcium 4%, iron 4%

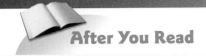

After You Read

CHAPTER SUMMARY

A wise consumer uses critical-thinking skills to evaluate food and nutrition information. Reliable information comes from qualified food, nutrition, and wellness experts. Advertisers use powerful techniques to influence your buying decisions. You must judge whether the advertising is true for you. Be alert for false, misleading, or exaggerated food or nutrition claims. The results of nutrition research studies often appear in the news. Remember that the study may not apply to you, and that a single study is not enough to change your food choices.

Vocabulary Review

1. Define each vocabulary term in your own words.

Content Vocabulary
- media literacy (p. 214)
- health fraud (p. 216)
- herbal supplement (p. 217)

Academic Vocabulary
- accurate (p. 214)
- conflict (p. 217)

Review Key Concepts

2. Identify sources of reliable food and nutrition information.

3. Evaluate food advertisements.

4. Recognize false health claims.

5. Interpret food and nutrition news.

Critical Thinking

6. Analyze a newspaper article about food and nutrition. Summarize the article, then determine if it offers reliable information.

7. Evaluate a Web site that has health claims about a new scientific study. How would you determine whether the site has reliable information?

8. Explain what questions you should ask in this situation: You see a TV news report stating that a certain food has been shown to increase the risk of heart disease. However, you have also read that the same food may help prevent cancer.

9. Hypothesize what might happen if you tried to eliminate carbohydrates from your meals and snacks because you heard that they would make you fat. Would this be a wise course of action? Why or why not?

Real-World Skills and Applications

Set Goals and Make Decisions

10. Health TV Imagine that you are on the staff of the school's television channel. You want to start a talk show with practical, reliable advice about health and nutrition for teens. Make an outline of the topics and guests you would have on the program.

Interpersonal and Collaborative

11. Advertise School Meals Plan an advertising campaign for your school's breakfast or lunch program. Work with a classmate to identify the campaign's goal and message. Create a slogan and visuals. Be creative, engaging, and honest.

Financial Literacy

12. Buy One, Get One Free This week, the 18-oz. box of your favorite whole-grain cereal is $0.50 off the regular $4.49 price. The smaller, 12.9-oz. box costs $3.79. You will buy just one box. How much will you pay per oz. for each size? Which box is less expensive per oz.?

Technology

13. Herbal Supplements Design a Web page with facts about an herbal supplement. Use reliable sources of information to research the benefits and risks of using the supplement. Footnote your sources, and include hyperlinks.

14. Food Advertising Count all the food advertisements you see or hear for one day. Find them from a variety of sources. Collect examples. As a class, discuss where the ads appeared, what advertising techniques were used, and the possible effects of these ads on teens' lives.

15. Consumer Protection The United States government has enacted legislation to protect consumers from fraud. Find out about a consumer's basic rights. If you were the victim of fraud, what steps might you take to get justice?

> **NCSS VI A Power, Authority, and Governance** Examine persistent issues involving the rights, roles, and status of the individual in relation to the general welfare.

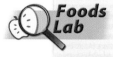

16. Test Product Claims Find several ads with claims for a food product, such as better tasting or ready in 10 minutes. Choose one product to taste-test or prepare in class. Does it fulfill the advertising promise? Document and share your findings in a visual presentation.

 Additional Activities For additional activities, go to this book's Online Learning Center at **glencoe.com**.

Academic Skills

 English Language Arts

17. Persuasive Ads Identify techniques used in persuasive writing. Find three advertisements that use these techniques. Then analyze the techniques used in each ad and explain whether each ad is persuasive, misleading, or both.

> **NCTE 6** Apply knowledge of language structure and conventions to discuss texts.

 Social Studies

18. New Ways to Advertise Many companies pay for their products or logos to appear on popular shows. This is called product placement. With the permission of a parent or teacher, watch a TV show and note the products you see. Write a paragraph to describe what these product placements tell you about the audience.

> **NCSS VII H Production, Distribution, and Consumption** Apply economic concepts and reasoning when evaluating historical and contemporary social developments and issues.

 Mathematics

19. Percents Some companies use infomercials to sell their products on TV. Infomercials are long commercials that look like informational shows. Of 191 infomercials broadcast during one month, 73 sold a weight-loss or health-care product. What percent of the infomercials does this represent?

Math Concept **Percentages** A fraction can be expressed as a percent by first converting the fraction to a decimal, and then converting the decimal to a percent by moving the decimal point two places to the right.

Starting Hint Set up a ratio, or fraction, with the number of health-care infomercials as the numerator, and the total number of infomercials as the denominator.

 For more math help, go to the Math Appendix

> **NCTM Number and Operations** Understand numbers, ways of representing numbers, relationships among numbers, and number systems.

STANDARDIZED TEST PRACTICE

ESSAY
Read the paragraph. Then read the writing prompt and write your essay on a separate piece of paper.

Test-Taking Tip Building your vocabulary will help you on many kinds of tests. Practice new vocabulary and concepts with your parents and other adults you know.

Knowing what sources of nutritional information to trust can be confusing. You may hear that a particular food is helpful, and then later hear that it also can be harmful. For example, one food may be known to help the heart, but hurt the liver.

20. Think about what you learned in this chapter. How do people usually make choices about what to eat and how to exercise? How can people make informed choices about food and health? Write an essay to explain your answer.

CHAPTER 16
Planning Nutritious Meals and Snacks

Explore the Photo ▶▶
Making a meal is more than following a recipe. You must plan what to serve, prepare it, and have it ready on time. *What management skills can help you plan a successful meal?*

Writing Activity
Character Analysis

Television Personalities Think about a chef in the media who you like. What does he or she say about meal times and food? Write a character analysis that describes the chef's personality, what kinds of foods he or she cooks, and how healthful his or her message is.

Writing Tips

1. **Describe** the character's appearance.

2. **Analyze** his or her words and actions.

3. **Explain** the reactions of others to the character.

Breakfast
Corn flakes with banana and milk
Orange juice

Packed Lunch
Turkey–Swiss cheese pita – lettuce, tomato
Grapes
2 Oatmeal cookies
Milk money (for chocolate lowfat milk)

Dinner
Tuna casserole
Steamed broccoli
Carrot salad
Whole wheat roll
Iced tea with lemon
Frozen yogurt topped with nuts

Snacks
Pretzels
Tangerine

Reading Guide

Before You Read

Helpful Memory Tools Successful readers use tricks to help them remember. Scan the headings in the chapter and think about memory tools you can use to help you to remember the information.

Read to Learn
Key Concepts
- **Identify** things to consider when you plan a meal.
- **Discuss** why it is important to eat breakfast.
- **Explain** how to pack a meal to eat away from home.
- **Describe** the components of a meal.
- **List** ways to make smart choices about snacking.

Main Idea
Learn to plan meals and snacks that are nourishing and appealing. For meals your family and friends will enjoy, consider individual needs and preferences, your resources, nutrition, and variety.

Content Vocabulary
◇ menu
◇ resources
◇ trade-off
◇ convenience food
◇ brunch
◇ appetizer

Academic Vocabulary
You will find these words in your reading and on your tests. Use the glossary to look up their definitions if necessary.
- affect
- valid

Graphic Organizer
As you read, indicate the reasons a person should eat each meal and an example of a food eaten at each meal time or snack.

	REASON	EXAMPLE
Breakfast		
Lunch		
Dinner		
Snacks		

 Graphic Organizer Go to this book's Online Learning Center at glencoe.com to print out this graphic organizer.

Academic Standards ■ ■ ■ ■ ■ ■ ■ ■ ■ ■ ■ ■ ■ ■ ■ ■

 English Language Arts
NCTE 1 Read texts to acquire new information.
NCTE 9 Develop an understanding of diversity in language use across cultures.
NCTE 12 Use language to accomplish individual purposes.

 Mathematics
NCTM Number and Operations Understand numbers, ways of representing numbers, relationships among numbers, and number systems.

 Science
NSES Content Standard A Develop abilities necessary to do scientific inquiry.
NSES Content Standard F Develop an understanding of personal and community health.

NCTE National Council of Teachers of English
NCTM National Council of Teachers of Mathematics
NSES National Science Education Standards
NCSS National Council of the Social Studies

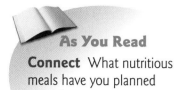

Vocabulary

You can find definitions in the glossary at the back of this book.

Plan Meals Wisely

There is no single correct pattern of eating. Your lifestyle, schedule, family, culture, and physical needs **affect**, or influence, when and how much you eat. Planning a menu takes management skills. A **menu** is a list of foods to be served.

As You Read

Connect What nutritious meals have you planned recently?

Plan Family Meals

Great meals provide nutrient-dense foods that look and taste good, and that go well together. Successful menus often start with the main dish. Other foods complement that dish. As you plan your menus, consider:

- **Food Preferences** Who will eat the meal? What do they like and dislike?

- **Nutrition** Use MyPyramid to include the right variety and food-group amounts each day to match the energy and nutrient needs of the people you are feeding.

- **Special Food Needs** Plan menu options for people with food allergies or other special needs so that everyone can enjoy the food.

- **Age** Teens and physically active adults may need larger portions or different foods than younger siblings or older grandparents. Small children may like simpler foods.

- **Meal Patterns** Will this be a light meal or the day's main meal? How do snacks fit in?

- **Schedules** Plan family meals as often as possible. Plan a menu that can be reheated easily to avoid stress and save time.

- **Your Resources** Consider your resources. **Resources** are the time, money, and energy needed to complete a task.

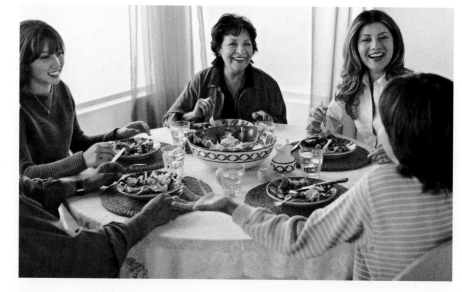

Meals Across the Lifespan Consider age, gender, special needs, and food preferences as you plan successful and healthful menus for your family. *Why might these family members have different calorie needs? How would you change this menu for your family?*

Manage Your Resources

Meal management helps you plan satisfying, healthful meals that match your schedule and resources. Resources include:

◆ **Time and Energy** Using resources often involves a trade-off. A **trade-off** is giving something up so you can have something else. If time and energy are short, choose a simple menu or convenience foods. A **convenience food** is a partly prepared or ready-to-eat food. Be careful when choosing convenience foods. They are often more expensive than foods you make from scratch.

◆ **Money** Consider your budget. Your food budget needs to cover the cost of all your food, including the food you eat away from home.

◆ **Food** Plan menus to use foods you already have at home. Add ingredients you still need to your shopping list.

◆ **Kitchen Skills** Consider your cooking skills. As you build your skills, you will be able to tackle more challenging recipes.

◆ **Kitchen Equipment** Make sure you have all the kitchen tools you need.

Consider Food Preferences

Your family members probably like different foods. Follow this advice when menu conflicts occur:

◆ **Look for compromises.** If you like green pepper but your sister does not, make a salad with green pepper on the side.

◆ **Take turns.** Prepare your favorite recipe this time and your brother's favorite next time.

◆ **Prepare less-favorite foods in different ways.** If a family member does not like cooked spinach, try serving a raw spinach salad instead.

◆ **Plan make-your-own meals occasionally.** Arrange ingredients for sandwiches and salads in serving dishes. Let everyone pick the ingredients they want.

✓ **Reading Check** **Discuss** Why do you need to consider your resources when you plan a meal?

Science in Action

Soda and Healthy Bones

Compare the ingredients and Nutrition Facts of soda and milk. Soda does not have the many bone-building nutrients milk has. Regular soda provides only calories and added sugars, and diet soda has no calories and few if any nutrients.

Procedure Research the possible effects of regularly drinking soda in place of milk or calcium-fortified soy milk with your meals.

Analysis Explain the effects of regularly substituting milk or fortified soy milk with sodas as a mealtime beverage. What are the possible effects of drinking soda for snacks, too? Describe how your body uses calcium for bone health and overall good health. List foods to include in meals and snacks that provide calcium.

NSES Content Standard A
Develop abilities necessary to do scientific inquiry.

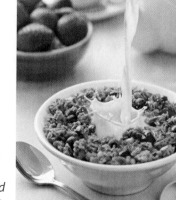

Breakfast Is a Healthy Start

Between dinner and breakfast, you may fast, or not eat, for 12 hours. The word *breakfast* means to break, or end, the fast. Breakfast refreshes your energy supply. Your body uses energy for breathing, growing, and other body processes while you sleep. By morning, your body cells need a new supply of energy for later in the day.

Breakfast also enhances mental and physical performance, helps control weight, and helps you avoid mid-morning hunger. People who skip breakfast may not get all the nutrients they miss in the morning.

Breakfast Choices

Breakfast refers to when you eat, not what you eat. It can supply up to one-third of your body's daily nutrient needs. Plan menus with foods from MyPyramid. Cereal topped with nuts, berries, and milk is a typical breakfast. Here are some other choices:

◆ A toaster waffle with strawberries and instant hot cocoa made with milk

◆ Ham and cheese on an English muffin with carrot sticks and grapefruit juice

◆ A blender shake (made with milk and sliced fruit) and whole-wheat toast

◆ A bagel and a yogurt-juice drink

Easy Breakfast Solutions

People give many excuses for skipping breakfast. These are not usually **valid**, or good, reasons. Each excuse has an easy solution:

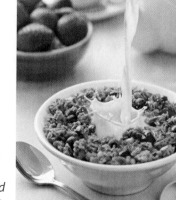

Nutrition & Wellness Tips

Save Time and Calories

✓ Plan one dish to serve twice: a bowl of chili today and leftover chili over a baked potato tomorrow, for example.

✓ Eat a baked potato with salsa instead of French fries as a side dish.

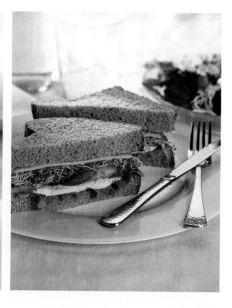

Start Your Day with Breakfast There are no strict rules about the foods you eat for breakfast, as long as they are healthful. *What foods could you eat before going to school?*

- **"I'm not hungry when I get up."** Get ready for your day first, and then eat breakfast.
- **"Eating a big breakfast makes me fat."** Breakfast helps control your appetite so you do not overeat later.
- **"I don't have time!"** Make breakfast the night before. Pack crackers, cheese, and grapes to eat on your way to school.
- **"I don't like breakfast foods."** Eat what you like. A sandwich or last night's leftovers are good choices.

✓ **Reading Check** **List** What are three reasons to eat a nutritious breakfast?

Pack Your Meals

Keep nutrition, ease, and food safety in mind when you pack a portable meal. Many salads and sandwiches are great for packed lunches. Even hot chili can be packed to go in a container that keeps food hot.

Pack a Lunch

A well-planned packed lunch contains nutrient-rich foods, including fruit, vegetables, and whole-grain products. It may have high-protein foods, such as lean meat, peanut butter, or soy nuts. Low-fat yogurt can add calcium-rich dairy foods to your meal. Be creative. Find different foods that provide the nutrients you need.

HOT JOBS!

Caterer
Caterers plan, prepare, and serve appealing menus for many different types of events. They work with their clients to develop menu plans while considering budget, equipment, and time.

Careers Find out more about careers. Go to this book's Online Learning Center at **glencoe.com**.

Discover International Foods

Mexico

Chicken, rice, tortillas, beans, avocados, tomatoes, and other foods found in Mexican cuisine add variety. They are loaded with nutrients. Corn and wheat tortillas are served as a wrap for burritos and soft tacos, or in mixed dishes such as enchiladas. From mild to spicy hot, more than a hundred different types of chili peppers add flavor. Mole ('mō-lā), a rich chile-chocolate sauce, is traditionally served over chicken or as a stew-like main dish. Flan (flän) is an egg custard often served for dessert.

Languages Across Cultures

arroz con pollo (ä-ros kon pō-yō) rice with chicken

queso blanco (kāsō blaṇ-kō) Mexican-style white cheese

Recipes Find out more about international recipes on this book's Online Learning Center at glencoe.com.

NCTE 9 Develop an understanding of diversity in language use across cultures.

How to Pack Food

Keep hot foods hot and cold foods cold. Harmful bacteria can multiply and make you sick if food is not kept at a safe temperature. Follow these guidelines to pack food safely:

◆ Pack foods in airtight containers to keep them fresh.

◆ Wash fresh fruits and vegetables before packing them.

◆ Refrigerate perishable lunch items until you pack them.

◆ Freeze your sandwich the night before. Sandwiches made with eggs, jelly, mayonnaise, or raw vegetables do not freeze well.

◆ Pack sandwich vegetables separately. Otherwise, they will wilt or make the bread soggy.

◆ Wait until morning to put cold foods into your lunch tote.

◆ Pack perishable foods in an insulated container with a frozen juice can, a bag of ice cubes, or a frozen gel pack.

◆ Wash, rinse, and dry your lunch tote after each use.

◆ Keep your lunch in a clean, cool place. Avoid sunny or warm areas, and dirty places such as inside a gym bag.

◆ Pack salad and dressing separately.

✓ **Reading Check** **List** What are three ways to keep your packed lunch safe to eat?

Light or Hearty Meals

Do you like to eat a big meal for breakfast, lunch, or dinner? Your body uses calories from meals in the same way no matter when you eat. You might plan a hearty brunch. **Brunch** is a breakfast-lunch combination. If your midday meal is big, you might prefer a light dinner. Use MyPyramid's guidelines to plan all of your meals, whether they are light or hearty. This will help you to ensure that your meals provide the nutrients your body needs. See **Figure 16.1** for ways to make a meal appealing.

Light Meals

Light meals often supply about one-third of the day's nutrients. Light meals should include foods from several food groups. Which food groups are in these healthful light meals?

◆ Grilled chicken salad with greens with a whole-grain roll, kiwifruit, and chocolate milk.

◆ Scrambled egg with berries, a rye bagel, and hot cocoa.

◆ Chicken burrito with sliced red peppers, zucchini sticks, and low-fat milk.

Hearty Meals

Many families eat hearty meals in the evening. Hearty meals are usually large meals. They provide lots of nutrients. The components of a hearty family meal may include:

◆ **Appetizer** An **appetizer** is a small portion of food, such as a soup or salad, served at the start of a meal.

◆ **Main Dish** A main dish is usually a meat, bean, or hearty mixed-food dish such as a shrimp and vegetable stir-fry.

◆ **Side Dishes** A side dish is a dish that accompanies and complements the main dish. Common side dishes include vegetables, rice, salad, or bread.

◆ **Beverage** A nutritious beverage such as milk, soy milk, or water goes with every meal.

◆ **Dessert** Many dinners end with dessert.

✓ **Reading Check**) **Discuss** How can MyPyramid help you plan a light or hearty meal?

Figure 16.1	Create Enticing Meals

Meals with Appeal You can use a variety of foods to create enticing and nourishing meals. *What makes this meal appealing? What food groups are represented?*

Color Include at least one brightly colored fruit or vegetable in each meal. You can also garnish the plate. A garnish is an edible decoration.

Texture Include crisp or chewy, smooth or chunky, hard or soft textures.

Flavor Include a variety of flavors—strong spicy flavors with milder flavors.

Temperature Include hot and cold foods.

Size and Shape Plan different sizes and shapes on the plate.

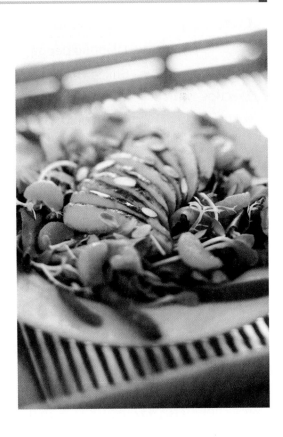

Smart Snacking

Snacks give you energy and provide nutrients you may have missed at mealtime. To make smart choices about snacking:

◆ Pick nutrient-dense, lower-fat snacks from the five food groups, such as fruit, vegetables, yogurt, or lean meat.

◆ Fill in food-group gaps with nutrient-dense food group snacks.

◆ Avoid higher-fat or high-calorie snacks, such as candy bars.

◆ Time small snacks two to three hours before mealtime.

◆ Use the Nutrition Facts on food labels to compare snack choices.

✓ **Reading Check** **Discuss** How can you get the most nutrition from your next snack?

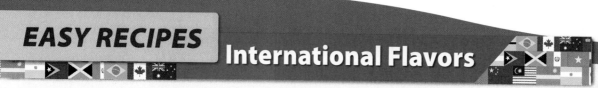

EASY RECIPES
International Flavors

Chicken Quesadillas

Customary	Ingredients	Metric
1	Jalapeno pepper	1
½ lb.	Grilled chicken breast, cut into cubes	250 g
1½ cups	Monterey Jack cheese, grated	375 mL
¼ cup	Green onion, chopped	60 mL
1 Tbsp.	Cilantro, chopped	15 mL
8 each	Corn tortillas	8 each
1 tsp.	Vegetable oil	5 mL

Try This!
Healthful Options
Serve with salsa. Add pinto or black beans to the quesadilla. You can also try it with beef or pork instead of chicken.

Yield: 4 servings, ⅓ pound, (150 g) each

❶ Cut open jalapeno pepper, remove and discard the seeds. Cut the pepper into tiny squares.
❷ Mix chicken, cheese, green onion, cilantro, and jalapeno in a bowl.
❸ Spread the mixture on the tops of four tortillas. Cover each with a second tortilla.
❹ Pour a little of the oil in a pan and cook the quesadilla until the cheese is melted and the two tortillas stick together. Flip the quesadilla once while cooking.
❺ Slice and serve.

Nutritional Information Per Serving: 301 calories, 12 g total fat, (6 g saturated fat), 55 mg cholesterol, 432 mg sodium, 26 g total carbohydrate (3 g fiber, 1 g total sugars), 23 g protein
Percent Daily Value: vitamin A 6%, vitamin C 4%, calcium 30%, iron 10%

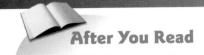

After You Read

CHAPTER SUMMARY

Successful meals and snacks should match your needs, preferences, resources, and skills. When you plan meals, you may need to make trade-offs to manage your time, energy, and budget. Breakfast provides food energy and nutrients for your day. Nutritious breakfasts can include easy-to-prepare, nutrient-dense foods you like. Meals can be light or hearty. Plan meals that provide enough food-group choices to meet your daily nutrient and energy needs. Appealing meals have a variety of colors, textures, temperatures, flavors, shapes, and sizes. Well-chosen snacks also provide nutrients and food energy.

Vocabulary Review

1. Use each of these vocabulary words in a sentence.

Content Vocabulary
- ◇ menu (p. 224)
- ◇ resources (p. 224)
- ◇ trade-off (p. 225)
- ◇ convenience food (p. 225)
- ◇ brunch (p. 228)
- ◇ appetizer (p. 229)

Academic Vocabulary
- ■ affect (p. 224)
- ■ valid (p. 226)

Review Key Concepts

2. Identify things to consider when you plan a meal.

3. Discuss why it is important to eat breakfast.

4. Explain how to pack a meal to eat away from home.

5. Describe the components of a meal.

6. List ways to make smart choices about snacking.

Critical Thinking

7. Compare and contrast the costs and benefits of making food from scratch versus using convenience foods.

8. Design a complete hearty dinner with roasted chicken as the main dish. Categorize the components of the meal and describe ways to make it nourishing and appealing.

9. Analyze the advantages of holding a potluck Thanksgiving dinner for 20 relatives of all ages. Explain strategies you could use to you reach your menu goals with the right variety of foods.

Real-World Skills and Applications

Set Goals and Make Decisions

10. Manage Resources Brainstorm three trade-offs you might make in managing resources for a meal. One example is cooking a side dish rather than buying it prepared. Explain why making trade-offs is important in good management.

Collaborative and Interpersonal

11. Interview a Meal Planner Interview someone who plans meals for large groups of people, such as the school's food-service director. What does he or she consider when planning meals? How are menus created? Summarize your interview.

Technology

12. Menu Costs Use a calculator to plan a nourishing dinner for your family for three different food budget levels. Plan each menu. Determine the costs for each ingredient. Figure the cost of the total menu. Then, figure the cost per person.

Financial Literacy

13. School Lunch Tyrell can buy lunch at the school cafeteria for $2. If he packs his own lunch at home, his average cost is $1.10. How much money could Tyrell save in a five-day week if he packs his lunch every day?

14. Ethnic Menus Using ethnic cookbooks or other sources, find a menu for a traditional meal from another culture. Create a visual presentation to show how it fits within the food groups. In what ways does it reflect the advice for meal appeal? How does it differ? What might explain the differences?

> **NCTE 1** Read texts to acquire new information.

15. Snack Record For three days, record what you eat for snacks and where, when, and with whom you eat them. Do you notice a pattern in your snacking? How often did you include food-group snacks in your eating plan? How could you improve your snack choices?

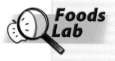

16. Popcorn Comparison Compare these different types of popcorn: popcorn popped on the stove top or in an air popper with no added butter or salt; and store-bought pre-bagged popcorn. Write a report describing the flavor, equipment and skills needed, cooking time, cost per serving, and fat and sodium content per serving. Prepare each type. Explain which popcorn you prefer, and why.

Additional Activities For additional activities go to this book's Online Learning Center at **glencoe.com**.

Academic Skills

English Language Arts

17. Healthful Breakfasts Create a public service announcement to promote smart breakfast eating. Include a catchy phrase that responds to common excuses for skipping breakfast. Record your announcement and present it to your class.

> **NCTE 12** Use language to accomplish individual purposes.

Science

18. Senses and the Menu Successful menus provide good nutrition and appeal to your senses. Your taste buds, nose, skin, and eyes evaluate food and send messages to your brain, which can signal saliva flow.

Procedure Track the sensory qualities in your meals over the next 2 to 3 days. What affects your desire to eat a meal?

Analysis Write a paragraph to describe how planning meals that appeal to your senses might help you eat for good nutrition, too.

> **NSES Content Standard F** Develop an understanding of personal and community health.

Mathematics

19. Make-Ahead Meals To save time and money, Brit's family cooks many meals in one day, then freezes them for later. Brit is making three meals of chili to freeze. She needs to increase the recipe for chili, which uses ⅔ cup of tomato sauce, by 3-fold. How much tomato sauce will she need?

Math Concept **Multiplying Rational Numbers** Whole numbers can be converted to fractions by using 1 as the denominator. Multiply the numerators and multiply the denominators, and simplify the answer.

Starting Hint Express the increase in the recipe as a fraction. Multiply the amount of tomato sauce needed for one recipe by this fraction. Then, simplify the answer in its lowest terms.

 For more math help, go to the Math Appendix

> **NCTM Number and Operations** Understand the meanings of operations and how they relate to one another.

STANDARDIZED TEST PRACTICE

ESSAY
Read the paragraph. Write your answer on a separate piece of paper.

> **Test-Taking Tip** In timed writing, you may feel the urge to rush. If you rush without a plan, you may lose focus. Instead, invest two or three minutes in planning.

Have you ever made an unhealthy eating choice because of convenience? Sometimes it seems easier to go through the drive-through than to buy the ingredients and make the meal. It takes planning to eat more healthfully, but it can be done!

20. Think about your own life and the choices you make about what to eat every day. How can you make healthful and practical choices? Write an essay describing a plan for your daily life.

CHAPTER 17
Shopping for Food

Explore the Photo ▶▶
You can use shopping skills to make smart decisions about flavor, nutrition, price, quality, safety, and convenience. *What affects your decisions when you shop for food?*

Writing Activity

"How-to" Paper

Business Communication Cooking for yourself requires preparation. Write a "How-to" paper that describes how to prepare for a shopping trip. Be detailed in your instructions and use clear, concise sentences.

Writing Tips

1. **List** all the steps in order.

2. **Name** all the materials you will need.

3. **Include** an introduction and a conclusion.

4. **Use** transition words and phrases.

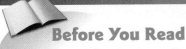

Before You Read

Prepare with a Partner Before you read, work with a partner. Read the headings and write down questions you both have about the chapter.

Read to Learn

Key Concepts

- **Outline** the components of a food shopping plan.
- **Identify** how to use food labels for smart shopping decisions.
- **Summarize** how to shop for value, quality, and food safety.
- **List** six ways to be a courteous customer when you shop.

Main Idea

Smart food shopping is important for wellness. Wise consumers choose foods for nutrition, quality, value, food safety, and their menu plan.

Content Vocabulary

- ◇ food budget
- ◇ impulse buying
- ◇ staples
- ◇ Nutrition Facts
- ◇ Daily Values
- ◇ nutrient content claim
- ◇ health claim
- ◇ comparison shopping
- ◇ unit price
- ◇ store brand
- ◇ generic brand
- ◇ national brand
- ◇ open dating

Academic Vocabulary

You will find these words in your reading and on your tests. Use the glossary to look up their definitions if necessary.

- ■ economic
- ■ estimate

Graphic Organizer

As you read, use a graphic organizer like the one below to list the six items that must be on a Nutrition Facts label.

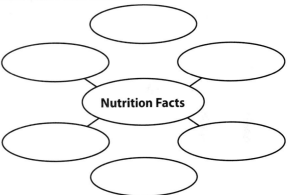

Nutrition Facts

 Graphic Organizer Go to this book's Online Learning Center at **glencoe.com** to print out this graphic organizer.

Academic Standards ■

 Mathematics

NCTM Number and Operations Compute fluently and make reasonable estimates.

NCTM Data Analysis and Probability Formulate questions that can be addressed with data and collect, organize, and display relevant data to answer them.

 English Language Arts

NCTE 4 Use written language to communicate effectively.

 Social Studies

NCSS IX D Global Connections Analyze the causes, consequences, and possible solutions to persistent, contemporary, and emerging global issues.

NCTE National Council of Teachers of English
NCTM National Council of Teachers of Mathematics

NSES National Science Education Standards
NCSS National Council for the Social Studies

Plan to Shop

A successful shopping plan starts by making decisions at home. How much can you spend? Where and when will you shop? Planning saves money, time, and effort.

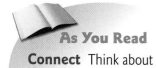

Vocabulary

You can find definitions in the glossary at the back of this book.

As You Read

Connect Think about how you make decisions when you go shopping.

Your Food Budget

Most families have a food budget. A **food budget** is an amount of money the family plans to spend on food. That may include food eaten at home and away from home. Plan menus within your budget, then make wise shopping decisions. You can plan appealing, nourishing menus on almost any budget.

Food prices depend on many **economic**, or cost-related, factors, such as processing, packaging, and transportation. Brand, product form and variety, packaging, and store type also affect price. Partly prepared or ready-to-eat foods may cost more. Fresh fruit and vegetables can cost more when they are out of season or when weather conditions result in smaller crop yields.

Check for food specials in newspapers and store flyers. Look for coupons, and plan menus around specially priced foods.

Your Shopping List

A shopping list is an important food budget management tool. A shopping list can help you:

◆ Shop faster and save money.

◆ Prevent impulse buying. **Impulse buying** is buying something you do not need just because it appeals to you.

◆ Avoid repeat trips to the store to buy items you forgot.

◆ Buy exactly what you need. Check your menu and list foods by amount and form. For example, do you need sliced or crushed canned pineapple?

◆ Ensure that you have enough staples. **Staples** are basic food items you keep on hand, such as rice or flour.

◆ Organize your shopping. You can group items according to store layout to save time.

Check Ahead Before You Shop A shopping list will help you save money and time. You will buy what you need for the menus you plan to prepare. *Why is it important to check what foods you have on hand before going to the store?*

Where to Shop

You have many choices when shopping for food. When deciding where to shop, consider location, prices, store hours, and the types of food sold. Choose clean stores that sell good-quality food, offer a good selection, and have helpful workers. Here are some examples of different types of places to shop for food:

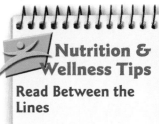

Nutrition & Wellness Tips

Read Between the Lines

✓ Read the Nutrition Facts on food labels to check the number of calories in foods promoted as fat-free.

- **Supermarkets** Supermarkets sell thousands of foods. They offer specials, food sampling, and coupons. Many also provide pharmacy, florist, or bank services.

- **Specialty Stores** These stores carry certain types of foods. Fish markets, butchers, bakeries, and ethnic food stores are specialty stores.

- **Convenience Stores** These small stores have a very limited selection of foods. Many sell lots of packaged snack foods. The price of food at convenience stores is usually much higher than at other types of food stores.

- **Food Cooperatives** Co-ops buy food in large quantities and sell to members at lower prices. Variety may be limited.

- **Farmers' Markets** These markets often sell locally grown and produced foods. Most are open for limited times during growing and harvest seasons. In some areas, farmers' markets are open year-round.

- **Warehouse or Discount Stores** These are similar to supermarkets, but food is often sold in larger quantities and at lower prices.

- **Online Stores** Some stores sell groceries online, including specialty and regional foods. Buying food from online stores can be very expensive because you are paying a higher fee for the convenience of having the food selected and delivered to you.

When to Shop

How often you buy food depends on your schedule, your storage space, and your personal preferences. Some people prefer to buy their food fresh every day. This requires more time. Other people prefer to shop just once a week. This saves time. You can also shop when the store is not crowded to save time.

Shop when you are not hungry. Hungry shoppers often buy more food than they need. A hungry shopper is much more likely to make impulse buys of snack foods, too.

✓ **Reading Check** **Recall** Where can you buy food?

Read Food Labels

By law, food labels must provide the food's name and its description, amount, ingredients, Nutrition Facts, manufacturer or distributor, and allergen labeling if allergens are present. (See **Figure 17.1**.) The U.S. Food and Drug Administration regulates food labels, except for those on meat and poultry. The U.S. Department of Agriculture regulates meat and poultry labels.

Food Labels list important information that will help you analyze the foods you may eat or drink. Use them to make decisions toward the most healthful choices for your nutritional needs.

Figure 17.1	Food Labels

Food Label Information Food labels provide valuable information to help you make wise food choices. *How might you use food labels to choose canned chicken broth with less sodium?*

DESCRIPTION	The description tells about the food and how it is prepared.
AMOUNT	This lists the quantity of the food by volume or by net weight without the weight of the container.
NUTRITION AND HEALTH INFORMATION	Information about the calories and nutrients is on the Nutrition Facts part of the label. This also may include health claims.
FOOD EXCHANGES	This information helps people with diabetes make food choices. It is based on Exchange Lists for Meal Planning from the American Diabetes Association and the American Dietetic Association.
INGREDIENTS	All ingredients, including additives, are listed by weight, from most to least.
ALLERGEN LABELING	The common allergens peanuts, eggs, wheat, tree nuts, soybeans, shellfish, fish, and milk are listed.
DIRECTIONS	This tells how to store or prepare the food. Sometimes there is a recipe.
MANUFACTURER/ DISTRIBUTOR	The name, address, and Web site of the company that makes or distributes the product appears on the label.
UNIVERSAL PRODUCT CODE (UPC)	The UPC identifies the item with a bar code. At checkout, a scanner reads the item and price. The UPC also helps track inventory.
FRESHNESS DATE	Some foods, especially perishable foods, are dated.

Check for Nutrition Information

Use food labels to find answers to these questions and choose foods that provide the calories and nutrients you need. The following is some of the information you may find on food packaging.

- ◆ **Nutrition Facts** provide specific information about the nutrition in one serving of the food. Use this information to compare the calories and nutrients in different foods. (See **Figure 17.2**.) Nutrition Facts are based on **Daily Values**, the recommended amounts in an eating plan. The Daily Values helps you judge how much of a nutrient each serving provides.

- ◆ A **nutrient content claim** states that a food has more or less of a nutrient or food substance: for example, that the food is low-fat. Foods must meet government criteria to carry these claims. (See **Figure 17.3** on page 241.)

- ◆ A **health claim** states that a food provides health benefits, for example, "lowers the risk of cancer." Claims must be based on scientific evidence.

- ◆ A structure or function claim states that a nutrient or food substance provides a benefit in the body, for example, "helps maintain bone health." These claims are also regulated.

Figure 17.2 Nutrition Facts

Nutrition Lists Nutrition Facts on labels can help you choose foods for the nutrients and calories they provide. *What if you ate two servings?*

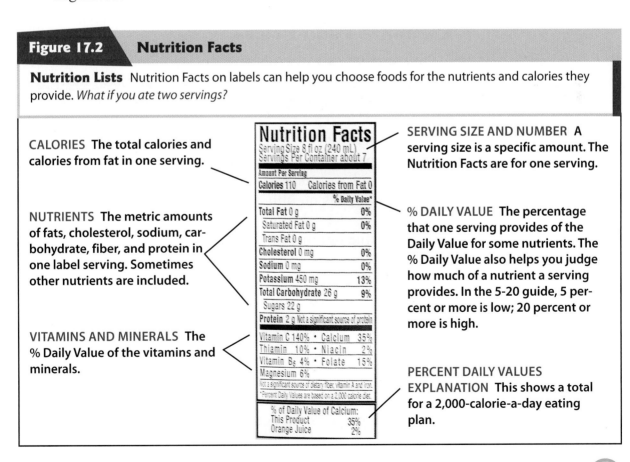

CALORIES The total calories and calories from fat in one serving.

NUTRIENTS The metric amounts of fats, cholesterol, sodium, carbohydrate, fiber, and protein in one label serving. Sometimes other nutrients are included.

VITAMINS AND MINERALS The % Daily Value of the vitamins and minerals.

SERVING SIZE AND NUMBER A serving size is a specific amount. The Nutrition Facts are for one serving.

% DAILY VALUE The percentage that one serving provides of the Daily Value for some nutrients. The % Daily Value also helps you judge how much of a nutrient a serving provides. In the 5-20 guide, 5 percent or more is low; 20 percent or more is high.

PERCENT DAILY VALUES EXPLANATION This shows a total for a 2,000-calorie-a-day eating plan.

Nutrition Facts
Serving Size 8 fl oz (240 mL)
Servings Per Container about 7

Amount Per Serving
Calories 110   Calories from Fat 0

	% Daily Value*
Total Fat 0 g	0%
Saturated Fat 0 g	0%
Trans Fat 0 g	
Cholesterol 0 mg	0%
Sodium 0 mg	0%
Potassium 450 mg	13%
Total Carbohydrate 26 g	9%
Sugars 22 g	
Protein 2 g Not a significant source of protein	

Vitamin C 140% • Calcium 35%
Thiamin 10% • Niacin 2%
Vitamin B₆ 4% • Folate 15%
Magnesium 6%

Not a significant source of dietary fiber, vitamin A and iron.
*Percent Daily Values are based on a 2,000 calorie diet.

% of Daily Value of Calcium:
This Product   35%
Orange Juice   2%

Grocery Store Worker

Grocery store workers stock shelves and help customers. Other jobs in grocery stores include butchers, bakers, checkout clerks, and produce and dairy managers.

Careers Find out more about careers. Go to this book's Online Learning Center at **glencoe.com**.

Other Label Information

Food labels provide other information to help you shop wisely and make informed decisions about your food choices. You may see these words on food packaging:

◆ **Organic** A food may be produced to be 100 percent organic, or it may be considered organic with 95 percent organic ingredients. These terms are regulated by the U.S. Department of Agriculture. Look for the USDA Organic seal.

◆ **Natural** This means that the food is not processed very much. The label must also explain why it is natural—for example, if it has no artificial ingredients.

◆ **Fresh** This term can be used only on raw food that has not been frozen, heated, or treated with preservatives.

✓ **Reading Check** **Identify** By law, what information must appear on a food label?

Shop for Value, Quality, and Food Safety

At the food store, you can put your shopping skills to work. Use your shopping list, and compare prices, amounts, and nutrition information.

Compare Food Prices

You have many ways to save money on food. One of the best ways is to use comparison shopping. **Comparison shopping** is comparing prices of different forms, container sizes, and brands in order to get the best value for your dollar.

You can use the unit price to compare costs for similar foods and different-size packages. The **unit price** on the shelf tag tells how much an ounce, pound, or other unit of the item costs. If the shelf tag has no unit price, **estimate**, or use your knowledge to guess, what the unit price would be. Divide the price of the item by the number of units.

To save money, you can use coupons and look for store specials. You can also buy store brands or generic brands. A **store brand** is used for a supermarket's own product. Store brands often cost less than national brands. A **generic brand** is a brand that usually has a plain label and no brand name. Generic brands usually cost the least. A **national brand** is a brand sold by major food companies. National brands are usually more expensive because they include the cost of promotions and advertising. Finally, you can sign up for frequent-customer cards. Some stores give customers with these cards special savings.

Buy the Right Amount

A larger container often costs less per unit, but not always. Check the unit price of each item. Buy a large size only if you can store it properly and use it all before it spoils. If not, you will waste food and money.

Buy only what you need of perishable foods, which may spoil quickly. Fresh fruits and vegetables, meat, chicken, fish, eggs, and milk are perishable.

If packages of meat or produce contain more than you want, ask a butcher or store clerk to package a smaller amount.

Figure 17.3	Nutrient Content Claims

Label Language Certain label terms are defined by the government. They can be used on the label only if the product meets the requirements. *How can nutrient content claims on labels help you?*

Nutrient Content Claims	What the Claims Mean	Other Terms
Free	An amount so small it probably has no effect. *For example:* Fat-free means less than 0.5 gram of fat per label serving.	no, zero, without, insignificant
Low	An amount defined as low for each nutrient or substance, or for calories. *For example:* Low-fat means 3 grams of fat (or less) per label serving.	few, little, contains a small amount of
Reduced	An amount describing a food with at least 25 percent less calories, fat, saturated fat, cholesterol, sugars, or sodium than a regular food.	fewer, lower, less
High	An amount that is 20 percent or more of the Daily Value for a nutrient. *For example:* High in calcium means at least 200 milligrams of calcium per label serving.	rich in, excellent source of
Good source	An amount that is 10 to 19 percent or more of the Daily Value for a nutrient. *For example:* Good source of calcium means 100 to 190 milligrams of calcium per label serving.	contains, provides
More	An amount that is 10 percent or more of the Daily Value for a nutrient. *For example:* More iron means at least 1.8 milligrams of iron per label serving.	enriched, fortified, added, extra, plus
Lean	Less than 10 grams of fat, 4.5 grams or less of saturated fat, and less than 95 milligrams of cholesterol per 3-ounce cooked serving.	Less fat
Light	One-third fewer calories or 50 percent less fat than the traditional version. Or, 50 percent less sodium than the traditional food. Sometimes, light also describes the food itself, such as light brown sugar. In these instances, it is not a nutrient content claim.	Lite

Choose the Right Form of Food

Many foods are sold fresh, frozen, or canned. Canned, frozen, and cooked fresh vegetables and fruits have about the same nutrient content. You can decide which is best for you by comparison shopping. Store them properly to keep their nutrients.

All forms of fruits and vegetables—fresh, frozen, and canned—provide important nutrients in a nutritious meal plan. The price of fresh fruits and vegetables may be lower or higher at different times of the year. Fresh fruits and vegetables are often more flavorful when they are in season—but they cannot be stored for long. Canned and frozen products are convenient. Canned foods are cooked already. They can be stored the longest.

Foods are also sold in different forms: for example, whole, sliced, or chopped. Read the description on the label. Choose the right form for the food you will prepare.

Sometimes you may choose to pay an additional amount as a trade-off for convenience. A frozen dinner probably costs more than the same homemade meal—unless you need to buy more ingredients than you will use in that meal.

Shop for Food Safety and Quality

Food bought at its peak contains the most nutrients. Follow these guidelines to shop with food safety and quality in mind:

♦ Look for undamaged containers. Give bulging, rusted, or dented cans or broken containers to a clerk. Check safety seals and buttons.

♦ Handle fresh fruits and vegetables gently. Bruised fruits and vegetables spoil faster.

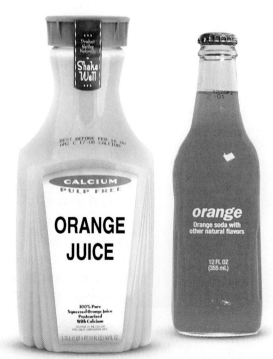

Which Would You Buy? Drinks with an orange flavor are not always juice. A product that is all juice will say 100% juice on the label. *Which of these beverages is all juice? What can you learn from the ingredient list?*

- Fill your cart and grocery bags carefully so fruits, vegetables, and other soft foods are not bruised or crushed.
- Buy refrigerated and frozen foods last or they may get warm.
- Be sure all refrigerated items feel cold.
- Be sure frozen food packages are frozen solid. Ice crystals or discoloration may mean that the package has thawed and been refrozen.
- Put raw meat, poultry, and fish in plastic bags. This will prevent their juices from leaking onto other foods.

Open Dating

Some foods have dates stamped on the package. **Open dating** means the packages are marked with dates that help consumers know about how long the product will be fresh. For example, the package may read "Sell by May 31" or "Best if used by June 8." A sell-by date means you can buy food by this date and still store it for a reasonable time. A best-if-used-by date tells when food is at its peak quality. Some foods, like bakery items, have packing dates. These dates relate to peak quality when foods were packed, not food safety.

After You Shop

The way food is handled and stored affects quality and safety. Take food home and store it right away. Milk, meat, and other perishable foods, as well as hot and cold take-out foods, need to be refrigerated. Frozen food must be kept frozen. Follow the safety information found on all of your packages.

✓ **Reading Check** **List** What are three ways you could save money at the supermarket?

Customer Courtesy

Courtesy from customers makes shopping more pleasant for everyone. Follow these guidelines to be courteous while shopping:
- **As You Shop** Return food you do not want to its proper place. Politely ask a clerk if you need help. Be patient when you wait your turn at the service counters. If you break something, get a clerk for clean-up. Do not block traffic by leaving your cart in the middle of the aisle.

- ◆ **At the Checkout Counter** Take your cart out of line if you have forgotten something so that you will not keep others waiting. Use the express checkout lane only if you have the number of items allowed. If you scan products yourself, follow directions. Have your coupons and payment ready.

- ◆ **In the Parking Lot** Take your shopping cart to the cart return so it will not damage cars or get in the way of traffic. Park in a handicapped space only if you are qualified to do so.

You can also make food shopping smoother and more fun by sharing the responsibility with friends and family members. Break your list into two or more parts, and each tackle one. You can help others by picking up groceries for an elderly or ill neighbor or a busy friend.

✓ **Reading Check** **Recall** What are three ways you can be courteous at the checkout counter?

EASY RECIPES — Everyday Favorites

Fruit Salad

Customary	Ingredients	Metric
1 cup	Green grapes, halved	250 mL
2 tsp.	Lemon juice	10 mL
2 each	Apples, cored, sliced	2 each
½ cup	Dried cranberries or raisins	½ cup
1 can (6 oz)	Mandarin oranges, drained	1 can (185 mL)
1	Banana	1 each

Try This!
Substitute other fresh and canned fruits.

Yield: 8 servings, ½ cup (125 g) each

1. Put apples in a medium bowl and mix with the lemon juice.
2. Carefully slice the grapes into halves and add to the bowl.
3. Add the grapes, mandarin oranges, and cranberries or raisins to the bowl.
4. Peel and slice the banana and add to the other fruit. Mix gently.

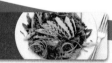

Nutritional Information Per Serving: 78 calories, 0 g total fat (0 g saturated fat), 0 mg cholesterol, 1 mg sodium, 20 g total carbohydrate (2 g fiber, 16 g total sugars), 1 g protein

Percent Daily Value: vitamin A 4%, vitamin C 20%, calcium 0%, iron 2%

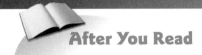

After You Read

CHAPTER SUMMARY

A shopping plan can help you save money, time, and effort. You may buy food in many places. Food labels provide information to compare foods. Use comparison shopping, unit pricing, open dating, coupons, and food specials to get more for your money. Buy the amount and form of food you will use. Remember food quality and safety. Be courteous as you shop.

Vocabulary Review

1. Use each of these vocabulary words in a sentence.

Content Vocabulary
- food budget (p. 236)
- impulse buying (p. 236)
- staples (p. 236)
- Nutrition Facts (p. 239)
- Daily Values (p. 239)
- nutrient content claim (p. 239)
- health claim (p. 239)
- comparison shopping (p. 240)
- unit price (p. 240)
- store brand (p. 240)
- generic brand (p. 240)
- national brand (p. 240)
- open dating (p. 243)

Academic Vocabulary
- economic (p. 236)
- estimate (p. 240)

Review Key Concepts

2. Outline the components of a food shopping plan.

3. Identify how to use food labels for smart shopping decisions.

4. Summarize how to shop for value, quality, and food safety.

5. List six ways to be a courteous customer when you shop.

Critical Thinking

6. Analyze the unit prices of two food items your family buys regularly. Conduct research to determine if your family is getting the best value.

7. Compare and contrast the label information on two different kinds of cereal.

8. Create a shopping plan for a family dinner menu. List smart shopping strategies.

9. Compare and contrast the time and resources involved in going on one major food shopping trip weekly, compared with several smaller ones.

Real-World Skills and Applications

Decision Making

10. Food Budgets Explain the factors that help a family decide how much money to spend on food. Why might one family need to spend a larger percentage of its income on food than another family? Write your answer in two or more paragraphs. Give specific examples.

Collaborative and Interpersonal

11. Label Information As a class, gather a variety of food labels. Include labels for all food groups and for several mixed foods. Using the Nutrition Facts, arrange the products from most to least per label serving for calories and then for different nutrients. Draw conclusions, and create a summary of your findings.

Technology

12. Electronic Shopping List Use spreadsheet software to create a checklist of foods for your family's shopping list. Include staples and items your family buys often. Categorize items by their store location where you usually shop. Use the list while shopping. Report any changes you would make and why.

Financial Literacy

13. Unit Pricing When you go shopping at the supermarket, you find that dry pasta costs $1.10 for a 12-ounce bag. Another bag of pasta costs $1.20 for a 16-ounce bag. Calculate the unit price, or price per ounce. Which is the best value? Show the calculations in your answer.

14. Price Comparison Compare the prices of the same food sold in several ways: national brand vs. store brand; economy size vs. regular size; supermarket vs. discount or warehouse store; canned vs. frozen. For each comparison, describe the pros and cons.

15. Supermarket Tour Tour a nearby supermarket. Find an unfamiliar food product. Use the package label, unit pricing, and other store resources, including store workers, to write a brief description of each product. Explain which of these foods you might buy and why.

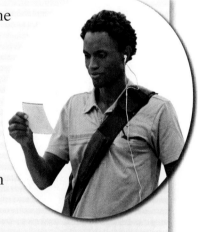

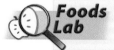

16. Compare Bread Conduct a taste test of four kinds of bread, with three having at least one whole-grain ingredient. Write a summary of the taste test that rates the breads for flavor, texture, appeal, and price. Analyze the label information. How do the breads compare nutritionally? Which would you buy, and why?

 Additional Activities For additional activities go to this book's Online Learning Center at glencoe.com.

Academic Skills

English Language Arts

17. Food Packaging Imagine that you work for a food company. Write the text for the packaging of a new healthful convenience food. Sketch the design. Include Nutrition Facts. Make appropriate factual claims that promote the product to people your age.

NCTE 4 Use written language to communicate effectively.

Social Studies

18. Shopping Frequency In many parts of the world, kitchens may have small refrigerators. In some places, electricity may not be readily available. Research how these factors might affect food shopping habits. Present your results in a report to your class.

NCSS IX D Global Connections Analyze the causes, consequences, and possible solutions to persistent, contemporary, and emerging global issues.

Mathematics

19. Food Budget Lin Bailey wants to compare the ways her family spends money on food. Create a pie chart to show the Bailey's weekly food budget. The family of four spends $250 per week, with $25 spent in restaurants, $20 on fast food, $10 on school meals, and $195 on groceries. Organize the pie chart by category.

Math Concept **Statistics** Statistics involves collecting, analyzing, and presenting data. The data can then be shown in tables and graphs.

Starting Hint Determine the percentage of each amount by dividing the category amount by the total amount. Use the percentages to create a pie chart.

 For more math help, go to the Math Appendix

NCTM Data Analysis and Probability Formulate questions that can be addressed with data and collect, organize, and display relevant data to answer them.

STANDARDIZED TEST PRACTICE

MULTIPLE CHOICE
Read the paragraph. Write your answer on a separate piece of paper.

Test-Taking Tip When you sit down to take a math test, jot down on your scrap paper important equations or formulas that you want to remember. This way, you will not worry about forgetting them during the test.

You could buy a head of lettuce for 79¢. Or you could buy an 8-oz. bag of lettuce for $3.19. The bag contains different varieties of prewashed lettuce, as well as shreds of radish and carrots.

20. Based on the paragraph, which of the following statements is true?
  a. Lettuce heads are not a good deal.
  b. Bags of salad are always a good deal.
  c. You may choose to pay for convenience as well as the food.
  d. Buying lettuce is too expensive.

CHAPTER 18
Eating Well When Away from Home

Explore the Photo ▶▶
On average, people in the United States eat about 25 percent of their meals away from home. *How does eating away from home affect your overall eating plan?*

Writing Activity

Cause-and-Effect Paragraph

Customer Comments Running a restaurant is a complex business. Write a cause-and-effect paragraph that explains a situation in a restaurant that has a consequence. If the service is excellent, for example, the business may become very successful.

Writing Tips

1. **Write** a clear introduction.
2. **Use** appropriate transitions to show the relation between the cause and the effect.
3. **Include** an introduction and a conclusion.

Before You Read

Use Notes Have a notepad on hand when you are reading the chapter. When you find unfamiliar ideas or terms, write them down. After you have finished reading, find answers for your questions.

Read to Learn

Key Concepts
- **Describe** factors to consider when choosing a restaurant.
- **Explain** how to make smart menu choices.
- **Describe** courteous behavior when you eat away from home.
- **Explain** how to handle a restaurant bill.

Main Idea

It is important to make wise choices when you eat away from home. Restaurant courtesy and menu knowledge are important.

Content Vocabulary

◇ entrée
◇ cuisine
◇ à la carte

 Graphic Organizer Go to this book's Online Learning Center at **glencoe.com** to print out this graphic organizer.

Academic Vocabulary

You will find these words in your reading and on your tests. Use the glossary to look up their definitions if necessary.

▪ regulation
▪ sequence

Graphic Organizer

As you read, fill in a web diagram like the one below. Fill in the surrounding circles with information you find in this chapter.

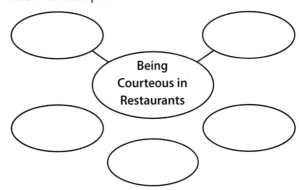

Being Courteous in Restaurants

Academic Standards ▪

 English Language Arts
NCTE 5 Use different writing process elements to communicate effectively.
NCTE 9 Develop an understanding of diversity in language use across cultures.
NCTE 12 Use language to accomplish individual purposes.

 Mathematics
NCTM Number and Operations Understand numbers, ways of representing numbers, relationships among numbers, and number systems.

 Science
NSES Content Standard F Develop an understanding of personal and community health.

 Social Studies
NCSS IA Culture Analyze and explain the ways groups, societies, and cultures address human needs and concerns.

NCTE	National Council of Teachers of English	**NSES**	National Science Education Standards
NCTM	National Council of Teachers of Mathematics	**NCSS**	National Council for the Social Studies

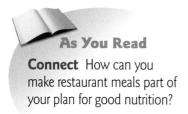

As You Read

Connect How can you make restaurant meals part of your plan for good nutrition?

Restaurant Choices

When you are away from home, you may choose where to eat depending on what you want to eat, where you are, how much time you have, and what you can afford. Be sure to know your options, needs, budget, and time. Before you pick a restaurant, consider the cost, the types of food served, variety on the menu, nutrition in the foods served, type of service, and cleanliness, as well as the restaurant's suitability for your special needs or preferences.

Cost, Speed, and Service

Table-service restaurants, where servers take orders at the table, often cost more than other places. Eating at these restaurants takes time, and you get personal service. If you have special food needs or preferences, servers are usually happy to accommodate you. It may be worth it to spend more for table service for special or relaxed meals.

Fast-food counters, cafeterias, self-service buffets, and delis have limited menus. This may mean that you have fewer choices for healthful living. Service is usually faster but less personal. Remember that quick may not mean inexpensive. Be sure to check prices carefully.

Cleanliness Counts

When you choose a place to eat, look around. Is everything clean? Public health **regulations**, or rules, require strict sanitation to prevent foodborne illness. If you see signs that food safety and cleanliness are neglected, talk to the manager.

✓ **Reading Check** **Explain** How would you choose a restaurant?

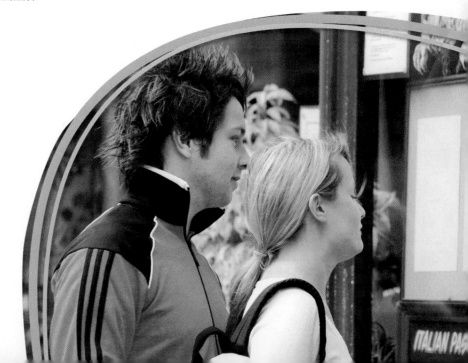

Check the Menu Some restaurants post menus outside to help you decide if you want to eat there. *If you had to choose between a fast-food and a table-service restaurant, what would influence your decision?*

Make Smart Menu Choices

Most menus are organized in a **sequence**, or specific order: appetizers or starters, salads, soups, entrées, side dishes, desserts, and drinks. An **entrée** is a main dish. To make smart menu choices, get information from the menu, order to match your nutrition needs, understand menu terms, and be careful about portion sizes and how much you eat.

Get Information

Learn about different cuisines and menu terms. **Cuisine** refers to specific foods and cooking styles. Make sure to:

◆ Check signs, leaflets, and Web sites for information about the food served.

◆ Ask the server. Most servers can describe ingredients, preparation techniques, and portion sizes.

◆ Read the menu thoroughly.

Order for Nutrition and Variety

Make an effort to make nutritional choices when eating away from home. Order sandwiches on whole-wheat bread. Add vegetables to burgers, sandwiches, and pizza. Choose salad, slaw, or another vegetable side dish. Order low-fat or fat-free milk.

Order Lighter Menu Options

Calories can add up quickly when you dine out. Understand preparation methods, side dishes, and toppings so that you can order to match your nutrition and calorie needs.

◆ **Preparation Methods** Choose baked or broiled fish, meat, or poultry for less fat and fewer calories. Buy nutrient-dense snacks.

◆ **Side Dishes** Ask about side dishes. Order a lower-calorie item à la carte when you can. **À la carte** means without side dishes.

◆ **Toppings** Salad dressing, butter, cream sauce, and gravy often have a lot of calories and fat. Order dressings and toppings on the side, food without the topping, or a lower-fat alternative.

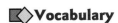

Vocabulary

You can find definitions in the glossary at the back of this book.

Science in Action

Evaluate Menu Options

Some menus carry nutrient content claims such as low-fat or low-sodium. Federal laws that apply to these terms on packaged food labels also apply to restaurant menus.

Procedure Get a menu from a restaurant or a restaurant's Web site that claims to have healthful menu options. Evaluate how much more healthful the healthful options are than similar items on the menu. You may need to do research on nutrition information to evaluate the healthfulness of the options.

Analysis Record your findings in a chart. Include how the ingredients differ and the nutrition information for each menu option. Write a paragraph about your observations. Reflect on how the more healthful options compared to the other options.

NSES Content Standard F
Develop an understanding of personal and community health.

Understand Menu Terms

The words used on menus can help you make healthful choices. These terms are clues to the nutrients and calories of menu items:

◆ Breaded, buttered, creamed, deep-fried, and rich suggest more calories and fat.

◆ Broiled, cooked in its own juices, grilled, steamed, and stir-fried suggest fewer calories and less fat.

◆ Cured, pickled, smoked, and prepared with soy sauce suggest more sodium.

◆ Au Gratin means topped with bread crumbs or grated cheese.

◆ Au Jus means the dish is served in the juices from roasting.

◆ Florentine means the dish is served with spinach.

◆ Primavera means the dish is prepared with fresh vegetables.

◆ Scalloped means the dish is baked in a cream sauce.

Restaurant Portions

Restaurant portions are often bigger than you need. Ask for a half portion, or split an order with someone. Order an appetizer and side dish without an entrée. If you are served a larger portion than you should eat, eat some food at the restaurant and take the rest home.

✓ **Reading Check** **Explain** How can you avoid eating too many calories when you dine out?

Use Good Restaurant Manners

Good manners and courtesy make eating together pleasant for everyone. Knowing what to do also keeps everyone comfortable. In a fast-food place, remove your tray from the table and discard any waste.

Get Your Table

When you plan to dine at a table-service restaurant, call ahead to reserve a table. Arrive on time. Give your name, the number of guests, and the time you prefer. Call to cancel the reservation if you cannot go.

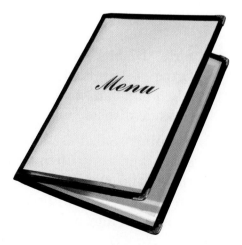

When arriving at a restaurant with or without a reservation, let the host or hostess lead you to a table unless a sign says to seat yourself.

Be Courteous

During your visit to a restaurant, be patient and considerate. Follow these other tips to be courteous:

◆ Catch the server's attention with eye contact and a smile.

◆ Tell your server politely if anything is wrong.

◆ Thank the server, especially for handling special requests.

◆ Leave a tip for service.

◆ Talk quietly. Do not talk to others at another table, unless you quietly go there. Conversations should not bother others.

✓ Reading Check **Describe** What are three ways to show courtesy to the server at a restaurant?

Pay the Bill

Handle the bill politely. If everyone will pay separately, ask for separate checks before ordering. You also can let one person pay, then settle the bill together later. When someone else is paying, be thoughtful of the cost.

Discover International Foods

Vietnam

The food of Vietnam reflects ingredients produced in Southeast Asia, and the Chinese and French who once ruled there. The cuisine uses vegetables, fruits, rice, and noodles. Noodles are made from wheat, rice, and mung beans. They are served in soup, salads, and stir-fries, and mixed with meat, fish, herbs, and vegetables. Nuoc mam (*nü-'äk 'mäm*), a reddish fish sauce made of fermented anchovies, adds flavor to many Vietnamese dishes. Most dishes are not spicy hot. Fruit is a popular dessert: oranges, bananas, starfruit, rambutans, and loquats are favorite fruits.

Languages Across Cultures

pho *(fō)* noodle dish; as translated "your own bowl." Pho bo is beef-noodle soup seasoned with cinnamon, cloves, and ginger and made with lime, bean sprouts, and onion.

goi cuon *(gòi cuốn)* mixed salad roll with pork, shrimp, herbs, and rice vermicelli wrapped in rice paper.

 Recipes Find out more about international recipes on this book's Online Learning Center at **glencoe.com**.

NCTE 9 Develop an understanding of diversity in language use across cultures.

Discuss any mistake on the bill quietly with the server. Place your money or credit card with the bill so the server sees it. Leave the tip on the table, or add it to you credit card bill. The standard tip for good service is 15 to 20 percent of the bill before tax. Leave at least 50 cents on small orders.

✓ **Reading Check** **Explain** How should you handle a bill if more than one person will pay?

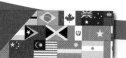

EASY RECIPES · International Flavors

Vietnamese Spring Rolls

Customary	Ingredients	Metric
4	Rice paper wrappers	4
½ cup	Rice vinegar	125 mL
½ cup	Sugar	125 mL
1 Tbsp.	Fresh mint	15 mL
½ Tbsp.	Fish sauce	8 mL
1 tsp.	Ginger, minced	5 mL
1 tsp.	Lemon juice	5 mL
2	Carrots, medium size	2
4	Green lettuce leaves	4
8	Cooked shrimp, cold	8

> **Vietnamese Flavors**
>
> Substitute cooked chicken or pork. Try using sprouts or cabbage instead of carrots.

Yield: 4 servings, one roll each.

1. Submerge rice paper wrappers in cold water to rehydrate them.
2. Combine rice vinegar, sugar, mint, fish sauce, ginger and lemon juice in a bowl. Chill for at least one hour.
3. Cut carrots into thin strips about 2 inches long.
4. Dry and spread out one of the rice paper wrappers. Lay down one of the lettuce leaves on top. Near one side, lay down two shrimp. Top with carrot strips and sprinkle with extra mint.
5. Roll up starting from the side with the shrimp. Stop halfway through, tuck in the sides and finish rolling up. Slice the roll diagonally across the middle. Repeat with the other three wrappers.
6. Serve cold with chilled sauce for dipping.

Nutritional Information Per Serving: 150 calories, 1 g total fat, (0 g saturated fat), 22 mg cholesterol, 236 mg sodium, 35 g total carbohydrate (2 g fiber, 28 g sugars), 4 g protein

Percent Daily Value: vitamin A 130%, vitamin C 10%, calcium 4%, iron 8%

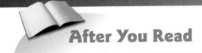

After You Read

CHAPTER SUMMARY

Where you dine out depends on what you want to eat, where you are, how much time you have, and your budget. Your knowledge of MyPyramid and the Dietary Guidelines can guide your food choices. Order a variety of nutrient-rich foods, be cautious about portion sizes, and understand preparation methods and menu terms so you can order carefully to control calories and fat. Good manners make eating out pleasant for everyone. During a visit to a restaurant, be patient and considerate. Paying the bill courteously is part of restaurant manners.

Vocabulary Review

1. Use each of these vocabulary words in a sentence.

Content Vocabulary
- ◇ entrée (p. 251)
- ◇ cuisine (p. 251)
- ◇ à la carte (p. 251)

Academic Vocabulary
- ■ regulation (p. 250)
- ■ sequence (p. 251)

Review Key Concepts

2. Describe factors to consider when choosing a restaurant.

3. Explain how to make smart menu choices.

4. Describe courteous behavior when you eat away from home.

5. Explain how to handle a restaurant bill.

Critical Thinking

6. Examine sources of information you would consult if you plan to go to a restaurant with someone who has a food allergy.

7. Compare and contrast how a teen can make healthful choices or unhealthful choices while eating at fast-food restaurants.

8. Evaluate how eating at school is different from eating in a restaurant.

9. Analyze why you might have a better dining experience at a restaurant if you are courteous to the server and to others around you.

Real-World Skills and Applications

Goal Setting and Decision Making

10. Restaurant Job Imagine that your goal is to be a server in a table-service restaurant for an after-school job. What steps might you take to prepare for the interview and the job to reach your goal? Write a paragraph outlining these steps.

Collaborative and Interpersonal

11. Restaurant Manners With your teacher's permission, form groups and discuss a negative or uncomfortable situation you may encounter in a resturant. Creatively present ways to resolve the problem in positive ways to your class. Role-play the situation for your class.

Technology

12. Create a Restaurant Menu Choose a name and theme for a new restaurant you would like to open. Design a menu using a graphics program. Include nutrition information. Share your menu with your class.

Financial Literacy

13. Split the Bill Three friends go out to eat and split the bill equally. The bill lists two entrées for $4.95, one entrée for $6.25, three drinks for $1.50, a dessert for $5.75, and a side order for $1.25. Each friend decides to tip 20%. How much does each friend owe?

14. Vending Machine Survey You can buy food away from home from vending machines. Conduct a vending machine survey to identify the types of foods and drinks sold. Include container sizes and prices. Analyze your findings for nutrition, variety, price, and other factors. Draw conclusions.

15. Ethnic Food Restaurants Get a menu from an ethnic restaurant. Go online if needed. Decide which menu items are your best choices for good nutrition. Explain how to get information about the menu. In class, list your options and explain your choices.

> **NCTE 12** Use language to accomplish individual purposes.

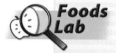

16. Analyze Fast Food Find a recipe for a taco salad and prepare it. Compare the recipe to a specific fast-food version of a taco salad. Use information from the fast-food restaurant chain to find out about the nutritional value of the fast food. Compare the taste, appeal, calories, nutrients, and cost. Identify ways to make the homemade version more healthful than the fast-food version. Share your analysis and conclusions in class.

Additional Activities For additional activities go to this book's Online Learning Center at glencoe.com.

Academic Skills

 English Language Arts

17. Menu Dictionary Using local and online restaurant menus, create a dictionary with at least 10 menu terms. Include pronunciation guides for unfamiliar terms. Note whether the term gives clues to the nutrient or calorie content. Compile a class menu dictionary.

> **NCTE 5** Use different writing process elements to communicate effectively.

 Social Studies

18. Ethnic Utensils In America, most dishes are eaten with forks, spoons, and knives. In some other countries, some dishes are eaten with bare hands or chopsticks. Choose an ethnic dish that is not eaten in the traditional American manner. Describe the dish, identify its place of origin, and describe how to eat it properly.

> **NCSS IA Culture** Analyze and explain the ways groups, societies, and cultures address human needs and concerns.

 Mathematics

19. Delivery Tipping Servers and deliverers count on tips to bring their pay up to minimum wage. If you order a pizza delivered to your home, figure a reasonable tip by estimating 15% of the cost of the pizza before any delivery fee. What would you tip a person bringing you a pizza costing $15.99, including a $1.00 delivery fee?

Math Concept **Percent** A percent (%) is a ratio that compares a number to 100. Convert a fraction to a decimal by dividing the numerator by the denominator.

Starting Hint Find first how much the pizza itself costs before the delivery fee. Then, find 15% of the pizza's cost for a tip. Round up to the nearest tenth.

 For more math help, go to the Math Appendix

> **NCTM Number and Operations** Understand numbers, ways of representing numbers, relationships among numbers, and number systems.

STANDARDIZED TEST PRACTICE

MULTIPLE CHOICE
Read the paragraph and choose the best answer to the question. Write your answer on a separate piece of paper:

> **Test-Taking Tip** Choose a vocabulary word you need to learn, write it on a sticky-note, then write its definition in your own words. Post the note in a place where you will see it throughout your day.

Most American restaurants serve overly large portions. This is often a way to promote the restaurant and make the meal look like a good value. Plan on bringing home excess food when you dine out so that you do not overeat.

20. Based on the paragraph, which of the following statements is true?
   a. Planning ahead can help keep you from overeating.
   b. All restaurants serve too much food.
   c. Restaurants want people to overeat.
   d. Restaurants rely on dietitians.

Unit 6 Thematic Project

Consider Nutritional Information

Nutritional information is factual information. Advertisements designed to sell food, however, do not always reveal the truth about the food. Being a critical consumer of information can help you make smart food choices.

My Journal

If you completed the journal entry from page 210, refer to it to see if the foods you ate on that particular day were smart food choices and how they could have been improved.

Project Assignment

In this project you will:
- Conduct research.
- Write a summary of your research.
- Create a poster displaying nutritional information about and advertisements for food items from a chain restaurant.
- Write interview questions.
- Interview someone in your community.
- While interviewing, take notes, and after interviewing, transcribe your notes.
- Make a presentation to your class.

Academic Skills You Will Use . . . .
English Language Arts

NCTE 1 Read texts to acquire new information
NCTE 8 Use information resources to gather information and create and communicate knowledge

STEP 1 Choose and Research a Topic

Conduct research about one of the following topics or another topic of your choice that is approved by your teacher. In addition, find examples of nutritional information from and advertisement about a chain restaurant. Write a summary of your research.
- Strategies marketers use to advertise food.
- How to make healthy nutritious choices at fast-food restaurants.
- Efforts to enact menu education and labeling laws.

STEP 2 Plan Your Interview

Use the results of your research to develop questions you will use to interview someone in your community who is qualified to discuss your research topic. Keep these writing skills in mind while you develop the questions.

Writing Skills
- Use complete sentences
- Use correct spelling and grammar
- Organize your questions in the order you want to ask them

STEP 3 Connect with Your Community

Interview someone in your community about your research and the information you found. You could interview a marketing professional, a dietician, or a restaurant owner, chef, or legislator about menu education and labeling laws.

Interviewing Skills
- Record responses and take notes.
- Listen attentively.
- When you transcribe your notes, write in complete sentences using correct spelling and grammar.

STEP 4 Create Your Final Report

Use the Unit Thematic Project Checklist to plan and give an oral report and create your poster comparing factual nutritional information with advertising information. Use these speaking skills as you present your final report.

Speaking Skills
- Speak clearly and concisely.
- Be sensitive to the needs of your audience.
- Use standard English to communicate.

STEP 5 Evaluate Your Presentation

Your project will be evaluated and reviewed based on:
- Depth of interview and questions
- Content of your presentation
- Mechanics—presentation and neatness

Evaluation Rubric Go to this book's Online Learning Center at glencoe.com for a rubric you can use to evaluate your final report.

Project Checklist

Plan	✓ Conduct research. ✓ Write a summary of your research. ✓ Write interview questions. ✓ Conduct an interview. ✓ Transcribe the notes from your interview. ✓ Create a poster displaying nutritional information about and advertisements for food items from a chain restaurant. ✓ Plan a five-minute presentation.
Present	✓ Make a five-minute presentation to your class that explains the results of your research and interview. ✓ Describe your poster, pointing out specific details about the nutritional information of various dishes sold by the restaurant, healthful and the types of information in and not in the advertisements. ✓ Invite the students of the class to ask any questions they may have. Answer these questions. ✓ When students ask questions, demonstrate in your answers that you respect their perspectives. ✓ Turn in your research summary, interview questions, interview notes, and poster to your teacher.
Academic Skills	✓ Conduct research to gather information. ✓ Communicate effectively. ✓ Organize your presentation so the audience can follow along easily. ✓ Thoroughly express your ideas.

Unit 7

From Kitchen to Table

Chapters in this Unit

Chapter 19 Kitchen Equipment
Chapter 20 Skills for Preparing Flavorful Food
Chapter 21 Cooking Basics
Chapter 22 Organizing the Kitchen
Chapter 23 Serving a Meal

Unit Thematic Project Preview

Plan Your Dream Kitchen

While studying this unit, you will learn about cooking utensils, kitchen appliances, and kitchen organization. In the unit thematic project at the end of this unit, you will conduct research about kitchen equipment and efficient kitchen design, then you will plan your ideal kitchen.

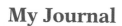

My Journal

What would your dream kitchen look like? Write a journal entry about the topics below.

- Describe an ideal kitchen.
- List the kitchen utensils and appliances you would have in your ideal kitchen.

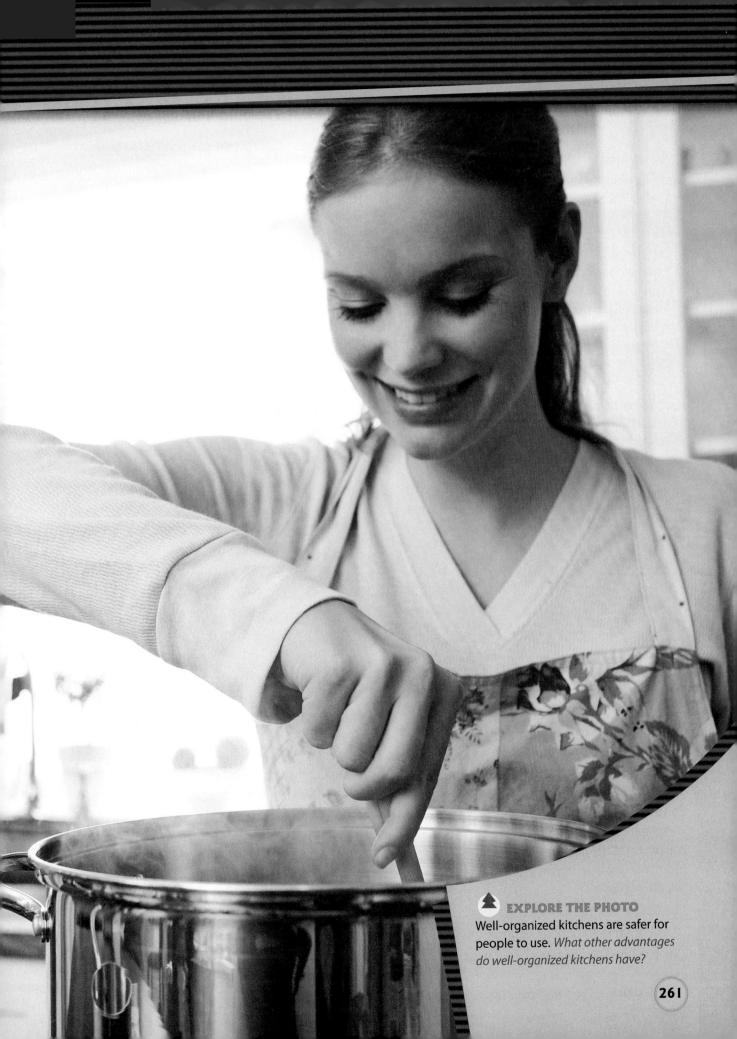

EXPLORE THE PHOTO
Well-organized kitchens are safer for people to use. *What other advantages do well-organized kitchens have?*

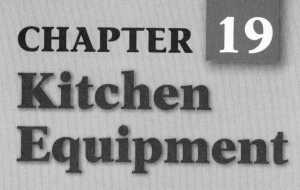

CHAPTER 19
Kitchen Equipment

Explore the Photo ▶▶
You need the right equipment to store, prepare, and cook food and to clean up afterward. *What kitchen equipment do you use most? How do you use it?*

Writing Activity

Persuasive Paragraph

Tools in Your Kitchen Which kitchen tool do you think is most useful? Write a persuasive paragraph explaining which tool or piece of equipment is the most important in the kitchen. Explain why it is so important.

Writing Tips

1. **State** your position clearly.
2. **Use facts** to back up your position.
3. **Explain** the benefits of your choice.

Reading Guide

 **Before You Read**

Pace Yourself Short blocks of concentrated reading, repeated frequently, are more effective than one long session. Focus on reading for 10 minutes. Take a short break. Then, read for another 10 minutes.

Read to Learn

Key Concepts

- **Discuss** how to choose, use, and care for kitchen appliances.
- **Identify** cookware and bakeware for different cooking and baking needs.
- **Select** appropriate kitchen tools for food preparation tasks.

Main Idea

Cooks use kitchen equipment to prepare healthful, flavorful meals. A well-equipped kitchen has large and small appliances, cookware and bakeware, and utensils for preparing food.

Content Vocabulary

◇ major appliance
◇ EnergyGuide label
◇ Energy Star
◇ range
◇ conventional oven
◇ convection oven
◇ microwave oven
◇ small appliance
◇ cookware
◇ bakeware

Academic Vocabulary

You will find these words in your reading and on your tests. Use the glossary to look up their definitions if necessary.

- indicate
- contribute

Graphic Organizer

As you read, list the four different categories of kitchen equipment in the second-tier boxes. Then, write specific types of equipment for each category in the third-tier boxes.

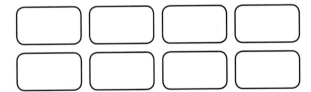

Kitchen Equipment

 Graphic Organizer Go to this book's Online Learning Center at **glencoe.com** to print out this graphic organizer.

Academic Standards ▪ ▪ ▪ ▪ ▪ ▪ ▪ ▪ ▪ ▪ ▪ ▪ ▪ ▪ ▪ ▪ ▪ ▪ ▪

 English Language Arts
NCTE 4 Use written language to communicate effectively.
NCTE 5 Use different writing process elements to communicate effectively.

 Social Studies
NCSS VIII A Science, Technology, and Society
Identify and describe both current and historical examples of the interaction and interdependence of science,

technology, and society in a variety of cultural settings.

 Mathematics
NCTM Algebra Represent and analyze mathematical situations and structures using algebraic symbols.
NCTM Measurement Understand measurable attributes of objects and the units, systems, and processes of measurement.

NCTE	National Council of Teachers of English	**NSES**	National Science Education Standards
NCTM	National Council of Teachers of Mathematics	**NCSS**	National Council for the Social Studies

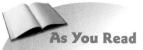

As You Read

Connect How would you teach someone how to shop for kitchen equipment?

Kitchen Appliances

Appliances add convenience, speed, and ease to the kitchen. Compare appliances before you buy them. Check the price, features, and energy efficiency of different models. Ask about the warranty and what it covers, and look for seals that indicate safety and energy cost.

Read the owner's manual first to learn how to safely use and care for an appliance. Manuals include safety guidelines and tips for getting the most benefit from an appliance. They also explain how each feature works, and what to do if the appliance stops working. Keep owner's manuals as handy references.

Vocabulary

You can find definitions in the glossary at the back of this book.

Major Appliances

A **major appliance** is a large appliance, such as a range, a refrigerator-freezer, or a dishwasher. Some are basic models, and others have special features. When shopping for an appliance, ask yourself: Are the special features worth the extra cost? Does the cost match my budget? The **EnergyGuide label** helps you compare the annual energy cost. The **Energy Star** label **indicates**, or shows, energy efficiency.

Energy-efficient appliances help kitchens meet LEED (Leadership in Energy and Environmental Design) standards. These standards are used to design buildings, including kitchens, that protect the environment.

| Figure 19.1 | EnergyGuide label, Energy Star logo |

Energy Check When you shop, compare appliances for energy efficiency. *How could you use the Energy-Guide label to make a smart appliance choice?*

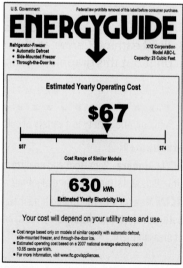

The EnergyGuide label estimates the appliance's annual energy cost.

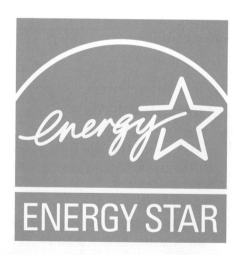

Appliances with the Energy Star label are energy-efficient. This mark may appear on the appliance, the packaging, or the EnergyGuide label.

Refrigerator-Freezers

Refrigerator-freezers keep perishable and frozen foods cold. Many have ice makers and water dispensers. Drawers for fruits, vegetables, and meat may have special temperature and humidity controls.

Most refrigerator-freezers have two or three outer doors. One or two doors are for the refrigerator. The last door is for the freezer. Some models have only one door with a small freezer section that has a lightweight inner door. This section can store already-frozen foods for up to two weeks. It is not cold enough to freeze fresh foods well.

If you have a lot of frozen food to store, you might consider purchasing a separate freezer. Before buying one ask yourself if it is worth the additional energy cost.

Using your refrigerator properly will prolong its life, keep food fresher, and make working in the kitchen easier and more pleasant. Follow these guidelines for energy efficiency, cleanliness, and food safety:

- Check inside temperatures with a refrigerator-freezer thermometer. A refrigerator should stay between 32°F and 40°F (0°C and 4°C)—and not below 32°F (0°C). If possible, keep your freezer at 0°F (-18°C) or less.

- Fill the refrigerator only about three-quarters full. An overloaded refrigerator has to work harder. It may not stay cold enough for food safety. Keep the freezer compartment full.

- Let air circulate properly. Do not cover wire shelves.

- Keep doors closed to save energy and keep food cold. Open the doors only to remove or put away food.

- Wipe up leaks and spills right away to prevent bacterial growth.

- Keep an open box of baking soda inside to absorb odors.

- Check refrigerator and freezer contents weekly. Discard spoiled food.

- Every few weeks, clean the refrigerator well—inside and out—with warm, soapy water.

- If the freezer is not self-defrosting, defrost it when ¼ inch to ½ inch (6 mm to 13 mm) of ice forms inside.

Is It Worth the Cost? Major appliances have many different features. Extra features usually add to the price. *How would you decide if extra features in an appliance are worth the cost?*

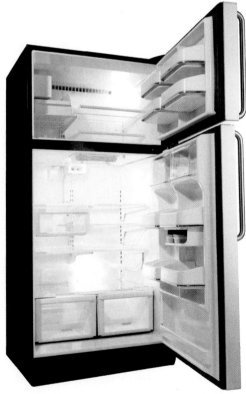

Major Cooking Appliances

The most important cooking appliance in most kitchens is the **range**—a large cooking stove. Ranges have cooktops, broilers, and ovens. Some are powered by gas, others by electricity. Controls for each unit let you adjust heat from low to high. Cooktops are burners or electric coils on the top surface and have a grill as well. An oven is an enclosed cooking compartment. A range may have one or more ovens. Broilers are usually inside the oven. They provide direct heat from the top to cook or brown food. You can usually adjust the broiler rack so the food is closer or further from the heat. Some kitchens have separate cooktop and oven units built into kitchen cabinets instead of ranges.

Kitchens may have up to three different types of ovens:

◆ A **conventional oven** cooks food by circulating hot air around food. You set the oven control to a specific temperature.

◆ A **convection oven** works like a conventional oven, except a fan circulates hot air at a high speed. It cooks many foods faster and more evenly than a conventional oven. It is not as fast as a microwave oven, however.

◆ A **microwave oven** cooks with waves of energy that produce heat inside food. Because most foods cook quickly, this method saves energy. Microwaves do not heat the whole oven, so the kitchen stays cool.

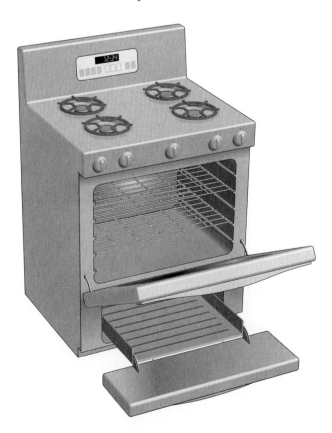

Cooking with a Range A basic range has three cooking areas: the cooktop, the broiler, and at least one oven. *What part of the range is used most often in your home?*

Safety is important when cooking with a range or oven. Follow the instructions in the owner's manual, and use these tips:

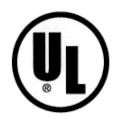

- Match the pan size to the size of the cooktop's heating element or burner flame.

- Use pans with flat bottoms. They will not tip over easily.

- Turn off the surface heating unit before removing cookware.

- Adjust oven racks to the desired positions before turning on the heat.

- When possible, bake several food items together for efficiency, such as meat loaf and a vegetable dish.

- Open the oven door as little as possible to keep heat in.

- When you open the oven door, stand to one side to avoid injury from hot air and escaping steam.

- After every use, clean the cooktop once the range cools. Use a cloth or non-scratch scrubber. Cleanup is easier before food dries. Immediate cleanup is important to food safety.

- Follow the owner's manual for cleaning. Some ranges have self-cleaning ovens, which use very high heat to turn residue to ashes.

How can you use this symbol to make decisions about the safety of appliances?

Dishwashers

A dishwasher saves time on clean-up. It also cleans and sanitizes dishes more effectively than hand-washing them. A dishwasher may use less water too.

For proper cleaning, a dishwasher needs enough water pressure, the right amount of detergent, and water that is at least 140°F (60°C). Hot air dries the dishes. Like other appliances, dishwashers have different features. Common features include delay settings, utensil holders, and movable racks.

Follow these guidelines to safely use and care for a dishwasher:

- Check the owner's manual for how to load dishes. An overloaded or improperly loaded dishwasher may not wash well.

- Use only detergent meant for a dishwasher. Use the right amount.

- Wash a full load to save energy and use water wisely.

- Use the right cycle: normal wash for regular soil, heavy wash for pots and pans, or a rinse-and-hold cycle.

- Pre-rinse dishes if the owner's manual says to do so. Scrape off large food particles and bones.

- Wait until the dishes cool down and the steam is gone to empty the dishwasher.

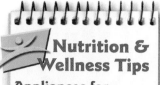
Small Appliances

A **small appliance** is a piece of portable electric equipment. Some are kitchen basics. Others, such as a waffle iron, do unique tasks. Weigh the appliance's cost against how often you will use it before you decide to buy.

Cooking with a small appliance may save energy when you cook small amounts of food. For example, you can bake a potato in a toaster oven rather than a conventional oven.

Small Cooking Appliances

◆ **Electric Skillet** To fry, simmer, steam, roast, and bake. Heat can be set at a specific temperature.

◆ **Slow Cooker** To slowly cook food, such as soups and stews, at a low temperature over many hours.

◆ **Toaster** To toast bread.

◆ **Toaster Oven** To toast, bake, and top-brown small amounts of food. Some models have a broiler.

Mixing and Cutting Appliances

◆ **Blender** To blend or cut food quickly. It can also grate, chop, puree, and mince. Blenders may be simple, two-speed types or have many speeds.

◆ **Food Processor** To slice, grate, shred, chop, grind, blend, or mix foods. It also can knead dough.

◆ **Mixer** To mix and beat. It can be a lightweight, hand-held model or a heavy-duty model on a stand.

Other Small Appliances

◆ **Garbage Disposal** To grind food waste so it is disposed through kitchen plumbing. Learn what can go in a disposer and how to use it safely and properly.

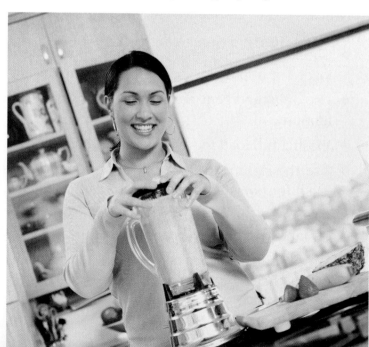

Kitchen Helpers Use small appliances to match your needs. *Which appliance(s) might you use to make a smoothie?*

How to Shop for Small Appliances

Most kitchens have basic appliances like toasters. Other appliances, like a food processor, may be nice to have, but are not always necessary. Before you buy a new kitchen appliance, ask yourself:

- Do I really need this appliance or tool? Can I use something else for the same task?
- Do I have space for this appliance?
- Can it handle the amount of food I usually prepare?
- Is it easy to use and clean? How will it **contribute**, or add, to my efficiency in the kitchen?
- Does the appliance have a safety seal and warranty? Is it energy efficient?
- How much does it cost? Is the cost worth the benefit?

Use and Care of Small Appliances

Misuse of a small appliance can cause an electric shock or start a fire. Always follow directions in the owner's manual carefully. Remember to follow these guidelines for using small appliances:

- Turn off the appliance before plugging it in or unplugging it.
- Unplug a mixer before putting in or removing the beaters. The mixer might accidentally start while your fingers are inside.
- Clean appliances after each use. Always remember to unplug them and let them cool before cleaning.
- Appliances that can be submerged in water are immersible. Unless appliances are labeled as immersible, do not put them in water. This may damage the appliance and create safety hazards.
- If an appliance sparks or shocks you, unplug it immediately. Have it repaired or replace it.

✓ **Reading Check** **Explain** Why should you unplug an appliance before cleaning it?

Math in Action

Electricity Savings

A customer pays a flat rate of $0.07 per kilowatt-hour for electricity. However, in the time-of-use savings plan, they could pay $5 per month plus a variable rate. Electricity costs $0.18 during the day, and $0.05 at other times. A family uses 380 kilowatt-hours during the day, and 620 kilowatt-hours during other times. Compare the flat rate cost and the time-of-use cost. Should the family sign up for the time-of-use plan?

Math Concept **Solve Equations with Grouping Symbols** Equations often contain grouping symbols such as parentheses to help separate functions in the equation. The first step in solving these equations is to resolve the equations inside the parentheses.

Starting Hint Find the flat rate amount by multiplying the total hours used by the cost per hour. Then, find the time-of-use rate by multiplying each type of hour by its respective cost. Add these totals to the fee for the plan. Then, compare the cost of the two plans.

NCTM Algebra Represent and analyze mathematical situations and structures using algebraic symbols.

 For more math help, go to the Math Appendix

Cookware and Bakeware

Cookware includes pots and pans used mostly on the cooktop. **Bakeware** is containers used for baking in the oven. Both cookware and bakeware are made from a variety of materials, including aluminum, stainless steel, cast iron, heat-resistant glass, enamel, and ceramic. Pottery and some glass cookware are for oven use only. Many have a nonstick finish. Cookware for the range includes:

◆ **Double Boiler** To gently heat delicate foods. This two-part saucepan can boil water in the lower compartment and heat food in the upper compartment.

◆ **Saucepan or Pot** To cook foods on the cooktop. Saucepans have one long handle. Pots have two small handles and are larger than saucepans.

◆ **Skillet** To brown and fry foods. Skillets are less deep than pots and saucepans. They usually have one long handle.

◆ **Steamer Basket** To hold food in a saucepan above boiling water. Small holes let steam pass to cook food.

◆ **Wok** To stir-fry. A wok is deeper than a skillet. Its slanted sides are wider at the top, and it has a rounded or flat bottom.

Cookware and bakeware for a conventional oven include:

◆ **Casserole Dish** To hold mixed dishes and some desserts while baking. Casserole dishes are made of heat-resistant glass, pottery, stoneware, or glass ceramic.

◆ **Baking Pan** To hold foods during baking. Baking pans are made of metal or heat-resistant glass and come in many shapes such as cake pans, baking sheets and pie pans.

◆ **Roasting Pan** To hold meat, poultry, fish, or vegetables during roasting. This shallow pan often has handles on both ends. It may have a rack to hold food above juices.

Cooktop Cookware Use cookware that is appropriate for your cooking method and the amount of food. *What are the similarities and differences among saucepans, pots, and skillets?*

Microwave Oven Cookware

Not all cookware used in conventional ranges is microwave-safe. Many types of paper and plastic products can be used for microwave cooking. Microwaves pass right through these materials to cook the food inside. Unsafe materials could get damaged, damage the oven, or even start a fire. Use microwave-safe cookware, and follow your microwave oven instructions.

Cookware that is generally safe in a microwave oven includes:
- Heatproof glass containers such as casserole dishes, baking dishes, and liquid measuring cups.
- Cookware especially designed for microwave oven use.
- Plastic items labeled as microwave-safe.
- Paper plates and towels labeled as microwave-safe.
- Wooden skewers for kabobs.

Cookware that is unsafe to use in a microwave oven includes:
- Metal cookware. Microwaves bounce off metal and create sparks that may damage the oven or start a fire.
- Pottery with metallic glazes.
- Plastic containers from prepared, dairy, or take-out foods.
- Brown paper bags or any products from recycled paper. They may contain chemicals that burn.
- Wooden containers. They dry out and get damaged over time.
- Paper towels or other containers made with synthetic or plastic fibers such as nylon. They may catch fire.
- Plastic wrap. It may melt and contaminate food.
- Aluminum foil, except in small amounts and used only according to oven instructions.

✓ **Reading Check** **List** What types of cookware are safe to use in the microwave oven?

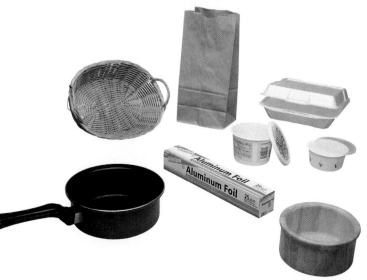

Safe or Unsafe for Microwaving? Not all containers are suitable for use in a microwave oven. *Which types of containers should you avoid using in a microwave?*

Kitchen Tools

Kitchen tools are as important to cooks as carpentry tools are to builders. You need the right tool for the job. Kitchen equipment does not have to be fancy to work, however.

Store tools close to where you will use them. Choose the tool designed for the job. Use kitchen tools correctly and safely. Clean and care for them properly so they last a long time. Put them back in their proper place so you can find them easily.

A variety of tools can help you with measuring, mixing, cutting, cooking, and draining.

Measuring Tools

Measuring cups and spoons are used to accurately measure amounts for recipes. Common measuring tools include:

- **Dry Measuring Cups** To measure dry and solid ingredients. A basic customary set includes 1-cup, ½-cup, ⅓-cup, and ¼-cup sizes. A metric set includes 250-mL, 125-mL, and 50-mL sizes.

- **Kitchen Scale** To measure the customary or metric weight of ingredients.

- **Liquid Measuring Cups** To measure liquids. These glass or plastic cups with a pouring spout come in 1 cup (250 mL), 2 cup (500 mL), and other sizes. They are usually marked with customary and metric measurements. Extra space at the top lets you carry liquids without spilling.

- **Measuring Spoons** To measure small amounts of liquid and dry ingredients. Most customary sets include 1 tablespoon, 1 teaspoon, ½ teaspoon , and ¼ teaspoon. A metric set includes 25 mL, 15 mL, 5 mL, 2 mL, and 1 mL.

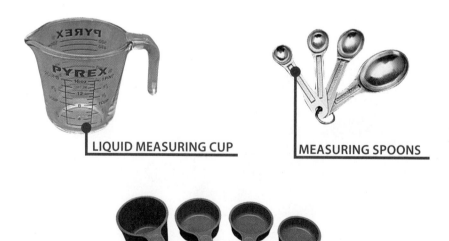

LIQUID MEASURING CUP

MEASURING SPOONS

DRY MEASURING CUPS

The Right Tools Cups and spoons used for eating are not meant for measuring. *What might happen if you used an eating spoon instead of a measuring spoon when following a recipe?*

Mixing Tools

Mixing tools help you prepare ingredients for cooking and baking recipes. Common mixing tools include:

- **Mixing Bowl** To hold foods as they are mixed. These bowls come in different sizes. They are made of glass, plastic, and metal.

- **Mixing Spoon** To beat, mix, and stir. It may be metal, wooden, or plastic.

- **Pastry Blender** To cut fat into flour when making pastry and biscuit dough. It has U-shaped wires capped with a handle.

- **Beater** To blend, whip, and lightly beat ingredients faster than you can with a spoon or whisk. It may be used for beating eggs or pancake batter.

- **Rubber Scraper** To remove food from spoons, sides of bowls, pans, jars, and cans.

- **Sifter** To add air to flour and other dry ingredients while mixing them, to mix ingredients well, and to remove lumps. A sifter is a container with a blade that forces dry ingredients, such as flour, through a fine wire screen.

- **Wire Whisk** To beat, stir, and blend. Its flexible wires are held together by the handle. Whisks with a rounder, bulb-like shape are especially good for beating egg whites.

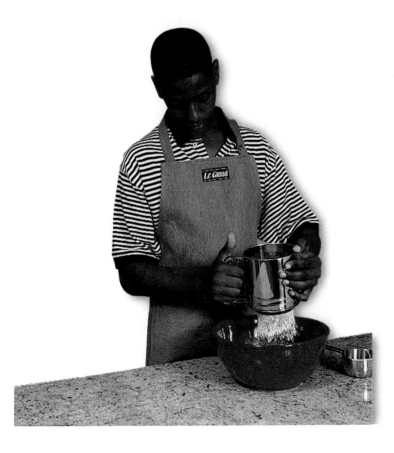

Mixing Tools This mixing equipment is used for hand-mixing. *Which type(s) of hand-mixing tool(s) would be most effective for beating eggs?*

Cutting Tools

Different cutting tools are designed for different tasks. Common cutting tools include:

◆ **Boning Knife** To easily separate meat or poultry from the bone. It has a strong tip and narrow, flexible blade.

◆ **Bread Knife** To cut bread, sandwiches, and cakes easily. It has a serrated, or sawtooth, edge.

◆ **Chef's Knife** To cut, slice, and chop. It has a long, triangle-shaped blade.

◆ **Paring Knife** To pare (remove) skin, and cut and slice fruits and vegetables.

◆ **Slicing Knife** To slice cheese, lettuce, cheese, meat, and poultry. It has a short blade.

◆ **Utility Knife** To cut and slice foods such as fruits and vegetables. It is an all-purpose knife.

◆ **Can Opener** To open cans by cutting through their metal lids. Some are electric appliances.

◆ **Cutting Board** To protect the counter or table while cutting. Cutting boards in different sizes are wooden, plastic, and ceramic, and come in different colors.

◆ **Grater** To shred cheese and vegetables and to grate citrus peel and other foods.

◆ **Kitchen Shears** To cut dried fruit and herbs and to snip away poultry skin and visible fat from meat and chicken.

◆ **Peeler** To remove the thin outer layer from vegetables and fruits, or to thinly slice them.

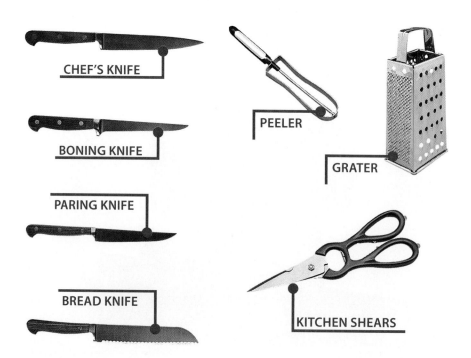

CHEF'S KNIFE

BONING KNIFE

PEELER

GRATER

PARING KNIFE

A Purpose for Each Tool
Each cutting tool is designed for a particular cutting task. *Which would you use to chop an onion?*

BREAD KNIFE

KITCHEN SHEARS

Cooking and Baking Tools

Common cooking and baking tools include:

- **Basting Spoon** To pour liquid over food, to stir, and to serve food. This large, shallow spoon has a long, heatproof handle.

- **Cooling Rack** To hold hot food as it cools.

- **Ladle** To dip liquid such as soup from a pan to a bowl.

- **Meat Thermometer** To measure the internal temperature of meat and poultry. Use the best thermometer:

    - **Oven-Proof** Place in sturdy foods, such as roasts or poultry, before cooking. Keep it there throughout cooking.

    - **Instant-Read** Place in food after cooking. Insert the thermometer's stem about 2 inches (5 cm) into the food.

    - **Microwave-Safe** This is the only type of thermometer safe to use when you microwave.

- **Metal Spatula** To level off dry or solid ingredients when measuring, to loosen baked goods from pans, and to spread or smooth frosting and spreads.

- **Pastry Brush** To brush oil, sauce, or glaze on food.

- **Rubber Scraper** To scrape batter and other foods from containers, and to fold one ingredient into another.

- **Rolling Pin and Cover** To roll out pastry, biscuit, or cookie dough. A cloth cover keeps dough from sticking.

- **Tongs** To lift or turn hot food without piercing it.

- **Turner** To lift and turn foods such as pancakes and hamburgers.

- **Utility Fork** To lift or turn food with long, strong tines.

Get a Grip These tools help you handle food when you cook and bake. *What tool would you use to turn chicken on a grill?*

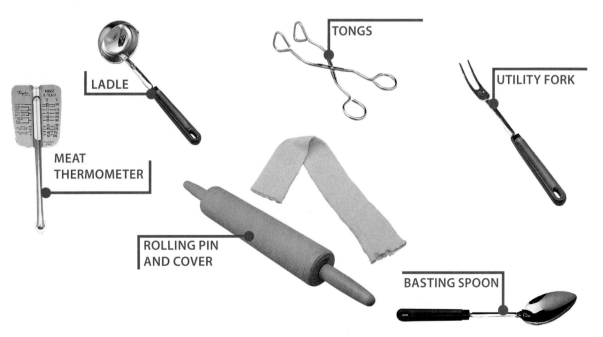

MEAT THERMOMETER · LADLE · TONGS · UTILITY FORK · ROLLING PIN AND COVER · BASTING SPOON

Draining Tools

Draining tools can help you drain foods from liquids before and after cooking:

◆ **Colander** To drain liquid from foods such as cooked pasta or washed fruit and vegetables.

◆ **Slotted Spoon** To lift solid food from liquid or sauce and to drain away liquid.

◆ **Strainer** To separate solids and liquids, such as seeds from fresh-squeezed juice.

✓ **Reading Check** **Recall** Can you use all meat thermometers in a microwave oven?

EASY RECIPES — Everyday Favorites

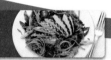

New England Clam Chowder

Customary	Ingredients	Metric
3 each	Red potatoes, medium	3
1	Sweet onion, large	1
3 slices	Bacon	3
8 oz.	Clam juice	250 mL
1 can (6.5 oz)	Clams, in water	200 mL
2½ cups	Whole milk	625 mL
1 Tbsp.	Parsley, chopped	3 mL

Flavor Options

Try this with corn and vegetable stock instead of clams and clam juice. Also, try replacing one cup of the milk with half-and-half.

Yield: 6 servings, 1 cup (250 mL) each

❶ Carefully wash and cut potatoes into ½-inch (1 cm) cubes. Dice onion and bacon.

❷ In a large saucepot on medium heat, cook bacon. When there is enough fat from the bacon, add onions and cook until bacon is done and onions are tender.

❸ Add potatoes, clam juice, and clams in their water. Simmer, covered, for 20 minutes.

❹ Add milk and simmer on low. Garnish with parsley and serve hot.

Nutritional Information Per Serving: 177 calories, 9 g total fat (4 g saturated fat), 25 mg cholesterol, 427 mg sodium, 17 g total carbohydrate, (1 g fiber, 6 g total sugars), 8 g protein

Percent Daily Value: vitamin A 6%, vitamin C 25%, calcium 15%, iron 6%

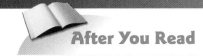

After You Read

CHAPTER SUMMARY

When you shop for appliances, compare the price, features, warranty, and energy efficiency. Choose major and small appliances to match your needs. Major appliances include the range, refrigerator-freezer, and dishwasher. To get the most use from your appliances, follow the owner's manual, keep them clean and well cared for, use them safely, and keep energy efficiency in mind. Choose cookware that is appropriate for use on the cooktop, oven, or microwave oven. To prepare foods easily and successfully, use the right kitchen tools for the job: for measuring, cutting, mixing, cooking, and draining.

Vocabulary Review

1. Use each of these vocabulary words in a sentence.

Content Vocabulary

◇ major appliance (p. 264)
◇ EnergyGuide label (p. 264)
◇ Energy Star (p. 264)
◇ range (p. 266)
◇ conventional oven (p. 266)
◇ convection oven (p. 266)

◇ microwave oven (p. 266)
◇ small appliance (p. 268)
◇ cookware (p. 270)
◇ bakeware (p. 270)

Academic Vocabulary

■ indicate (p. 264)
■ contribute (p. 269)

Review Key Concepts

2. Discuss how to choose, use, and care for kitchen appliances.

3. Identify cookware and bakeware for different cooking and baking needs.

4. Select appropriate kitchen tools for food preparation tasks.

Critical Thinking

5. Organize a list of equipment and tools you would need to bake a fruit pie.

6. Devise a step-by-step plan for shopping for a refrigerator-freezer.

7. Prioritize the top ten kitchen tools that you think are most important to have.

8. Explain the factors you should look at when choosing knives?

9. Describe what to do if a kitchen appliance stops working or does not work properly.

Real-World Skills and Applications

Goal Setting and Decision Making

10. Major Purchase Imagine that you are buying a new microwave oven. Identify factors that would affect your decision. Compare power levels, features, prices, and warranties. Provide a written comparison.

Interpersonal and Collaborative

11. Refrigerator Safety Imagine that family members open the refrigerator frequently and sometimes forget to close it. The refrigerator is too full. They do not always wipe up spilled food inside. Role-play safe and efficient use of the refrigerator with your classmates

Technology

12. Training Video Develop a training video to demonstrate the safe and appropriate use of a kitchen appliance or tool, and its features. If available, use equipment from your foods lab. Play the video in class.

Financial Literacy

13. Stockpile or Toss? It is not always cost-efficient to keep a large supply of food on hand. You spend $21.95 on 5 pounds of beef at the grocery store, and store it in your refrigerator. You eat only 3.5 pounds of beef before the rest spoils. How much money was wasted on the extra beef?

14. Tools of the Trade Find four recipes that require measuring, cutting, mixing, and cooking or baking. Explain the tools you would use for each of the recipe tasks, and why. Make a three-column chart, showing the recipe tasks, your tool of choice, and the reasons for your choice.

15. Energy-Efficient Appliances Visit a store to learn about an energy-efficient appliance, such as an induction cooktop. Prepare a written report explaining the appliance, its technology, and why it is energy efficient. Include information about the EnergyGuide and Energy Star mark. Explain its pros and cons.

> **NCTE 4** Use written language to communicate effectively.

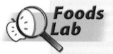

16. By Hand or Appliance? Find a recipe that needs mixing and cutting. Prepare it twice: first with hand tools, such as a rotary beater and knife. Then, follow the same recipe using small appliances, such as a blender and food processor. Compare the advantages and disadvantages of the two methods. Explain your preference.

Additional Activities For additional activities go to this book's Online Learning Center at glencoe.com.

Academic Skills

 English Language Arts

17. Owner's Manual Write an owner's manual for a kitchen tool. Provide a description and instructions for use, for cleaning, and storage. Make your information clear for a first-time owner. Use diagrams and how-to tips for clarity.

> **NCTE 5** Use different writing process elements to communicate effectively.

 Social Studies

18. Other Appliances People in many cultures use rice cookers every day. In some rice cookers, rice cooks in the bottom and other foods can be kept warm in baskets on top. Think of another small appliance. What recipes could you use the appliance for? Write your answer in a two-paragraph report.

> **NCSS VIII A Science, Technology, and Society** Identify and describe both current and historical examples of the interaction and interdependence of science, technology, and society in a variety of cultural settings.

 Mathematics

19. Pitcher Sizes When she opened her refrigerator Lucy noticed milk leaking from the milk carton. In order to save the remainder from the milk carton, she must transfer the remaining milk into her own containers. She bought a ½ gallon of milk. She lost about 1 cup of milk. She has a 1-quart pitcher and three 1-pint thermoses. Which should she use to store the remaining milk?

Math Concept **Customary Measurement System** The United States uses the customary system of measurement. In this system, 1 gallon = 4 quarts, 1 quart = 2 pints, and 1 pint = 2 cups.

Starting Hint Convert the measurements of Lucy's remaining milk into measurements that will compare with the containers she has available.

> **NCTM Measurement** Understand measurable attributes of objects and the units, systems, and processes of measurement.

STANDARDIZED TEST PRACTICE

ESSAY
Read the paragraph. Write your answer on a separate piece of paper:

> **Test-Taking Tip** Study for tests over a few days or weeks, and continually review class material. Do not wait until the night before and try to learn everything at once.

Here are some more tips on how you can make your kitchen energy efficient. Twice a year, have someone help you move the refrigerator so you can vacuum the coils in the back. If possible, do not place the oven and the refrigerator next to each other. Use the burner on the stove that best matches the pot size. This saves on heat loss and make spills easier to clean.

20. Think about what you learned in the chapter and from the paragraph above. Write a paragraph about what can be done to make a kitchen more energy-efficient.

CHAPTER 20
Skills for Preparing Flavorful Food

Explore the Photo ▶▶
Have you ever made a taco with too much hot pepper? The secret to successful food preparation is knowing how to use recipes correctly and measure accurately. *Why are recipes useful?*

Writing Activity

Write an Advertisement

Open a Restaurant Imagine you are opening a new restaurant and want to advertise it on TV. Write a 30-second advertisement inviting customers to your restaurant. Describe the atmosphere and the menu.

Writing Tips

1. **Identify** the audience for whom you will write.

2. **Write** your ad so that it draws attention, arouses interest, and causes action.

3. **Appeal** to people's feelings while being truthful.

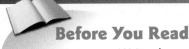

Before You Read

Use Diagrams Write down the main idea of the chapter. Then review the headings and create a diagram that outlines the main topics in the chapter.

Read to Learn

Key Concepts
- **Compare** scratch and convenience cooking.
- **Explain** the information in a recipe.
- **Describe** how to measure dry and liquid ingredients accurately.
- **Describe** cutting and combining techniques.
- **Discuss** the use of herbs, spices, and other flavorings.
- **Suggest** additions to a recipe's ingredients for better nutrition.

Main Idea

Recipes tell you how to combine food and seasonings in the right amounts and in the right way. Good food preparation skills make food appealing and keep it nourishing.

Academic Vocabulary

You will find these words in your reading and on your tests. Use the glossary to look up their definitions if necessary.

- transfer
- project

Content Vocabulary

- scratch cooking
- convenience cooking
- recipe
- ingredient
- yield
- customary measurement system
- metric system
- volume
- weight
- level off
- heaping
- herb
- spice
- rub
- condiment

Graphic Organizer

Use a chart like the one below to record the seven steps in following a recipe.

1.
2.
3.

 Graphic Organizer Go to this book's Online Learning Center at **glencoe.com** to print out this graphic organizer.

Academic Standards ■

 English Language Arts
NCTE 8 Use information resources to gather information and create and communicate knowledge.
NCTE 9 Develop an understanding of diversity in language use across cultures.

 Mathematics
NCTM Measurement Apply appropriate techniques, tools, and formulas to determine measurements.

NCTM Number and Operations Understand the meanings of operations and how they relate to one another.

 Social Studies
NCSS I E Culture Demonstrate the value of cultural diversity, as well as cohesion, within and across groups.

 Science
NSES Content Standard B Develop an understanding of the structure and properties of matter.

NCTE National Council of Teachers of English
NCTM National Council of Teachers of Mathematics

NSES National Science Education Standards
NCSS National Council for the Social Studies

◆**Vocabulary**
You can find definitions in
the glossary at the back of
this book.

Scratch or Convenience Cooking?

Modern appliances and convenience foods allow you to make most meals very quickly. However, you can also prepare food from scratch. **Scratch cooking** is preparing a dish from unprepared foods. You control the ingredients and how the dish is made. Scratch cooking often costs less than using convenience foods. Scratch cooking usually takes more time, energy, and kitchen skills.

Convenience cooking is cooking using convenience foods, or partially or fully prepared or processed foods. You can create a meal quickly with less effort. For instance, you might top a store-bought unbaked pizza shell with marinara sauce, packaged shredded cheese, and pre-sliced vegetables or meat. You have less control over the ingredients with convenience cooking.

✓ **Reading Check**) **Apply** Which cooking approach would you use if you wanted to have the most control over the outcome?

Recipe Use

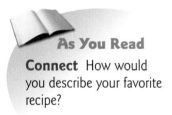

As You Read

Connect How would you describe your favorite recipe?

A **recipe** lists ingredients and instructions for preparing a dish. (See **Figure 20.1**.) You can find recipes in magazines and cookbooks, on the Internet, on cooking shows, and by talking to other cooks.

Food preparation in recipes changes food in many ways. For example, you might change the form of the food (mixing), apply heat (cooking), add air (beating), remove moisture (toasting), remove heat (chilling), or heat with moisture (steaming).

Parts of a Recipe

A well-written recipe should contain these parts:

◆ **Headnote** The headnote provides key information about the recipe.

◆ **Ingredients** An **ingredient** is one of the items of food needed to create a recipe. Ingredients should be listed in the order in which they are used.

◆ **Amounts** The amounts of each ingredient you need.

◆ **Pre-Preparation** The pre-preparation steps describe what must be done before measuring, such as shredding cheese.

◆ **Directions** The directions are the step-by-step instructions for preparation.

◆ **Equipment** The appliances and tools needed to make the recipe are listed.

- ◆ **Temperature** The temperature describes the control settings for cooking equipment used during preparation.
- ◆ **Time** The time specifies how long to cook or chill the food.
- ◆ **Yield** The **yield** is how much the recipe makes, or the number of servings.
- ◆ **Nutrient/Calorie Information** This lists nutritional information per serving.

Figure 20.1 **The Parts of a Recipe**

What Recipes Tell You Recipes are written in different styles. All good recipes have the basic elements listed below. *What pre-preparation steps are needed for this recipe?*

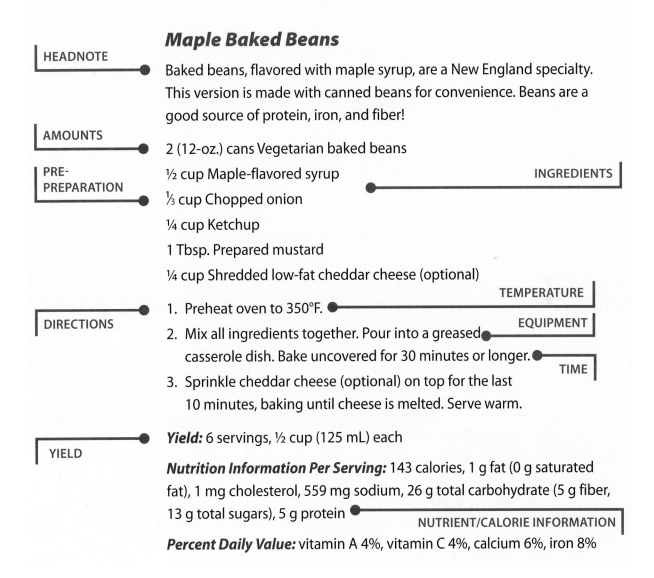

HEADNOTE

Maple Baked Beans

Baked beans, flavored with maple syrup, are a New England specialty. This version is made with canned beans for convenience. Beans are a good source of protein, iron, and fiber!

AMOUNTS

PRE-PREPARATION

2 (12-oz.) cans Vegetarian baked beans

½ cup Maple-flavored syrup

⅓ cup Chopped onion

¼ cup Ketchup

1 Tbsp. Prepared mustard

¼ cup Shredded low-fat cheddar cheese (optional)

INGREDIENTS

TEMPERATURE

DIRECTIONS

1. Preheat oven to 350°F.

EQUIPMENT

2. Mix all ingredients together. Pour into a greased casserole dish. Bake uncovered for 30 minutes or longer.

TIME

3. Sprinkle cheddar cheese (optional) on top for the last 10 minutes, baking until cheese is melted. Serve warm.

YIELD

Yield: 6 servings, ½ cup (125 mL) each

Nutrition Information Per Serving: 143 calories, 1 g fat (0 g saturated fat), 1 mg cholesterol, 559 mg sodium, 26 g total carbohydrate (5 g fiber, 13 g total sugars), 5 g protein

NUTRIENT/CALORIE INFORMATION

Percent Daily Value: vitamin A 4%, vitamin C 4%, calcium 6%, iron 8%

Following Recipes

Experienced cooks may not need recipes for everything they prepare. Recipes are very helpful for beginning cooks, however. Read a recipe carefully. Ask yourself:

◆ Are the directions clear and complete?

◆ Do I have the skills and equipment needed?

◆ Which ingredients do I have? Do I have the time and money to buy missing ingredients? Can I substitute others?

◆ How long will the recipe take to prepare?

◆ How does this dish fit into my meal and eating plan?

Use these guidelines to follow recipes effectively and get best results:

◆ Read the recipe carefully before starting. Learn what any unfamiliar terms mean.

◆ Assemble all the ingredients and equipment first.

◆ Measure carefully, especially for baked goods.

◆ Use the exact equipment named in the recipe.

◆ Follow the recipe exactly. When you have more cooking experience, you can vary recipes.

◆ Reread the recipe as you work to be sure you do not leave anything out.

◆ Pay attention. Check the progress of your food and use a thermometer to ensure food safety.

Figure 20.2	Ingredient Substitutions

Easy Substitutions These substitutions lower fat and cholesterol. *What other nutrition benefits could you get by using plain yogurt in place of sour cream?*

Ingredient:	Substitution:
Cream	Evaporated fat-free milk
Sour cream	Plain yogurt, light or nonfat sour cream, or cottage cheese (blended until smooth)
Whole milk	Fat-free, low-fat, or reduced-fat milk
Cheese	Reduced-fat or fat-free cheese
Ground beef or sausage	Lean or extra-lean ground beef, lean ground turkey or chicken, or 95% fat-free sausage
Bacon	Ham, smoked turkey, or Canadian bacon
1 whole egg	2 egg whites or ¼ cup (60 mL) egg substitute
1 ounce baking chocolate	3 Tbsp. (45 mL) cocoa powder plus 1 Tbsp. (15 mL) oil

Ingredient Substitutions

Some recipes are flexible. In a stew, for example, you might want more onion and fewer spices. You might also adjust the recipe for less fat or salt, or to add more vegetables and dairy foods. (See **Figure 20.2**.) When you bake foods such as breads, cakes, and cookies, follow recipes exactly. Substitutions may change the results of baked goods.

Measuring Basics

Recipe success depends on accurate measuring. Too much or too little of an ingredient can make a big difference!

The **customary measurement system** is the measurement system commonly used in the United States. The **metric system** is a system of weights and measures based on multiples of 10. The metric system is used in most other countries. Scientists and health professionals use the metric system. **Figure 20.3** shows the equivalents for different units of measure.

Figure 20.3	Equivalent Measures

Customary and Metric Some measuring equipment has customary and metric measures. Sometimes you may need to convert measurements. *If you need 360 mL of rice, how much rice do you need in customary measurements?*

Customary Units	Customary Equivalents	Approximate Metric Equivalents
Volume		
¼ teaspoon (tsp. or t.)		1 mL
½ tsp.		2 or 3 mL
1 tsp.		5 mL
1 tablespoon (Tbsp. or T.)	3 tsp.	15 mL
1 fluid ounce (fl. oz.)	2 Tbsp.	30 mL
¼ cup (C. or c.)		60 mL
⅓ cup		80 mL
½ cup		120 mL
⅔ cup		160 mL
¾ cup		180 mL
1 cup	8 fl. oz. or 16 Tbsp.	250 mL
1 pint (pt.)	2 cups or 16 fl. oz.	500 mL
1 quart (qt.)	2 pt. or 4 cups or 32 fl. oz.	1,000 mL or 1 liter (L)
1 gallon	4 qt. or 8 pt. or 128 fl. oz.	4 L
Weight		
1 ounce (oz.)		28 grams (g)
1 pound (lb.)	16 oz.	500 g
2 lb.	32 oz.	1,000 g or 1 kilogram (kg)

Units of Measure

Ingredient amounts are usually given in these three ways:

◆ **Volume** refers to how much space the ingredient takes up.

◆ **Weight** refers to how heavy or light the ingredient is. Scales measure weight.

◆ The number of items, such as two bananas.

The term ounce is used for weight (dry ounce) and for volume (fluid ounce). When a recipe calls for ounces, you need to know if you need to measure by weight or by volume.

Measure Dry Ingredients

Equipment for measuring volume includes liquid measuring cups, dry measuring cups, and measuring spoons. Measuring cups and spoons come in many sizes. Here are some examples:

◆ **Customary** 1 cup, ½ cup, ⅓ cup, ¼ cup, 1 Tbsp., 1 tsp., ½ tsp., ¼ tsp.

◆ **Metric** 250 mL, 125 mL, 50 mL, 25 mL, 15 mL, 5 mL, 2 mL, 1 mL

Dry ingredients include flour, sugar, rice, and spices. Choose the exact size of measuring tool for the amount you need. You should level off dry ingredients. To **level off** is to scrape any extra off the top of the measuring cup or spoon, using a straight edge. Sometimes recipes call for a heaping measurement. A **heaping** measurement is above the top of the cup or spoon.

Food Prep How To

MEASURE DRY INGREDIENTS

1 Hold the cup or spoon over the ingredient's container, wax paper, or a separate plate. If any spills over, it will be caught without going into the other ingredients.

2 Fill the cup or spoon slightly over the top.

TIP   Do not shake or tap the cup to make more room. Do not pack the ingredient into the measuring utensil unless the recipe says to do so or unless you are measuring brown sugar.

3 Use a straight edge, such as a straight-edge spatula or the back of a knife, to level off the ingredient.

Measure Sugar

◆ **Brown Sugar** Pack sugar firmly into the exact-size cup. Press it in with a rubber scraper or the back of a spoon. Leave no air holes. Overfill the cup a little, then level it off.

◆ **Granulated Sugar** Put it through a strainer or press it with a spoon if it is lumpy before you measure it. Overfill the cup a little, then level it off.

Measure Flour

◆ **Sifted Flour** Put the flour through a sifter to separate the particles of flour and add air. Sift before measuring. Place wax paper under the measuring cup. Spoon flour into the sifter, then sift into the measuring cup. Use the wax paper to transfer any excess flour back into the flour bag.

◆ **Unsifted Flour** If the recipe does not call for sifted flour, stir the flour with a spoon before measuring.

Measure Liquid

Use a liquid measuring cup for liquids such as water or honey. It has a pouring spout and extra space at the top to help prevent spills. Use measuring spoons for small amounts.

Before measuring syrup or honey, coat the measuring cup with oil so they flow out of the cup more easily. Use a rubber scraper to get all the syrup or honey out.

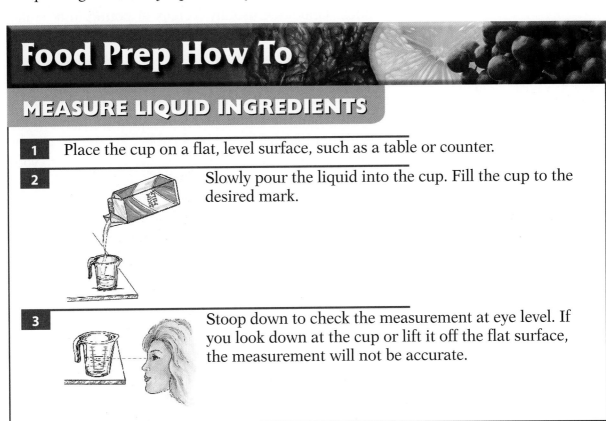

Food Prep How To

MEASURE LIQUID INGREDIENTS

1 Place the cup on a flat, level surface, such as a table or counter.

2 Slowly pour the liquid into the cup. Fill the cup to the desired mark.

3 Stoop down to check the measurement at eye level. If you look down at the cup or lift it off the flat surface, the measurement will not be accurate.

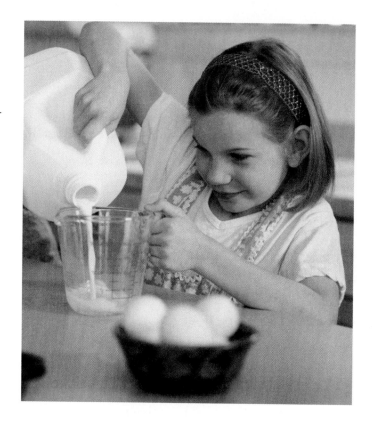

Accurate Measurement
Taking the time to measure ingredients carefully can help make a recipe a success. *Why is it important to use the right tools for measuring different ingredients?*

Measure Solid Fat

Solid fats, such as butter, margarine, and shortening, are measured in several different ways. Here are two easy ways:

◆ **Stick Method**   Butter and margarine are often sold by the stick. One stick usually weighs ¼ pound and equals ½ cup. Wrappers are usually marked in tablespoons. Cut off the amount you need.

◆ **Dry Measuring Cup Method**   Spoon shortening into a dry measuring cup. Pack the cup firmly, but slightly more than full. Then level it off. Work out all air bubbles so the measurement is accurate. Use a rubber scraper to get the shortening out of the cup and **transfer**, or move, it to your mixing bowl.

Other Measurements

◆ **Temperature** The customary system measures temperature in degrees Fahrenheit (°F). The metric system measures in degrees Celsius (°C). Many thermometers show both.

◆ **Length** Recipes sometimes include length measurements, such as the length and width of a pan or the size of a vegetable. The customary system measures length in inches (in.), while metrics uses millimeters (mm) or centimeters (cm).

Increasing or Decreasing Recipe Yield

If you want more or fewer servings than the recipe provides, you must **project**, or estimate, the needed number of servings and then increase or decrease the ingredient amounts. These steps tell you how:

1. **Decide the yield you want.** Yield is the number of servings a recipe makes. For example, you need pasta salad for seven people. The recipe yields four servings. Plan for eight. That is easier to calculate.

2. **Calculate new amounts.** After you know how much you need, divide the desired yield by the original yield to find the adjustment. For example, eight servings of pasta salad divided by four servings of pasta salad equals two, or an adjustment of twice as much pasta salad.

3. **Change each ingredient amount.** The original amount of each ingredient multiplied by the adjustment equals the new amount for the ingredient. For example, for eight servings of pasta salad instead of four, multiply the original amount of each ingredient by two.

Use a similar formula to decrease a recipe. If a recipe makes 12 servings and you need to make four, multiply each ingredient amount by ⅓ (4 divided by 12 equals ⅓). You can use these equations for nearly every recipe.

Discover International Foods

Egypt

The people of Egypt, a large country in northern Africa, enjoy foods that are part of their Arab culture and their available food supply. Important ingredients include lamb, yogurt, goat's milk cheese, chickpeas and other beans, nuts, flatbread, bulgur, and vegetables such as tomatoes, cucumbers, and eggplant. Beans are eaten alone or as part of many dishes. A common breakfast is *ful*, bread, olives, cheese *(mish)*, and sweet tea or coffee. Roasted or grilled pigeon, stuffed with seasoned rice or corn, is a delicacy.

Languages Across Cultures

baba ghanoush *(bä-bə-gə-'nüsh)* puree of eggplant, tahini (sesame seed paste), olive oil, lemon juice, and garlic. It is often eaten as a spread.

ful *(fül)* slow, simmered beans, which may be mashed with tomatoes and onion. Mashed beans are made into fried patties called *tamiya*.

 Recipes Find out more about international recipes on this book's Online Learning Center at **glencoe.com**.

NCTE 9 Develop an understanding of diversity in language use across cultures.

Tips for Changing the Yield

Here are some guidelines for changing the yield of a recipe:

♦ Calculate and write down all new amounts before starting to prepare a recipe.

♦ Use **Figure 20.3** to convert between customary and metric measurements, if necessary. Convert hard-to-measure amounts to easier ones, too. For example, ⅛ cup is 2 tablespoons.

♦ If the amount cannot be decreased easily, estimate. For most casserole, stew, soup, and salad recipes, exact amounts are not essential. A whole egg instead of half in a casserole would probably still give good results.

♦ Baked goods such as breads, cookies, and cakes depend on exact amounts. If you round off amounts or change only some of them, the recipe may not work. For example, a cake may not rise properly or a cheesecake may not cook uniformly.

♦ If a recipe cannot be increased or decreased easily, find a different solution. Prepare the whole amount and freeze half for later, for example.

♦ Consider the sizes of the equipment you are using. If you use a larger baking pan with an increased yield, for example, brownies will take longer to bake. Instead, divide the mixture into two pans of the original size and shape. When decreasing a recipe, cook in a smaller pan. Otherwise, food may cook too quickly or dry out.

✓ **Reading Check**) **Calculate** In what three ways are ingredient amounts usually given?

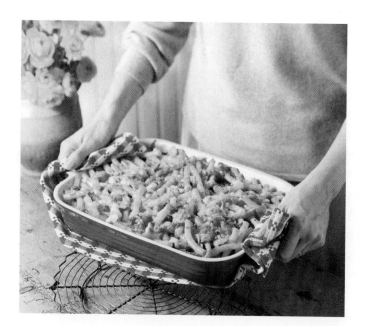

The Right Amount Recipes for salads, soups, and casseroles are more flexible than recipes for baked goods. *What should you do if you cannot easily change a recipe's yield?*

Basic Food Preparation Terms

Recipes use certain terms for food preparation techniques. Each term has its own specific meaning. You need to use the right technique to get the results you expect from a recipe. It is helpful to become familiar with the most widely used cutting and combining terms, as well as other common recipe terms.

Cutting Skills

Good knife skills help you cut food properly and safely. Learn to hold the knife and food properly. Use sharp tools and a clean cutting board. Cutting directly on a kitchen counter or table can damage the surface and may cause the knife to slip. This can cause injury. Remember to wash the knife and cutting board with hot, soapy water after each use. You should understand these basic cutting terms:

- **Chop** Cut food into small, irregular pieces using up-and-down motions. Use a knife, food chopper, kitchen shears, or food processor.
- **Cube** Cut into ½-inch square pieces.
- **Julienne** Cut into match-like strips.
- **Cut In** Divide food into pieces with a knife or scissors.
- **Dice** Cut into small, square pieces that are ¼ inch (or smaller) per side.
- **Mince** Cut into very fine pieces using an up-and-down motion. Use a knife, food chopper, or food processor with a fine blade.
- **Peel** Strip off the outside skin or peel, as with oranges. Some foods can be peeled with your fingers. Other foods require a hand peeler to remove skin.

Combining Skills

Mixing properly is essential. Different terms indicate what tool to use and how quickly and completely to combine ingredients.

- **Beat** Make a mixture smooth using a brisk over-and-over motion with a spoon or a wire whisk, or using a rotary motion with an electric or hand mixer.
- **Cream** Soften fat with a spoon or mixer, either before or while mixing it with another food (usually sugar), to make the mixture soft, smooth, and creamy.
- **Cut In** Distribute solid fat in small pieces evenly through dry ingredients, using a cutting motion with two knives, a fork, or a pastry blender.

HOT JOBS!

Cookbook Author

Cookbook authors create or gather recipes, test them, and prepare manuscripts for cookbooks. They also write about food and often plan and sometimes shoot the photos or graphics.

Careers Find out more about careers. Go to this book's Online Learning Center at **glencoe.com.**

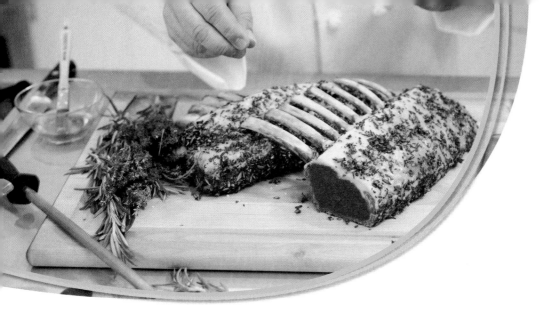

A Flavor Experience Herbs and spices give ethnic foods their unique flavors. *What herbs are popular in your house?*

◆ **Fold In** Blend delicate ingredients, such as beaten egg whites and whipped cream, gently using two motions. Use one motion to cut straight down through the mixture and another to turn the mixture up and over. Rotate the bowl by about one-quarter and repeat until the whole mixture is lightly blended. Fold carefully with a wooden spoon or a rubber scraper so air bubbles do not break and decrease volume.

◆ **Knead** Work dough with the hands by repeatedly folding, pressing, and turning it.

◆ **Mix** Combine ingredients to evenly distribute them.

◆ **Stir** Mix ingredients with a spoon using a circular or figure-8 motion to combine them or to distribute heat evenly.

◆ **Whip** Beat rapidly with a beater, mixer, or wire whisk to incorporate air and increase volume.

Other Recipe Terms

Here are some other recipe terms that you should know:

◆ **Drain** Pour off liquid from a food, or place food in a strainer or colander.

◆ **Garnish** Decorate a food or dish with a small amount of colorful food such as parsley.

◆ **Marinate** Let food stand in marinade for a length of time to tenderize it and develop flavor. Marinade is a flavorful liquid such as Italian dressing.

◆ **Season** Add ingredients, such as herbs and spices, for more flavor.

✓ **Reading Check** **Interpret** Why is it important to know the different terms for cutting and combining ingredients?

Cooking with More Flavor

Skilled cooks enhance flavor without adding too much salt or sugar. They know how to use spices, herbs, condiments, and other flavorful ingredients.

Herb and Spice Use

An **herb** is a fragrant, edible leaf, used to season food. Herbs are either fresh or dried. A **spice** is a seasoning from the bark, buds, seeds, roots, or stems of plants and trees. Spices are usually dried. **Figure 20.4** on page 295 lists several of the most common herbs and spices and how to use them.

Follow these guidelines to use herbs and spices skillfully:

- **Choose herbs and spices that complement other ingredients.** You often can substitute or add herbs and spices in recipes.

- **Substitute fresh for dried herbs.** In general, 1 teaspoon of dried herbs equals about 1 tablespoon of fresh herbs.

- **Use methods to release full flavor.** For soups and stews, add herbs and spices toward the end of the cooking time. Add seasonings to chilled foods several hours before serving so flavors can blend. Crumble dry herbs between your fingers to release the flavor. Chop fresh herbs finely.

- **Use seasoning blends and rubs.** Buy herb and spice blends, or make your own. A **rub** is an herb or spice mixture applied to meat, poultry, or fish before cooking. For example, an Italian blend is dried basil, marjoram, and oregano.

- **Store herbs and spices carefully.** Store dried herbs and spices in airtight containers in a cool, dry place. They keep their peak flavor for up to a year. Keep fresh herbs in the refrigerator. Wrap them in damp paper toweling, then in an airtight plastic bag.

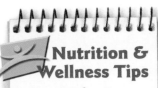

Nutrition & Wellness Tips

Recipe Makeovers

✓ Write down recipe substitutions so you know how to make your adapted version again.

Science in Action

Beating Egg Whites

Beat egg whites for a light and fluffy omelet or soufflé. Beating egg whites forms air bubbles, creating foam that has up to eight times the volume than before beating. Once you combine and cook the beaten egg whites with other ingredients, the extra volume will be baked in!

Procedure Try beating egg whites at home. Are small bubbles stronger or weaker than bigger bubbles? Do you want strong or weak bubbles when cooking? Compare bubbles to balloons—when are balloons stronger?

Analysis Create a one-page written report about your observations. Conduct research on the structure of bubbles, and add your findings to your report.

NSES Content Standard B Develop an understanding of the structure and properties of matter.

Condiment Use

A **condiment** is a substance added in small amounts to food, often at the table, to improve, adjust, or complement the food's flavor. Ketchup, relish, mustard, and tartar sauce are common condiments. So are soy sauce, tamari, and worcestershire sauce. You can buy or make condiments. Here are some examples of other common condiments:

- **Salsa** This is usually a mixture of chopped tomatoes, onion, peppers, and herbs. It is a popular condiment to Mexican, and Central and South American dishes. It can be mild or hot. Try salsa with poultry, fish, meat, and egg dishes.

- **Chutney** This is a mild, spicy, or sweet mixture of fruit or tomatoes, vinegar, sugar, and spices. It has its origins in India, and sometimes includes mango, coconut, or curry powder. Serve chutney with meat, poultry, or fish or as a spread for bread.

- **Vinegar** This is a tart condiment that comes in many varieties, such as cider vinegar, balsamic vinegar, and rice vinegar. Vinegar is often used in salad dressings.

- **Pesto** This is a finely chopped mixture of basil, garlic, pine nuts, cheese, and olive oil. It is bright green in color and often served with Italian dishes. It can also be enjoyed on sliced bread.

Other Flavor Boosters

Many other ingredients can also add flavor to food. Here are just a few examples:

- Sun-dried tomatoes add tang to pizza and pasta. They also taste great in salads.

- Chili peppers add spicy flavor. You can add chili peppers to almost any dish to give it some kick. Handle chilies carefully, because they can irritate your eyes and skin. Remember to wash your hands after handling chili peppers.

- Citrus zest, or grated citrus rind, can add fresh flavor to fruit salads. It is often used as flavoring in baking breads and cakes. Try it with grilled chicken.

- Flavoring extracts, such as vanilla or almond extract, add flavor to baked goods such as cakes and cookies. You can also find mint and lemon extract in the spice aisle at the supermarket.

✓ **Reading Check** **Recall** How and when should you add dried rosemary to beef stew for the best flavor?

Figure 20.4   **Herb and Spice Guide**

Adding Flavor Herbs and spices lead the way to new taste experiences. *Instead of seasoning with salt, what herbs or spices might taste good on potatoes or green beans?*

Herb or Spice		Forms Available	Tastes Good With
Basil		Fresh or dried leaves, ground	Tomato dishes, peas, green beans, eggplant, zucchini, soups, eggs
Black pepper		Whole peppercorns, ground	Vegetables, stews, meat, poultry, fish, soups, salads
Celery seed		Dried	Potato, egg, and tuna salads; soups, sauces, fish, vegetables
Chili powder		Ground	Mexican-style dishes, barbecue sauce, meat loaf, stews
Cinnamon		Ground, stick, with sugar, in blends such as pumpkin pie spice	Baked goods such as cakes, buns, breads, pies, and cookies; apples, hot chocolate
Cloves		Whole, ground	Whole ham, roast pork, stews, pickled fruit, baked goods, chocolate desserts, sweet vegetables
Garlic		Cloves, powdered, minced, salt	Meat dishes, sauces, dressings, vegetables, butter spread, salads
Ginger		Fresh, ground	Baked goods, stews, chicken, carrots, squash, sweet potatoes, pears, stir-fries, beverages
Nutmeg		Whole, ground	Baked goods, custard, puddings, apples, carrots, squash, eggnog
Oregano		Fresh or dried leaves, ground	Tomato dishes, Italian and Mexican foods, lamb, pork, poultry, peas, green beans, onions, zucchini
Paprika		Ground	Salads, cream sauces for vegetables, potatoes, eggs, poultry
Parsley		Fresh or dried leaves	Soups, salads, slaws, meat, fish, poultry, all vegetables, sauces, omelets, rice
Rosemary		Fresh or dried leaves	Beef, lamb, and chicken dishes; fruits
Sage		Fresh or dried leaves, rubbed, ground	Pork dishes, meat, fish, poultry stuffing, consommé, cream soups, fish chowder, salad dressing
Thyme		Fresh or dried leaves	Eggs, fish, stews, salads, tomato sauces, legumes, vegetables

Nutritional Recipe Makeovers

You can modify many dishes for nutrition without giving up flavor. You might adjust a recipe to lower the calories or fat or to increase the fiber, calcium, iron, and other nutrients. Recipes for many dishes, such as salads, soups, stir-fries, and casseroles, are flexible and can be modified for better nutrition.

◆ Add beans, cut-up vegetables, or tofu to mixed dishes.

◆ Use less of high-fat ingredients such as butter, margarine, salad dressing, and peanut butter.

✓ **Reading Check** **Apply** What could you add to a stir-fry to increase the amount of calcium or fiber in the dish?

EASY RECIPES

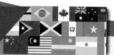

International Flavors

Ful Mesdames

Customary	Ingredients	Metric
2 Tbsp.	Olive oil	30 mL
2 cups	Canned or cooked fava beans*	500 mL
3 cloves	Garlic, finely chopped	3 cloves
To taste	Salt and pepper	To taste
4	Hard-cooked eggs	4
¼ cup	Parsley	60 mL
1	Lemon, quartered	1

Try This!

Add fresh, diced tomatoes to the recipe. Feta cheese makes a good garnish.

* Substitute any cooked beans (legumes) if fava beans are not available.

Yield: 4 servings, about ¾ cup (200 mL) each

❶ Heat oil in a medium saucepan over medium heat.

❷ Add beans and garlic. Add salt and pepper to taste. Mix gently.

❸ Cook to heat through, about 5 to 8 minutes. Add a little more oil if beans seem dry.

❹ Put 1 peeled, hard-cooked egg in each of 4 bowls. Cover with beans. Garnish with parsley and lemon quarters.

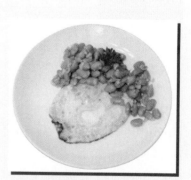

Nutritional Information Per Serving: 250 calories, 12 g total fat (2 g saturated fat), 212 mg cholesterol, 397 mg sodium, 23 g total carbohydrate (5 g fiber, 1 g total sugars), 13 g protein

Percent Daily Value: vitamin A 10%, vitamin C 20%, calcium 6%, iron 15%

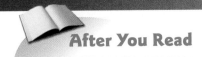

After You Read

CHAPTER SUMMARY
Food can be prepared from scratch or with partly or fully prepared foods. Recipes are instructions for preparing food. They list ingredients and amounts, directions, and how much they serve. To successfully follow a recipe: measure accurately, follow directions and learn cooking terms and techniques. You can change a recipe's yield to make more or fewer servings. Herbs, spices, and condiments can add flavor to your dishes. You can also modify many recipes to improve nutritional value.

Vocabulary Review

1. Define each vocabulary term in your own words.

Content Vocabulary
- scratch cooking (p. 282)
- convenience cooking (p. 282)
- recipe (p. 282)
- ingredient (p. 282)
- yield (p. 283)
- customary measurement system (p. 285)
- metric system (p. 285)
- volume (p. 286)
- weight (p. 286)
- level off (p. 286)
- heaping (p. 286)
- herb (p. 293)
- spice (p. 293)
- rub (p. 293)
- condiment (p. 294)

Academic Vocabulary
- transfer (p. 288)
- project (p. 289)

Review Key Concepts

2. Compare scratch and convenience cooking.

3. Explain the information in a recipe.

4. Describe how to measure dry and liquid ingredients accurately.

5. Describe cutting and combining techniques.

6. Discuss the use of herbs, spices, and other flavorings.

7. Suggest additions to a recipe's ingredients for better nutrition.

Critical Thinking

8. Propose reasons why the metric system is not commonly used in food preparation in the United States. What are the advantages of using the customary measurement system? What are the advantages of the metric system?

9. Analyze a cookbook recipe. Photocopy it and label each recipe part. Note any missing or additional information. Highlight food preparation terms in the recipe.

Real-World Skills and Applications

Goal Setting and Decision Making

10. Recipe Makeover Identify a personal goal for healthier eating, such as eating less fat, sodium, added sugar, or calories. Modify a favorite recipe to match your goal. Rewrite the recipe. Write a paragraph to describe and evaluate the differences in flavor and nutrition.

Interpersonal and Collaborative

11. Classroom Recipe Collection Collect four recipes you like or want to try. Gather them from family, friends, or other sources. Organize your recipes for easy use, perhaps on small cards, computer files, a notebook, or file drawer. Work with your classmates to compile all of your recipes into one recipe book.

Technology

12. Computing Recipe Yields Use a computer spreadsheet, recipe software, or hand calculator to change the yield of a recipe and adjust the ingredient amounts. Demonstrate the process you used in class. Explain the advantages and limitations of using various types of technology.

Financial Literacy

13. Crumbing Bread You can make your own breading for coating fish or chicken before cooking by saving and crushing cereal, cracker, and even nut crumbs. Find what packaged bread crumbs cost at the grocery store. Then, calculate how much you can save by crumbing your own bread.

14. The Right Measuring Equipment Fill several different mugs and glasses with water. Measure the contents of each using a liquid measuring cup. Fill several different flatware teaspoons with sugar. Measure the sugar again using a measuring teaspoon. What can you conclude about using standard measuring equipment? Write a two-paragraph report about your findings.

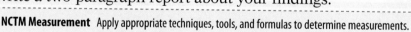

NCTM Measurement Apply appropriate techniques, tools, and formulas to determine measurements.

15. Sensory Evaluation Prepare two samples of pancakes: one from scratch and one from a mix. Compare textures, flavors, appearance, nutritional value, and cost per serving. Which is most appealing? Why? Create a chart or spreadsheet to show the results.

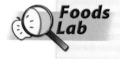

16. Knife Skills Use raw potatoes to safely practice techniques for cutting and slicing: chop, cube, dice, julienne, mince, pare, and slice. Identify and use the correct tools. Make a chart with photos to show each type of knife cut and the tool needed to make the knife cut.

Additional Activities For additional activities, go to this book's Online Learning Center at glencoe.com.

Academic Skills

English Language Arts

17. Recipes from the Past Conduct research to find a recipe that is at least 100 years old. How does it differ from today's recipes? Rewrite the recipe to follow today's recipe style and explain the differences on your updated recipe.

> **NCTE 8** Use information resources to gather information and create and communicate knowledge.

Social Studies

18. Ethnic Recipes Research a recipe from outside your culture. Write a report that analyzes the culture from which the recipe originates, the ingredients in the recipe, and the preparation techniques used. Explain if the recipe is written differently than a typical American recipe. Share your findings with the class.

> **NCSS I E Culture** Demonstrate the value of cultural diversity, as well as cohesion, within and across groups.

Mathematics

19. Changing Recipe Amounts Imagine that you want to make the Ful Mesdames recipe in this chapter for seven people. How would you change the recipe to make sure you have enough? Rewrite the customary measurements to show the changes.

Math Concept **Multiply Integers** Positive numbers, negative numbers, and zero are all integers. They can be represented as points on a number line, and can be multiplied.

Starting Hint The written recipe is for four servings. Increase the yield to eight servings, which is easier to measure. Divide the desired yield by the original yield to find the adjustment. Multiply the adjustment with the original amount of each ingredient to find the new ingredient amounts.

 For more math help, go to the Math Appendix

> **NCTM Number and Operations** Understand the meanings of operations and how they relate to one another.

STANDARDIZED TEST PRACTICE

MULTIPLE CHOICE
Read the paragraph. Write your answer on a separate piece of paper.

> **Test-Taking Tip** Use the Chapter Summary, Vocabulary Review, and Review Key Concepts at the end of each chapter to study for your test.

Some recipes call for sifted flour or for other ingredients to be sifted with flour. But many modern cooks ask if sifting is still necessary. Why? Because pre-sifted flour is common today. For some recipes, additional sifting may not be necessary.

20. Based on the paragraph, which of the following statements is true?
  a. Sifting flour is required when baking.
  b. No one needs to use a sifter anymore.
  c. Sifting is used only for mixing flour.
  d. Sifting will improve the results for some recipes.

CHAPTER 21
Cooking Basics

Explore the Photo ▶▶
Food can be cooked in many different ways. The cooking method you choose depends on the food and the results you want. *What cooking method is used for your favorite food?*

Writing Activity
Personal Narrative

Cook the Way You Like Have you ever eaten something that was not as good as you hoped it would be? Write a short story about a time you ate something you could have improved by changing the ingredients, the seasonings, or the way it was cooked. Include descriptive words.

Writing Tips

1. **Gather** ideas by freewriting.
2. **Ask** yourself questions to fill out details of the narrative.
3. **Construct** a graphic organizer as a visual map for your narrative.

Reading Guide

Before You Read

Two-Column Notes Two-column notes are a useful way to study and organize what you have read. Divide a piece of paper into two columns. In the left column, write down main ideas. In the right column, list supporting details.

Read to Learn

Key Concepts

- **Discuss** how food science applies to cooking and preparing food.
- **Compare** moist-heat cooking, dry-heat cooking, and frying.
- **Summarize** the steps for microwave cooking.
- **Outline** how to prepare food to save nutrients and enhance flavor.

Main Idea

When food is prepared, physical and chemical changes take place. The cooking method chosen depends on the types of foods, your time and equipment, and the results you want.

Content Vocabulary

- ◇ food science
- ◇ physical change
- ◇ chemical change
- ◇ conduction
- ◇ convection
- ◇ radiation
- ◇ dry-heat cooking
- ◇ moist-heat cooking
- ◇ frying
- ◇ microwave oven
- ◇ cooking power
- ◇ standing time

Academic Vocabulary

You will find these words in your reading and on your tests. Use the glossary to look up their definitions if necessary.

- ■ relate
- ■ differentiate

Graphic Organizer

As you read, fill in a web diagram like the one below to show similar ways heat affects food.

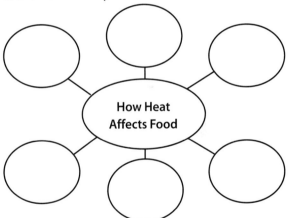

How Heat Affects Food

 Graphic Organizer Go to this book's Online Learning Center at **glencoe.com** to print out this graphic organizer.

Academic Standards ▪

 English Language Arts
NCTE 5 Use different writing process elements to communicate effectively.

 Science
NSES Content Standard B Develop an understanding of the structure and properties of matter.

 Mathematics
NCTM Number and Operations Understand the meanings of operations and how they relate to each other.

NCTM Data Analysis and Probability Select and use appropriate statistical methods to analyze data.

NCTE National Council of Teachers of English
NCTM National Council of Teachers of Mathematics

NSES National Science Education Standards
NCSS National Council for the Social Studies

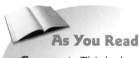

Vocabulary

You can find definitions in the glossary at the back of this book.

As You Read

Connect Think about the cooking methods you have used in class and at home.

The Science of Food Preparation

When food is prepared and cooked, it changes form physically and chemically. **Food science** is the study of the nature of foods and the changes that occur in them naturally and as a result of handling and processing.

What Is Food?

Food is a form of matter made of many different chemicals that can be ingested and used by an organism for nutrients and energy. Chemicals in food can be natural or manufactured.

A beef steak has many chemicals. It has fats such as stearic, palmitic, oleic, and linoleic acids. It has carbohydrates such as glycogen and pectin. It has proteins such as collagen, myosin, and myglobin. **Figure 21.1** shows the chemical makeup of water, proteins, carbohydrates, and fats—all found in animal-based and plant-based foods.

How Foods Can Be Changed

Foods can change physically and chemically. Slicing bread is a physical change. A **physical change** is a change in the shape or size, but not the basic chemical structure. Slicing bread does not change its taste or nutrient value.

Toasting bread, however, produces a chemical change. A **chemical change** is a change in the substances of the food. When you toast bread, it looks, smells, and tastes different.

What Ingredients Do

Each ingredient in a food mixture has a unique job in the chemical processes that change food. For example:

- ◆ **Leavening agents** (baking powder, baking soda, and yeast) make batter and dough rise and get lighter.
- ◆ **Eggs** give structure, flavor, and color to food. They also thicken food and add air.
- ◆ **Fats and oils** give tenderness, flakiness, and flavor.
- ◆ **Flour** thickens mixtures and holds other ingredients together.
- ◆ **Liquids** give moisture for blending and help leavening agents start their work.
- ◆ **Sweeteners** add sweetness and tenderness and promote browning.
- ◆ **Seasonings and flavorings** add interest and flavor.

Figure 21.1 | **Building Blocks of Food**

Food Ingredients All the ingredients in foods are made of elements from nature: carbohydrate, hydrogen, oxygen, nitrogen, iron, calcium, and many other elements. *Why is water called H_2O?*

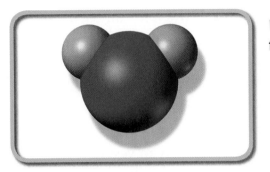

Water is a compound. A water molecule is made from two hydrogen atoms and one oxygen atom.

Proteins are made up of many small units called amino acids. Each amino acid contains four elements: carbon, hydrogen, oxygen, and nitrogen. About 20 common amino acids are arranged in different ways to make all food proteins. One protein molecule might contain thousands of amino acids.

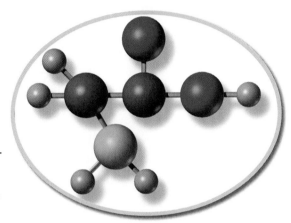

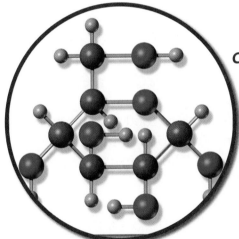

Carbohydrates contain simple sugars, such as glucose. Each simple sugar contains three elements: carbohydrate, hydrogen, and oxygen. Simple sugars are arranged in chains to make complex carbohydrates, or starches, and fiber.

Fats are made up of one glycerol molecule and three fatty-acid molecules. A fatty-acid molecule is a chain of molecules made of carbon, oxygen, and hydrogen. These diagrams show the middle of two fatty acids. Fats that are solid at room temperature have fatty acids with more hydrogen. Liquid oils have less hydrogen in their fatty acids.

Saturated Fatty Acid

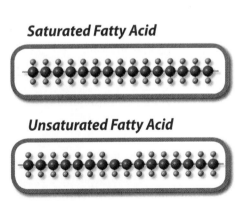

Unsaturated Fatty Acid

How Cooking Affects Food

Imagine a world without cooked food! People learned long ago that many foods taste better when cooked. Heat from cooking also has these effects:

- ◆ **Heat speeds up chemical reactions in food.** This causes the food to change, and it destroys harmful bacteria.

- ◆ **Heat helps the body digest some food substances better.** As oatmeal grains heat in water, they absorb water and soften, so they become easier to digest.

- ◆ **Heat affects texture.** Cooking makes potatoes soft and bacon crispy.

- ◆ **Heat affects color and flavor.** Green vegetables cooked for a short time become a brighter green. Their flavor also changes. Overcooked vegetables may not be as tasty.

- ◆ **Heat tenderizes protein-rich foods.** This makes them easier and more appealing to eat.

- ◆ **Heat can cause some nutrient loss.** For example, some vitamin C dissolves into cooking water. If this solution, or mixture, is poured down the drain, some vitamins go with it.

How Heat Transfers to Food

Cooking transfers heat to food. Heat is a form of energy. It makes food molecules move very quickly. They are too tiny to see, but you notice their vibration as heat.

Heat transfers from a heat source to food through conduction, convection, and radiation. The more surface area a food has, the faster heat transfers to it. The temperature and heat source also affect cooking speed.

Cooking Changes Food Heat changes food in many ways. *How does cooking change an uncooked pizza?*

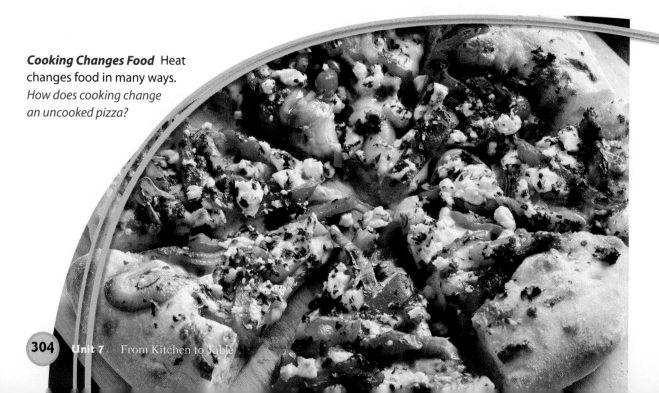

Conduction

Conduction is transfer of heat energy through direct contact between a hot surface and the food. Molecules transfer heat energy by bumping into each other. Pan-frying or sautéing are common forms of conduction.

When an egg fries in a skillet, the cooktop heats up first. Its molecules begin to vibrate. These molecules touch molecules on the bottom of the skillet. They start to vibrate. These vibrations cause heat through friction when the molecules bump into each other. Heated molecules in the skillet bump into molecules in the egg. The result? The egg cooks.

Convection

Convection cooking is the transfer of heat through the circulation or flow of heated molecules of hot liquid or hot air. With boiling, steaming, and frying, heat transfers through liquid. In baking and roasting, the heating elements within the conventional oven heat the air, which comes in contact with and cooks the food. In a convection oven, a fan moves hot air around the food.

When soup boils, heat first transfers to the pot through conduction. Convection starts as molecules in the bottom of the soup heat up. Hot soup molecules spread apart and become less dense. Heated liquid weighs less than cooler liquid above it. That makes hot liquid rise. Cooler liquid sinks to the bottom, where it heats up. This continues until all the liquid reaches the same temperature.

Radiation

Radiation is energy that is transmitted through air waves. When you hold your hand near a stovetop burner, the heat you feel comes from radiation. When the energy reaches food, molecules in the food vibrate and the food heats up. Grilling and broiling transfer heat by radiation. When you use a grill, the heat is below the food. The heat is above the food when you use a broiler.

Combination Methods

Some cooking methods involve a combination of conduction, convection, or radiation. Grilling or broiling cooks food primarily through radiation from a heat source, but there is also conduction of energy from the cooking grate and convection of energy through heated air. Baking and roasting cook food primarily through convection energy from heated air, but also through radiation from oven walls and conduction from the baking pan to the food.

Nutrition & Wellness Tips

Cook for Flavor and Nutrition

✓ Grill or roast eggplant, bell peppers, and zucchini to bring out their flavor without added fat.

✓ Thicken soups and stews with drained and mashed canned beans for more fiber and protein.

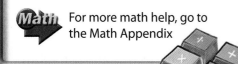
How Altitude Affects Cooking

Cooking or baking at high altitudes takes longer than at low altitudes. Higher altitudes have lower air pressure. As air pressure decreases, water molecules escape into the air more easily. In Denver, a mile above sea level, water boils at about 202°F (95°C). In sea-level Miami, water boils at about 212°F (100°C).

How does altitude **relate**, or connect to, cooking? At high altitudes, you need to cook or bake food longer. Since water boils at a lower temperature, it takes longer to kill bacteria, too. Most cookbooks show cooking and baking times for sea level.

✓ **Reading Check** **Compare** What are the differences among conduction, convection, and radiation in transferring heat?

Cooking Methods

Most food is cooked by dry heat, moist heat, or frying. The method you use depends on the type of food and the results you want.

Dry-Heat Cooking

Dry-heat cooking is cooking food uncovered without adding liquid or fat. Broiling, roasting, and baking are dry-heat methods.

Cooking in dry heat improves the flavor, texture, and appearance of many foods. Food usually turns brown and develops a crisp or tender crust on the outside. It stays moist and tender inside. Be careful not to overcook foods with dry heat. This can dry them out.

Baking and Roasting

Baking and roasting use dry heat. Breads, cakes, pies, cookies, and similar foods are baked. Fish, tender meat and poultry, and some fruits and vegetables can be baked or roasted. Preheat the oven when baking or roasting. When roasting meat or poultry, set it on a rack to drain fat away from food.

Broiling

Broiling is cooking with direct heat from above. Tender cuts of meat, poultry, fish, and some fruits and vegetables can be broiled. Place food in a broiler pan under the broiler unit.

You control how fast food cooks by its distance from the heat. For the best results, place thick foods farther from the heat and increase the cooking time.

Use tongs instead of a fork to turn foods while broiling. A fork can puncture the meat, releasing flavorful juices.

Do not line the broiler pan grid with foil. Fat will not be able to drain away. The food will fry and could even catch fire.

Pan-Broiling

Use the pan-broiling method for thin, tender cuts of meat. The meat's natural fat provides all the fat you need. To pan-broil, place food in a hot, ungreased skillet. Cook uncovered until it browns on one side. Turn and continue cooking until done. Pour off any fat that accumulates as you cook.

Moist-Heat Cooking

Moist-heat cooking is a cooking method that uses hot liquid, steam, or both. Moist-heat cooking can tenderize less tender cuts of meat and poultry. It also blends flavors and helps keep food from drying out. Foods cooked in moist heat do not brown. Canning is moist-heat cooking done right in the can.

You cook with moist heat when:

◆ The food is a liquid, such as soup or hot cocoa.

◆ The food is covered in liquid, such as rice, dry beans, and pasta.

◆ The pan or container is covered so that steam and moisture stay inside.

You can use several different types of appliances for moist-heat cooking. In a conventional oven, you can cook food in a covered dish, a foil package, or a special plastic cooking bag. In a microwave oven, you can cook or steam food in a vented covered dish. On a cooktop, you can boil, steam, or simmer in cookware on the top of the range. You can also use a small appliance like a slow cooker or a covered electric skillet to cook in liquid.

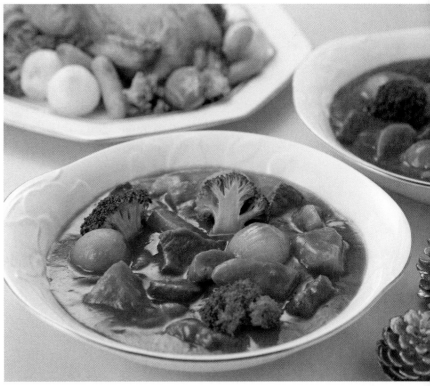

Blend the Flavors Moist heat allows flavors to blend together. *What foods, other than stew, use moist heat to blend flavors?*

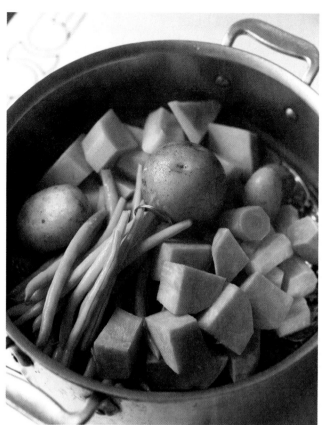

Steamed Foods A steamer holds food above boiling water for moist cooking. *What types of foods might you steam?*

Boiling and Simmering

When liquid boils, bubbles constantly rise to the surface and break. The boiling point of liquid is the temperature at which it turns to steam. The boiling point of water is 212°F (100°C). To boil, use a big enough pot to hold both the liquid and the food. Bring the liquid to the boiling point, then add the food.

Simmering gently cooks food in liquid slightly below the boiling point. Bubbles form slowly and break before they reach the surface. Simmering is better than boiling for most foods except noodles. Foods lose more nutrients, flavor, and texture when boiled. Boiling also toughens protein-rich foods.

Steaming

Many foods, such as vegetables, can be cooked in steam. Use a steamer basket or an electric steamer. Place the basket inside a pan with a small amount of boiling water and cover the pan to keep the steam inside. The basket holds food above the water, but has holes to let steam flow through and cook the food.

Frying

Frying is cooking in small or large amounts of fat. Fat can be heated to a higher temperature than water. Frying gives the food a brown and crispy surface.

Frying causes food to soak up fat, so you should use as little fat or oil as possible when pan frying. Liquid vegetable oil is lower in saturated fat than solid fat. For better nutrition, choose other cooking methods, such as pan-broiling.

Pan-Frying and Sautéing

Pan-frying uses less fat than deep frying so less fat gets soaked up. Some tender or quick-cooking foods can be pan-fried in a skillet in a small amount of fat. Using a cooking oil spray or a non-stick skillet allows you to use even less fat. Pan-frying is often used to precook foods like onions before they are used in a recipe. This is called sautéing (sä-'tā-ŋ). The foods are chopped or sliced so they cook or soften quickly.

Deep-Fat Frying

Deep-fat frying, also called French frying, is when food is completely covered in a large amount of fat. Deep-fat frying adds a lot of fat to food. When deep-fat frying, follow the recipe directions carefully. Do not overheat the fat. Check the temperature of the fat with a deep fat thermometer. Also, be sure food is dry before frying it. Moisture can cause hot fat to spatter, which can cause serious burns.

Combination Cooking Methods

Braising and stir-frying are two methods that combine frying with moist heat. Braising is browning food in a small amount of fat, followed by long, slow, moist-heat cooking. It tenderizes tougher meats that take a while to cook. Stir-frying is a quick way to fry then steam vegetables, tofu, or tender cuts of meat, poultry, or fish using a small amount of oil at a high temperature followed by steaming.

More Cooking and Heating Terms

Here are some other common cooking and heating terms:

- **Baste** Brush or pour liquid over food, such as turkey, as it cooks.
- **Blanch** Cook quickly, but not completely, in boiling liquid.
- **Brown** Cook briefly until the surface turns brown.
- **Preheat** Heat an appliance before you put food in it.
- **Reduce** Simmer or boil liquid until it is less than its original volume to concentrate flavor.
- **Sear** Brown meat's surface quickly with very high heat.
- **Toast** Brown food by direct heat or in the oven.

✓ **Reading Check** **Compare** Which cooking methods add no fat to dishes?

Microwave Cooking

A microwave oven can defrost, heat, reheat, and cook food quickly. Frozen and canned foods, many convenience foods, many leftovers, liquids, and fresh vegetables cook or heat well in a microwave oven. Microwaving is not as suitable for many baked foods or foods that should be crisp or browned.

How Microwave Ovens Work

A **microwave oven** uses electromagnetic radiation to cook food. (See **Figure 21.2.**) Microwaves bounce off the oven walls and enter food, causing water molecules in the food to vibrate.

The heat transfers to other molecules in the food. Microwave ovens cook food in one-quarter to one-half the time of other methods.

The amount of electricity that a microwave oven uses to generate microwaves is its **cooking power**. Cooking power is measured in watts of electricity. Most microwave ovens have about 500 to 700 watts. The higher the wattage, the faster food cooks. Microwave ovens have power settings—for example, High, Medium High, Medium Low, and Defrost/Low.

Choose a Microwave-Safe Container

Follow microwave instructions on convenience food packages. Learn to **differentiate**, or recognize a difference, between microwave-safe containers and unsafe ones.

Round, oval, or ring-shaped pans allow microwave energy to strike the food from all angles. Food in the corners of square or rectangular containers tends to overcook.

Arrange Food for Even Cooking and Cover Food

Arrange food carefully for even microwave cooking. Read the recipe and arrange the food as specified by the recipe. Cut the foods into pieces that are about the same size. Place thicker or tougher parts of food toward the outside edges of the container.

Figure 21.2	Microwave Technology

Microwaves at Work The magnetron changes electricity to microwaves. A fan circulates microwaves. They also bounce off the sides of the oven. Food heats or cooks quickly. *Why should you never turn on a microwave oven when it is empty?*

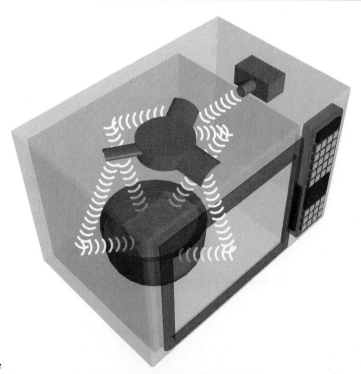

Covering food helps keep moisture in and prevent spattering. Use a microwave-safe cover.

Consider Cooking Time and Power Level

Good microwave cooking skills result in moist, flavorful foods. If food cooks too long or is not covered properly, it gets tough and too chewy. Cooking time depends on several factors:

- **Amount of Moisture, Sugar, or Fat** Drier food, and foods with more sugar or fat, heat faster.
- **Amount of Food** More food takes more cooking time.
- **Placement of Food** Food in the oven's center cooks more slowly.
- **Food Size** Smaller pieces of food cook faster.

Choose the minimum time in the recipe or package directions. If you need to add more cooking time, cook for another 30 seconds and check again.

Use the power level suggested in the recipe or instructions. If the oven uses less than 625 to 700 watts, you may need a little extra time or a higher power setting.

Rotate Food for Even Cooking

Many microwave ovens have hot spots where food cooks faster. You may need to rotate food, stir it, or rearrange or turn food over. Do this after half the cooking time.

Allow Standing Time

When the microwave oven shuts off, molecules still vibrate. **Standing time** is a period of time when food continues to cook after microwaving. If instructions say to let food stand, cover it for the time specified. Test it with a thermometer.

Microwave Oven Safety

Be careful not to start a fire or burn yourself. Never use metal containers. Eggs in their shells can burst in the microwave oven. Pierce potatoes and egg yolks, with a fork before cooking them.

Prevent Burns

Follow these guidelines to prevent burns:

- Use pot holders to remove food from the oven.
- Do not use containers with tight-fitting covers.
- Watch out for steam when you remove the covers from cooking containers or open a bag of microwave popcorn.
- Let food cool slightly before eating it.

✓ **Reading Check** **Recall** How can you help food cook evenly when microwaved?

Cooking for Nutrition and Flavor

Use proper techniques to help keep more nutrients and flavor in food. Some nutrients can be destroyed by heat or oxygen or lost in cooking liquids. Retain nutrients by:

◆ Pare or trim as little from fruits and vegetables as possible.

◆ Keep food whole or in large pieces when possible.

◆ Cook food for the right length of time.

◆ Use cooking liquids from vegetables in soups and stews.

✓ Reading Check **Explain** How can you help retain nutrients in food?

EASY RECIPES
Everyday Favorites

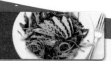

Quick and Hearty Chili

Customary	Ingredients	Metric
1 Tbsp.	Vegetable oil	15 mL
1	Large white onion, diced	1
1 pound	Ground turkey	500 g
3	Garlic cloves, finely chopped	3
1 large can (28 oz)	Peeled, crushed tomatoes	800 g
1 jar (16 oz)	Salsa, mild or hot	450 g
1 can (15 oz)	Kidney or black beans, drained	425 g
½ tsp.	Cumin	3 mL
2 tsp.	Chili powder	10 mL

Try This!
Try mixing two or three different kinds of beans. Add fresh or frozen corn. You can also adjust to your own taste with more or less chili powder.

Yield: 8 servings, 1¼ cup (375 mL) each

❶ In a large pot, heat the oil on medium heat. Add onions and cook until tender. Add the turkey and garlic and cook until brown.

❷ Drain off excess fat and add the tomatoes, salsa, beans and cumin. Simmer, stirring occasionally, for 25 minutes.

❸ Add chili powder, simmer another five minutes, and serve in bowls.

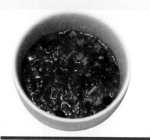

Nutritional Information Per Serving: 208 calories, 7 g total fat (2 g saturated fat), 45 mg cholesterol, 542 mg sodium, 22 g total carbohydrate (7 g fiber, 4 g total sugars), 16 g protein

Percent Daily Value: vitamin A 25%, vitamin C 30%, calcium 8%, iron 15%

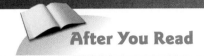

After You Read

CHAPTER SUMMARY

When food is prepared, physical and chemical changes take place. During cooking, heat energy transfers to and within food. You can cook food with moist or dry heat, by frying, or by microwaving. The type of cooking method you choose depends on the types of food, your time and equipment, and the results you want. Proper cooking techniques help retain nutrients and flavor.

Vocabulary Review

1. Use each of these vocabulary words in a sentence.

Content Vocabulary
- food science (p. 302)
- physical change (p. 302)
- chemical change (p. 302)
- conduction (p. 305)
- convection (p. 305)
- radiation (p. 305)
- dry-heat cooking (p. 306)
- moist-heat cooking (p. 307)
- frying (p. 308)
- microwave oven (p. 309)
- cooking power (p. 310)
- standing time (p. 311)

Academic Vocabulary
- relate (p. 306)
- differentiate (p. 310)

Review Key Concepts

2. Discuss how food science applies to cooking and preparing food.

3. Compare moist-heat cooking, dry-heat cooking, and frying.

4. Summarize the steps for microwave cooking.

5. Outline how to prepare food to save nutrients and enhance flavor.

Critical Thinking

6. Analyze why it is important to know the different ways in which heat is transferred to food? In your analysis, describe the three main ways heat transfers to food.

7. Explain the differences between physical and chemical changes in food. Give examples of dishes that show each type of change.

8. Analyze this situation: You are cooking chicken breasts in a skillet. Why might you need to move the pan away from the heat? How can you safely do this?

9. Explain why stir-frying or microwaving instead of simmering can help retain nutrients in green beans and broccoli.

Real-World Skills and Applications

Decision Making and Goal Setting

10. Quick and Nutritious Meal You have 30 minutes to prepare dinner. You have chicken breasts. What cooking methods could you use to prepare dinner? What could you add to the meal to increase its nutritional value? Explain your answer in a two-paragraph report.

Interpersonal and Collaborative

11. Healthful Cooking Web Page As a class, create a Web page showing creative, flavorful, and healthful ways to prepare food. Include recipes, cooking tips, and photos. Arrange to have the page added to your school's Web site.

Technology

12. Watch a Cooking Show Watch a cooking show on television or the Internet to learn about a specific cooking technique. Take detailed notes and write a description of what you learned. Give an oral presentation to your class to explain the cooking technique.

Financial Literacy

13. Pre-Cooked vs. Home-Cooked You can buy a roasted 3-pound chicken at the supermarket for $7.99. You can also buy a 3-pound uncooked chicken for $1.79 per pound, then roast it yourself. How much might you save by cooking it yourself?

14. Different Cooking Methods Identify six ways to prepare potatoes. Classify them according to their basic cooking method. Follow your teacher's instructions to form teams, and prepare potatoes using one of the methods. What were the advantages and drawbacks of your cooking method? Present your findings in an oral report.

15. Microwave Hot Spots Cover the inside bottom of a microwave oven with waxed paper. Evenly space several large marshmallows on top. Microwave on 100% power for 60 seconds without any rotation. Identify any microwave hot spots. How does rotation prevent them? Document your findings in a written report with pictures.

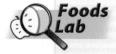

16. Time to Microwave Peel two large potatoes. Cut them into both big and small pieces. Microwave the pieces on high for one minute. Check to see whether they are done. If necessary, add extra time in 30-second increments. Rotate the pieces frequently. Which pieces are done first? Last? Draw conclusions and summarize your findings in a paragraph.

Additional Activities For additional activities go to this book's Online Learning Center at glencoe.com.

Academic Skills

English Language Arts

17. Culinary Advice Write an advice column for the school newspaper. Ask and answer two questions about boosting flavor and nutrition in everyday recipes. Share your column in class.

> **NCTE 5** Use different writing process elements to communicate effectively.

Science

18. Carmelizing Cooking carmelizes the natural sugars in food.

Procedure Research what happens to onions when they are cooked for a while. Why does the color and aroma change?

Analysis Write your answer in a paragraph. Discuss how carmelization affects the appeal of many foods.

> **NSES Content Standard B** Develop an understanding of the structure and properties of matter.

Mathematics

19. Cooking Times Microwaving four large potatoes takes about one-sixth the time needed to bake them in a conventional oven. If it will take you 1½ hours to bake theses potatoes in a conventional oven, how long will it take you to cook them in a microwave oven?

Math Concept **Dividing Rational Numbers** To divide a number by a rational number (such as a fraction), multiply the first number by the multiplicative inverse of the second. A multiplicative inverse is a reciprocal: ½ x ²⁄₁ = 1.

Starting Hint Begin by converting the time to minutes. Then, multiply the minutes by the fraction ⅙ to find your answer.

 For more math help, go to the Math Appendix

> **NCTM Number and Operations** Understand the meanings of operations and how they relate to one another.

STANDARDIZED TEST PRACTICE

ESSAY
Read the paragraph and think about what you learned in the chapter. Write your answer on a separate piece of paper.

Test-Taking Tip Once you learn a new word, try to use it right away—verbally in a conversation or on paper in a sentence. For example, how can you use the word *conversation* in a conversation with someone?

You can add flavor, different textures, and nutrients to foods without adding too much fat. For example, top a casserole with croutons or bran flakes. Add sliced banana to a peanut butter sandwich or put beans in an omelet. Substitute one food for another. Use fresh spinach instead of iceberg lettuce or mash sweet potatoes instead of white potatoes.

20. Write an essay about how you can change a standard family recipe or meal to add more flavor, texture, and nutrients.

CHAPTER 22

Organizing the Kitchen

Explore the Photo ▶▶
You can learn to be organized when you work in the kitchen. *In what ways do good chefs organize their work? How might you do the same?*

Writing Activity

Identify Purpose and Audience

Get Ready! Imagine that you need to explain how to make a dish to someone. Choose an audience and explain how to make the dish, highlighting the most important part of your instructions for that audience.

Writing Tips

1. **Determine** if your purpose is to inform, persuade, entertain, or describe.

2. **Consider** the aspects of a topic suitable for your audience.

3. **Explain** how to make the dish.

Reading Guide

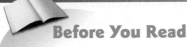

Before You Read

Think of an Example Look over the Key Concepts for this chapter. Think of an example of how or when you could use one of the skills from the Key Concepts. Think about why the skills are important.

Read to Learn

Key Concepts

- **Describe** how to organize a kitchen for efficiency.
- **Illustrate** a work plan for preparing a meal or recipe.
- **Discuss** how to work efficiently as a team in a foods lab.
- **Explain** ways to reduce, reuse, and recycle.

Main Idea

An organized kitchen, a good work plan, and efficient work skills are essential for successful meals. They also make food preparation enjoyable.

Content Vocabulary

◇ work center
◇ work triangle
◇ work plan
◇ pre-preparation step
◇ dovetailing
◇ recycling

Academic Vocabulary

You will find these words in your reading and on your tests. Use the glossary to look up their definitions if necessary.

- ▪ simultaneous
- ▪ establish

Graphic Organizer

As you read, use a chart like the one below to show the four steps you need to remember when you make a work plan.

1.
2.
3.
4.

 Graphic Organizer Go to this book's Online Learning Center at glencoe.com to print out this graphic organizer.

Academic Standards • • • • • • • • • • • • • • • • • • •

 English Language Arts
NCTE 9 Develop an understanding of diversity in language use across cultures.
NCTE 12 Use language to accomplish individual purposes.

 Science
NSES Content Standard F Develop an understanding of natural resources.

NSES Content Standard F Develop an understanding of personal and community health.

 Mathematics
NCTM Measurement Understand measurable attributes of objects and the units, systems, and processes of measurement.

NCTE National Council of Teachers of English
NCTM National Council of Teachers of Mathematics

NSES National Science Education Standards
NCSS National Council for the Social Studies

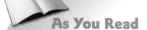

Vocabulary

You can find definitions in the glossary at the back of this book.

Organize the Kitchen

A well-organized kitchen helps you manage the tasks of storage, preparation, and cleanup. Good management saves much time and energy.

Organized work centers make good use of kitchen space. A **work center** is an area devoted to a certain type of task. Equipment and supplies are within easy reach. Work centers have a flat and clutter-free surface for working. Work centers may overlap.

Your kitchen layout determines your work centers. **Figure 22.1** describes three common types of work centers. The imaginary lines connecting these work centers form the **work triangle**. In an efficient work triangle, the three sides total 12 to 22 feet (4 to 7 meters).

As You Read

Connect Think about the different areas in your kitchen and how they are used.

Organize for Physical Challenges

A little planning can help you organize a kitchen for common physical challenges. Here are some examples:

- **Impaired Vision** Improve lighting. Relabel containers in large letters. Apply contrasting paint or tape to counter edges.

- **Limited Hand Strength** Install large, easy-to-grip handles on doors. Put wet dishcloths under mixing bowls and cutting boards to avoid slipping.

- **Difficulty Standing or Walking** Provide a stool for sitting. Eliminate throw rugs. Provide a sturdy rolling cart.

- **Wheelchair Use** Make room for wheelchairs to roll under countertops and the sink. Insulate hot water pipes to avoid leg burns. Store food and equipment within easy reach. Provide a work surface at wheelchair height.

✓ **Reading Check** **Describe** What are the advantages of a well-organized kitchen?

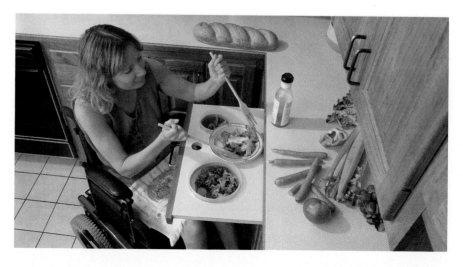

Clutter-Free Convenience This kitchen work surface is at a convenient height for a seated user. *What other features does it offer?*

Make a Work Plan

Work plans can help you prepare a simple recipe or a whole dinner—without forgetting a single step. A **work plan** is a list of all the steps for preparing a recipe or meal. It includes identifying preparation tasks, making a schedule, planning how to work efficiently, and finishing the job, and cleaning up. A well-thought-out work plan also shows who will do each task.

Even experienced cooks often make work plans when they prepare a new dish or special meal. As you gain kitchen experience, you may not need a work plan every time you prepare a meal.

Figure 22.1	Kitchen Work Centers

A Place for Everything Most kitchens have three basic work centers for storing, cooking and serving food, and for cleaning up. *What other work centers might a kitchen have?*

Work Center	Location	Activities	Items to Store There
Storage Center	Around the refrigerator-freezer, with cabinets nearby	• Storing fresh and frozen foods • Storing nonperishable foods • Storing leftovers	• Food • Foil, plastic wrap, storage containers, and bags
Cooking and Serving Center	Around the range and microwave oven	• Cooking food • Serving food	• Pots and pans • Cooking tools such as spatulas, ladles, wooden spoons, and tongs • Small appliances • Potholders and oven mitts • Serving bowls and platters
Cleanup Center	Around the sink and dishwasher	• Washing fresh fruits and vegetables • Rinsing and washing dishes, pots, pans, and utensils	• Vegetable brush, colander, peeler, and cutting boards • Soaps and detergents • Dishtowels and dishcloths • Other cleaning supplies For convenience, dishes, glassware, and eating utensils may be stored here after they are cleaned.

Identify Preparation Tasks

A combined work plan has all the steps for preparing a meal. A recipe may call for a **pre-preparation step**. This is a step to get food and equipment ready. For example, if a recipe requires 2 cups of cooked rice, cooking the rice is a pre-preparation step.

Consider how to dovetail tasks. **Dovetailing** is doing two tasks simultaneously. **Simultaneous** means taking place at the same time. For example, for the complete meal described in **Figure 22.2**, while the couscous cooks, you can season and cook the chicken. Do not try to dovetail tasks that require your full attention.

Figure 22.2	Preparation Tasks

Have a Plan Your work plan lists all the tasks for each recipe and the meal. *Would you do all the tasks here in the order listed? Why or why not?*

Food	Tasks	Time
	• Wash your hands. Get ready to cook.	5 minutes
	• Gather ingredients and equipment.	5 to 10 minutes
Broiled Chicken	• Thaw chicken breasts in the refrigerator.	overnight
	• Season chicken with herbs. Put chicken on broiler rack.	2 minutes
	• Broil in oven.	7 to 10 minutes
	• Place chicken on plate.	1 minute
Frozen Broccoli	• Remove broccoli from package, put in microwave-safe container.	5 minutes
	• Microwave on medium power.	10 minutes
	• Let stand.	1 to 2 minutes
	• Put broccoli in a bowl.	1 minute
Orange Mint Couscous	• Wash and chop mint leaves.	5 minutes
	• Measure and toast pine nuts.	5 minutes
	• Measure orange juice. Bring to boil in a medium saucepan.	5 minutes
	• Measure couscous and mint. Add to orange juice. Let stand.	5 to 10 minutes
	• Measure and add raisins and pine nuts to cooked couscous. Fluff with a fork.	1 minute
	• Put couscous in a bowl.	1 minute
Frozen Strawberry Yogurt	• Fill individual bowls with yogurt.	3 minutes
Fat-Free Milk	• Pour milk.	1 minute
	• Set table.	5 minutes
	• Serve food.	1 minute
	• Put leftovers away.	5 minutes
	• Clean kitchen.	15 minutes

Make a Schedule

Schedules are important—especially for a beginning cook. **Figure 22.3** shows a schedule for preparing the meal described in Figure 22.2. Schedules help you think ahead so all the food is ready at the same time. You can plan time to enjoy what you prepare and to clean up afterward. People work at different speeds and may do tasks in a different order. The best schedules are flexible. Consider these factors in your overall schedule:

- ◆ **Time to prepare the food.** Write in your work plan how long each task will take. Cooking times usually appear in the recipe or package directions. Estimate for other tasks. Allowing too much time is better than too little.

- ◆ **Time to serve the food.** Work back from your meal time. For example, if you want to serve lunch at noon and you estimate 45 minutes of preparaton, start at 11:15 a.m.

- ◆ **Time to eat and clean up.** Remember to leave time for a relaxed meal and for cleaning up afterward.

Figure 22.3	Make Your Schedule

On Schedule Once you have a combined work plan, turn it into a schedule with all the tasks. *What would you add to this schedule if you were cooking with someone else?*

Time	Tasks
Night Before	Thaw chicken breasts in the refrigerator.
5:15	Wash hands. Get ready to cook.
5:20	Set table.
5:25	Gather ingredients and equipment.
5:33	Wash mint. Let drain.
5:35	Remove broccoli from package, put in microwave-safe container.
5:40	Measure and toast pine nuts for couscous.
5:45	Measure orange juice. Bring to boil in a medium saucepan.
5:55	Chop mint. Measure couscous and mint. Add couscous and mint to hot orange juice. Let stand.
6:00	Season chicken with herbs. Put chicken on broiler rack.
6:02	Broil chicken in oven.
6:12	Microwave broccoli on medium power. Let stand.
6:22	Pour milk.
6:23	Measure and add raisins and pine nuts to cooked couscous. Fluff with a fork. Put couscous in a bowl.
6:25	Put broccoli in a bowl. Place chicken on a plate. Serve food.
After the Main Course	Remove dishes from table. Fill individual bowls with frozen yogurt. Serve yogurt.
After Dinner	Clear table. Put leftovers away. Clean kitchen.

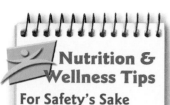
With these factors in mind, follow these steps to make your final meal or recipe schedule:

◆ Put tasks in a logical order.

◆ Write down the starting time for each task.

◆ Determine which tasks can be dovetailed.

Work Efficiently

As you work in the kitchen, always think about how you can be more efficient and still follow safety and cleanliness rules. Do not take shortcuts that may endanger you or the people who eat the food. Follow these guidelines to save time and energy and be efficient when working in the kitchen:

◆ Start with a clean, orderly area. Always put things back when you are done.

◆ Gather and arrange equipment and ingredients first.

◆ Use the most efficient equipment. For example, you can chop onions with a food processor. With practice, using a chef's knife is just as fast and easier to clean.

◆ Set a timer for tasks that take a specific time. Do not rely on your memory.

◆ Dovetail tasks. Divide the work into specific tasks if someone is helping you.

◆ Do tasks ahead if you can.

◆ Check off completed tasks on your work plan.

◆ Clean up as you work. Have a clean, wet dishcloth handy to wipe up spills.

Between tasks, wash used equipment with hot, sudsy water.

Efficiency Saves Effort When you schedule your work plan, remember that some tasks can be dovetailed, and some menu items can be prepared ahead. *Which foods for this dinner could you prepare the day before?*

Finish the Job and Clean Up

After the meal is over, you still have work to do. The final step after preparing and serving a meal is cleaning up. The leftovers need to be stored properly and right away. Pots, pans, and dishes need to be washed. Wipe up crumbs and spills from the table and counters. Sweep the floor. Once the kitchen is clean, the job is done! Follow these tips to speed the process of cleaning up:

◆ Scrape or rinse food from pots and pans, dishes, and utensils into the garbage container or disposer. If food is stuck, soak the dish in hot water.

◆ Wipe greasy pans with paper towels before washing to remove excess oil.

◆ Arrange the dishes in the order they will be washed: glassware, dishes, flatware, pots, pans, and other cooking utensils.

◆ Fill the sink or dishpan with hot, soapy water. Immerse a few dishes at a time.

◆ Wash dishes with a clean dishcloth or sponge.

◆ Rinse all washed dishes in hot water.

◆ Let clean dishes air-dry in a dish drainer, or dry them with a clean towel.

◆ Follow the directions for using a dishwasher. Some items may be damaged by a dishwasher.

◆ Clean the countertops and cooktop with hot, soapy water. Wipe off the dining table.

◆ Clean any food from the sink.

◆ Make sure there are no spills on the floor.

◆ Dispose of garbage properly.

✓ Reading Check) Recognize Why might a beginning cook need a work plan for preparing a meal?

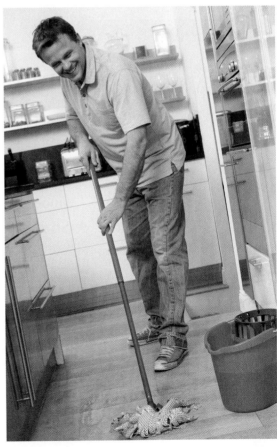

Clean As You Go Cleaning up as you finish each task saves time and effort after a meal. *What cleanup tasks can become a habit as you prepare food?*

Evaluate Green Methods

Today, many people are using green methods in their kitchens. Green methods are ways of doing tasks that help conserve energy, water, and food. There are many steps in a work plan that can be done in a green manner.

Procedure Research green methods for the kitchen, then evaluate your foods lab. How well does your class conserve energy, water, and food? What can you do as a class to improve conservation and reduce waste and pollution?

Analysis Write a checklist of actions you can take as a class to conserve. Rate each action on a scale of 1 to 3, with 3 representing actions you almost always take, 2 representing actions you sometimes take, and 1 representing actions you almost never take. Write a paragraph to explain how this evaluation might affect your future actions in the foods lab.

NSES Content Standard F Develop an understanding of natural resources.

Work as a Team

Cooking successfully with others, either at home or in your foods lab, takes teamwork. Teamwork in the kitchen requires a common goal and a team plan. It also takes cooperation and a willingness to assist each other. Remember to stay patient and resolve problems calmly.

Plan in Your Foods Lab

Planning a menu and creating a work plan will make your experience in the foods lab go smoothly. Follow these guidelines to make a plan for a team:

◆ Prepare your work plan together. Write a person's name beside each task.

◆ Look for ways to work efficiently as you plan. Your foods lab time is limited.

◆ Determine when you want to serve the food, how much time you need to eat, and how long cleanup will take. The rest of the lab time is for organizing and preparing the food. If food cannot be prepared in the amount of time you have, you will need to either choose another recipe. You may also need to prepare part of the dish on another day.

◆ Divide tasks equally among team members. For example, one person might gather the ingredients while the other sets the table. For larger tasks, you might share preparation steps. Making one person do most of the work is unfair and slows down the whole group.

◆ Review the schedule. Time tasks so that the work flows smoothly.

◆ Stick to the plan, but be prepared to make changes if an unexpected problem arises.

◆ Take responsibility for your share of work. Complete the tasks that are assigned to you in a timely manner.

◆ When you finish your tasks, ask how you can help others.

✓ **Reading Check** **Describe** What are three signs that a foods lab group is using good teamwork?

Evaluate Your Foods Lab

Evaluate your meal and your experience in the foods lab after the cleanup is done. Rate the food for appearance, texture, and flavor. Judge how well you worked together. That will help you work better as a team next time. As a team, ask:

◆ Did your work plan go as you expected? Were you done on time?

◆ Did you work as a team? Did everyone help?

◆ Was the food prepared properly? How did it look and taste?

◆ Was the table set correctly? Was the food served properly?

◆ Did you leave the area clean and orderly?

◆ Did any unexpected problems arise? If so, how did you handle them?

◆ How might you change your plan next time? Why?

✓ **Reading Check** **Recall** How can you determine if your foods lab was successful?

Conserve and Recycle

Our planet has a limited supply of natural resources. The way you handle the resources affects your health, the health of others, and the health of the environment. A good goal for any home is to **establish**, or bring into existence, an earth-friendly kitchen. You can do this by conserving energy, water, and food and by reducing, reusing, and recycling. **Recycling** means sorting and disposing of reusable items so their materials can be made into new products.

Rate the Foods Lab As part of your foods lab, you should rate the food and how well you worked together. *Why is it important to evaluate the food and your team?*

Conserve Energy

Follow these guidelines to conserve energy and control pollution.

◆ Keep appliances clean and in good condition. Dirty or damaged appliances often use more energy.

◆ Turn on appliances only when you need them.

◆ Get energy efficient appliances.

◆ Use a microwave oven or small appliances, such as a toaster oven, when you can. They may use less energy than a cooktop or large oven.

◆ Cook the whole meal in the oven at the same time.

◆ Keep the oven and the refrigerator doors closed. Energy is wasted when appliances need to regain their temperature.

◆ Preheat an oven just before you need it.

◆ Plan your shopping trips to use less fuel.

Conserve Water

Communities depend on clean water. In some areas water is limited. Droughts, or unusually long periods without rain or snow, can create water shortages. Pollution can ruin the water supply.

Discover International Foods

North Africa

Algeria, Morocco, and Tunisia combine nutrient-dense foods in similar dishes. Couscous, a North African pasta, is mixed with milk for breakfast and fruit for dessert and is steamed with meat, vegetables, chickpeas, raisins, and spices. Spice and herb blends, including cumin, cinnamon, ginger, chiles, saffron, and mint, add delicate to peppery-hot flavors. Peppery *harissa* is popular in Tunisia. Algerians often use tomatoes. Moroccans like saffron. North Africa is famous for paper-thin pancakes, tagines, cold vegetable appetizers, and fish dishes, too.

Languages Across Cultures

couscous (ʹküs-ˌküs) a granular pasta popular in North Africa

tagines (ʹtä-jēnz) savory Moroccan stews with meat or chicken, simmered with vegetables, olives, lemons, garlic and spices. They are often served with couscous. They are typically cooked in cone-shaped pots.

 Recipes Find out more about international recipes on this book's Online Learning Center at glencoe.com.

NCTE 9 Develop an understanding of language use across cultures.

Follow these guidelines to conserve water.

- ◆ Have dripping faucets repaired. One drop a second can waste 700 gallons of water in a year.

- ◆ Run the dishwasher only when it is full.

- ◆ Do not leave water running when you are not actively using it.

- ◆ Turn off the faucet when you have enough water.

- ◆ As you wash dishes, turn water off and on as you rinse.

Reduce, Reuse, and Recycle

Discarded items and packaging contribute to waste. Waste not only uses resources, such as fuel for transport, but also takes up space in landfills. Product packaging makes up a third or more of the trash people create.

- ◆ Try to buy items with less packaging. Another option: buy in bulk with reusable packaging.

- ◆ When possible, avoid single-serve containers, which use more packaging per serving.

- ◆ Use fewer disposables, which are used once or twice and then thrown away. For example, bring water in your own, clean, refillable water bottle, rather than buying a new bottle of water each time.

- ◆ Try to reuse some packaging. For example, wash empty jars and use them to store bulk foods or leftovers.

- ◆ Take old plastic and paper bags back to the store to recycle, if possible.

Making new items from recycled ones often takes fewer resources than using new materials. Recyclable items carry the recycling symbol on the right. Here is how to do your part to recycle:

- ◆ Try to buy foods sold in recyclable packaging.

- ◆ Learn how community and school recycling programs work and what items they take. Cardboard, aluminum and steel cans, glass bottles and jars, plastic bags and bottles, and newspapers are recyclable.

- ◆ Rinse containers to remove food residue first. You may need to remove labels from cans or sort items.

- ◆ Look for places to recycle drink cans and plastic bottles in public places.

Follow the Arrows
Many common consumer products contain recycled content. Choose products that bear this symbol whenever possible. *What everyday products do you use that contain recycled materials?*

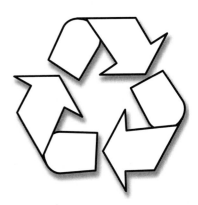

Conserve Food

Food is scarce in many parts of the world. Yet a large amount of food in the United States is discarded. How can you help?

◆ Buy only the amount of food you can use before it loses quality and spoils. Store it properly.

◆ Prepare food properly. Poorly prepared food may end up in the garbage can.

◆ Take only as much food as you know you will eat.

◆ Use leftovers creatively and safely. Store them properly.

◆ If you have a garden, make a compost bin. Add kitchen waste like corn husks.

✓ Reading Check **Compare** What is the difference between recycling and reusing an item?

EASY RECIPES   International Flavors

Orange-Mint Couscous

Customary	Ingredients	Metric
1 cup	Orange juice	250 mL
½ cup	Zucchini	125 mL
½ cup	Red onion	125 mL
¾ cup	Uncooked couscous	185 mL
2 Tbsp.	Fresh, chopped mint leaves	30 mL
½ cup	Raisins	125 mL
¼ cup	Chopped toasted pine nuts	60 mL

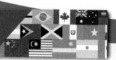

Try This!
Couscous is also often served like rice, and used to catch the sauce from a main dish. To make it plain, steam equal parts couscous and water.

Yield: 4 servings, ½ cup (125 mL) each

❶ In a tightly covered medium saucepan, bring orange juice, zucchini, and onion to a boil.

❷ Stir in the couscous and mint. Remove from heat and cover pan. Let stand five minutes.

❸ Add raisins and pine nuts, and fluff couscous with a fork before serving.

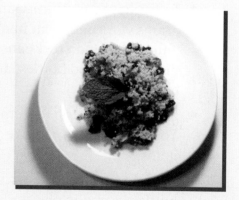

Nutritional Information Per Serving: 336 calories, 10 g total fat (1 g saturated fat), 0 mg cholesterol, 112 mg sodium, 55 g total carbohydrate (4 g fiber, 9 g total sugars), 7 g protein

Percent Daily Value: vitamin A 6%, vitamin C 60%, calcium 6%, iron 30%

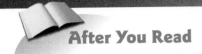

After You Read

CHAPTER SUMMARY

A well-organized kitchen has three basic work centers—for storage, cooking and serving, and cleanup. Equipment and ingredients are kept where they are handy to use. Basic management skills save time and energy in the kitchen. This allows time to prepare, serve, eat, and clean up a meal. Using a work plan helps you identify preparation tasks, make a schedule, work efficiently, and finish the job well. Cooking successfully with others takes cooperation. As a team in a foods lab, you can apply good kitchen management principles. Good management also includes reducing, reusing, and recycling as you buy, store, and cook food. That is important for conserving the earth's resources.

Vocabulary Review

1. Use each of these vocabulary words in a sentence.

Content Vocabulary
◇ work center (p. 318)
◇ work triangle (p. 318)
◇ work plan (p. 319)
◇ pre-preparation step (p. 320)
◇ dovetailing (p. 320)
◇ recycling (p. 325)

Academic Vocabulary
■ simultaneous (p. 320)
■ establish (p. 325)

Review Key Concepts

2. Describe how to organize a kitchen for efficiency.

3. Illustrate a work plan for preparing a meal or recipe.

4. Discuss how to work efficiently as a team in a foods lab.

5. Explain ways to reduce, reuse, and recycle.

Critical Thinking

6. Analyze a cooking demonstration on television, on the Internet, or at a community event. Record all the examples of efficiency and teamwork that you notice.

7. Evaluate how waste created in the kitchen can be reduced, reused, or recycled.

8. Predict how long it would take to safely and correctly prepare a specific recipe. Test your prediction. Evaluate your findings.

9. Conclude what might happen in a disorganized foods lab.

Real-World Skills and Applications

Goal Setting and Decision Making

10. Work Together Follow your teacher's instructions to form teams. Imagine that your team has been asked to create a work plan for creating a turkey sandwich. Create a work plan that includes all steps in preparation, serving, eating and cleanup.

Interpersonal and Collaborative

11. Time-and-Motion Study Do a time-and-motion study for a common kitchen task, such as making a salad or washing dishes. Count the motions, such as the number of trips to the refrigerator, and time the entire task. Summarize and evaluate your findings in a one-page report. How could you use less time and fewer motions?

Technology

12. Kitchen Design Imagine that you are a kitchen planner, hired to design a new kitchen. Use a computer drafting or design program to create the floor plan. Label the work centers. Label where equipment and food should be stored. Write an explanation of why your plan is efficient.

Financial Literacy

13. Value Comparison You have enough time to use fresh garlic in your planned dish, however, you are also considering the convenience option. A 32-oz. jar of minced garlic costs $4.99. Fresh garlic is on sale for $0.50 lb. Each bulb weighs about 8 ounces. How much could you save by mincing 32 ounces of fresh garlic rather than purchasing the jar?

14. Family Teamwork Pick a recipe to make in your foods lab. Make two work plans to prepare the recipe: by yourself and with two lab partners using teamwork. Make the recipe using both work plans. Which plan was more efficient? More enjoyable? Explain your answers in a brief essay.

15. Time Management Most managers look for ways to save time and increase productivity. Conduct research to find out about time management techniques used in the workplace. How might you use these techniques in the foods lab? Share your findings in a five-minute oral report.

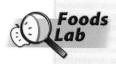

16. Your Foods Lab As a kitchen team, evaluate the design of your foods lab. Identify the kitchen's shape, its work centers, and the types of equipment stored in each. Name the type of tasks done in each work center. Brainstorm ways to prepare food in this kitchen efficiently.

Additional Activities For additional activities go to this book's Online Learning Center at **glencoe.com**.

Academic Skills

 English Language Arts

17. Promote Conservation Design a poster, magazine ad, radio or television commercial, or Web page that encourages other teens to conserve resouces. Include specific reasons for conserving and ways to conserve.

> **NCTE 12** Use language to accomplish individual purposes.

 Science

18. Labeling Frozen Foods No food can be refrigerated or frozen permanently. You should always label food.

Procedure Research what can happen to foods that have been refrozen, and to foods that are frozen for too long.

Analysis Describe the results of your research in a report. Include recommendations for labeling frozen food.

> **NSES Content Standard F** Develop an understanding of personal and community health.

 Mathematics

19. Estimate Dinner Time You are preparing tuna casserole for dinner. It takes you 1 minute to wash your hands, 10 minutes to gather ingredients and tools, 10 minutes to boil the noodles, 12 minutes to combine the ingredients, 25 minutes to bake the casserole, 5 minutes to set the table, and 2 minutes to serve the casserole. What time will you need to start to eat at 6:30?

Math Concept **Units of Measurement** You may need to decide which measurement units, including measurements of time, are needed to find a solution.

Starting Hint Find the total minutes required to make the casserole. Convert this number into hours and minutes. Work backward from the planned eating time.

 For more math help, go to the Math Appendix

> **NCTM Measurement** Understand measurable attributes of objects and the units, systems, and processes of measurement.

STANDARDIZED TEST PRACTICE

MULTIPLE CHOICE

Read the paragraph. Then read the question and choose the correct answer.

Here is a tip for efficient cooking: Set out all your ingredients before you start cooking. Then put each one away as you use it. You can tell before you start cooking if you are missing an ingredient. You can decide on a substitute or a different recipe.

20. Based on the paragraph, which of the following best completes the following sentence? Efficient cooking might include

_____ .

  a. going to the store for missing ingredients

  b. cooking with someone else

  c. adding extra ingredients to a recipe

  d. assembling all the ingredients first

> **Test-Taking Tip** Pay close attention to the words and phrases around an unfamiliar word. Putting a word in context will often give you clues to its meaning.

CHAPTER 23
Serving a Meal

Explore the Photo ▶▶
A table that is set properly and a meal that is served properly make a meal more pleasant. *Besides good food, what makes a meal enjoyable for you? Why?*

Writing Activity

Compare and Contrast Paper

Cultural Dishes Indian food is known for its curry, while Japanese food is famous for sushi and tempura. Write a compare and contrast paper that identifies what is the same and what is different about foods from two different cultures. Describe the dishes clearly with ingredients, preparation, and style of serving and eating.

Writing Tips

1. **Use** a Venn Diagram to map your ideas.
2. **Organize** your paper with a subject-by-subject or feature-by-feature analysis.
3. **Use** appropriate transitions.

Reading Guide

Before You Read

Buddy Up for Success Find a buddy to share your notes. You can compare notes and fill in gaps in each other's information. You can also quiz each other.

Read to Learn

Key Concepts

- **Describe** three types of meal service.
- **Describe** how to set a table properly.
- **Identify** good table manners.
- **Explain** how to use variety, presentation, and garnishes to make meals appealing.
- **Provide** guidelines for successful entertaining.

Main Idea

Meal service, table setting, and table manners are customs that make mealtime and entertaining pleasant. Serving food attractively is important, too.

Content Vocabulary

◇ family style   ◇ place setting
◇ plate service   ◇ cover
◇ buffet service   ◇ etiquette
◇ tumbler   ◇ garnish
◇ stemware   ◇ R.S.V.P.
◇ flatware

Academic Vocabulary

You will find these words in your reading and on your tests. Use the glossary to look up their definitions if necessary.

■ sequence
■ conduct

Graphic Organizer

As you read, use a chart like the one below to write notes about the three basic types of meal service.

Type of Meal Service	Description
Family Style	
Plate Service	
Buffet Service	

 Graphic Organizer Go to this book's Online Learning Center at **glencoe.com** to print out this graphic organizer.

Academic Standards ■

 English Language Arts
NCTE 11 Participate as members of literacy communities.

 Social Studies
NCSS I F Culture Interpret patterns of behavior reflecting values and attitudes that contribute or pose obstacles to cross-cultural understanding.

 Mathematics
NCTM Geometry Analyze characteristics of two- and three-dimensional geometric shapes and develop mathematical arguments about geometric relationships.
NCTM Number and Operations Compute fluently and make reasonable estimates.

NCTE   National Council of Teachers of English
NCTM   National Council of Teachers of Mathematics

NSES   National Science Education Standards
NCSS   National Council for the Social Studies

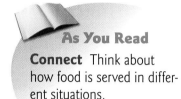

Vocabulary

You can find definitions in the glossary at the back of this book.

As You Read

Connect Think about how food is served in different situations.

Types of Meal Service

Around the world, mealtime is for sharing. Every family has customs for who sits where and how meals are served. Specific customs for serving and eating meals vary from family to family and culture to culture. Whatever the customs, being thoughtful of others matters most.

A well-planned routine makes mealtime orderly, relaxed, and comfortable. Meals in the United States are usually served in one of three ways:

♦ **Family Style** Food is placed in serving dishes on the table. People help themselves and pass serving dishes to each other.

♦ **Plate Service** Food is served on each person's plate. Then, plates are brought to the table. A formal meal is often served this way, in several courses.

♦ **Buffet Service** Serving dishes of food are arranged on a table or counter. People serve themselves. Then, they carry their food to an eating area. Buffet service is common for larger gatherings.

Even within a meal, food may be served in several ways. For instance, for a buffet-style meal, individual salads may be on the table already. Bread may be passed at the table. Dessert may be served on individual plates after the main course is cleared.

✓ Reading Check **Discuss** Which serving style would you choose for a dinner party? Why?

The Table Setting

A properly set table makes eating pleasant and convenient. How you set the table depends in part on the type of meal service.

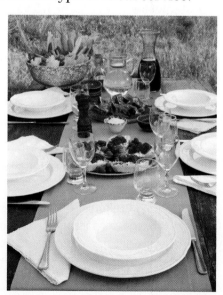

Pick the Right Plate Nice tableware makes food look appealing and can help carry out a theme. *How else can you make food appealing on the plate?*

Tableware

Dishes, flatware, glasses, and linens for serving food and eating are called tableware. The tableware you need depends on your menu, how you serve it, and how casual or formal your meal is. Tableware includes:

- **Plates** The main course is usually served on dinner plates. Smaller plates are used for salad, bread, and dessert.

- **Cups and Saucers, or Mugs** Hot drinks are served in mugs or cups with saucers.

- **Glasses** A **tumbler** is a glass without a stem. **Stemware** is glassware with a stem between the flat bottom of the glass and its bowl.

- **Other Dishes** Cereal, soup, stew, and some salads and desserts are served in bowls. You may also need larger serving bowls and platters for family-style service.

- **Flatware** The knives, forks, and spoons for eating are called **flatware**. This includes a dinner knife for cutting meat, dinner and salad forks, teaspoons for beverages and some desserts, and a larger spoon for soups and stews.

- **Table Linens** These include napkins, place mats, and tablecloths.

Set the Table

Each type of tableware has a specific place. The arrangement of tableware for one person is a **place setting** or a **cover**. **Figure 23.1** shows where tableware goes.

Setting a table is easiest when done in this **sequence**, or order:

1. Decide what tableware each person will need.

2. Cover the table with a tablecloth or place mats. Add a table decoration or centerpiece, if desired.

3. Put the dinner plate in the center of each place setting. If possible, allow 20 inches (50 cm) in width for each place setting so people can sit comfortably.

4. Arrange the flatware. Place it so the utensil used first is farthest from the plate.

5. Finally, add other tableware around the dinner plate and flatware.

Table Decorations

No matter how simple, a table decoration is the final touch for a beautiful table. Centerpieces may be ordinary things from your home or something created just for the occasion. Consider these easy ideas:

◆ Fresh fruit in a bowl or basket that could be served for dessert.

◆ Fresh flowers or herbs in an attractive container.

◆ One or more candles.

✓ Reading Check **Identify** What types of tableware do you need to remember when setting a table?

Figure 23.1 **The Place Setting**

Set a Place Correctly Each place setting is arranged for convenience during the meal. *If you do not serve a salad course, which of these items do you not need?*

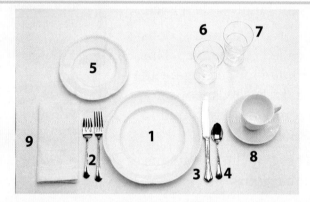

1. Place the dinner plate in the center, about 1 inch (2.5 cm) from the table's edge.
2. Place the forks to the left of the dinner plate. If the salad will be eaten before the main course, put the salad fork on the outside and the dinner fork near the plate.
3. Place the knife to the right of the dinner plate with the blade facing the plate.
4. Put the spoon to the right of the knife. For more than one spoon, place the spoon used first farthest from the dinner plate. Line up the utensils with the bottom edge of the dinner plate.
5. Put the salad plate above the forks.
6. Place the water glass just above the tip of the knife.
7. Place additional glasses to the right and slightly in front of the water glass.
8. Put the cup and saucer to the right of the spoons, with the cup's handle facing the right.
9. Put the napkin to the left of the forks. The napkin's folded edge should be away from the forks. That way, the napkin can be picked up by the corner edge and unfolded easily.

Make Meals Enjoyable

Eating together is more enjoyable with pleasant surroundings and considerate behavior. Positive attitudes also contribute to healthful eating. To create a pleasant tone around the table:

- Use a table decoration.
- Serve food in bowls or on plates, not from packages or jars.
- Have serving spoons and forks ready.
- Present food attractively, perhaps with a simple garnish.
- Play pleasing music. Turn off the television and cell phones.
- Include everyone in conversations. Keep them positive.

Table Manners

Table manners, or etiquette, are a reflection of you. **Etiquette** is polite behavior that shows respect and consideration for others. When you demonstrate appropriate behavior, or **conduct**, you display good manners. Table manners:

- Show courtesy and respect for everyone eating with you.
- Make meals pleasant and relaxed.
- Help others feel at ease and valued.
- Help you feel good about yourself.

Good table manners differ from culture to culture. For example, in southern China, it is polite to lift a bowl close to your mouth so that rice is not spilled. Here are some simple guidelines for good table manners.

Sit at the Table

- Come to the table when food is ready.
- Sit with good posture, instead of slouching.
- Keep your elbows off the table as you eat.

Serve Food

- Take food from a serving dish with a serving fork or spoon.
- Do not reach too far or in front of someone for food.
- Politely ask others to pass food you cannot reach.
- Wait until everyone is served before starting to eat.

Use Tableware

- Unfold your napkin on your lap. Keep it there.
- Use the outside spoon or fork first.
- Rest your flatware on the plate, not the table. Place the knife across the top of the plate.

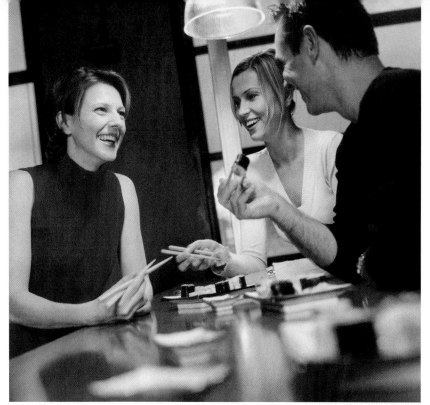

Manners at Work In the world of work, good manners are important for success. A business meal may start with introductions. *How would you introduce people properly?*

As You Eat

◆ Let hot food cool before taking a bite. Do not blow on it.

◆ Cut just one or two small pieces of food at a time.

◆ Lift food to your mouth rather than lowering your head toward the plate.

◆ Eat everything on your utensil at one time.

◆ Use a piece of bread to push food onto a spoon or fork. Do not use your fingers.

◆ Take small bites. Chew quietly with your mouth closed.

◆ Sip rather than gulp beverages.

◆ Do not talk or drink with food in your mouth.

◆ During a family-style meal service.

Master Awkward Moments

◆ Remove fruit pits and fish bones from your mouth discreetly. Cover your mouth with a napkin.

◆ Use a napkin to blot your mouth if needed. Do not use it to blow your nose.

◆ If you must cough or burp, cover your mouth and turn your head away from the table. Quietly excuse yourself. If you must cough, sneeze, or must blow your nose, excuse yourself and leave the table.

◆ If you spill something, apologize. Help clean up. Then forget it so the accident does not stay in the conversation.

After You Eat

◆ Place your napkin neatly to the left of your plate.

◆ Place your knife and fork parallel across the center of your plate, with the handles in the 4 o'clock position.

◆ Offer to help with cleanup.

◆ If you must leave before others are done, excuse yourself.

◆ Thank anyone who prepared the meal.

Clear the Table

After everyone finishes eating, it is time to clear the table. Stand to the side of someone who is seated as you clear tableware from each place setting. Then, carry it to the cleanup area. Do not scrape or stack dishes at the table.

✓ **Reading Check** **Recall** Why is mealtime etiquette important?

Serve Meals with Appeal

Serving a pleasant meal also involves art and skill. Make nourishing meals and snacks appealing with the foods you choose, the way you arrange them, and the touches you add before serving. Remember to add variety to your meals: colors, textures, shapes and sizes, flavors, and food temperatures.

Food with Flair

Create a feast for the eyes! Delicious-looking food is arranged carefully and artistically. Take cues from food photos in magazines or the ways TV chefs display their food.

◆ **Decide if you need more than one plate.** Some foods need a small bowl so their juices will not run. If your main course is hot, serve chilled foods on a side plate.

◆ **Know the basics.** Avoid overcrowding a plate. Use tongs or other utensils to arrange food. Avoid using your fingers.

◆ **Use your imagination.** Arranging food attractively takes thought, but not necessarily extra time.

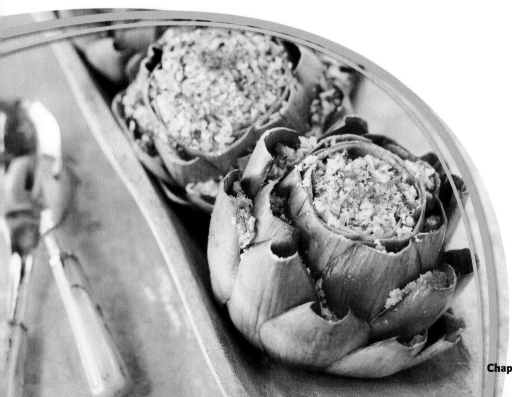

Be Artistic Attractive presentation is not only for restaurant meals. With some simple artistic touches, you can serve a meal that will make you proud. *What makes this meal look so appealing?*

Garnishes

A **garnish** is an edible decoration that adds a contrasting color, texture, flavor, temperature, or shape to food. A garnish can be fancy or simple. It should enhance your food, not overpower it. Simple garnishes include:

◆ Carrot shreds on a green salad.

◆ Crunchy slivered almonds on grilled chicken.

◆ Garlic croutons on tomato soup.

◆ Citrus slices or a few small berries beside broiled fish.

◆ A sprig of a fresh herb on almost any main dish.

◆ Edible flowers on salads, appetizers, or desserts.

✓ **Reading Check** **List** What function does a garnish serve?

Easy Entertaining

Whenever people gather to share activities, celebrate, or just enjoy each other's company, food usually plays a part.

Plan a Get-Together

As the host, you are responsible for planning and organization. Follow these guidelines to plan a get-together:

◆ **Pick a Theme** You may have a built-in theme, such as a graduation or holiday. You can also invent a theme if you like, such as a make-a-pizza party.

◆ **Choose a Place** Choose a convenient date and time for you, other family members, and your guests.

◆ **Plan a Menu** Plan a menu to match your skills. Choose foods you have prepared before. Pick foods you can make ahead. Know how you will keep food at safe temperatures.

◆ **Plan the Guest List** Decide how many people you can serve comfortably. Then, plan the guest list. Your guests can enjoy each other's company even if they are not yet friends.

◆ **Invite Your Guests** Ask guests a few days or weeks ahead of time so they can plan to attend. Invite them in person, by phone, in writing, or by e-mail. Give the basics in the invitation: date, time, place, occasion, and whether food will be served. Give a reply date. Use the abbreviation R.S.V.P. **R.S.V.P.** is an acronym for a French phrase that means please reply. Include your contact information.

◆ **Decorate** Create a pleasant atmosphere with tableware, a tablecloth or place mats, and a table decoration.

- **Make a Work Plan** List everything you need to do and gather. Make a schedule. Follow your plan.
- **Thank Your Guests** After the get-together, thank your guests for coming.

Serve Buffet Style

Buffet service is easy, especially for a crowd. To arrange a buffet table, see **Figure 23.2.** Follow these guidelines:

- **Choose Easy-to-Manage Foods** This is especially important when guests must eat from plates in their laps or while standing.
- **Plan the Traffic Flow** Guests approaching the buffet should not get in the way of those leaving it with food.

Figure 23.2 **Buffet Style Service**

Your Buffet Table Arrange the buffet so guests can serve themselves easily. *What types of food might you serve on a casual buffet?*

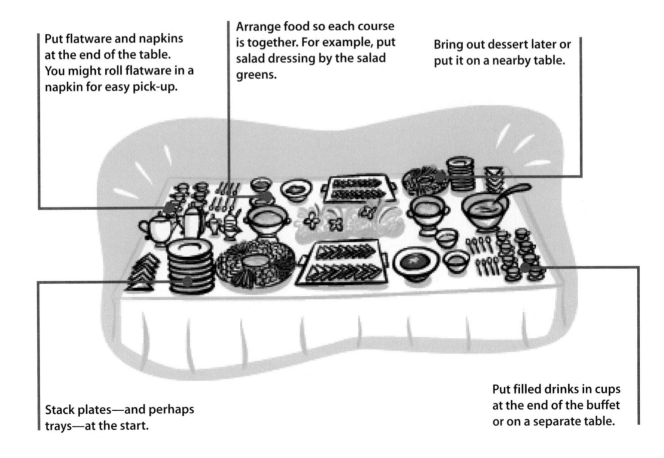

Put flatware and napkins at the end of the table. You might roll flatware in a napkin for easy pick-up.

Arrange food so each course is together. For example, put salad dressing by the salad greens.

Bring out dessert later or put it on a nearby table.

Stack plates—and perhaps trays—at the start.

Put filled drinks in cups at the end of the buffet or on a separate table.

◆ **Keep Hot Foods Hot and Cold Foods Cold** Set out smaller amounts. Refill the buffet as needed. You can also use warming trays, slow cookers, or trays of ice.

Be a Thoughtful Guest

Being a courteous guest is as important as being a gracious host. Follow these guidelines to be a thoughtful guest:

◆ **Before the Party** Reply to the invitation right away. Offer to bring food or other things. Tell your host if you have special food needs. Perhaps bring food you can eat.

◆ **At the Party** Arrive on time. Use good manners. Spend time with other guests.

◆ **After the Party** Thank the host. Offer to help clean up.

✓ **Reading Check** **List** If you want to have a party, what should you do to prepare?

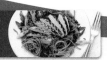

EASY RECIPES

Everyday Favorites

Party Guacamole

Customary	Ingredients	Metric
2	Avocados, whole	2
½ cup	Red onion	125 mL
1	Roma tomato	1
1 tsp.	Cilantro (optional)	5 mL
1	Serrano chili pepper	1
2	Limes	2

Try This!
Adjust level of spice with more or less Serrano pepper, or try different peppers.

Yield: Six servings, ½ cup (125 g) each

➊ Cut avocados in half and remove the pit and skin. Put in a bowl and mash with a fork.
➋ Chop the onion and cilantro. Remove seeds and skin from tomato and chop.
➌ Remove seeds from Serrano pepper and chop. Add all to bowl.
➍ Squeeze juice from limes into bowl and stir to combine everything.
➎ Serve with chips or vegetables.

Nutritional Information Per Serving: 122 calories, 10 g total fat (1 g saturated fat), 0 mg cholesterol, 6 mg sodium, 10 g total carbohydrate (6 g fiber, 1 g total sugars), 2 g protein

Percent Daily Value: vitamin A 4%, vitamin C 25%, calcium 2%, iron 2%

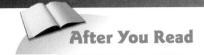

After You Read

CHAPTER SUMMARY

Different families and different cultures have different ways of serving food and eating meals. Most meals in the United States are served family style, or with plate or buffet service, or a combination. Meals are more pleasant when attention is paid to the surroundings, the table setting, and table manners. Each type of tableware has a specific place. Table manners show respect and consideration for others. An artistically served meal is visually appealing. Planning and organization are keys to successful entertaining. Buffet service is an easy entertaining option.

Vocabulary Review

1. Use each of these vocabulary words in a sentence.

Content Vocabulary
◇ family style (p. 334)
◇ plate service (p. 334)
◇ buffet service (p. 334)
◇ tumbler (p. 335)
◇ stemware (p. 335)

◇ flatware (p. 335)
◇ place setting (p. 335)
◇ cover (p. 335)
◇ etiquette (p. 337)
◇ garnish (p. 340)
◇ R.S.V.P. (p. 340)

Academic Vocabulary
■ sequence (p. 335)
■ conduct (p. 337)

Review Key Concepts

2. Describe three types of meal service.

3. Describe how to set a table properly.

4. Identify good table manners.

5. Explain how to use variety, presentation, and garnishes to make meals appealing.

6. Provide guidelines for successful entertaining.

Critical Thinking

7. Analyze why some topics are not appropriate for general conversation at the table

8. Design a plan for an attractive table decoration made from items you already have around the house.

9. Determine how to arrange the seating for guests at your table if one of your guests or family members is left-handed.

Real-World Skills and Applications

Problem-Solving

10. Making Decisions You plan to make a turkey-mushroom casserole for a dinner party you are having tonight. Which style of meal service will you use to serve the casserole? What factors will affect your decision? Write your answers in a paragraph.

Interpersonal and Collaborative

11. Table Manners With classmates, role-play these three situations: 1) You just finished dinner and need to leave for a school event, while others are still eating. 2) You are attending a formal dinner party, a piece of food gets stuck between your teeth. 3) The meal customs of your hosts differ from the customs of your culture.

Technology

12. Chopsticks Research how chopsticks are used in Japan, China, and other Asian countries. Then create a video, showing how to use chopsticks appropriately. Share your video. Give your classmates the opportunity to practice using chopsticks.

Financial Literacy

13. Price Comparison Mae went to the store and found a bouquet of flowers for $24.99. Then she found fresh apples she could use for a centerpiece instead. The red apples were $1.36 per lb. The green apples were $1.69 per lb. If she buys 6 pounds of each type of apple instead of a floral centerpiece, will she spend more or less money?

14. Table for Two Design a table setting for two people. Include the menu, theme, and dishes and flatware needed. Suggest linens and table decorations. Create a poster or other visual display to show your table design.

15. Choosing Tableware Visit a store that sells tableware. Look at the different types, designs, costs, and materials. Decide what flatware, dishes, glasses, and linens you would buy for everyday use for a family of four. Write a short essay explaining your choices.

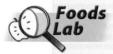

16. Place Setting Using tableware in your foods lab, correctly arrange a place setting. Use a dinner plate, salad plate, water glass, teaspoon, soup spoon, dinner fork, dinner knife, dessert fork, napkin, and place mat. Explain the placement of each item.

Additional Activities For additional activities go to this book's Online Learning Center at glencoe.com.

Academic Skills

English Language Arts

17. Interview an Exchange Student Using interviewing skills, talk with an exchange student in your community about meal and eating customs in his or her country. Find out how food is served and learn about table manners. Write a brief article about what you learned.

> **NCTE 11** Participate as members of literacy communities.

Social Studies

18. Utensils from Other Cultures Conduct research on utensils used in other cultures besides the standard fork, knife, and spoon. Write a paragraph to describe the use of one or more of these utensils.

> **NCSS I F Culture** Interpret patterns of behavior reflecting values and attitudes that contribute or pose obstacles to cross-cultural understanding.

Mathematics

19. Meal Service Decision Hassan's parents are planning a party. It would cost them $15 per guest for a catered buffet dinner for 85 people. A catered sit-down meal for 50 people would cost $25 per person. Which option is cheaper?

Math Concept **Word Problems** The first step in tackling a word problem is to understand the question, or questions that are asked. Restate the questions in your own words.

Starting Hint Multiply each pair of numbers, then compare to find which is the cheapest.

 For more math help, go to the Math Appendix

> **NCTM Number and Operations** Compute fluently and make reasonable estimates.

STANDARDIZED TEST PRACTICE

MULTIPLE CHOICE
Read the paragraph. Write your answer on a separate piece of paper.

Some party hosts ask guests to bring certain things to contribute, such as a dessert or salad. Others prefer potluck, where each guest brings something of his or her choice to share. Even if you prefer a potluck dinner party, you can still plan ahead. For example, ask some guests to bring a dessert and others to bring a salad of their choice.

20. Based on the paragraph, which of the following statements is true?
  a. Potluck dinner parties are rare.
  b. Plan ahead for a less stressful party.
  c. Planning for parties is always stressful.
  d. Too many desserts can spoil a party.

> **Test-Taking Tip** When taking a test, do not use a mechanical pencil, ink pen, or correction fluid. Use a soft lead No. 2 pencil to mark your answers, and make changes with a good eraser.

Unit 7 Thematic Project

Plan Your Dream Kitchen

Everyone has their own vision of a dream kitchen. Some people might visualize a small, efficiently organized kitchen with convenient work centers and only basic appliances. Other people might prefer a larger kitchen with more counter space and lots of appliances, utensils, and other gadgets. In this project, you will plan your dream kitchen.

My Journal

If you completed the journal entry from page 260, refer to it to see if you have different ideas about how you visualize your ideal kitchen after reading the unit.

Project Assignment

In this project you will:

- Conduct research on kitchen equipment and appliances you would include in your ideal kitchen.
- Summarize your research.
- Write interview questions.
- Interview someone in your community who is knowledgeable about kitchen equipment and kitchen design.
- While interviewing, take notes, and after interviewing, transcribe your notes.
- Create a poster showing the layout of and equipment in your ideal kitchen.
- Make a presentation to your class.

Academic Skills You Will Use ....

English Language Arts

NCTE 3 Apply strategies to interpret texts.
NCTE 12 Use language to accomplish individual purposes.

STEP 1 Choose and Research Kitchen Equipment

Conduct research on basic kitchen utensils and appliances that you would include in your ideal home kitchen. As you conduct your research, print out photos of the various types of equipment. Write a summary of your research that:

- Describes the kitchen utensils and appliances you would include in your ideal kitchen
- Includes information about how you would use each utensil or appliance

STEP 2 Plan Your Interview

Write a list of questions to ask someone in your community who is knowledgeable about kitchen equipment or kitchen design.

Writing Skills

- Use complete sentences.
- Use correct spelling and grammar.
- Organize your questions according to your list of utensils and small appliances.

STEP 3 Connect with Your Community

Using the questions you wrote in Step 2, interview someone in your community who is knowledgeable about kitchen equipment and kitchen design, such as a kitchen equipment salesperson, an avid home cook, or a chef.

Interviewing Skills

- Record responses and take notes.
- Listen attentively.
- When you transcribe your notes, write in complete sentences using correct spelling and grammar.

STEP 4 Create Your Final Report

Use the Unit Thematic Project Checklist to plan and give an oral report and create your poster. Use these speaking skills as you present your final report.

Speaking Skills

- Speak clearly and concisely.
- Be sensitive to the needs of your audience.
- Use standard English to communicate.

STEP 5 Evaluate Your Presentation

Your project will be reviewed and evaluated based on:

- Depth and diversity of research
- Content of your presentation
- Mechanics—presentation and neatness

 Evaluation Rubric Go to this book's Online Learning Center at **glencoe.com** for a rubric you can use to evaluate your final report.

Project Checklist	
Plan	✓ Research kitchen equipment and small appliances. ✓ Write a summary of your research. ✓ Write interview questions. ✓ Conduct an interview. ✓ Transcribe the notes from your interview. ✓ Design a poster showing the design of your ideal kitchen. Include photos of the kitchen utensils and equipment you researched. ✓ Plan a five-minute oral presentation.
Present	✓ Make a presentation to your class to discuss the results of your research and interview. ✓ Display your poster, explaining how the kitchen design is efficient and describing the essential utensils and equipment you would include in it. ✓ Invite the students of the class to ask any questions they may have. Answer these questions. ✓ When students ask questions, demonstrate in your answers that you respect their perspectives. ✓ Turn in your research summary, interview questions, interview notes, and poster to your teacher.
Academic Skills	✓ Conduct research to gather information. ✓ Communicate effectively. ✓ Organize your presentation so the audience can follow along easily. ✓ Thoroughly express your ideas.

Unit 8

Learning About Foods

Chapters in this Unit

Chapter 24 Grains
Chapter 25 Vegetables
Chapter 26 Fruits
Chapter 27 Milk
Chapter 28 Meat, Poultry, and Fish
Chapter 29 Eggs, Beans and Nuts
Chapter 30 Fats and Oils

Unit Thematic Project Preview

Discover Organic Foods

While studying this unit, you will learn about the many different types of foods. In the unit thematic project at the end of this unit, you will conduct research about organic foods and interview someone in your community who is knowledgeable about organic foods.

My Journal

Organically grown and raised foods are becoming a popular option. Write a journal entry to answer the questions below.

- What do I know about organic foods?
- What would I like to know about organic foods?

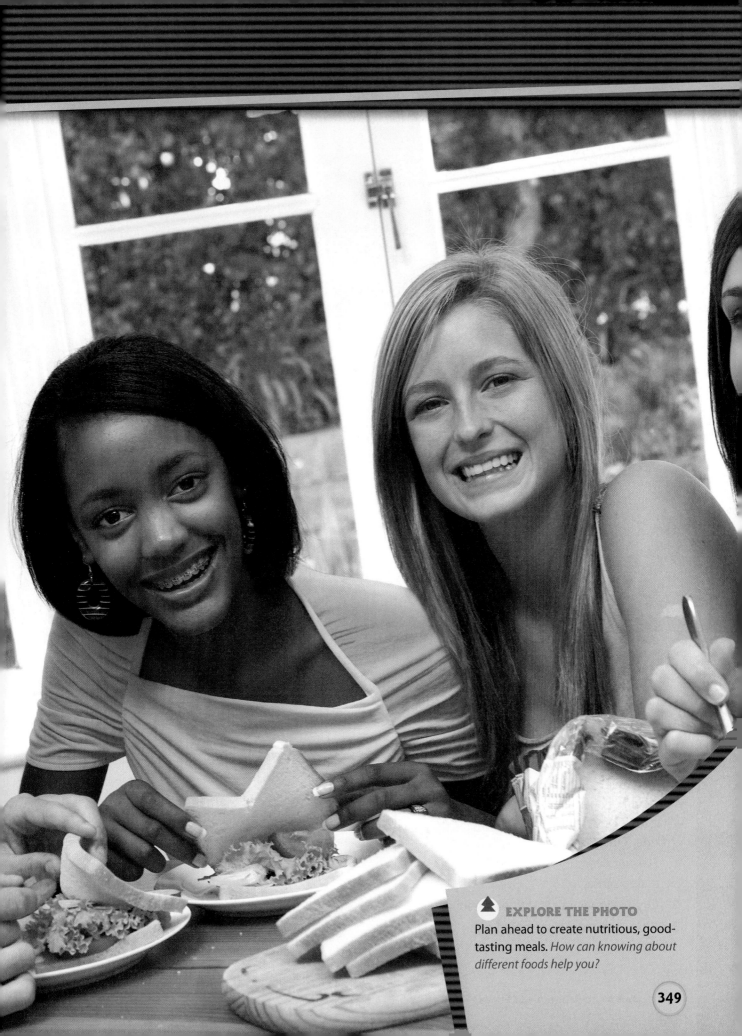

EXPLORE THE PHOTO
Plan ahead to create nutritious, good-tasting meals. *How can knowing about different foods help you?*

CHAPTER 24
Grains

Explore the Photo ▶▶
Bread, cereal, rice, and pasta all fit in MyPyramid's Grains Group. *What grain foods made with grains have you eaten?*

Writing Activity

Write a First Draft

Plan a Party Planning a party is fun, and part of the fun is picking the location, the entertainment, the type of food to be served, and how to serve it. Write the first draft of an essay about your dream birthday party. What kind of entertainment would you have? What food would you serve?

Writing Tips

1. **Arrange** your ideas in an order that makes sense.

2. **Organize** your draft into paragraphs.

3. **Plan** each paragraph around one main idea.

Reading Guide

Before You Read

How Can You Improve? Think about the last exam you took on material you had to read. What reading strategies helped you on the test? Make a list of ways to succeed on your next exam.

Read to Learn

Key Concepts

- **Identify** the health benefits of grain foods, especially whole grains.
- **Explain** how a variety of grain foods can fit in everyday meals and snacks.
- **Discuss** how food science applies to grain products.
- **Summarize** smart tips for buying and storing grain products.
- **Describe** how to prepare grain foods for quality, nutritional value, and appeal.

Main Idea

Grain products deliver satisfying flavors, hearty textures, and health benefits. Whole grains are especially healthful.

Content Vocabulary

◇ whole grain
◇ endosperm
◇ germ
◇ bran
◇ refined grain
◇ starch
◇ cereal grain
◇ al dente

Academic Vocabulary

You will find these words in your reading and on your tests. Use the glossary to look up their definitions if necessary.

- process
- develop

Graphic Organizer

As you read, use a table like the one below to write notes about the two main types of grains. Include examples of types of foods for each.

Whole Grains	Refined Grains

 Graphic Organizer Go to this book's Online Learning Center at **glencoe.com** to print out this graphic organizer.

Academic Standards

 English Language Arts
NCTE 4 Use written language to communicate effectively.
NCTE 9 Develop an understanding of diversity in language use across cultures.

 Mathematics
NCTM Number and Operations Understand the meanings of operations and how they relate to one another.

 Science
NSES Content Standard F Develop an understanding of personal and community health.

 Social Studies
NCSS I E Demonstrate the value of cultural diversity, as well as cohesion, within and across groups.

NCTE National Council of Teachers of English
NCTM National Council of Teachers of Mathematics

NSES National Science Education Standards
NCSS National Council of the Social Studies

Grains for Good Nutrition

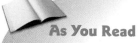

As You Read

Connect Think about the ways you can incorporate grains into your eating plan.

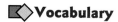

Vocabulary

You can find definitions in the glossary at the back of this book.

Grains are either whole and refined. A **whole grain** is a grain that has the entire grain kernel. A grain kernel has three parts. (See **Figure 24.1.**) The **endosperm** is the inner part of the grain. The endosperm is mostly carbohydrate and some protein. The **germ** is the small base of the seed. The germ sprouts when planted. It contains protein, some fat, B vitamins, vitamin E, and minerals. The **bran**, the coarse, outer layer, supplies most of the fiber, plus B vitamins and minerals. Whole-wheat flour, oatmeal, and brown rice are whole grains.

A **Refined grain** is a grain that is milled to remove the bran and the germ. This **process**, or action, gives the grain a finer texture and improves shelf life. It also removes nutrients, phytonutrients, and fiber. Refined grains are often enriched. To enrich is to add back lost nutrients. Enrichment adds back iron and certain B vitamins. White flour, white bread, cornflakes, and white rice are refined grain products.

Grain foods provide many nutrients, including:

◆ **Carbohydrates** Grains are excellent sources of starches. A **starch** is a complex carbohydrate. Grains also provide sugars, or simple carbohydrates.

◆ **Fiber** Fiber, a non-digestible complex carbohydrate, helps your digestive tract work properly. It may offer protection from heart disease and some cancers. Whole grains are plentiful in fiber. Most refined grains contain little fiber.

Figure 24.1	Parts of a Grain Kernel

What Is in a Grain Kernel? Whole-grain foods are very nourishing. *What are the nutrition benefits of choosing more whole-grain products?*

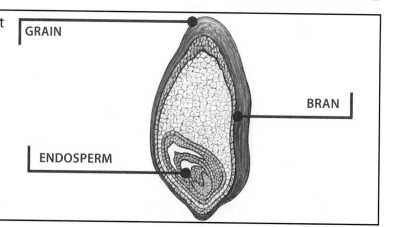

The grain kernel, or seed, is the part of the plant that is eaten. Whole-grain products are made from all three parts of the grain kernel. Refining separates these parts so each can be used individually.

GRAIN

BRAN

ENDOSPERM

- **Low-Fat and Cholesterol** Grains naturally have no cholesterol and little fat. Ingredients that boost fat and calories may be added during preparation.

- **B Vitamins and Iron** Many grain products are also fortified with folic acid, and other vitamins and minerals.

- **Amino Acids** Grains provide some amino acids, but are not complete proteins.

MyPyramid Advice

What does the wide orange band of MyPyramid mean? Eat more from the Grain Group than from other food groups! Grain products are perfect partners for vegetables, fruits, cheese, meat, chicken, fish, and beans.

If you need about 2,000 calories daily, you need 6 ounces (170 g) from the Grain Group daily. Eat more if your energy needs are higher. Make at least half of your grain choices whole grain. The following are food equivalents of an ounce of grains:

- One slice of bread
- One cup (250 mL) of ready-to-eat cereal
- One half-cup (125 mL) of cooked cereal, rice, or pasta
- One 6-inch (15-cm) tortilla
- One mini-bagel
- Three cups of popped popcorn
- Five whole-wheat crackers

✓ **Reading Check** **Recall** If you need 2,000 calories a day, how many ounces of whole-grain foods should you try to eat daily?

Fit in Grains

Grains fit in every meal—snacks, too. Think about the many different foods you would miss if there were no grains! Make your grain choices count for good nutrition with nutrient-dense whole-grain and enriched-grain products. Go easy on grain products with added sugars and fats, such as doughnuts and cakes.

Whole Grains Breads come in many shapes, sizes, and flavors. Many, including whole-wheat bagels, are made with whole grains. *Can you think of breads made with whole grains that you might try?*

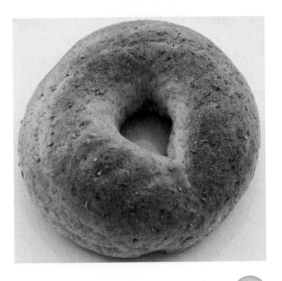

Many Kinds of Grains

Wheat, oats, and rice are common grains, but there are many others you can try for variety, such as:

- **Corn** Hominy is dried, hulled corn without the germ. It is ground for grits.

- **Barley** This mild-flavored grain adds flavor to soups and stews. Whole barley is a whole grain. Pearl barley is not.

- **Buckwheat** This makes a nutty-flavored flour. Hulled, crushed, and roasted buckwheat is used for kasha.

- **Bulgur** Bulgur is cracked wheat made from cooked, dried whole wheat. It has a nutty flavor and chewy texture.

- **Quinoa** ('kēn-,wä) This is a small, bead-shaped grain that is sweet and nutty. Use it as a rice substitute.

Go Whole with Grains

You can add more whole grains to your meals and snacks:

- Snack on plain popcorn or whole-grain chips.

- Mix your own cereals with toasted oats.

- Use rolled oats or crushed cereal as a breading.

- Enjoy grain dishes, like polenta, from other cultures.

✓ **Reading Check** **Describe** How can you add more whole grains to your meals?

Discover International Foods

Russia

Russia spans from Eastern Europe to Siberia in northern Asia. Much of its vast land mass is too cold or too dry for farming. Russia is a major producer of grains (wheat, barley, oats, rye, buckwheat), potatoes, and caviar, or fish eggs. Hearty grains are used for dumplings, soups, pancakes, breads, other baked goods, and kasha (cooked porridge). Vegetables such as beets, cabbage, mushrooms, and potatoes are part of soups, salads, casseroles, and dumplings. Fruits are mostly cooked. Meat, chicken, goose, duck, or fish often are served for dinner.

Languages Across Cultures

blini ('blē-nē) small pancakes, typically made with buckwheat flour, and eaten with ingredients such as smoked salmon, fruit preserves, and sour cream.

borscht ('bòrsh(t)) cold or hot soup made with beets, and sometimes vegetables and meat. It is topped with sour cream.

 Recipes Find out more about International recipes on this book's Online Learning Center at glencoe.com.

NCTE 9 Develop an understanding of diversity in language use across cultures.

Grain Products in Science

A **cereal grain** is a seed from a grass such as wheat, rice, oats, corn, rye, or barley. The grain is processed, perhaps ground for flour, and then cooked to become edible. As grain products bake or cook, their starch molecules change.

Starch molecules come in two forms: highly-branched amylopectin, and long, chain-like amylase. Most starch in food is amylopectin. The ability of starch to thicken depends on the ratio of these two starch molecules

What Happens When Oatmeal Cooks?

Cooking oatmeal in water creates a chemical change in its starch. Some bonds between the atoms of carbohydrate molecules break. They form new bonds with atoms of different molecules. As starch granules, or clusters, absorb water molecules, they swell and soften. Eventually, they break apart, releasing the nutrients inside. The oatmeal gets softer and easier to digest.

Oatmeal that starts cooking in cold water is creamier than oatmeal that starts cooking in boiling water. Because it takes time to heat the water, the oatmeal has more time to absorb liquid.

What Makes Pasta Sticky?

Pasta needs to be cooked properly. Otherwise it may stick together, becoming a large, unappetizing lump.

When pasta cooks, its starch dissolves into the cooking water. As the starchy water cools, it gets glue-like. Gluey starch attaches to the noodles, making them sticky.

✓ **Reading Check** **Explain** When cooked oatmeal goes from dry to soft and creamy, is this a physical or chemical change?

The Science of Starch Sometimes pasta sticks together when you cook it. *Why does this happen?*

Buy and Store Grain Products

Choose grain products that match your resources, recipes, and nutritional needs. Follow these guidelines when choosing grains:

- Check Nutrition Facts on food labels. A higher-percent Daily Value for fiber signals more whole grain or bran. Choose refined grain products labeled as enriched. Whole-grain ingredients are on the ingredient list first: brown rice, bulgur, graham flour, oatmeal, whole-grain corn, oats, whole rye, whole wheat, and wild rice. Products labeled as multi-grain, stone-ground, 100% wheat, cracked wheat, seven-grain, and bran do not mean whole-grain.

- Check the ingredient list for added sugars (sucrose, high-fructose corn syrup, honey, and molasses) and oils (partially hydrogenated vegetable oils). They add calories. Choose mostly foods with few added sugars, solid fats, or oils.

- Check the freshness date on the package.

Use the unit price for the best value. Grain products with many added ingredients may cost more than simpler products.

Shop for Bread

Bread is sold in many ways: already baked, as well as in baking mixes, refrigerated dough and batter, and frozen dough. Bagels, tortillas, rolls, and pitas are breads, too.

Be aware that dark-colored bread does not always contain whole-grain flour. It may be enriched bread with color added. There are also some whole-grain breads that are white! They are made with flour from a white-wheat grain.

Shop for Breakfast Cereals

When shopping for breakfast cereals, compare them for their nutritional value, price, and convenience.

- Ready-to-eat cereals need no preparation. Some are made with several grains.

- Packaged cereals may be sweetened with added sugars, or can be combined with dried fruit or nuts.

- Oatmeal, grits, and cream of wheat need cooking. You can buy regular, quick-cooking, and instant varieties.

- Cereals with dried fruits and nuts often cost more. Add your own to reduce the cost.

- Some breakfast cereals are fortified with large amounts of vitamins and minerals.

Read the Nutrition Facts to decide which products are right for you.

Shop for Pasta

Pasta refers to spaghetti, macaroni, and similar products. Pasta is sold dried, refrigerated fresh, fresh-frozen, frozen-cooked, and mixed in packaged foods. Pasta comes in hundreds of shapes and sizes. (See **Figure 24.2.**)

Most pasta is made from enriched or whole-wheat flour and water. Some noodles also contain eggs. Noodles can be made with other grains. For example, Thai noodles are made from rice and Japanese soba noodles are made from buckwheat.

Figure 24.2	Pasta Shapes

Pasta Shapes Pasta has many different names. Common types are made from refined wheat or whole grains. *What other pasta shapes can you name and describe?*

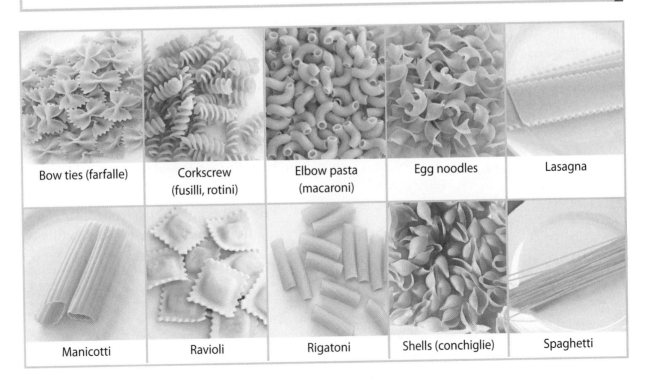

Bow ties (farfalle) | Corkscrew (fusilli, rotini) | Elbow pasta (macaroni) | Egg noodles | Lasagna

Manicotti | Ravioli | Rigatoni | Shells (conchiglie) | Spaghetti

Shop for Rice

There are many rice options. Rice is sold in boxes and bags, and in convenience foods such as frozen dishes and canned soup.

- **Brown Rice** This whole grain is chewier than white rice, and it has a rich, nutty flavor. It cooks more slowly than white rice.

- **White Rice** White rice has been processed, leaving just the endosperm. If enriched, white rice has B vitamins and iron. Arborio (a short-grain rice), basmati (a long-grain rice), and jasmine rice have unique flavors.

- **Different-Size Grains (White and Brown)** Cooked long-grain rice is dry and fluffy. Short-grain rice is moist and sticks together when cooked. That makes it easy to pick up with chopsticks. Medium-grain rice is in between.

- **Par-Boiled, or Converted, Rice** This is a white rice that is processed so the cooked grains are fluffy and separate when cooked. The process also helps rice retain more nutrients from the bran and germ. It takes longer to cook than other types of white rice.

- **Instant Rice (Brown and White)** Instant rice is pre-cooked, rinsed, and dried. It cooks faster than regular rice.

- **Wild Rice** Wild rice is really a seed, not rice. It has a savory flavor and is often prepared in the same way as rice.

Store Grain Products Properly

Follow these guidelines to store grain products properly and keep them fresh.

- Keep bread in the store wrapper and in a cool, dry place. Fresh bakery breads may stay longer in an air-tight plastic bag. Freeze bread for longer storage.

- If the kitchen is hot and humid, or if the label tells you to, refrigerate bread so that mold will not **develop**, or grow.

Nutrition & Wellness Tips

Shop for Convenience

✓ Buy frozen whole wheat waffles or pancakes to heat in the microwave oven or toaster for quick, easy meals.

✓ Use cornbread mix, refrigerated bread-stick dough, and pre-made pizza shells for quick bread baking.

Versatile Grains Grain-based dishes are common in cultures all over the world. Paella, made with rice and seafood, comes from Spain. *What grains are popular in other cultures? How are they prepared?*

◆ Store dry grain products in a covered container in a cool, dry place. Most will keep for about a year.

◆ Refrigerate whole grains unless you are going to use them right away. They contain some oils that can turn rancid, or go bad, at room temperature.

✓ Reading Check) **Recall** What is the best way to store whole grains and uncooked rice?

Cook Grain Products

Grain products like rice, pasta, and oatmeal are cooked in water. As they cook, they absorb water and swell to double or triple their original size.

Different grain products require different cooking times and methods. Follow the instructions on the package. Cook pasta just until it is al dente. **Al dente** is tender but slightly firm.

When properly cooked, grain products are tender. Undercooked grains are hard or chewy. Overcooked grains become soft and sticky.

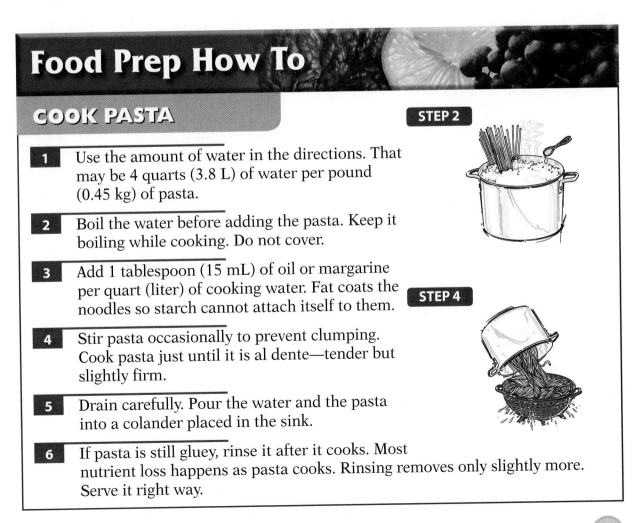

Food Prep How To

COOK PASTA

STEP 2

1. Use the amount of water in the directions. That may be 4 quarts (3.8 L) of water per pound (0.45 kg) of pasta.

2. Boil the water before adding the pasta. Keep it boiling while cooking. Do not cover.

3. Add 1 tablespoon (15 mL) of oil or margarine per quart (liter) of cooking water. Fat coats the noodles so starch cannot attach itself to them.

STEP 4

4. Stir pasta occasionally to prevent clumping. Cook pasta just until it is al dente—tender but slightly firm.

5. Drain carefully. Pour the water and the pasta into a colander placed in the sink.

6. If pasta is still gluey, rinse it after it cooks. Most nutrient loss happens as pasta cooks. Rinsing removes only slightly more. Serve it right way.

Cook Rice and Other Grains

![Nutrition & Wellness Tips]

Nutrition & Wellness Tips

✓ Use unsalted broth or fruit juice as the liquid when cooking grains. Experiment with herbs and spices to enhance flavors.

Follow these guidelines to cook rice and other cereals:

◆ Use only the amount of liquid that rice will absorb. When all the liquid is absorbed and the rice is tender, it is done.

◆ Allow more cooking time for brown rice and wild rice.

◆ Do not rinse rice; rinsing removes nutrients.

◆ Stir rice as little as possible. Stirring scrapes starch off the grains, making rice sticky.

◆ Use a large enough container. Grains double or triple in size as they cook.

✓ **Reading Check** **Explain** How much liquid should you use when cooking rice?

EASY RECIPES

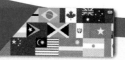

International Flavors

Blini

Customary	Ingredients	Metric
2	Eggs	2
1 ¼ cups	Whole milk	315 mL
¾ cup	Flour	190 mL
½ cup	Buckwheat flour	125 mL
½ tsp.	Sugar	3 mL
¼ tsp.	Salt	1 mL
1 Tbsp.	Butter	15 mL

Try This!

Blini are traditionally used to scoop and eat caviar, but you can enjoy them with fish, particularly salmon, and sour cream.

Yield: 6 servings of 10 bite-size pancakes each

❶ Combine dry ingredients in a large bowl and mix well.

❷ In another bowl, beat eggs and add to milk. Combine wet ingredients with dry ingredients and mix thoroughly.

❸ Use a little of the butter to grease a skillet or large frying pan.

❹ Pour tablespoon-sized drops of batter onto the hot skillet and cook until edges brown and bubbles appear on surface, about one minute. Turn and cook an additional minute.

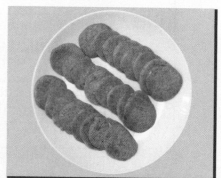

Nutritional Information Per Serving: 167 calories, 6 g total fat (3 g saturated fat), 92 mg cholesterol, 146 mg sodium, 22 g total carbohydrate (1 g fiber, 3 g sugars), 7 g protein

Percent Daily Value: vitamin A 4%, vitamin C 0%, calcium 8%, iron 8%

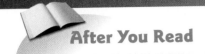

After You Read

CHAPTER SUMMARY

Grain products are made from wheat, rice, oats, cornmeal, barley, and other grains. Grains especially whole grains, provide important nutrients and health benefits. Many grains fit in meals and snacks. Cooking changes starch in grain, making it soft and easier to digest. Food labels and unit prices help you spot whole grain and enriched grain products. Store grain products for freshness. Use the right amount of liquid and time listed on the package or recipe when cooking. Grain products are also used in baking.

Vocabulary Review

1. Use each of these vocabulary words in a sentence.

Content Vocabulary
◇ whole grain (p. 352)
◇ endosperm (p. 352)
◇ germ (p. 352)
◇ bran (p. 352)
◇ refined grain (p. 352)
◇ starch (p. 352)
◇ cereal grain (p. 355)
◇ al dente (p. 359)

Academic Vocabulary
■ process (p. 352)
■ develop (p. 358)

Review Key Concepts

2. Identify the health benefits of grain foods, especially whole grains.

3. Explain how a variety of grain foods can fit in everyday meals and snacks.

4. Discuss how food science applies to grain products.

5. Summarize smart tips for buying and storing grain products.

6. Describe how to prepare grain foods for quality, nutritional value, and appeal.

Critical Thinking

7. Interpret the meaning of the phrase, "Make your carbs count for good nutrition." Give examples of how to make carbs count.

8. Identify the foods that would be missing from a typical day if you did not eat any grains. Then, project the consequences of eliminating foods from the Grain Group from your meals and snacks.

9. Explain the nutrition reasons for making at least half your grain food choices whole grains. Think of five ways you could fit more whole grains into your meals and snacks.

Real-World Skills and Applications

Interpersonal and Collaborative

10. School Menus Follow your teacher's instructions to form a group. Imagine you are a school meal advisory group. Suggest five nourishing menus with different grain foods. Agree on your group's goals, ideas, and menus. Choose some whole grain foods. Share your menus with the class.

Solve Problems

11. Make Substitutions Write the grain foods someone might eat in a typical week. Suggest substitutions for more variety. For example, decide on an alternative to sandwich bread, a different breakfast cereal, or an alternative to rice or pasta. Create a chart to show your substitutions, and compare the calorie and nutrient content of your choices.

Technology

12. Grains Online Get your teacher's permission to research unfamiliar grains on the Internet. Find out about their appearance, their processing, their taste and texture, and how they are cooked or prepared. Use a word processing program to write a report about them in your own words.

Financial Literacy

13. Bake or Buy Croutons? Bethany and Jesse are making a greens salad for dinner, and would like to add croutons. Making croutons from bread heels is usually less expensive than buying a box of them. If homemade croutons are $.03 cents each, and a box of 40 croutons is $2.20 at the store, how much money will they save by making their own?

14. Grain Labeling Browse food labels at the supermarket to learn about nutrition in grain products. Find at least five products with claims such as made with whole grains, good fiber source, fortified with, enriched with, or fewer calories. Record each product name in a chart, and explain its claims.

15. Compare Costs Compare the cost and preparation time for the same grain product in different forms—for example, instant, quick-cooking, and regular oatmeal. Determine the cost per one half cup (125 mL) after cooking. Write an explanation of which one you might buy and why.

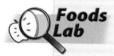
16. Experiment with Pasta Prepare two samples of spaghetti. Cook one sample according to the package directions. Cook the other for seven minutes longer than the directions specify. Compare their appearance, texture, and taste. Write your observations and conclusions.

Additional Activities For additional activities go to this book's Online Learning Center through glencoe.com.

Academic Skills

 English Language Arts

17. Advertise Grain Products Create an advertisement about a grain product. Identify your product, audience, and medium (print, TV, radio, online) first. Share the product's benefits. Be convincing, clear, and accurate. Present the ad in class.

> **NCTE 4** Use written language to communicate effectively.

 Social Studies

18. Grains Around the World Different cultures have different breads. For example, naan from India is a flatbread baked in a tandoori oven. Research breads from around the world. Note the culture each type of bread comes from.

> **NCSS I E Culture** Demonstrate the value of cultural diversity, as well as cohesion, within and across groups.

 Mathematics

19. Finding Years Archaeologists have found evidence that Egyptians used yeast 4,000 years ago for baking breads. What year would that be? Explain how you would make your calculation.

Math Concept **Subtracting Integers** To subtract an integer, add its additive inverse. For example, to find $2 - 5$, add the additive inverse of 5 to 2. In this case $2 + (-5) = -3$.

Starting Hint The calendar we use is called the Gregorian calendar. In this calendar, there is no year 0. The year that precedes 1 CE is 1 BCE. Start by subtracting 4,000 from the current year. Add back 1 to account for the lack of a year 0.

 For more math help, go to the Math Appendix.

> **NCTM Number and Operations** Understand meanings of operations and how they relate to one another.

STANDARDIZED TEST PRACTICE

MULTIPLE CHOICE
Read the paragraph. Write your answer on a separate piece of paper.

Test-Taking Tip Use familiar word parts to help you figure out unfamiliar vocabulary. Any part of the word may help. For example, the term al dente may not look familiar, but dente could remind you of the word dental. The term means firm to the bite. The term's literal Italian translation is "to the tooth."

Some people are allergic to wheat or wheat gluten. But people with this problem can still get plenty of healthful grains in their diets if they plan carefully. For example, some bakeries substitute the wheat in bread with a grain called spelt. Corn flour is also a nourishing alternative to wheat flour.

20. Based on the paragraph, which of the following best completes the following sentence?
People who are allergic to wheat ____ .
a. cannot eat corn tortillas
b. can substitute other grains for wheat
c. can eat wheat if they pair it with another grain
d. cannot tolerate bread

CHAPTER 25
Vegetables

Explore the Photo ▶▶
Vegetables come in an amazing variety of shapes, colors, textures, sizes, and flavors. *What are the most unusual vegetables you have ever tried?*

Writing Activity

Edit a First Draft

Rewrite and Improve The first draft of an essay is rarely in good enough shape to turn in to the teacher. Look at the first draft you wrote for Chapter 24 and revise it. Try to find spelling and grammar mistakes. You may think of a better way to phrase some of your sentences. You may also think of details you forgot before.

Writing Tips

1. **Edit** your sentences so they make sense.

2. **Be objective** when editing your own work.

3. **Proofread** carefully to find errors.

Reading Guide

Before You Read

Get Your Rest The more well rested and alert you are when you sit down to study, the more likely you will be to remember the information later.

Read to Learn

Key Concepts

- **Explain** why vegetables are good for your health.
- **Explain** where vegetables come from, how they get their colors, and how they react to heat, water, and air.
- **Summarize** smart ways to buy and store vegetables.
- **Describe** how to clean and prepare vegetables.

Main Idea

Vegetables provide nutrients, as well as flavor, color, and appeal, to your meals and snacks. Learn to buy, store, and prepare them properly.

Content Vocabulary

- ◇ chlorophyll
- ◇ flavonoid
- ◇ carotenoid
- ◇ enzyme
- ◇ produce
- ◇ in season
- ◇ tender-crisp

Academic Vocabulary

You will find these words in your reading and on your tests. Use the glossary to look up their definitions if necessary.

- ■ community
- ■ significant

Graphic Organizer

Vegetables come from many different parts of plants. Use a diagram like the one below to name seven different plant parts that vegetables come from.

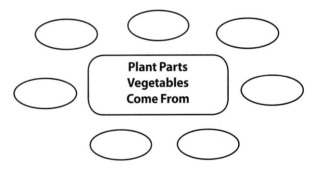

Plant Parts Vegetables Come From

 Graphic Organizer Go to this book's Online Learning Center at **glencoe.com** to print out this graphic organizer.

Academic Standards ▪ ▪ ▪ ▪ ▪ ▪ ▪ ▪ ▪ ▪ ▪ ▪ ▪ ▪ ▪ ▪ ▪ ▪ ▪

 English Language Arts
NCTE 4 Use written language to communicate effectively.

 Social Studies
NCSS I A Culture Analyze and explain the ways groups, societies, and cultures address human needs and concerns.

 Mathematics
NCTM Number and Operations Understand the meanings of operations and how they relate to one another.
NCTM Algebra Understand patterns, relations, and functions.

NCTE National Council of Teachers of English
NCTM National Council of Teachers of Mathematics

NSES National Science Education Standards
NCSS National Council for the Social Studies

Eat Vegetables for Health

Vegetables taste good—especially if prepared properly. Vegetables also provide many nutrients that are vital to your health. No matter what their form—fresh, frozen, canned, or dried vegetables can be nutrient-dense. Here are reasons to eat vegetables:

As You Read

Connect How wide of a variety of vegetables are in your eating plan?

- ◆ **Fewer Calories** Most vegetables are low in calories. They can help you lower your calorie intake if you eat more vegetables and fewer high-calorie foods.

- ◆ **Carbs for Energy** Most of your food energy should come from carbohydrates. Vegetables provide starches and some sugars. Corn, green peas, potatoes, squash, and turnips are popular starchy vegetables.

- ◆ **Fiber** Fiber gives shape to vegetables. It can be found in celery stalks, potato skins, and the stems of lettuce leaves. Fiber helps your digestive system work properly and helps you feel full with fewer calories.

- ◆ **Low Fat, No Cholesterol** Almost all vegetables naturally contain little or no fat unless fat is added in processing, cooking, or serving. Also, all vegetables are cholesterol-free.

- ◆ **Vitamins and Minerals** Different vegetables provide different vitamins and minerals. (See **Figure 25.1** for the vitamins and minerals found in some common vegetables.) This is one reason why eating a variety is so important.

- ◆ **Phytonutrients** Vegetables provide more than nutrients. Phytonutrients—substances found naturally in plants—may help protect you from cancer, heart disease, and other health problems.

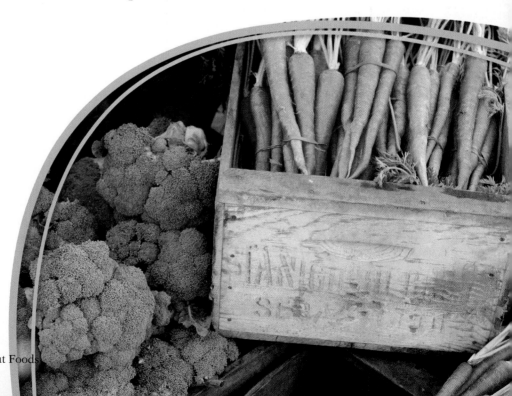

Fiber for Health Many vegetable snacks are good sources of fiber. *What are the benefits of snacking on foods with more fiber?*

Figure 25.1 — Vegetable Vitamins and Minerals

Vegetable Nutrition Eating a good mix of vegetables provides a variety of vitamins and minerals. *Did you eat any of these vegetables this week? What nutrients did they provide?*

Vegetable	Vitamin A	Vitamin C	Folate	Calcium	Magnesium	Potassium
Bok choy	X	X				
Broccoli	X	X	X			
Cabbage		X				
Carrots	X					
Green Peppers		X				
Lentils			X			X
Okra		X			X	
Peas, green		X	X			X
Potato		X				X
Spinach	X	X	X	X	X	X
Sweet Potato	X	X				X
Tomato	X	X				X
Turnip greens	X	X	X			
Winter squash	X	X				X

Contains at least 10 percent of the Daily Value (DV) of that vitamin or mineral. Calculations are based on ½ cup (125 mL), except for potato, sweet potato, and tomato, which are one medium-sized vegetable.

MyPyramid Advice

Someone who needs 2,000 calories per day needs about 2½ cups (625 mL) from the Vegetable Group daily. The equivalent of one cup (250 mL) of vegetables includes:

◆ Two cups (500 mL) raw leafy vegetables

◆ One cup (250 mL) cooked, canned, or chopped raw vegetables

◆ One cup (250 mL) cooked dry beans, peas, or lentils

Vegetables have five subgroups, based on their nutrient content. Divide your choices among dark-green vegetables, orange vegetables, dry beans and peas, starchy vegetables, and other vegetables. Dry beans and peas belong in both the Vegetable Group and the Meat and Beans Group. You should count them in just one group.

Vegetables should not substitute for other food-group foods. For example, if you decide to get calcium from spinach and skip milk, you may miss other benefits that the Milk Group provides.

More Vegetables, More Variety

Some ways to add more vegetables to your meals are:

◆ Eat a variety of different-colored vegetables. Different colors offer different health benefits.

- Create a tasty mixed salad with vegetables.
- Add more vegetables—including beans—to foods you eat often, such as sandwiches, burritos, or scrambled eggs.
- Try vegetables that are new to you.
- Try to eat one more vegetable serving each day for the next month.

✓ Reading Check **Discuss** How can you get more vegetables, with more variety, into your eating plan?

Vegetables and Food Science

Besides their nutrition, science can help you understand where vegetables come from, how they get their colors, and how they react to heat, water, and air.

Fruits, Flowers, Roots, and More

Did you know that vegetables come from many different parts of plants? Vegetables can be:

- Fruits, such as tomatoes, eggplants, and peppers.
- Flowers, such as broccoli and cauliflower.
- Stems, such as asparagus and celery.
- Roots and tubers, such as beets, carrots, and turnips.
- Bulbs, such as onions.
- Leaves, such as cabbage, greens, kale, and spinach.
- Seeds, such as beans, corn, and peas.

Vegetable Colors

Not all vegetables are green. Thanks to different pigments, vegetables come in a rainbow of colors. Pigments that add color also work as phytonutrients.

Chlorophyll

Chlorophyll is the pigment that makes vegetables green. When green vegetables are cooked, acids can dull their color. Acid in the vegetables' cells leaks out and comes in contact with the chlorophyll. Chlorophyll also comes in contact with the acids in tap water. A chemical reaction turns green vegetables a drab olive-green or yellow-green color.

Proper cooking can help prevent dull-colored vegetables. Put them directly into boiling water and keep cooking time short. Steaming keeps vegetables above water, away from any acids.

◆Vocabulary

You can find definitions in the glossary at the back of this book.

Flavonoids

Flavonoids are the pigments that give vegetables like eggplant, purple potatoes, and red cabbage their red, purple, and blue colors. These pigments leak out of vegetables and dissolve in water. Adding an acid helps flavonoids to keep their color. For example, red cabbage sometimes turns blue during cooking. If it is cooked with an apple or a tablespoon of vinegar—which both have acids—it stays red.

Carotenoids

Carotenoids give many vegetables, such as tomatoes, winter squash, carrots, and sweet potatoes, their deep-yellow, orange, and red colors. These pigments are stable. These colors stay vibrant in vegetables unless they are badly overheated. One form of a carotenoid is used as food coloring. It is called Lycopene and is found in tomatoes and other red fruits.

More Vegetable Science

Three substances can affect, and sometimes dull, the colors of vegetables: acids, bases, and enzymes. Good cooks try to retain vegetables' natural colors.

- ◆ **Acids** In food, these substances taste sour. Fruits such as oranges and apples contain weak acids, such as citric acid. Many vegetables have acids, too.

- ◆ **Bases** These are the chemical opposites of acids. They often feel slippery, and they have a bitter taste. Baking soda is a base.

- ◆ **Enzymes** An **enzyme** is a special protein that helps chemical reactions happen. Enzymatic browning occurs when the cells of cut, peeled, or bruised vegetables, such as potatoes, are exposed to oxygen. The darkened vegetable is safe to eat, but unappetizing. Cooking destroys enzymes that cause enzymatic browning. You can soak potatoes in water or toss them with a little acidic ingredient, such as lemon juice, to stop browning.

✓ Reading Check **Describe** What are the pigments that give vegetables their color?

Math in Action

Veggies-of-the-Month Club

The Jones family decided that not only would they try a new vegetable or vegetable dish this month, but next month they would try two. The month after that, they would try three new vegetables. If the Jones family continues in this pattern, how many new vegetable dishes will they have sampled after six months?

Math Concept **Determining Patterns**
An arithmetic pattern is one in which a value is added each time. In this case, the value added is $n + 1$ where n is the numerical sequence 0, 1, 2, 3, and so on.

Starting Hint Determine the pattern for adding vegetables, and write an equation to help you find the answer. Then, solve the equation.

NCTM Algebra Understand patterns, relations, and functions.

 For more math help, go to the Math Appendix

Buy and Store Vegetables

Do you pick out vegetables at the store, or help put them away at home? Knowing how to shop for vegetables and store them properly is essential. Quality vegetables look and taste better. When they are stored properly, they retain their nutrients and are safer to eat.

Supermarkets sell fresh vegetables in their produce departments. **Produce** includes fresh vegetables, fruits, and herbs. Vegetables may be sold loose, in packages, or bound together with a band or tape. Your community, or local area, may also have farmers' markets where fresh vegetables are sold.

Look for fresh vegetables that are solid, have a good color, and are crisp or firm. Avoid vegetables that are bruised, damaged, or decayed, that are too pale, soft, or wilted, or that are unusually small or large.

Buy in Season

Produce is grown locally and shipped from all over the world to stores and restaurants. That allows you to buy many varieties of fresh vegetables all year. Many vegetables are more plentiful **in season**. In season means harvested at the time of year when ripe. That is when their quality is highest and when they often are lowest in cost. For example, vine-ripened tomatoes and corn are in season in the summer.

Buy What You Need

Fresh vegetables are perishable. They keep their peak quality for only a short time and may spoil quickly. To avoid waste, buy only the amount of fresh vegetables you need.

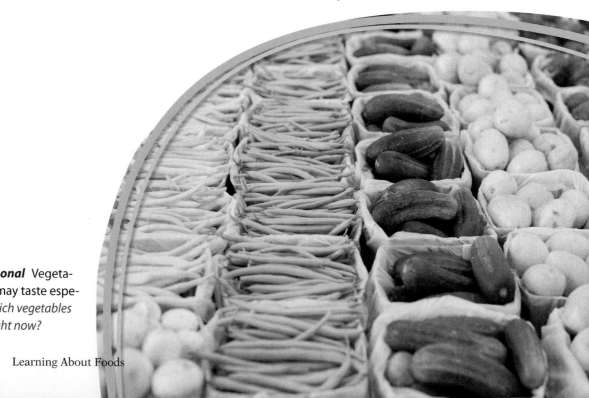

Fresh and Seasonal Vegetables in season may taste especially good. *Which vegetables are in season right now?*

Buy for Convenience

Frozen and canned vegetables are convenient. Because they are partly or fully prepared, frozen vegetables may cost more than fresh vegetables. Canned vegetables often cost less. Saving time may be worth any added cost. You can find convenience vegetables in several areas of the supermarket:

- **Grocery Aisles** Canned vegetables are sold whole, sliced, or as sauces. They may cost less than fresh or frozen vegetables. You also may find canned vegetable juices and dried vegetables, such as instant mashed potatoes.

- **Freezer Case** Frozen vegetables are sold whole, chopped, mixed with other vegetables, or frozen in a sauce.

- **Produce Department** Produce is sold just picked, already cleaned, or even sliced. Also, look for salad mixes, stir-fry vegetable mixes, washed veggie snacks, and fresh salsa.

- **Deli** You may find pre-made salads or heat-and-eat vegetables at the deli counter.

- **Salad Bar** Prepared vegetables for salads, snacks, and other vegetable dishes are sold at a salad bar.

Nutrition & Wellness Tips

Shop Safely

✓ While you shop, keep fresh vegetables away from chemicals and meats.

✓ Bag fresh vegetables separately from cleaning supplies, raw meat, poultry, and seafood.

✓ Only buy pre-cut vegetables that are refrigerated or surrounded by ice.

Store for Quality

Proper storage keeps vegetables at peak quality for flavor, appearance, and nutrition. To store vegetables:

- Refrigerate them as soon as you unpack your grocery bags.

- Shake off moisture, which makes vegetables spoil faster. Do not wash vegetables until you are ready to prepare them.

- Place vegetables in plastic bags, covered containers, or the crisper bin of your refrigerator.

- Store fresh vegetables away from raw meat, poultry, and seafood.

- Keep onions, potatoes, and winter squash in a cool, dark, dry place—not in the refrigerator.

- Store frozen vegetables in the freezer. Thaw them in the refrigerator or microwave oven just before use. Do not refreeze.

- Keep unopened, canned vegetables in a cool, dry place. Store leftovers in the refrigerator.

- Keep dried vegetables in an airtight container in a cool, dry place.

✓ Reading Check Describe How do high-quality fresh vegetables look and feel?

Agricultural Scientist

Agricultural scientists research and apply sciences of food, plants, soil, and animal production. Their work helps ensure an adequate, safe food supply.

Careers Find out more about careers. Visit this book's Online Learning Center at **glencoe.com**.

Prepare Healthful Vegetables

Vegetables can fit into your eating plan in many ways. Serve them in side dishes, salads, and garnishes. Prepare them in main dishes or sandwiches. Use them in breads and desserts. No matter how you eat them, prepare vegetables with care.

Clean Fresh Vegetables

Follow these guidelines to clean vegetables before preparing or eating them:

◆ Wash your hands with warm water and soap for at least 20 seconds before and after handling fresh vegetables.

◆ Wash vegetables under cold, running water to remove dirt and surface microorganisms. Rub them briskly with your hands. Do not soak them or use any soap.

◆ Use a clean brush to scrub firm vegetables, such as potatoes and squash.

◆ Dry produce with a clean towel.

◆ Trim away parts you cannot eat, such as tough stems. Cut out rough spots or soft spots.

◆ Remove outer leaves of greens such as lettuce and cabbage.

◆ Wash unused vegetables from an opened package.

Vegetable Food Safety

Some bacteria can pose a **significant**, or important, threat to health. Keep vegetables that will be eaten raw separate from raw meat, poultry and seafood and the utensils used to prepare them. Clean all surfaces and utensils that touch fresh vegetables with hot water and soap before and after preparation.

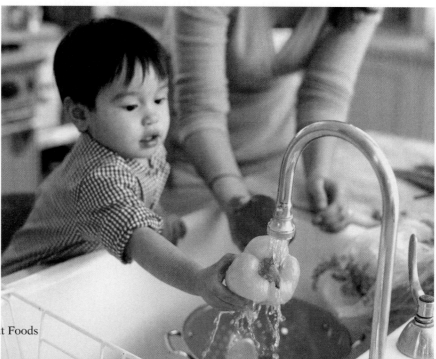

Tasty and Safe Cleaning vegetables removes dirt, residues, and bacteria that can cause foodborne illness. *What else should be done to fresh vegetables to prepare them for eating or cooking?*

Food Prep How To

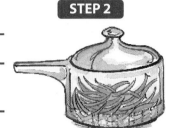

STEP 2

1	Bring a small amount of water to a boil.
2	Add the vegetables. Cover the pan with a tight-fitting cover. Turn down the heat.
3	Simmer the vegetables just until they are tender-crisp.
4	Serve the vegetables in their cooking liquid.

TIP The cooking liquid contains some of the nutrients that were lost from the vegetables. It will also help keep the simmered vegetables warm.

Vegetable Cooking

Cooking softens vegetables and makes them easier to chew and digest. It also changes their flavors and sometimes their colors. Some vegetables, such as potatoes, winter squash, and artichokes, must be cooked before you can eat them.

Cooking Methods

Vegetables can be cooked in many ways:

- **Steam** Cook many fresh vegetables in a steamer basket. Let the vegetables steam until they are **tender-crisp**—tender, but still firm and slightly crisp.

- **Bake or Roast** Bake vegetables such as potatoes, sweet potatoes, and squash in their skins. You can roast many vegetables to brown the outside.

- **Simmer** Simmer fresh or frozen vegetables in a small amount of water. Use just enough water to cover the bottom of the pan, and cover with a lid.

- **Grill** Grilling until tender-crisp gives vegetables a char-broiled flavor. Spear an assortment of cut vegetables on skewers.

- **Microwave** Place vegetables in a covered, microwave-safe container with a small amount of water. Pierce large vegetables like potatoes and squash with a fork.

- **Stir-Fry** Stir-frying adds a small amount of fat. Use a healthful oil. Combine different kinds of vegetables for color, flavor, and nutrition.

- **Heat** Canned vegetables are pre-cooked, so they need only to be heated.

Preserve Nutrients, Texture, and Color

Cooked properly, vegetables keep their color, flavor, texture, and nutrients. Follow these guidelines to cook vegetables:

◆ Leave edible skins on vegetables like carrots, potatoes, or zucchini. The skin provides fiber and nutrients.

◆ Use just a small amount of water for simmering vegetables. If you cut vegetables for cooking, leave the pieces as large as possible. They will lose fewer vitamins in the water.

◆ Avoid overcooking. The shorter the cooking time, the better!

◆ Cover vegetables when you simmer, steam, or microwave them to speed cooking time and preserve nutrients.

Add Flavor Without Fat and Salt

Add herbs or lemon juice to enhance the flavor of vegetables. Salt can mask a vegetable's natural flavor. Toss vegetables with a small amount of butter or margarine for a buttery flavor. The flavor is more intense if it is added just before serving.

✓ **Reading Check** **Analyze** How should you simmer vegetables to preserve nutrients, color, texture?

EASY RECIPES

Everyday Favorites

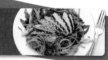

Vegetable Cole Slaw

Customary	Ingredients	Metric
3 stalks	Celery	3
3	Carrots, medium	3
½ head	Cabbage (Napa or other)	½
½ head	Red cabbage	½
½ each	Green apple	½
2 Tbsp.	Olive oil	30 mL
1 Tbsp.	Apple cider vinegar	15 mL

Try This!
Add fresh bell peppers of various colors for a tasty alternative.

Yield: Six servings, 1 cup (250 mL) each

❶ Wash and, with paper towel, pat dry the vegetables and apple. Cut the vegetables and apple into thin matchstick-sized strips.

❷ Mix oil and vinegar and toss with cut vegetables.

❸ Chill and serve cold.

Nutritional Information Per Serving: 97 calories, 5 g total fat (1 g saturated fat), 0 mg cholesterol, 71 mg sodium, 13 g total carbohydrate (4 g fiber, 7 g total sugars), 2 g protein

Percent Daily Value: vitamin A 150%, vitamin C 100%, calcium 8%, iron 6%

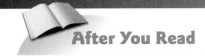

After You Read

CHAPTER SUMMARY

Colorful vegetables are packed with nutrition, texture, and flavor. Vegetables are nutrient dense with little fat and few calories. A variety of vegetables adds interest and appeal. Vegetables come from different parts of a plant. Proper food handling and preparation can help vegetables keep their natural color, texture, and flavor and nutrients. Vegetables are sold fresh, canned, frozen, dried, and juiced. All forms of vegetables should be stored and prepared to keep their safety and quality. Vegetables can be cooked using many methods. Proper cooking helps retain nutrients, quality, and appeal.

Vocabulary Review

1. Use each of these vocabulary words in a sentence.

Content Vocabulary
◇ chlorophyll (p. 368)
◇ flavonoid (p. 369)
◇ carotenoid (p. 369)
◇ enzyme (p. 369)
◇ produce (p. 370)
◇ in season (p. 370)
◇ tender-crisp (p. 373)

Academic Vocabulary
■ community (p. 370)
■ significant (p. 372)

Review Key Concepts

2. Explain why vegetables are good for your health.

3. Explain where vegetables come from, how they get their colors, and how they react to heat, water, and air.

4. Summarize smart ways to buy and store vegetables.

5. Describe how to clean and prepare vegetables.

Critical Thinking

6. Evaluate how seasonal vegetables can complement a nutritious eating plan. How could you add them to your meals and snacks? What are some of the advantages of using seasonal vegetables?

7. Analyze the consequences of an eating plan with too few vegetables.

8. Design changes that a family can make in the way it shops for vegetables. What can different family members do to get more variety in their Vegetable Group choices? How will smart shopping choices benefit the family's nutrition?

9. Explain how you can add vegetables to a food or recipe you already make or eat. Describe if they will be raw, or cooked before or after adding them. If cooked, which methods might you use to cook them?

Real-World Skills and Applications

Interpersonal and Collaborative

10. Global Vegetables Follow your teacher's instructions to break into teams. Imagine you are the staff of a new restaurant that specializes in international vegetable dishes. Research five vegetable-based dishes from other cultures. Create a menu with the names of the dishes, their ingredients, some nutritional benefits, and an illustration. Share your menu with the class.

Decision Making and Problem Solving

11. Plan Ahead Imagine that you have been asked to bring a fresh vegetable tray to a party. What six kinds of vegetables would you include? Aim for variety. Identify the major nutrients and their sources. Draw a diagram of your tray.

Technology

12. Create a Spreadsheet Show how you can include vegetables in breakfast, lunch, dinner, and snacks for one week. Create a computer spreadsheet for seven days showing your meals and snacks for each day. Show vegetables you could eat, their form, and how to prepare them.

Financial Literacy

13. Loose or Bagged Salad? Many produce shoppers choose bagged salad. The bags contain lettuce and other vegetables that are already cut and washed. Visit the produce section of your supermarket and choose a bagged salad. Note the contents. Find the same products in the loose section, and compare costs. Which is more cost-effective: loose or bagged salads?

14. Freshness Experiment How much longer do fresh vegetables keep their quality when stored properly? Plan and carry out an experiment to find out. Choose one specific storage guideline to test. Write a report with your hypothesis, procedure, observations, and conclusions.

15. Evaluate Cooking Methods Cook the same type of vegetable using three different cooking methods. Judge each for its flavor, color, and texture. Write your results. Share them in class. Which cooking method do you prefer for the type of vegetable selected? Why?

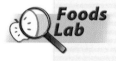

16. Texture Testing Prepare two samples of fresh or frozen broccoli: one cooked just until tender-crisp, the other cooked until very soft. Compare the texture, color, and flavor of each. Which one is more appealing to you? Why? How do you think they compare nutritionally? Why?

Additional Activities For additional activities go to this book's Online Learning Center at glencoe.com.

Academic Skills

 English Language Arts

17. Research a Vegetable Choose one vegetable that grows in your region. Research its nutritional value; when it is in season; what plant part it is; how to store and prepare it; and what pigment it has. Describe its flavor and texture. Write a one-page report with an image.

> **NCTE 4** Use written language to communicate effectively.

 Social Studies

18. Vegetables in Ethnic Cuisine Find out about a vegetable commonly used in another country. Locate it at a supermarket, a farmers' market, or a specialty store. Learn where it comes from and how to prepare it. Prepare it if you can.

> **NCSS I A Culture** Analyze and explain the ways groups, societies, and cultures address human needs and concerns.

 Mathematics

19. Got Vegetables? MyPyramid recommends eating at least 2½ cups of vegetables every day. Cory has eaten 1 cup of sweet potato, ¼ cup of carrots, and ⅓ cup of tomato juice. How much more should he eat today?

Math Concept **Adding Unlike Fractions** To add unlike fractions, convert them to like fractions with the same denominator. Look for the least common multiple of their denominators, and rename the fractions with a common denominator

Starting Hint Look for the least common multiple of the denominators of the food Cory has eaten today. Then, add the fractions and change the total MyPyramid recommendation to a like fraction. Find the difference.

 For more math help, go to the Math Appendix

> **NCTM Number and Operations** Understand the meanings of operations and how they relate to one another.

STANDARDIZED TEST PRACTICE

MULTIPLE CHOICE
Read the paragraph, then write an answer to the following question on a separate piece of paper.

> **Test-Taking Tip** When performing a matching exercise, match the easiest, most recognizable words first. The number of choices left may make finding the remaining pairs much easier.

Some people base their meals on in-season foods grown locally. This ensures that their food is extremely fresh. They can also support local farmers. These consumers know that other precious resources like oil or extra packaging are not wasted.

20. Based on the paragraph, which of the following statements is true?
   a. If you do not buy locally, the environment may be damaged.
   b. The term in-season refers to food grown organically.
   c. Buying locally helps ensure freshness.
   d. Small farmers never use pesticides.

CHAPTER 26
Fruits

Explore the Photo ▶▶

The bright colors, natural sweetness, and refreshing juiciness of fruits make them appealing to eat alone or with other foods. *How much fruit should a person eat each day?*

🖊 Writing Activity

Essay Question and Answer

Fruits of the World Fruits come in many shapes, sizes, and colors. Some such as bananas and apples are familiar. Others such as pomegranates or persimmons may seem unusual. Write a question and a corresponding answer in an essay about fruits in different cultures.

Writing Tips

1. **Develop** a question that is challenging.

2. **Plan** an answer that connects to the key words of the question.

3. **Organize** your answer with an introduction, a body, and a conclusion.

Reading Guide

Before You Read

Use Color Get three different colored pens to use to take notes. You could use red for vocabulary words, blue for explanations, and green for examples.

Read to Learn
Key Concepts

- **Explain** how eating a variety of fruits can contribute to good health.
- **Discuss** how fruit gets and keeps its color.
- **Summarize** smart ways to buy and store fruit.
- **Describe** how to prepare fruits in safe, nutritious, and appealing ways.

Main Idea

Fruits add color, flavor, and nutrition to meals and make delicious snacks. They are easy to find, simple to prepare, and can be low in cost. Enjoy a variety of fruit.

Content Vocabulary

- ◇ citrus fruit
- ◇ acid
- ◇ pome
- ◇ drupe
- ◇ ripe
- ◇ fruit nectar
- ◇ cider
- ◇ fruit juice concentrate

Academic Vocabulary

You will find these words in your reading and on your tests. Use the glossary to look up their definitions if necessary.

- ■ minimize
- ■ economical

Graphic Organizer

As you read, use a chart like the one below to list the six types of fruit and describe the characteristics of each type.

Type of Fruit	Characteristics

 Graphic Organizer Go to this book's Online Learning Center at glencoe.com to print out this graphic organizer.

Academic Standards •

 English Language Arts
NCTE 12 Use language to accomplish individual purposes.

 Mathematics
NCTM Algebra Represent and analyze mathematical situations and structures using algebraic symbols.

 Science
NSES Content Standard C Develop an understanding of matter, energy, and organization in living systems.

NCTE National Council of Teachers of English	**NSES** National Science Education Standards
NCTM National Council of Teachers of Mathematics	**NCSS** National Council for the Social Studies

Vocabulary

You can find definitions in the glossary at the back of this book.

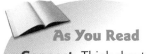

As You Read

Connect Think about the nutrients in the fruits you like best.

Fruit Is Good for You

Fruits have many health benefits:

◆ **Energy** Fresh fruits have sugars that supply energy.

◆ **Fiber** Fiber is in the edible skins. It is also part of the pulp in citrus fruits. A **citrus fruit** is a fruit that has a thick rind and juicy pulp. Oranges and tangerines are citrus fruits.

◆ **No Fat or Cholesterol** Most fruits contain no fat. All fruits are cholesterol-free.

◆ **Vitamins and Minerals** Fruits have an array of vitamins and minerals. (See **Figure 26.1.**)

◆ **Phytonutrients** Phytonutrients in fruits help protect against cancer, heart disease, and other health problems.

MyPyramid Advice

Someone who eats 2,000 calories daily needs about two cups (500 mL) from the Fruit Group daily. Fruit comes in a variety of forms—fresh, frozen, canned, dried, and juice. Choose whole or cut-up fresh fruit rather than juice or sweetened products when possible to **minimize**, or reduce, added sugar.

| Figure 26.1 | Vitamins and Minerals in Fruits |

Naturally Nutritious Different fruits are higher in different vitamins or minerals. *Which fruits listed below contain the most different vitamins and minerals?*

Fruit	Vitamin A	Vitamin C	Folate	Potassium
Apricot	x	x		x
Avacado			x	x
Banana*		x		x
Cantaloupe	x	x		x
Guava	x	x		
Mango	x	x		
Orange*		x	x	
Papaya		x		
Peach*	x	x		
Pear*		x		
Pomegranate*		x		x
Raspberries		x		
Starfruit		x		

Contains at least 10 percent of the Daily Value (DV) of that vitamin or mineral. Calculations are based on ½ cup (125 mL) servings, except where noted by an asterisk (*), which denotes a medium piece of fruit.

Fruit Variety

Take advantage of the array of colors, shapes, and textures of fruits. Eat a vitamin C-rich fruit or juice every day. Try a fruit you have never tasted. Use dried, canned, and frozen fruit when fresh fruits are costly or not available. Choose fruits with edible skins for extra fiber.

✓ **Reading Check**) **Discuss** What are the benefits of adding enough fruit to your meals and snacks?

Fruit in Food Science

Fruit changes its look, texture, and taste when exposed to heat, water, and air. Food science explains why.

Acids can affect the color of cooked and cut fruit. An **acid** is a chemical that tastes sour. Many fruits contain weak acids. Oranges, lemons, limes, and grapefruits contain citric acid.

Fruit Groupings

There are six basic types of fruits:

♦ A **pome**, like an apple or a pear, has a core with seeds and grows on trees.

♦ A **drupe**, like a peach or a cherry, has a large pit and grows on trees.

♦ Berries, like strawberries and grapes, are small fruits that grow on vines, trees, or bushes.

♦ Citrus, like oranges and grapefruits, have segments and grow on trees.

♦ Melons, like cantaloupes and watermelons, grow on vines.

♦ Tropical fruits, like avocados and bananas, grow in warm climates.

Fruit Colorings

Most fruit colors come from pigments. Pigments are also phytonutrients.

Green fruits like kiwifruit and limes get their color from chlorophyll.

Flavonoids give cherries, blueberries, and blackberries their red, purple, and blue colors.

Carotenoids are mostly yellow and orange. Oranges and peaches have carotenoids.

Browning from Enzymes

Some fruits contain a colorless compound. When cut or peeled surfaces are exposed to oxygen, an enzyme turns this compound gray, brown, or black. An enzyme is a protein that helps chemical reactions happen. The darkened fruit looks unappealing, but it is safe to eat.

Cooking destroys these enzymes. Sprinkle fruit with lemon or orange juice, which has citric acid, to slow the browning.

✓ **Reading Check** **Apply** How can you prevent cut bananas and pears from turning brown?

Buy and Store Fruit

Do you know how to shop for and store fruits and fruit juices? Getting the best quality and nutrition from your fruit choices should be your goal.

Fresh Fruit

You can find many varieties of fresh fruits. **Ripe** fruit is generally flavorful, colorful, and firm but not hard. Unripe fruit is usually hard to the touch and less flavorful.

◆ Apples, berries, cherries, grapes, and citrus fruits should be ripe when you buy them. They stop ripening when they are picked.

◆ Apricots, avocados, bananas, peaches, and pears continue to ripen after they are picked.

Nutrition & Wellness Tips

Snack Ideas

✓ Mix fresh or canned fruit pieces with plain low-fat yogurt and top with granola or cereal.

✓ To make a fruit smoothie, blend cut fruit, plain low-fat yogurt, ice cubes, and juice.

Discover International Foods

Countries of the Caribbean

Caribbean foods reflect those who settled in the area: British, Chinese, Dutch, East Indians, French, Spanish, and West Africans. Barbecuing was popular with native Arawaks, who called it *barbacoa*. The subtropical climate is suited to many fruits (banana, breadfruit, cherimoya, citrus, mango, guava, papaya, passion fruit, and pineapple) and vegetables (akee, calabaza, chayote, plantain, okra, sweet potatoes, taro, and yautia). Fish dishes, such as *escabeche* and codfish cakes, are popular on the Caribbean islands. Other popular foods include cassava bread, rice and beans, curried goat, and callaloo soup.

Languages Across Cultures

arroz con gandules (ä-'ròth-(,)kòn-gän-'dü-lēz) Puerto Rican dish made by cooking rice, pigeon peas, and sofrito (paste of annatto seeds and lard).

jerk ('jərk) Spicy-hot seasoning blend rubbed on chicken, fish, or meat before grilling.

 Recipes Find out more about Caribbean recipes on this book's Online Learning Center at **glencoe.com**.

Shop for Quality

High-quality fresh fruits have the best flavor and nutrition. Look for fruits that have these qualities:

- **Full Size** Fruits that are smaller than normal were picked too soon and will not ripen properly.

- **Bright and Fresh** Avoid those with dark spots.

- **Plump and Heavy** This usually means they are juicy.

- **Free of Dents, Bruises, or Decay** Avoid fruits with mushy brown spots or powdery areas.

- **Firm** Press fruit gently so you do not damage it. Some ripe fruit will be slightly soft. Very soft fruit may be over-ripe. Hard fruit may not ripen.

- **Pleasant Aroma** Some fruits such as peaches, nectarines, and melons smell sweet when ripe.

When buying fresh-cut fruit, choose fruit that is refrigerated or surrounded by ice. Keep fresh fruit separate from meat, poultry, and seafood.

Buy in Season

Some fruits are in season, or plentiful, ripe, and high in quality, at a certain time of the year. Fruits in season cost less, offering an **economical**, or financial, benefit to buying them. (See **Figure 26.2.**)

Fruit is shipped from many parts of the world. That is why you can buy many varieties all year long.

Fruit Juice

Juice comes in many different forms.

- Beverages labeled as juice must be 100 percent juice. They may be bottled, concentrated, or ready-to-serve.

- **Fruit nectar** is a thick, sugar-sweetened beverage of fruit juice and pulp, which contains fiber.

- Products labeled as fruit punch, fruit drink, juice blend, or juice cocktail contain only a portion of juice. The rest is water, added flavorings, and added sugar.

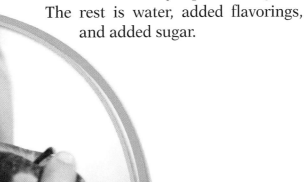

Just Right Choose fresh fruits that are not bruised or too soft. *How do you know the apple this girl is eating is ripe?*

Figure 26.2 **Seasonal Fruit**

Prime-Time Fruits Each season is ideal for certain fruits. Fruits are in season when they are most plentiful and highest in quality. *When are the best seasons to make fresh apple pie, fresh-squeezed orange juice, and strawberry shortcake?*

	Jan.	Feb.	Mar.	Apr.	May	Jun.	Jul.	Aug.	Sep.	Oct.	Nov.	Dec.
Apple									x	x	x	
Apricot						x	x					
Avocado	x	x	x	x	x	x	x	x	x	x	x	x
Cherry					x	x	x	x				
Grapefruit	x	x	x	x	x	x	x	x	x	x	x	x
Mango					x	x	x	x	x			
Melon								x	x	x		
Orange (navel)	x	x	x	x	x						x	x
Peach					x	x	x	x	x	x		
Pear	x	x	x				x	x	x	x	x	x
Plum					x	x	x	x	x	x		
Strawberry				x	x	x						

Some fruit juices and drinks are fortified with calcium, but they should not replace calcium-rich choices from the Milk Group. All food groups are important to good health.

Look for pasteurized fruit juice and cider. **Cider** is a beverage made by pressing juice from fruit. Unpasteurized juice or cider must be refrigerated. It must also have a food safety warning attached to it, unless the juice comes from a farmer's market.

Convenience Shopping

There are many convenient fruit options in your supermarket.

◆ **Produce Department/Salad Bar** Look for pre-cut fruit and pre-made fruit salads.

◆ **Grocery Aisles** Canned or jarred fruits may be whole, sliced, halved, or crushed. Look for bottled and boxed juices. Dried fruits are sold in packages or as bulk foods.

◆ **Dairy Case** Look for cartons of chilled, ready-to-serve fruit juices and juice drinks.

◆ **Freezer Case** Frozen fruits are whole, sliced, or crushed. Some have sugar added. Look for juice with most of the water removed, called **fruit juice concentrate**.

Store Fruit for Quality

Follow these guidelines to store fruit properly:

◆ Let slightly underripe fruits stand at room temperature. Put them into a paper bag to speed ripening.

◆ Refrigerate ripe fruits and eat within several days to slow further ripening and spoilage. Do not refrigerate bananas.

◆ Keep fruit separate from raw meat, poultry, or fish.

◆ Store cut or peeled fruits in an airtight container in the refrigerator at 40°F (4°C) or less.

◆ Keep frozen fruit and fruit juice in the freezer until needed. Thaw them in the refrigerator.

◆ Store dried fruits and unopened cans of fruit and juice in a cool, dry place. Refrigerate leftover canned fruit in an airtight container, not in the can.

◆ Store refrigerated juice in the refrigerator.

✓ **Reading Check** **Explain** What qualities would you look for when buying fresh fruit?

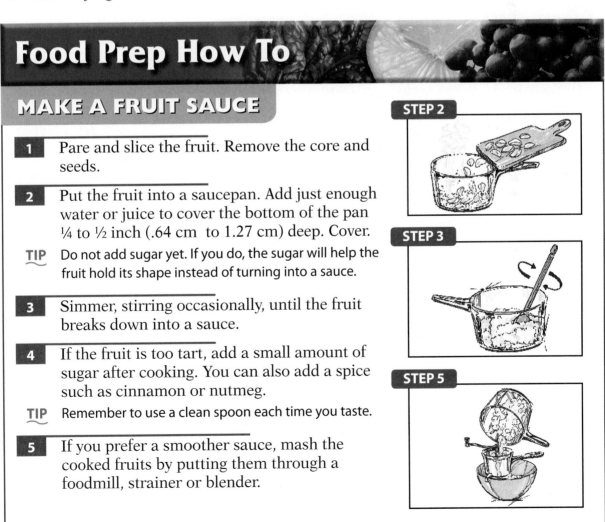

Food Prep How To

MAKE A FRUIT SAUCE

1 Pare and slice the fruit. Remove the core and seeds.

2 Put the fruit into a saucepan. Add just enough water or juice to cover the bottom of the pan ¼ to ½ inch (.64 cm to 1.27 cm) deep. Cover.

TIP Do not add sugar yet. If you do, the sugar will help the fruit hold its shape instead of turning into a sauce.

3 Simmer, stirring occasionally, until the fruit breaks down into a sauce.

4 If the fruit is too tart, add a small amount of sugar after cooking. You can also add a spice such as cinnamon or nutmeg.

TIP Remember to use a clean spoon each time you taste.

5 If you prefer a smoother sauce, mash the cooked fruits by putting them through a foodmill, strainer or blender.

STEP 2

STEP 3

STEP 5

Healthful Fruit Preparation

The proper preparation of fruit preserves its nutrients, flavor, and quality. Frozen fruit is best served before it thaws completely so that it feels firm, not mushy or rubbery. Fresh fruit needs to be rinsed under cold running water just before eating to remove dirt and pesticides. Scrub firm, whole fruit with a clean, soft-bristled brush. Cut out any bruised spots.

Once your fruit is properly cleaned, it is ready to be eaten—or simmered, steamed, baked, broiled, sautéed, or microwaved.

- ◆ **Cook whole fruits** with the core or pit removed. Bake or microwave in a small amount of liquid.

- ◆ **Microwave whole fruit** quickly to keep nutrients and flavor. Pierce the skin of unpared fruit so it will not burst.

- ◆ **Cook cut, sliced, or dried fruits** by simmering in liquid. Add a little sugar to help fruit keep its shape.

✓ Reading Check **Discuss** How can you cook fruit?

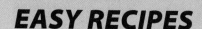

EASY RECIPES — International Flavors

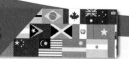

Roasted Pineapple

Customary	Ingredients	Metric
1	Pineapple	1
2 Tbsp.	Butter	30 mL
¼ cup	Brown sugar	65 mL
¼ tsp.	Cinnamon	1 mL

Try This!
Serve with ice cream for a special dessert. This can also be grilled, brushing the grill with the melted butter before adding the pineapple slices.

Yield: Four servings, ½ cup (125 mL) each

❶ Preheat oven to 400 degrees. Remove the top, bottom, skin and core from the pineapple

❷ Cut pineapple into circular pieces.

❸ Melt the butter and spread it over the bottom of a roasting pan. Sprinkle half the brown sugar over the bottom of the pan and arrange pineapple slices on top.

❹ Sprinkle remaining brown sugar and cinnamon over the top of the pineapple and bake. Remove from oven when juices begin to bubble and darken.

Nutritional Information Per Serving: 159 calories, 6 g total fat (4 g saturated fat), 15 mg cholesterol, 7 mg sodium, 28 g total carbohydrate (2 g fiber, 24 g total sugars), 1 g protein

Percent Daily Value: vitamin A 4%, vitamin C 70%, calcium 2%, iron 4%

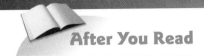

After You Read

CHAPTER SUMMARY

Fruit, which makes up MyPyramid's Fruit Group, is part of a healthful eating plan. Different fruits and fruit juices add color, flavor, nutrition, and interest to meals and snacks. Fruit gets its color from pigments. The natural color can change as it is prepared and cooked. Fruit is sold fresh, frozen, canned, dried, and as juice. When buying fresh fruit, look for signs of ripeness and quality. Fruit retains nutrients, flavor, and quality when stored and prepared properly. Fresh fruits can be washed and eaten raw or cooked using many methods.

Vocabulary Review

1. Use each of these vocabulary words in a sentence.

Content Vocabulary
- citrus fruit (p. 380)
- acid (p. 381)
- pome (p. 381)
- drupe (p. 381)
- ripe (p. 382)
- fruit nectar (p. 383)
- cider (p. 384)
- fruit juice concentrate (p. 384)

Academic Vocabulary
- minimize (p. 380)
- economical (p. 383)

Review Key Concepts

2. Explain how eating a variety of fruits can contribute to good health.

3. Discuss how fruit gets and keeps its color.

4. Summarize smart ways to buy and store fruit.

5. Describe how to prepare fruits in safe, nutritious, and appealing ways.

Critical Thinking

6. Examine ways to encourage more people to replace sugary snacks or desserts with fruit. How can you suggest adding more fruits to current recipes?

7. Imagine you are throwing a party, and you want to serve dishes that are interesting and appealing. Suggest creative ways to use fruit in your menu.

8. Critique homemade blueberry sauce and store-bought syrup. Which has better nutrition? What are the advantages and disadvantages of each?

9. Judge an eating plan. Jorge plans to eat at least 2 cups of fruit per day and to drink calcium-fortified orange juice instead of milk. Is this a good eating plan?

Real-World Skills and Applications

Interpersonal and Collaborative

10. Start a Fruit Smoothie Business Follow your teacher's instructions to form a business team. Divide into chefs, marketers, and dietitians. Chefs will create five smoothie recipes using different fruits. Marketers will create names for the smoothie recipes. Dietitians will describe the health benefits of each smoothie. Share your work in class.

Problem-Solving

11. Making Fruit Juice You must make enough orange juice to provide four people with 6 ounces each. Find out how to make freshly-squeezed juice. Estimate how many oranges you need. Write your results in a two-paragraph report.

Technology

12. Fruit Recipe PowerPoint Find a fruit recipe on the Internet. Prepare the recipe if possible. Present the recipe in a PowerPoint presentation with its name, ingredients, preparation, yield, and nutrition information. Use words, graphics, and/or photos. Share the presentation in class.

Financial Literacy

13. By the Ounce Comparison shopping is more difficult when package sizes do not match. Which is the best bargain on Mandarin oranges: a 7-ounce cup for $1.15, an 11-ounce can for $0.99, or a 15-ounce can for $1.25? Divide to find the price per ounce to find the better deal.

14. Read Fruit Labels In your supermarket, examine beverages labeled as juice, juice drink, juice cocktail, fruit drink, juice blend, and fruit-flavored soda. What percent of juice do they contain? Which have added sugars, colors, or flavors? How does the nutrition compare? Write your findings and conclusions in a chart. Share them in class.

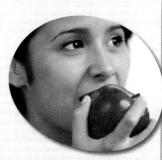

15. Fruit Storage Test Get three unripe pears or peaches. Put one into a loosely-closed paper bag on the counter, one in an airtight container in the refrigerator, and one uncovered on a refrigerator shelf. After three to four days, compare the texture, color, and flavor, and write a one-page report on your observations.

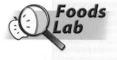

16. Conduct a Taste Test Different types of the same fruit have different qualities. Gather several types of apples, such as Red or Golden Delicious, Rome Beauty, Granny Smith, and Winesap. Compare the flavors, colors, and textures. Write your comparisons and conclusions. Find out which types of apples are best for baking.

Additional Activities For additional activities go to this book's Online Learning Center at glencoe.com.

Academic Skills

 English Language Arts

17. Write a Letter Write a letter to someone who has a sweet tooth. Persuade him or her that fruit is an easy, healthful, and convenient substitute for candy or cookies. Use information from this chapter, but write in your own words.

> **NCTE 12** Use language to accomplish individual purposes.

 Science

18. Edible Fruit Products Some fruits have medicinal uses. For example, papaya can be used to settle the stomach.

Procedure Research a fruit that is used medicinally. Find out how the fruit is used. Research evidence to support its use.

Analysis Create a five-minute oral presentation on your findings, and turn in your notes.

> **NSES Content Standard C** Develop an understanding of matter, energy, and organization in living systems.

 Mathematics

19. Counting Calories A medium-size banana contains 70 calories, a cup of blackberries contains 75 calories, ½ cup of raisins contains 250 calories, and a small bunch of grapes contains 75 calories. You plan to eat ½ cup of blackberries, ½ banana, ¼ cup raisins, and 2 bunches of grapes. How many calories are contained in your choices?

Math Concept **Solve Equations with Grouping Symbols** Equations often contain grouping symbols such as parentheses. Solve the equations within the parentheses first.

Starting Hint Group each fruit amount within parentheses (for example, ½ of a banana would be $70 \div 2$). String them together using addition signs.

 For more math help, go to the Math Appendix

> **NCTM Algebra** Represent and analyze mathematical situations and structures using algebraic symbols.

STANDARDIZED TEST PRACTICE

MULTIPLE CHOICE
Read the paragraph. Write your answer on a separate piece of paper.

> **Test-Taking Tip** Key terms sometimes contain individual words that are familiar separately, but may lose their meaning when combined, such as the term *fruit nectar*. First, try to puzzle out the meaning of a new term by using what you already know about the words. Then, check the glossary. Figuring out the meaning yourself will help you remember it better.

Many fruits are sweet. Maybe that is why most people do not realize that olives and tomatoes are also fruit. Fruit is the ripened ovary containing the seeds of a flowering plant. Some things that you may think are nuts, grains, and "vegetables" are actually fruit.

20. Based on the paragraph, which best completes the following sentence? The term fruit can refer to _____ .
   a. the flowers of plants
   b. any sweet part of a plant
   c. many foods that are considered vegetables
   d. just about any food in the kitchen

CHAPTER 27
Milk

Explore the Photo ▶▶
Milk and milk foods are great-tasting, versatile, and packed with nutrients. *In what forms do you enjoy milk?*

Writing Activity

Write a Step-by-Step Guide

How to Enjoy Milk Many teenagers drink less milk than children do. They may think milk is for kids. Write a step-by-step guide to how milk foods might be prepared in a way that would appeal to teenagers. Remember to keep the finished product nutrient dense.

Writing Tips

1. **Explain** terms the reader may not know.

2. **Write** the steps in chronological order and use transition words.

3. **Use** precise verbs to make your explanation clear.

Reading Guide

Before You Read

Study with a Buddy It can be difficult to review your own notes and quiz yourself on your reading. According to research, studying with a partner for just twelve minutes can help you learn better.

Read to Learn
Key Concepts
- **Describe** the nutrients in milk and summarize how much teens should eat from the Milk Group.
- **Identify** ways to enjoy milk, yogurt, and cheese in meals and snacks.
- **Discuss** how food science applies to milk products.
- **Summarize** ways to buy dairy foods.
- **Describe** how to store and prepare milk, yogurt, and cheese.

Main Idea
Milk, yogurt, and cheese add flavor and nutrition to meals and snacks. Buy and store them wisely. Prepare them in recipes, served hot and cold!

Content Vocabulary
- ◇ lactose
- ◇ cultured product
- ◇ fermentation
- ◇ coagulate
- ◇ denaturing
- ◇ curdle
- ◇ pasteurized
- ◇ homogenized
- ◇ curd
- ◇ whey

Academic Vocabulary
You will find these words in your reading and on your tests. Use the glossary to look up their definitions if necessary.
- ■ affect
- ■ develop

Graphic Organizer
In a graphic organizer like the one below, write down five things that you already know about foods from the Milk Group in the first column. Use the second column to make notes about new information as you read the chapter.

What I Know	What I Learned

 Graphic Organizer Go to this book's Online Learning Center at **glencoe.com** to print out this graphic organizer.

Academic Standards ∙

 English Language Arts
NCTE 4 Use written language to communicate effectively.

 Mathematics
NCTM Number and Operations Understand numbers, ways of representing numbers, relationships among numbers, and number systems.

NCTM Number and Operations Compute fluently and make reasonable estimates.

 Science
NSES Content Standard F Develop an understanding of personal and community health.

NCTE National Council of Teachers of English	**NSES** National Science Education Standards
NCTM National Council of Teachers of Mathematics	**NCSS** National Council for the Social Studies

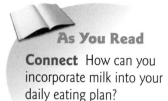

Vocabulary

You can find definitions in the glossary at the back of this book.

As You Read

Connect How can you incorporate milk into your daily eating plan?

Milk—Good for You and Your Bones

Foods from the Milk Group not only build your growing body, they also provide energy and maintain your good health. These are the main nutrients in milk:

♦ **Bone-Building Nutrients** Milk Group foods are the main calcium sources for most Americans. Most milk and some yogurt are fortified with vitamin D. This vitamin helps your body use calcium.

♦ **Other Vitamins and Minerals** Besides bone-building nutrients, most milk products provide riboflavin (a B vitamin), vitamin A, potassium, and other vitamins and minerals for good health.

♦ **Protein Power** The complete protein in milk foods helps to build, repair, and maintain your body's tissues. Just 1 cup (250 mL) of milk provides about 16 percent of the protein you need for the day!

♦ **Carbohydrates for Energy** Milk and milk products contain natural sugar. **Lactose** is the sugar in milk and many other milk products.

♦ **Variable Fat** The fat content of Milk Group foods varies. Many are reduced fat or fat free. Whole milk and many products made from it are high in fat, and in saturated fat.

♦ **Water** Cow's milk is 87 percent water.

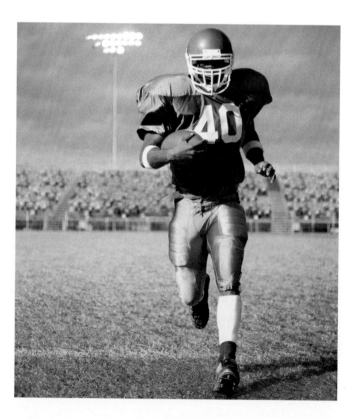

Strength from Milk Milk can help you build strong bones and tissues. Most people need the equivalent of 3 cups (750 mL) of milk daily. *How can someone fit calcium-rich milk products into a busy day?*

MyPyramid Advice

Most people need the equivalent of 3 cups (750 mL) from the Milk Group daily. That provides about 70 percent of the 1,300 mg of calcium that teenagers need daily. Most children ages 2 to 8 years need about 2 cups (500 mL) from the Milk Group daily. Choose mostly low-fat and fat-free milk products.

One cup (250 mL) from the Milk Group equals:

- 1 cup (250 mL) milk or yogurt.
- 1½ ounces (42 g) natural cheese, such as cheddar, Swiss, Monterey Jack, or mozzarella.
- 2 ounces (56 g) processed cheese.
- ⅓ cup (80 mL) shredded cheese.
- 2 cups (500 mL) cottage cheese.
- 1 cup (250 mL) pudding made with milk.
- 1 cup (250 mL) frozen yogurt.
- 1½ cups (375 mL) ice cream.

Soy milk fortified with calcium and vitamin D is not made from cow's milk. It is made from soybeans and does not have all the nutrients in cow's milk. If fortified, soy milk can provide calcium and vitamin D for those who have trouble digesting lactose and for people who do not consume milk products.

Butter, cream, sour cream, and cream cheese are mostly fat. They have little or no calcium. They do not fit in the Milk Group. Use them in small amounts as part of your discretionary calories.

✓ **Reading Check** **Discuss** How much should a person generally eat from the Milk Group each day?

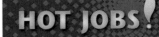

Food Processing Occupations

People who work in food processing turn raw foods into food products you can buy. Dairy processors, butchers, and cheese makers are among those who work in food processing.

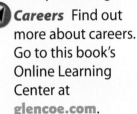

Careers Find out more about careers. Go to this book's Online Learning Center at **glencoe.com**.

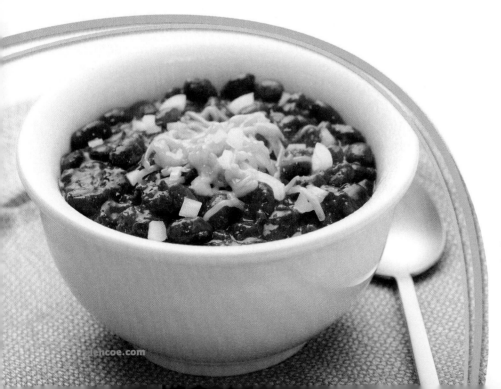

Say Cheese! Shredded cheese as a chili topper or in a mixed dish adds flavor and nutrition. *What other foods can you top with shredded cheese?*

Fitting In Milk Products

Adding flavorful milk products to your meals and snacks can be easy and tasty!

◆ Choose fat-free or low-fat milk at mealtime.

◆ Top crunchy cereal with fruit yogurt.

◆ Put cheese and apple slices on crackers.

◆ Whirl yogurt with fruit and ice in a blender to make a smoothie.

◆ Stir herbs into ricotta cheese, plain yogurt, or whipped cottage cheese to make a dip.

◆ Sip hot cocoa made with milk.

◆ Use plain yogurt as a calcium-rich substitute for sour cream.

◆ Add cheese to a sandwich.

◆ Make oatmeal and condensed cream soups with low-fat milk, not water.

✓ **Reading Check** **Discuss** Besides drinking low-fat milk, what other ways could you get the nutrients in milk?

Milk in Food Science

Food science explains why fluid milk changes to become solid dairy products.

How Is Yogurt Made?

Yogurt is a cultured product. A **cultured product** in the Milk Group is made by fermenting fluid milk with friendly bacteria cultures. **Fermentation** is a chemical reaction that slowly splits complex compounds into simpler substances. Fermentation changes sugars to carbon dioxide and to alcohol or other acids.

To make yogurt, cottage cheese, and sour cream, bacteria are added to milk that change lactose to lactic acid. Milk is first heated to kill unwanted bacteria and change protein, then helpful bacteria are added. Lactic acid is very sour. It gives cultured dairy foods their unique flavors. Fermentation with different types of bacteria is used to make other dairy foods.

Making Milk Products
Some milk products like cheese are made when proteins in liquid milk coagulate, or form solid masses. *What other products are made from liquid milk?*

What Makes Milk Coagulate and Curdle?

Both heat and acids coagulate milk. To **coagulate** means to thicken. Proteins in fluid milk are arranged in tight coils or loops. Heat and exposure to acidic ingredients **affect**, or act on, protein molecules by straightening them. They bump into each other and bind together in tight clumps. This process of breaking down proteins' structure is called **denaturing**. As a result, fluid milk changes to a soft semisolid or solid mass, like cheese.

Curdled milk is fine for making cheese, but not for making sauces, puddings, or creamy soups. To **curdle** means to separate into small lumps (curds) and a watery liquid (whey) as proteins coagulate. Milk that is added too quickly to a hot or acidic mixture, like tomato soup, can curdle. Compounds in fruit and vegetables, and salt, can also cause curdling. Once milk curdles, no amount of stirring will get the lumps out.

✓ **Reading Check** **Explain** What chemical reaction is involved in making yogurt?

Milk Product Variety

The dairy case and freezer are not the only places in the store to find milk products. Milk is sold in many different forms and used in many ways.

Milk

The type of milk you buy depends on its use. If several types suit your purpose, compare label information and prices. Then decide.

Fresh Milk

Most milk in the United States is cow's milk. Grade A on the label means that milk meets quality standards set by the U.S. Food and Drug Administration. You will also see these terms:

- **Pasteurized** means heat-treated to kill bacteria that could cause disease or spoil milk.

- **Homogenized** means processed to break fat globules into tiny drops and mix them permanently and evenly in milk. Otherwise, fat would rise to the top as cream.

Milk is sold as whole, reduced fat, low-fat, and fat-free. Whole milk has about 3.3 percent milk fat. Skim milk is fat free. **Figure 27.1** compares types of milk.

Math in Action

Cream Cheese

Neufchâtel is often called light cream cheese because it is a close substitute for cream cheese. Cream cheese has 6 to 9 grams of fat per serving. Neufchâtel has ⅓ less fat than cream cheese. About how many grams of fat does Neufchâtel contain?

Math Concept **Divide with Fractions** Find part of a whole by working with fractions.

Starting Hint Find the range: What is one-third less than six? What is one-third less than nine?

NCTM Number and Operations Compute fluently and make reasonable estimates.

Math For more math help, go to the Math Appendix

Figure 27.1	Shop for Milk Products

Choose from Many Milk Options! When shopping for milk, compare the price and advantages of each type. *How do the nutrients in different types of milk compare? Would you choose fat-free milk, whole milk, or something in between?*

Product	Calories per 1 cup (250 mL)	Fat (g)	Calories from fat	Protein (g)	Calcium (mg)
Whole milk	150	8	72	8	291
Reduced-fat milk (2% milk)	120	4.5	40	8	297
Low-fat milk (1% milk)	100	2.5	22	8	300
Fat-free, or nonfat, milk (skim milk)	80	0	0	8	302
Chocolate whole milk	210	8.5	76	8	280
Low-fat chocolate milk	10	2.5	22	8	288

Shop Wisely for Fresh Milk

Fresh milk is sold in paper cartons, plastic jugs, and glass bottles. As you shop:

♦ Check the listed sell-by date. Milk can keep in your refrigerator for several more days after that date. Be sure to keep milk at the proper temperature.

♦ Use the label to compare nutrients. Most milk is vitamin D fortified. Vitamin A is always added to fat-free and low-fat milk. It replaces the vitamin A that was removed with the fat. Sometimes extra protein is added. Look at the Nutrition Facts for all the nutrient information.

Milk for Convenience

Milk is sold in non-refrigerated grocery aisles, too!

♦ **Nonfat dry milk** is powder with water and fat removed. Mix it with water to use it like fresh fat-free milk, or use it dry in creamy soups or casseroles.

♦ **UHT milk** is processed at an ultra-high temperature to kill all bacteria. Unopened, it can be kept at room temperature for up to six months.

♦ **Evaporated milk (whole or fat-free)** is concentrated milk sold in a can. More than half the water has been removed. Use it full strength in soups and sauces and as a substitute for cream.

♦ **Sweetened condensed milk** is similar to evaporated milk but with a lot of added sugar. Many recipes call for this type of milk.

Yogurt

Yogurt was invented centuries ago to preserve milk. Stores sell many kinds of yogurt today:

♦ **Fat-Free, Low-Fat, and Whole-Milk Yogurt**

♦ **Plain and Flavored Yogurt** Flavored yogurts are sweetened with fruit, added sugar, or a sugar substitute. With plain yogurt you can add fruit without adding sugar.

♦ **Yogurt with Live, Active Cultures** The friendly bacteria are still alive and active. They may offer health benefits, such as aiding your digestive system and promoting immunity. These live cultures are also called probiotics.

Shop Wisely for Yogurt

Use Nutrient Facts and ingredient lists on cartons to compare nutrition as you shop. Use unit prices to compare costs. Look for a label statement for live, active yogurt cultures. Remember to check the carton's freshness date.

Cheese

Cheese preserves milk's nutrients. Cheeses vary in color, texture, and flavor. They can be soft, mild, and creamy or hard, pungent, and crumbly. Differences come from processing and the type of milk that is used.

The same basic steps produce every type of cheese. First, ingredients are added to coagulate casein (a protein) in milk, causing it to thicken and separate. Then the solid part, or **curd**, is separated from the liquid, or **whey**. Curds are made into cheese. Hard cheeses such as cheddar contain mostly curds. Soft cheeses such as mozzarella have some whey.

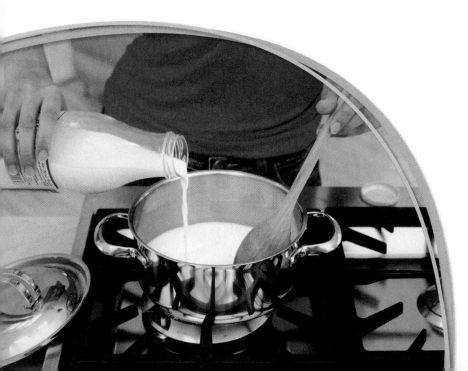

Warm Milk Use low heat to warm milk without burning it. Stir constantly. *What recipes might call for milk that has been warmed?*

Many cheeses are aged, or ripened, at a special temperature and humidity for two months or longer. Aging processes help cheese **develop**, or slowly create, unique flavors and textures.

Three Main Types of Cheese

- **Unripened (fresh) cheeses** are not aged. Cottage cheese, ricotta cheese, and cream cheese are examples. They are soft and stay fresh only a few days after purchase.

- **Ripened cheeses** are aged. These include very hard cheeses (Parmesan, or Romano), hard cheeses (cheddar, or Swiss), semisoft cheese (Muenster), and soft cheese (mozzarella). Veined cheeses (blue cheeses) are made with an edible mold. You can store ripened cheese longer than unripened cheese.

- **Process and cold-pack cheeses** are blends of ripened cheeses. They are smooth, melt quickly, and can be stored longer. Process American cheese is one example.

Shop Wisely for Cheese

Be an informed consumer when you buy cheese:

- Pick the cheese type that matches the recipe you are preparing.

- Compare fat and calories by reading food labels.

- Decide if sliced, shredded, or grated cheese is worth the extra cost.

- Check the freshness date.

- Compare prices. Some ripened and specialty cheeses are very expensive.

Frozen Milk Products

Ice cream, frozen yogurt, and other frozen dairy desserts are milk products, too. Use the Nutrition Facts to compare nutrient information. Look for solidly frozen cartons that are not dented or discolored.

Cream and Sour Cream

Cream has much more fat than milk. Heavy whipping cream, used for whipped toppings, has the most fat, followed by light cream. Half-and-half is half milk and half cream, with half the fat (or less) of heavy cream. Thick, creamy sour cream is cultured.

✓ **Reading Check** **Discuss** How can you tell if the milk or yogurt you buy is low-fat or fat-free?

Store and Prepare Milk Products

Proper storage and preparation ensure the best flavor, texture, and nutrition from milk products.

Store Milk Products

Store milk products properly to keep them fresh and safe.

◆ Keep perishable milk products refrigerated. Use fresh milk and unripened cheese within a week, and yogurt within two weeks. Ripened cheeses can be stored longer.

◆ Refrigerate liquid milk in its original container.

◆ Keep milk products tightly closed, covered, or wrapped for safety and appeal.

◆ Store unopened canned, powdered, or UHT milk in a cool, dry place. Once opened, put powdered milk into an airtight container.

◆ After opening canned or UHT milk or after adding water to powdered milk, store them like fresh milk. Store open canned milk in a clean, covered pitcher.

Prepare Milk Products

Milk products are used in many recipes. They provide rich flavor and creamy texture to beverages, soups, sauces, casseroles, desserts, baked foods, and more.

Many dips and spreads are made with cream cheese or sour cream. Both are high in fat. Make yogurt cheese as a low-fat substitute.

Food Prep How To

MAKE YOGURT CHEESE

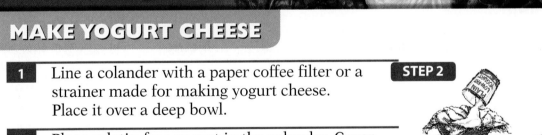

1	Line a colander with a paper coffee filter or a strainer made for making yogurt cheese. Place it over a deep bowl.
2	Place gelatin-free yogurt in the colander. Cover.
3	Refrigerate. Allow the whey to drain away for 2 to 24 hours. The longer it drains, the thicker the cheese gets.
4	Put the yogurt cheese into a storage container. Add flavorings such as herbs, nuts, or dried fruit.
5	Cover tightly and refrigerate. Discard the whey.

STEP 2

Cook with Milk

Keep milk from scorching, curdling, and foaming.

- ◆ **To avoid scorching,** use low heat. Stir frequently. Watch carefully. Heat just until the milk begins to steam.

- ◆ **To avoid curdling,** add acidic ingredients, like lemon juice or tomato sauce, slowly while stirring.

- ◆ **To avoid foaming,** stir milk as it cooks.

- ◆ **To keep skin from forming,** put plastic wrap on the surface of cooked milk products as they cool.

Cook with Cheese

Cheese needs to melt, not cook. Ripened and process cheeses melt well. Process cheese melts very quickly.

- ◆ Heat cheese at a low temperatures for a short time. High heat and long cooking make cheese tough and rubbery.

- ◆ Add cheese to hot white sauce near the end of cooking.

- ◆ Layer cheese between other ingredients to protect it from direct heat.

- ◆ Add cheese toppings at the end of baking or broiling.

- ◆ Use medium power when microwaving cheese.

✓ Reading Check **Describe** What are two problems that can occur when you cook with milk?

EASY RECIPES — Everyday Favorites

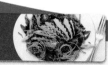

Egg Cream

Customary	Ingredients	Metric
2 Tbsp.	Chocolate syrup	30 mL
½ cup	Low-fat milk	120 mL
½ cup	Seltzer water	125 mL

Yield: 1 serving, ¾ cup (375 mL) each

1. Pour syrup into a tall, chilled, 8 oz glass.
2. Add milk.
3. Add cold seltzer water and stir.

Nutritional Information Per Serving: 161 calories, 2 g total fat, (1 g saturated fat), 10 mg cholesterol, 75 mg sodium, 30 g total carbohydrate, (0 g fiber, 26 g sugars), 5 g protein

Percent Daily Value: vitamin A 4%, vitamin C 0%, calcium 15%, iron 2%

Did You Know?
An egg cream does not contain eggs. The drink is believed to have been invented in Brooklyn in the late 1800s. It can be flavored with vanilla or strawberry syrup.

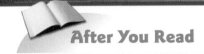

After You Read

CHAPTER SUMMARY

Milk and milk products are good sources of many nutrients, including protein, calcium, and vitamin D. Most people need the equivalent of 3 cups (750 mL) of milk daily. Milk, yogurt, and cheese come in different forms and flavors. They can be eaten as they are or mixed in beverages and dishes. Friendly bacteria, heat, and acidic ingredients change milk and help create products like yogurt and cheese. Stores sell many fresh and convenience dairy products. Shop wisely. Store milk products properly. Cook milk products carefully to keep their texture and flavor.

Vocabulary Review

1. Use each of these vocabulary words in a sentence.

Content Vocabulary
- lactose (p. 392)
- cultured product (p. 394)
- fermentation (p. 394)
- coagulate (p. 395)
- denaturing (p. 395)
- curdle (p. 395)
- pasteurized (p. 395)
- homogenized (p. 395)
- curd (p. 397)
- whey (p. 397)

Academic Vocabulary
- affect (p. 395)
- develop (p. 398)

Review Key Concepts

2. Describe the nutrients in milk and summarize how much teens should eat from the Milk Group.

3. Identify ways to enjoy milk, yogurt, and cheese in meals and snacks.

4. Discuss how food science applies to milk products.

5. Summarize ways to buy dairy foods.

6. Describe how to store and prepare milk, yogurt, and cheese.

Critical Thinking

7. Identify the foods that would be missing from a typical day if you did not eat any milk products. Then, project the consequences of eliminating these foods from your meals and snacks.

8. Suggest changes that a family can make in the way it shops for milk products. What effect will smart shopping choices have on the family's nutrition?

9. Design a meal that uses milk products efficiently to maximize nutrition and minimize fat content.

Real-World Skills and Applications

Technology

10. Dairy Around the World Get your teacher's permission to use the Internet to research milk and milk products in three cultures other than yours. Learn about the animal source of their milk. Describe their milk products and use in the culture's meals and snacks. Share your findings orally in class.

Interpersonal and Collaborative

11. Promote Dairy Foods Follow your teacher's instructions to break into teams. Imagine that your team is an ad agency developing a print ad for a new milk product. Describe the product, its qualities, its nutritional benefits, and its uses in your ad. Display the ad in your classroom.

Problem-Solving

12. Trim the Fat Your friend often spreads cream cheese on a breakfast bagel, eats a grilled cheese sandwich for lunch, snacks on chips and sour cream dip, and finishes dinner with ice cream. He drinks whole milk with meals. Suggest ways he could trim fat and still enjoy milk products. Write your answers in a paragraph.

Financial Literacy

13. Freeze Cheese Roberta bought a 1-lb brick of cheddar cheese for $4.99 and kept it in her refrigerator. She used only ¾ of the cheese before it had to be thrown away. Tien bought a 16-oz bag of shredded cheddar for $5.99. She froze the bag and eventually used all of the cheese. Who made the more cost-effective choice?

14. Milk Processing Find out about the steps in producing and processing milk or cheese. Contact a dairy farmer, a dairy processing plant, a cheese maker, or your state agriculture department. Create a flowchart, with your sources, to share your findings in class.

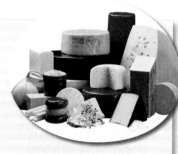

15. Compare Yogurt Products Visit your local supermarket. Choose at least five types of yogurt, such as plain, regular fruit-flavored, low-fat, sugar-free, and fat-free. Compare unit prices, ingredients, and Nutrition Facts. Compile your findings in a chart. Why are so many varieties produced? Which would you choose?

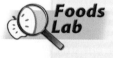

16. Ripened or Process Cheese? Cut two small, same-size slices: one of ripened cheese, such as natural cheddar, and one of process cheese, such as American. Place each on a cracker or a crusty bread slice. Put both in a toaster oven at 300°F (176°C). Watch closely until both melt. Write your comparisons and conclusions.

Additional Activities For additional activities go to this book's Online Learning Center at glencoe.com.

Academic Skills

 English Language Arts

17. Milk Myths Write a dialogue between two teens. One teen is misinformed about milk. In the dialogue, refute at least one misconception and provide at least three facts about milk.

> **NCTE 4** Use written language to communicate effectively.

 Science

18. Soy vs. Cow's Milk Both cow's milk and soy milk are nourishing. They are usually fortified during processing.

Procedure Use the **Nutritive Values of Foods Appendix** at the back of this book. List the nutrients that fat-free, 2%, whole milk and fortified soy milk provide.

Analysis Compare the nutritional values of 1 cup (250 mL) of each type of milk to a brand of soy milk. Graph the data.

> **NSES Content Standard F** Develop an understanding of personal and community health.

 Mathematics

19. Yogurt Cheese You want to make a low-fat, calcium-rich dip for a party. You decide to make yogurt cheese, which you will mix with herbs. One cup (250 mL) of yogurt can make 4 oz (113 g) of yogurt cheese. If you want to make 16 oz (450 g) of yogurt cheese, how much more plain yogurt will you need to buy to make enough dip for the party?

Math Concept **Find Equivalent Ratios**
Equivalent ratios have the same meaning. To find an equivalent ratio, multiply or divide both sides by the same number.

Starting Hint Begin by creating a ratio for cups of yogurt to ounces of yogurt cheese for the original recipe (1:4). Then, create a ratio using the new ounce total (x:16). Solve for x.

 For more math help, go to the Math Appendix

> **NCTM Number and Operations** Compute fluently and make reasonable estimates.

STANDARDIZED TEST PRACTICE

MULTIPLE CHOICE
Read the paragraph. Write your answer on a separate piece of paper.

> **Test-Taking Tip** Use familiar word parts to help you remember new definitions. Any part of the word may help. For example, the suffix ose in lactose means sugar.

In the past, buttermilk was the liquid left after cream was churned to make butter. Today, buttermilk is made by fermenting milk with helpful bacteria, as yogurt is made. Buttermilk is usually made with fat-free or low-fat milk. It has a tangy flavor and thick consistency.

20. Based on the paragraph, which of the following statements is true?
   a. The thick consistency comes from buttermilk's high fat content.
   b. Buttermilk is made by adding butter to milk.
   c. Yogurt and buttermilk are both fermented dairy products.
   d. Buttermilk does not provide as much nutrition as milk does.

CHAPTER 28
Meat, Poultry, and Fish

Explore the Photo ▶▶

Think of how versatile meat, poultry, and fish are! They take center stage in lunch and dinner menus or make tasty ingredients in mixed dishes. *What meat, poultry, or fish dishes have you eaten?*

🖊 *Writing Activity*

Write a Persuasive Paragraph

Regional Dishes Different regions of the country feature different meats, poultry, and fish in their cuisine. Maine, for example, is famous for its lobster, while Texas is famous for beef. Write a persuasive paragraph about trying meat, fish, or poultry dishes from the region where you live.

Writing Tips

1. **State** your position clearly.

2. **Use** facts to back up your position.

Reading Guide

Before You Read

Take Guilt-Free Rest Breaks Feeling guilty about resting creates more stress. The brain has a hard time absorbing new data when it is stressed. Your reading skills will be better if you are relaxed and ready to learn.

Read to Learn

Key Concepts

- **Explain** how lean meat, poultry, and fish fit into a healthful eating plan.
- **Discuss** how food science applies to cooking meat, poultry, and fish.
- **Summarize** tips for buying lean meat, poultry, and fish.
- **Describe** how to prepare meat, poultry, and fish to keep them lean, tender, and safe.

Main Idea

Meat, poultry, and fish provide nutrition, flavor, and satisfaction. Learn to buy and store them wisely. Cook them properly to keep them moist, tender, lean, safe, and appealing.

Content Vocabulary

◇ poultry
◇ lean meat
◇ marbling
◇ organ meat
◇ meat cut
◇ score
◇ marinade
◇ Maillard reaction
◇ giblet
◇ finfish
◇ shellfish
◇ fillet
◇ surimi
◇ cured meat

Academic Vocabulary

You will find these words in your reading and on your tests. Use the glossary to look up their definitions if necessary.

▪ logical
▪ effect

Graphic Organizer

As you read, use a graphic organizer like the one below to list types of meat, poultry, and fish.

Types of Meat, Poultry, and Fish		
Types of Meat	**Types of Poultry**	**Types of Fish**

  Graphic Organizer Go to this book's Online Learning Center at glencoe.com to print out this graphic organizer.

Academic Standards •

 English Language Arts
NCTE 3 Apply strategies to interpret texts.
NCTE 9 Develop an understanding of diversity in language use across cultures.

 Science
NSES Content Standard A Develop abilities necessary to do scientific inquiry.

 Mathematics
NCTM Data Analysis and Probability Formulate questions that can be addressed with data and collect, organize, and display relevant data to answer them.

 Social Studies
NCSS I A Culture Analyze and explain the ways groups, societies, and cultures address human needs and concerns.

NCTE National Council of Teachers of English
NCTM National Council of Teachers of Mathematics

NSES National Science Education Standards
NCSS National Council for the Social Studies

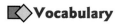

Vocabulary

You can find definitions in the glossary at the back of this book.

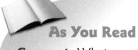

As You Read

Connect What are some of the nutrients you can find in a meat sandwich?

Meat, Poultry, and Fish— Packed with Protein

Roast beef, stuffed pork chop, chicken stir-fry, baked ham, grilled shrimp, and broiled salmon all provide important nutrients:

◆ **Protein** Meat, poultry, and fish provide high-quality protein. **Poultry** is a term used to describe chicken, turkey, or other birds raised as food. Protein helps build and repair tissues in your body. It also promotes growth in your teenage years.

◆ **Vitamins and Minerals** They supply B vitamins, including thiamin, niacin, vitamin B_6, and vitamin B_{12}. These vitamins help your body produce energy and keep your nervous system healthy. Meat, poultry, and fish also provide iron for red blood cells, zinc for immunity, and vitamin E and potassium for a healthy heart. Fish supplies iodine. Fish with edible bones, like sardines and canned salmon, supply calcium.

◆ **Fat and Cholesterol—Meat** Fat and cholesterol in meat, poultry, and fish varies. Too much saturated fat and cholesterol is not heart healthy. **Lean meat** from beef, pork, or lamb has less fat, saturated fat, and cholesterol than fatty meats. Flecks of fat throughout these meats are called **marbling**. Fatty meats such as processed meats (sausages, hot dogs) and bacon are high in saturated fat. **Organ meat**, which includes liver, heart, kidney, and tongue, is high in cholesterol.

◆ **Fat and Cholesterol—Poultry** Poultry contains less total fat and saturated fat than many meats. Its fat is mostly in—and just under—the skin.

◆ **Fat and Cholesterol—Fish** Most fish is low in fat. Most of the fat it does have is unsaturated. Fattier fish, such as salmon, is a good source of heart-healthful omega-3 fatty acids.

Everyday Choices Meals are often planned around meat, fish, or poultry. *What are some important nutrients they provide?*

MyPyramid Advice

Meat, poultry, and fish are part of the Meat and Beans Group. A person who needs 2,000 calories per day should have about 5½ ounces (156 g) from this food group daily. You may need 5 to 7 ounces (140 to 196 g), depending on your calorie needs.

Choose mostly lean meat and poultry. It is **logical**, or sensible, to vary your protein choices. Fish contain healthy oils, so eat them often. Use low-fat cooking methods such as broiling, roasting, or grilling.

Three ounces (84 g) of cooked meat, poultry, or fish is about the size of a deck of playing cards. Three ounces (84 g) is:

◆ 1 medium pork chop (about ½ in. or 13 mm thick)

◆ ½ of a small chicken breast

◆ 1 small lean, cooked hamburger patty (3 ounces or 84 g)

◆ 1 bun-size fish fillet

Two ounces (56 g) is:

◆ ½ cup (125 mL) canned tuna or ground beef

◆ 1 small chicken leg or thigh

◆ 2 pieces thinly sliced sandwich-size meat

✓ **Reading Check** **Estimate** What visual clue can you use to judge the portion size of meat, poultry, and fish?

Discover International Foods

Argentina

Argentine cuisine is influenced heavily by European immigrants, especially those from Spain and Italy. Unlike the cuisine of other Latin American countries, it has limited Native American influence. Argentina is a major producer of beef, wheat, corn, milk, and soybeans. Red meat is a common part of the Argentine diet. Wheat products, which are dietary staples, are used to make wheat-based pastries and pasta dishes. *Asado* (barbecued beef) and empanadas are common. Dulce de leche, a caramel-like mixture of milk and sugar, is used to fill pancakes, cookies, and cakes and as a spread on bread.

Languages Across Cultures

chimichurri *(ˌchi-mē-ˈchu̇-rē)* popular thick herb sauce, made of olive oil, vinegar, parsley, oregano, onion, garlic, and salt and pepper, served with meat

empanada *(ˌem-pə-ˈnä-də)* pastry filled with meat, chicken, ham and cheese, or vegetable mixtures

🔎 *Recipes* Find out more about international recipes on this book's Online Learning Center at glencoe.com.

NCTE 9 Develop an understanding of diversity in language use across cultures.

The Food Science of Protein

Many recipes feature meat, poultry, or fish. Science explains browning and why some meats are tender and others are tough.

Connective Tissue and Tenderness

Meat, poultry, and fish have muscle, fat, bone, and connective tissue. (See **Figure 28.1**.) Protein molecules in connective tissue are shaped like coiled springs. Their strong, rope-like fibers support and hold muscles together.

Connective tissue forms as cattle and poultry exercise their skeletal muscles. Exercise has an **effect**, or influence, on the amount of connective tissue that develops. Meat and poultry from leg, wing, and shoulder muscles have more connective tissue. This makes it less tender. Fish has little connective tissue, so it is very tender.

Elastin and collagen are two types of connective tissue.

◆ **Elastin** also is called gristle. It does not break down during cooking. Meat from young animals has less elastin than meat from older animals, so it is more tender.

◆ **Collagen** disperses when heated. Once cooled, it becomes a semisolid called gelatin, which is more tender than collagen. Gelatin helps give cooked meat its plump appearance.

Figure 28.1 **Composition of Meat**

Choosing Meat Meat has four types of tissue. *What would you look for if you were shopping for a lean steak to serve for dinner?*

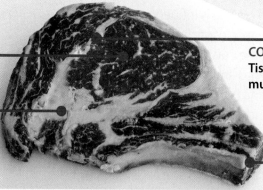

MUSCLE
This is the lean, red, or pinkish part of meat.

CONNECTIVE TISSUE
Tissue surrounds sections of muscle, holding it together.

FAT
Layers of fat are found between the muscles. In addition, marbling, or flecks of fat, are found throughout the muscle. Marbling adds moisture—and calories.

BONE
Many retail cuts have one or more bones.

Tenderizing: Get Physical!

You can tenderize tough meat cuts by cutting or tearing their fibers. A **meat cut** is a slice or portion from a specific part of the animal. Grinding, scoring, and pounding meat also tenderize. To **score** is to make shallow cuts.

Tenderizing: Marinades and Enzymes

Acids and enzymes tenderize tough meat cuts through chemical reactions.

◆ **Acids** The acids in a marinade help break and unwind large proteins in meat. A **marinade** is a mixture of an acidic ingredient, like citrus juice or vinegar, and seasonings. Soak meat in a marinade before cooking it. Then discard the marinade.

◆ **Enzymes** Fruit like papaya, and figs contain enzymes, or special proteins, that break down muscle fiber and collagen during cooking. You can also buy enzyme meat tenderizers.

Tenderizing: Cooking Techniques

Meat cuts and poultry vary in tenderness. Tender choices cook well in dry heat; less tender choices in moist heat. **Figure 28.2** shows how to cook tender and less tender meats.

The secret to tender meat, poultry, and fish is careful heat control. When cooked, proteins unwind and coagulate, or get firm. Fats melt and connective tissue softens. If you overcook meat or poultry in dry heat, proteins shrink and become tough.

Why Do Meat and Poultry Turn Brown?

Have you noticed that the outside of roasted meat or poultry is browner and more flavorful than the inside? Browning is caused by the **Maillard reaction**. During this reaction, protein changes as it reacts with sugar at high temperatures. The result is a deep brown color and rich flavor.

Why does the inside of meat not get as brown? The inside is moist and does not get as hot as the outside. Meat does not brown when microwaved because the air in a microwave oven never gets hot enough for the Maillard reaction to take place!

✓ **Reading Check** **Describe** How do you tenderize tough meat?

Science in Action

White and Dark Meat

Myoglobin is a compound in muscles that holds oxygen. Muscles that move constantly need oxygen and have more myoglobin. The red color in many meats comes from its myoglobin. These meats are from animals, such as cattle—or from parts of animals—that move a lot. Chicken thighs and legs come from a part of a bird that moves more than the breast and wings do.

Procedure Think about turkey, pork, and lamb. Describe the color of raw poultry and meat cuts.

Analysis Explain why a turkey drumstick is considered dark meat, and why a turkey breast is considered white meat. Explain why some cuts of raw pork, such as chops, are lighter in color than raw beef or lamb.

NSES Content Standard A
Develop abilities necessary to do scientific inquiry.

Figure 28.2   **Tenderness and Cooking Methods**

Cooking Meat, Poultry, and Fish The cooking method you choose depends in part on tenderness. *How might you cook ribs? Why?*

Tender Cuts of Meat and Poultry	Cooking Methods

Beef
Loin, sirloin, and short loin cuts, rib cuts, ground meat
Pork
Ham, all cuts of pork
Poultry
Broiler, fryer
	Dry Heat Methods*
	    Baking
	    Broiling
	    Grilling
	    Roasting
	    Stir-frying***
	Pan-frying, Frying

Less Tender Cuts of Meat and Poultry	**Cooking Methods**

Beef/ Pork
Brisket, chuck, flank**, round**, shoulder, stew meat
Poultry
Stewing chicken
	Moist Heat Methods
	    Braising***
	    Simmering
	    Stewing

Fish	**Cooking Methods**
Fillet, steak	**Dry Heat Methods*** **Moist Heat Methods** **Pan-frying, Frying**

* Dry heat cookery produces a browning reaction on the surface, which results in a distinct flavor.

** May be cooked with dry heat if tenderized first.

*** Braising and stir-frying are a combination of dry and moist heat cooking.

Shop for Meat, Poultry, and Fish

Consider cost, nutrition, and cooking methods as you shop for meat, poultry, and fish. Pick well-wrapped packages that do not leak. Frozen packages should be frozen solid and free of ice crystals. Check the sell-by date for freshness. These foods should also show that they have passed government inspection.

Buy Meat

Most supermarkets carry four kinds of fresh or frozen meat, or red meat:

- ◆ **Beef** Comes from mature cattle over one year old. It has a rich, hearty flavor.
- ◆ **Veal** Comes from young cattle about three months old. It has a mild flavor.
- ◆ **Lamb** Comes from young sheep. It has a delicate but distinctive flavor.
- ◆ **Pork** Comes from pigs or hogs. It has a mild flavor.

Meat Cuts

Meat is sold in different cuts. First, the meat carcass is divided into large wholesale cuts. (See **Figure 28.3**.) Then, they are cut again into retail cuts. Meat cuts differ in tenderness, leanness, and price. The package label shows the kind of meat, wholesale cut, and retail cut. (See **Figure 28.4** on next page.)

Buy Fresh Meat

◆ Look for lean cuts. They have less marbling and very little fat around the edges. Beef cuts labeled round and loin are lean. Pork and lamb labeled loin or leg are lean.

◆ Choose ground beef that is at least 90% lean.

◆ Look for U.S. Department of Agriculture voluntary grading on beef, veal, or lamb. The top three grades are Prime (top grade; most marbling; expensive), Choice (high quality; less marbling; less expensive), and Select (for beef) or Good (for veal and lamb) (least marbling; least expensive). Pork is not graded.

◆ Choose bright-red beef, grayish-pink veal and pork, and light- to dark-pink lamb. Do not buy packages with an odor.

Figure 28.3 **Beef Cuts**

Wholesale Cuts Different meat cuts come from different parts of the animal. *Round steak and bottom round roast are retail cuts of beef. What wholesale cut do they come from?*

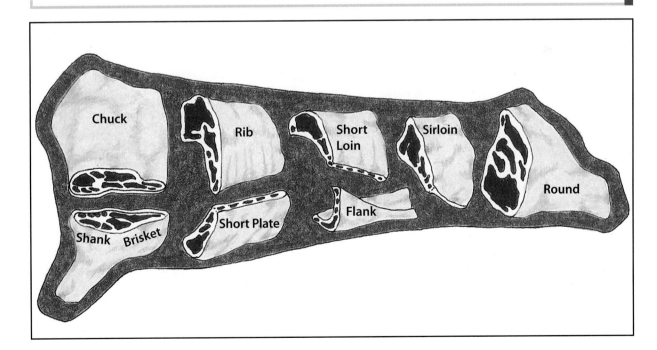

Figure 28.4 Meat, Poultry, and Fish Labeling

Label Lingo Check meat, poultry, and fish labels for buying information. *How can label information help you get value when you buy meat?*

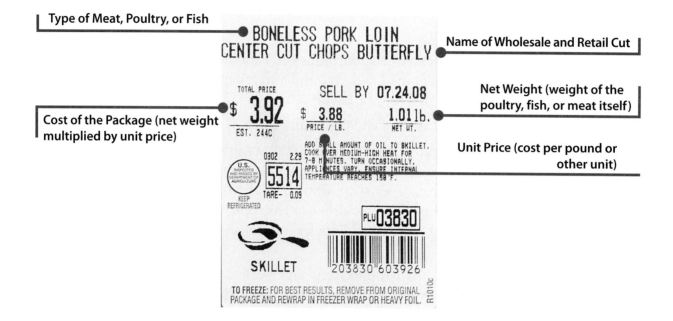

Type of Meat, Poultry, or Fish

BONELESS PORK LOIN
CENTER CUT CHOPS BUTTERFLY

Name of Wholesale and Retail Cut

TOTAL PRICE
$ 3.92
EST. 244C

SELL BY 07.24.08
$ 3.88
PRICE / LB.
1.01 lb.
NET WT.

Net Weight (weight of the poultry, fish, or meat itself)

Cost of the Package (net weight multiplied by unit price)

Unit Price (cost per pound or other unit)

ADD SMALL AMOUNT OF OIL TO SKILLET.
COOK OVER MEDIUM-HIGH HEAT FOR
7-8 MINUTES. TURN OCCASIONALLY.
APPLIANCES VARY. ENSURE INTERNAL
TEMPERATURE REACHES 150°F.

U.S. INSPECTED AND PASSED BY DEPARTMENT OF AGRICULTURE

0302   2.29
5514
TARE- 0.09
KEEP REFRIGERATED

PLU 03830

SKILLET   203830 603926

TO FREEZE: FOR BEST RESULTS, REMOVE FROM ORIGINAL
PACKAGE AND REWRAP IN FREEZER WRAP OR HEAVY FOIL.

Buy Poultry

Both chicken and turkey have white and dark meat. White meat comes from the breast. It is more tender, milder in flavor, and lower in fat than dark meat. Turkey has a stronger flavor than chicken. Duck, Cornish hen, and goose are poultry, too.

You can buy uncooked chicken and turkey, fresh or frozen:

◆ **Whole** May include giblets. A **giblet** is the edible internal organ of poultry, such as the heart, liver, or gizzard. Broiler and fryer chickens are tender. Stewing chickens or hens are less tender.

◆ **Parts** Can be a cut-up whole chicken or specific parts, such as wings, legs, or thighs.

◆ **Boneless, Skinless** Poultry breasts with bone and skin removed; also called cutlets. This is a lean choice.

◆ **Ground Poultry** Read the label. Some ground poultry contains skin, which adds fat.

Look for poultry with creamy white to yellow skin. The skin should be free of bruises, tiny feathers, cuts, and discoloration. These are the qualities of Grade A poultry. Grading is not required. Frozen poultry should be frozen solid.

Buy Fish

Finfish have fins, backbones, and gills. Catfish, red snapper, and perch are mild, light-colored finfish. Trout, tuna, and salmon are darker and have more healthy fats. **Shellfish** have shells instead of bones and fins. Crabmeat, lobster, shrimp, clams, oysters, scallops, and mussels are shellfish.

Read labels carefully. Inspected products carry an inspection seal. Some fish products are graded for quality. Grade A fish is the highest quality.

Buy Finfish

Finfish—fresh and frozen—are sold as:

- **Whole** as caught.
- **Drawn** with the insides removed.
- **Dressed** with the head, tail, fins, scales, and internal organs removed.
- **Steaks,** or cross sections cut from a dressed fish. They may have bones.
- **Fillets**, or sides of fish cut from the bones and backbone. They are usually boneless.

Fresh finfish have firm, moist flesh, shiny skin, and no browning around the edges. They have a mild aroma. Whole or drawn fish have clear, bulging eyes. Frozen fish should be solid with little or no frost. Avoid frozen fish that looks discolored or dry.

Buy Shellfish

Shellfish are sold fresh or frozen, uncooked or cooked, canned, or prepared in frozen dishes. Fresh shellfish are often sold live. When you tap the shells of fresh, live clams, mussels, and oysters, they should close tightly. When touched, crabs should move. Lobsters should curl their tails when picked up.

Surimi contains chopped fish plus other ingredients for flavor. It is shaped and colored to look like shellfish. Surimi is fully cooked and sold refrigerated or frozen.

Buy Processed and Convenience Products

Find convenience meat, poultry, and fish on store shelves, refrigerated, or frozen. Cut-up meat for stews and other ready-to-cook foods are sold at the meat and fish counters. The deli department sells precooked, ready-to-heat products.

Cured meat is treated with salt, sugar, or sodium nitrate to slow spoilage and add distinctive flavors. Some are pre-cooked. Ham, cold cuts, bacon, corned beef, and hot dogs are popular cured meats. Since curing adds sodium, eat these foods in moderation. Lower-fat versions of many processed meats are available.

Plan to Save Money

Meat, poultry, and fish can be expensive. To save money:

◆ Buy less-tender cuts, which often cost less.

◆ Combine a smaller amount of protein-rich foods with less-costly grains and vegetables. For instance, stir-fry chicken strips with vegetables. This also reduces fat and adds variety.

◆ Buy meat on sale or in large quantities. Freeze portions.

Compare Costs

How much to buy depends on how many are eating, if you want leftovers, and how much lean meat and bone a cut has. (See **Figure 28.5**.)

Figure cost per serving—not cost per pound. Cost per pound includes bones and fat you trim off and discard. Cost per serving is only what you eat. To figure cost per serving:

1. Find the number of servings per pound in **Figure 28.5**.

2. Multiply by the number of pounds in the package. This gives the number of servings per package.

3. Divide the total price by the number of servings in the package.

Comparing cost per serving helps you find bargains. For example, a whole chicken may cost less than cut-up parts.

Figure 28.5	Purchasing Meat, Poultry, and Fish

Buy the Right Amount The number of portions per pound depends on the type of meat, poultry, or fish. *You plan to braise a pork roast for eight. How large a roast do you buy if it has a bone? If boneless?*

One pound (450 g) of uncooked ...	Will provide this many 3-ounce (84 g) cooked portions.
Boneless or ground meat or poultry, fish fillets, scallops, peeled shrimp	4
Meat with a small amount of bone (steaks, roast, chops)	2 to 3
Meat with a large amount of bone (shoulder cuts, short ribs)	1 to 2
Whole chicken or turkey, most poultry with bones	2
Whole fish	1
Drawn fish (insides removed)	2
Shrimp in shell	3
Live clams and oysters	2 to 3

Store Meat, Poultry, and Fish for Safety

Store fresh meat, poultry, and fish in the refrigerator if you plan to use it right away. Wrap it tightly. Place it in a pan or on a plate to keep juices from spreading bacteria to other foods. Use cuts of meat within 3 to 5 days and poultry and ground meat within 1 to 2 days.

Freeze fresh meat, poultry, and fish for longer storage. Wrap them tightly in airtight plastic bags, containers, or freezer paper. Label and date each package.

Refrigerate cooked leftovers within two hours. Use them within 3 to 4 days. Freeze for longer storage. Remove the dressing from stuffed chicken or turkey. Refrigerate it separately.

✓ **Reading Check** **Describe** What are three ways to make the most of your food dollar when buying meat, fish, or poultry?

Cook Meat, Poultry, and Fish

Properly cooked meat, poultry, and fish is juicy, tender, and full of flavor. Cooking tenderizes meat muscle and brings out natural flavors. It browns the surface, providing a pleasant color and aroma. Most importantly, cooking kills harmful bacteria that might cause foodborne illness.

Keep It Lean

◆ Broil, grill, roast, braise, or stew meat, poultry, or fish. Frying adds fat and calories.

◆ Trim visible fat. Remove poultry skin before or after cooking. Drain off fat drippings.

◆ Skip or limit breading on meat, poultry, or fish. Breading adds fat and calories. It also causes food to soak up more fat during frying.

◆ Use less gravy. Switch to vegetable salsas, fruit sauces, or other low-fat sauces.

Cook for Safety and Doneness

Raw meat, poultry, and fish must be handled carefully to prevent foodborne illness. Follow food safety rules in Chapter 5. A few reminders:

◆ Thaw in the refrigerator, in an airtight package in cold tap water, or on low power in the microwave oven—never at room temperature!

Food Prep How To

BRAISE MEAT

1 Brown the meat well in a large, heavy pan or pot using a small amount of oil.

2 Remove the meat to a clean plate. Drain the fat from the pan.

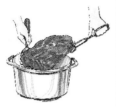

TIP With a heat-resistant spoon, loosen the browned bits of meat from the pan. They add flavor and color to the cooking liquid.

3 Return the meat to the pan. Add a small amount of liquid, such as water, broth, or vegetable juice.

4 Cover the pan. Cook over low heat on the cooktop or in the oven at about 325°F (163°C).

5 During cooking, skim the fat off the top of the cooking liquid. Turn the meat several times.

6 Cook until the internal temperature reaches at least 160°F (71°C).

7 Reduce the cooking liquid over low heat to make a thick sauce.

Food Prep How To

ROAST MEAT, POULTRY, AND FISH

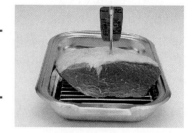

1 Place the meat fat side up on a rack in a large roasting pan. The rack allows fat to drain away as it melts.

2 Insert an oven-safe meat thermometer into the thickest part of the meat, away from bone and fat.

3 Roast, uncovered and without liquid until the internal temperature of the meat reaches the appropriate temperature. Roast tender cuts of meat quickly at a high temperature. Roast tougher cuts slowly at a lower temperature.

4 When the meat is done, remove it from the pan. Let it stand for 15 to 20 minutes. The meat will carve more easily after standing. Serve immediately after carving.

- Check labels of frozen convenience foods. Some must be thawed; others should be cooked while frozen.
- Separate raw meat, poultry, and fish from cooked and ready-to-eat foods.
- Do not wash or rinse meat or poultry.
- Cook thoroughly to a safe internal temperature.
- Wash cutting boards, knives, utensils, and countertops with hot soapy water.

Cook Meat

The cooking method you choose depends on the meat's tenderness and its retail cut. Cooking time depends on the size and shape of the meat and the cooking temperature.

- **Braise** less tender cuts of meat.
- **Roast** only large, tender cuts. A thin fat layer on the meat keeps it from drying out.
- **Broil** tender cuts such as ground beef, beef steaks, lamb chops, and ham slices. The meat should be at least ¾-inch (1.9 cm) thick so it does not dry out. Cooking time depends on meat's distance from the heat and its thickness.
- **Panbroil** meats less than 1 inch (2.54 cm) thick, such as hamburgers and pork chops.

Check Meat for Doneness

Using a meat thermometer is the only accurate way to check for doneness. Meat must reach an internal temperature of at least 160°F (71°C) for safety. Insert the thermometer into the thickest part of the meat, without touching bone or fat. Insert the meat thermometer sideways into a hamburger patty's center.

Cook Poultry

Properly cooked poultry is tender, moist, and flavorful. Poultry is cooked in many ways. A large, whole bird must cook for a long time. Roasting chicken or turkey pieces is faster. Braising tenderizes older poultry such as stewing chickens.

A whole turkey or chicken can be stuffed just before roasting. Cooking dressing or stuffing separately is safer, however.

Undercooked poultry may have harmful bacteria. Place an oven-safe meat thermometer in the thickest place, such as the thigh for whole poultry, without touching bone. A whole chicken or turkey should reach 180°F (82°C); poultry breasts and ground chicken should reach 170°F (77°C). Stuffing should reach 165°F (74°C).

Nutrition & Wellness Tips

Flavorful Meat, Poultry, and Fish

✓ Gently rub the surface with an herb or spice blend before cooking.

✓ Baste with sauce such as barbecue or soy sauce, mustard, or chutney.

Cook Fish

Broiling, baking, grilling, and microwaving are easy ways to cook fish. Often, the same recipe works with different kinds and forms of fish and shellfish. Being naturally tender, fish needs only a short cooking time at moderate temperatures.

Raw fish is translucent, or semi-clear. As it cooks, it becomes opaque, or solid in color. Properly cooked fish is opaque throughout. The flesh flakes easily with a fork. Overcooked fish is dry and mealy, and falls apart.

Use the 10-minute rule for cooking finfish. Measure the thickest part of the fish, including any stuffing. Bake fish 10 minutes for every 1 inch (2.5 cm) of thickness. If the fish is more than ½-inch (1 cm) thick, turn it after half the cooking time. Cooking times for shellfish vary.

✓ **Reading Check** **List** What are five ways to cook and keep meat, poultry, and fish lean?

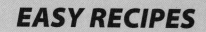

EASY RECIPES
International Flavors

Chimichurri Sauce

Customary	Ingredients	Metric
2 cloves	Garlic	2
½ cup	Fresh chopped cilantro	125 mL
1 cup	Fresh chopped parsley	250 mL
⅓ cup	Olive oil	80 mL
¼ cup	Red wine vinegar	60 mL
½ tsp.	Salt	2 mL
1	Lemon	1

Try This!

This sauce can be used as a marinade, but its fresh taste makes it best on top of roasted or grilled meats. Try spicing it up with finely chopped jalapenos or cayenne pepper.

Yield: 6 servings, ⅓ cup (80 mL) each

1. Mince the garlic and put it into a medium bowl with the cilantro, parsley, olive oil, vinegar and salt.
2. Squeeze juice from the lemon and combine all with a fork or whisk.
3. Refrigerate for up to two hours to blend flavors, and spread over freshly baked, sautéed or grilled meat.

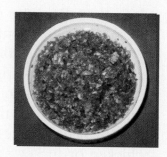

Nutritional Information Per Serving: 120 calories, 13 g total fat, (2 g saturated fat) 0 mg cholesterol, 201 mg sodium, 2 g total carbohydrate (1 g fiber, 0 g total sugars), 0 g protein

Percent Daily Value: vitamin A 20%, vitamin C 30%, calcium 2%, iron 4%

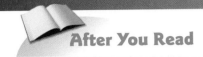

After You Read

CHAPTER SUMMARY

Meat, poultry, and fish offer high-quality protein, along with B vitamins, iron, zinc, and some other nutrients. Poultry and fish have less saturated fat than red meat. Choose mostly lean protein foods, vary your choices, and consume sensible amounts. Plan ahead and shop wisely to make the best meat, poultry, and fish choices for your nutrition needs, budget, and recipe. Consider the retail cut, its tenderness, and its planned use. Store and prepare meat, poultry, and fish properly to ensure quality, good taste, and food safety.

Vocabulary Review

1. Use each of these vocabulary words in a sentence.

Content Vocabulary
- ◇ poultry (p. 406)
- ◇ lean meat (p. 406)
- ◇ marbling (p. 406)
- ◇ organ meat (p. 406)
- ◇ meat cut (p. 409)
- ◇ score (p. 409)
- ◇ marinade (p. 409)
- ◇ Maillard reaction (p. 409)
- ◇ giblet (p. 412)
- ◇ finfish (p. 413)
- ◇ shellfish (p. 413)
- ◇ fillet (p. 413)
- ◇ surimi (p. 413)
- ◇ cured meat (p. 413)

Academic Vocabulary
- ■ logical (p. 407)
- ■ effect (p. 408)

Review Key Concepts

2. Explain how lean meat, poultry, and fish fit into a healthful eating plan.

3. Discuss how food science applies to cooking meat, poultry, and fish.

4. Summarize tips for buying finfish and shellfish.

5. Describe how to prepare meat, poultry, and fish to keep them lean, tender, and safe.

Critical Thinking

6. Evaluate a current fad diet from a magazine that involves meat. What do they say about eating meat? Do you find the diet to be healthful?

7. Evaluate the possible effects of eating too little from the Meat and Beans Group.

8. Explain the health reasons for choosing lean cuts of meat, fish and poultry.

9. Imagine you are making dinner for your family. Suggest creative ways to serve meat, poultry, or fish as part of an appealing complete meal.

Real-World Skills and Applications

Decision Making

10. Stay Within Budget You are giving a good-bye party to an old friend. You bought two pounds of boneless chicken breasts to grill for six people. Now your guest list is ten! How can you adapt the menu to feed four more people? What will you decide to do? Be specific. Explain the reasons for your decision.

Technology

11. Demonstrating Doneness Create a two-minute video that shows viewers how to check the doneness of roast beef, a hamburger, whole chicken, or finfish. In the audio, explain what you are doing and why, and give doneness temperatures. Remember that the tools you use are important.

Interpersonal and Collaboration

12. Keep Poultry Safe Work in a small group. Imagine you all belong to a service club that helps support a homeless shelter. You decide to sponsor a chicken lasagna dinner for 100 people to raise funds. Identify food safety issues for purchasing, storing, cooking, and serving chicken lasagna.

Financial Literacy

13. Stretching Your Food Dollar Steak is $7.99 a pound. You bought an 8-oz. steak for yourself for dinner, but just found out you will have a guest. You can purchase a second steak to serve your guest, or stretch the steak you have with rice and vegetables you can buy for $2.09. Compare the cost of each option.

14. Menu Planning Plan a meal for four people. Use local store advertisements or coupon inserts to make an economical meat, poultry, or fish choice. Identify the meat cut or type of poultry or fish. Find an appropriate recipe and include cost-per-serving and the cooking method.

15. Environment Research environmental issues on finfish and shellfish safety. Go online or interview experts to learn about the issues and groups that protect the safety of the fish supply. Discuss why a clean environment for fish and shellfish is important. Write a two-page report.

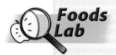

16. Compare Ground Beef Shape two 4-ounce (112 g) patties: one from regular ground beef, another from extra lean ground beef. Panbroil patties separately in a nonstick pan, with no added fat. Cook for the same time. Weigh the cooked patties and drippings. Compare. Draw conclusions.

Additional Activities For additional activities go to this book's Online Learning Center at glencoe.com.

Academic Skills

 English Language Arts

17. Design a Restaurant Menu Use the Internet to find creative menu items using meat, poultry, and fish. Then create a clear, descriptive, and creative menu that includes at least two items made with meat, poultry, or fish in each category: appetizers, soups, salads, sandwiches, and entrees.

> **NCTE 3** Apply strategies to interpret texts.

 Social Studies

18. Meat around the World People in other parts of the world eat meat dishes that are less known here. Haggis is a dish popular in Scotland. It is made with sheep stomach. Research a dish from a culture other than your own that contains a type of meat you do not eat. Include a recipe, the country of origin, a description, and explain why that dish is eaten.

> **NCSS I A Culture** Analyze and explain the ways groups, societies, and cultures address human needs and concerns.

 Mathematics

19. Compare Calories, Fat, and Protein Create a histogram chart to compare the nutritional value of 3½ oz. of these protein foods.

- Boneless chicken breast, roasted: 165 calories, 31 g protein, 4 g fat
- Chicken breast with skin, roasted: 197 calories, 30 g protein, 8 g fat
- Pork chop (lean and fat), boneless, broiled: 260 calories, 28 g protein, 16 g fat
- Pork loin (lean only), roasted: 214 calories, 29 g protein, 10 g fat

Math Concept **Histogram** A histogram uses bars to show the distribution of data.

Starting Hint Find the information that is the same, and make it into a row or column.

 For more math help, go to the Math Appendix

> **NCTM Data Analysis and Probability** Fomulate questions that can be addressed with data and collect, organize, and display relevant data to answer them.

 ## STANDARDIZED TEST PRACTICE

MULTIPLE CHOICE
Read the paragraph. Write your answer on a separate piece of paper.

Test-Taking Tip When answering multiple-choice questions, look for answers that use words such as *always, none,* or *never.* They are usually not the correct answers.

You can cook chicken in the microwave oven. Season it first to help achieve a brown color. A microwave cookbook gives tips on cooking favorite and new dishes.

20. Based on the paragraph, which of the following is true?
a. Chicken is everyone's favorite food.
b. Meat does not brown in the microwave.
c. You can cook meat in the microwave oven.
d. A whole chicken is never cost-effective for a family.

CHAPTER 29
Eggs, Beans, and Nuts

Explore the Photo ▶▶
Eggs, beans, and nuts taste great eaten alone. They also add flavor, function, and nutrition to many mixed dishes. *How do eggs, beans, and nuts fit into your meals and snacks?*

Writing Activity
Descriptive Paragraph

Breakfast, Lunch, or Dinner Write a descriptive paragraph about how you like eggs, beans, and nuts prepared. At which meal do you usually eat them? What seasonings do you like? Is it a cultural, family or ethnic dish, or one that you have created?

Writing Tips

1. **Decide** what mood you want to create in the paragraph.
2. **Write** a strong topic sentence.
3. **Present** details in a logical order.

Reading Guide

Before You Read

Predict Before starting the chapter, browse the content by reading headings, bold terms, and photo captions. Do they help you predict the information in the chapter?

Read to Learn

Key Concepts

- **Explain** how eggs, beans, and nuts fit into a healthful eating plan.
- **Summarize** tips for buying and storing eggs, beans, and nuts.
- **Discuss** how food science applies to preparing eggs.
- **Compare** the many ways to safely cook eggs.
- **Describe** how to prepare beans and nuts for flavor, quality, and nutrition.

Main Idea

Nutrient-packed eggs, beans, and nuts are good protein sources. They are prepared in many ways and featured in main dishes, side dishes, desserts, and snacks.

Content Vocabulary

◇ legume
◇ tofu
◇ egg substitute
◇ quiche
◇ omelet

Academic Vocabulary

You will find these words in your reading and on your tests. Use the glossary to look up their definitions if necessary.

■ promote
■ convenient

Graphic Organizer

Use a web diagram like the one shown below to identify the six ways an egg can be cooked alone.

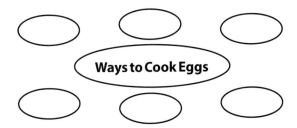

Ways to Cook Eggs

 Graphic Organizer Go to this book's Online Learning Center at glencoe.com to print out this graphic organizer.

Academic Standards ●

 Mathematics

NCTM Measurement Apply appropriate techniques, tools, and formulas to determine measurements.

NCTM Number and Operations Compute fluently and make reasonable estimates.

 English Language Arts

NCTE 12 Use language to accomplish individual purposes.

 Social Studies

NCSS I A Culture Analyze and explain the ways groups, societies, and cultures address human needs and concerns.

NCTE National Council of Teachers of English	**NSES** National Science Education Standards
NCTM National Council of Teachers of Mathematics	**NCSS** National Council for the Social Studies

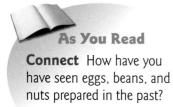

Vocabulary

You can find definitions in the glossary at the back of this book.

As You Read

Connect How have you have seen eggs, beans, and nuts prepared in the past?

Eggs, Beans, and Nuts— Nourishing Choices

Eggs, beans (legumes), and nuts belong to the Meat and Beans Group of MyPyramid. A **legume** is an edible seed grown in a pod. Legumes include dry beans, dry peas, lentils, peanuts, and soybeans. As peas and beans mature, they dry out. Eggs, beans, and nuts provide many beneficial nutrients:

◆ **Protein** Eggs—like meat, poultry, and fish—are good sources of all essential amino acids. Soybeans are, too. Soy protein has unique heart health benefits. The protein in legumes, nuts, and seeds is excellent, but limited in some essential amino acids.

◆ **Vitamins and Minerals** Eggs supply folate and other B vitamins, iron, and phosphorus. Legumes provide folate and other B vitamins, iron, potassium, and small amounts of calcium. Nuts offer folate and phosphorus. Both legumes and nuts supply small amounts of zinc. Sunflower seeds, almonds, and hazelnuts are good vitamin E sources.

◆ **Carbohydrates** Legumes provide complex carbohydrates from starches. Legumes and nuts also provide fiber.

◆ **Fat and Cholesterol** Except for peanuts and soybeans, most legumes are nearly fat free. Nuts and seeds are fairly high in fat, but it is mostly unsaturated. Because they come from plants, legumes and nuts are cholesterol free. Egg yolks are high in cholesterol and contain some fat.

◆ **Phytonutrients** Eggs have lutein, which may **promote**, or help, vision. Legumes, nuts, and seeds contain other highly beneficial phytonutrients.

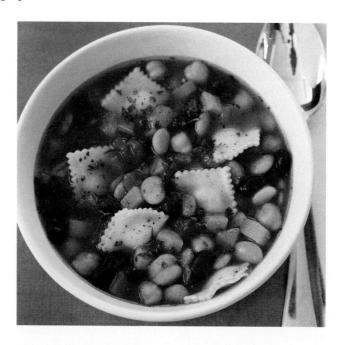

Beans—A Source of Plant Proteins Many protein-rich soups are made with beans. *What other ways could you feature beans as the main protein source in a meal?*

MyPyramid Advice

Eggs, beans, nuts, and seeds are an important part of your daily intake. If you eat 2,000 calories a day, you need about 5½ ounces (156 g) from the Meat and Beans Group. Remember that egg yolks are high in cholesterol. These foods count as 1 ounce (28 g) from the Meat and Beans Group:

◆ 1 egg

◆ ¼ cup (60 mL) cooked dry beans or peas

◆ ½ ounce (14 g) nuts or seeds

◆ 1 Tbsp. (15 mL) peanut butter

◆ ¼ cup (60 mL) tofu

◆ 2 Tbsp. (30 mL) hummus

◆ One half of a soy or garden burger

Dry beans and other legumes can also count as ½ cup (125 mL) from the vegetable group, but one serving cannot count for two food groups.

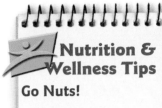

Nutrition & Wellness Tips

Go Nuts!

✓ Add slivered almonds to steamed vegetables.

✓ Add toasted peanuts or cashews to a vegetable stir-fry instead of meat.

✓ Add walnuts or pecans to a green salad.

Choices for Variety and Nutrition

Eggs, beans, and nuts can take center stage in a meal. They can also add variety and nutrition to side dishes and snacks.

◆ Eat legumes several times a week. Try chili with beans, bean burritos, or garbanzo beans on a chef's salad.

◆ Try **tofu**, a cheese-like curd made from soybeans. Use it in soups, stir-fries, dips, and casseroles.

◆ Try tempeh, a fermented soybean patty with a nutty or smoky flavor. Grill it or crumble it into soup or chili.

◆ Prepare egg dishes with egg substitutes. An **egg substitute** is made from egg whites, which have no fat or cholesterol.

◆ Snack on a hard-cooked egg, edamame (soybeans in the pod), hummus, or a small handful of nuts or peanuts. Try nuts or peanut butter in place of meat or poultry.

✓ **Reading Check**

Identify How many ounces does a person need daily from the Meat and Beans Group?

Try Tofu in Stir-Fries Tofu, made from soybeans, is rich in protein and low in fat and sodium. *What other foods provide soy protein?*

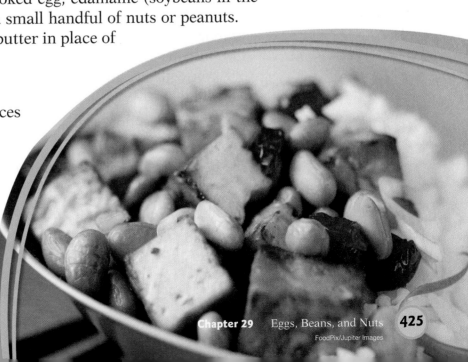

FoodPix/Jupiter Images

Buy and Store Eggs, Beans, and Nuts

Eggs and legumes are usually a nutrition bargain. Along with nuts, they are also **convenient**, or easy to use, for everyday meals.

Buy and Store Eggs

A carton usually contains one dozen eggs. The shell's color has no effect on taste or nutrition. Eggs are inspected for safety and graded for quality. To buy and store eggs wisely:

◆ Buy only uncracked refrigerated eggs.

◆ Compare prices for different sizes. Eggs usually are sold as pee wee, medium, large, extra large, and jumbo. Size does not affect quality, though most recipes are tested using large eggs.

◆ Look for the sell-by date for freshness.

◆ Look for pasteurized liquid eggs in the refrigerator or freezer case.

◆ Buy egg substitutes for less or no cholesterol. They may be refrigerated, frozen, or dried.

◆ Consider specialty eggs. Some have more omega-3 fats or vitamin E, or less cholesterol. Check nutrition facts.

◆ Refrigerate uncooked whole eggs in their original carton and use within five weeks. Do not wash before storage.

◆ Keep unopened pasteurized eggs and egg substitutes refrigerated for up to 10 days or frozen for up to one year. Once opened, use them within three days.

Buy and Store Legumes

Legumes come in many varieties. Check **Figure 29.1** for common types. To buy and store legumes wisely:

◆ Buy uncooked legumes, which are sold in boxes or bags. You will save money, though soaking and cooking them will take several hours.

◆ Try fresh legumes, such as edamame.

◆ Buy canned or frozen legumes for convenience. Canned beans are cooked and ready to eat.

◆ Choose canned beans with less salt, or rinse canned beans after opening them to reduce sodium in your diet.

◆ Keep uncooked dry beans in airtight containers in a cool, dry place. Store canned beans in a cool place, too.

◆ Refrigerate or freeze leftover cooked beans promptly.

Figure 29.1 **A Rainbow of Legumes**

Vary the Colors, Sizes, and Shapes! Dry beans and peas come in many different varieties. These are popular ones. *In what dishes have you eaten these different types of beans and peas?*

Split Peas Yellow or green. Mild flavor. Used mainly in soups.

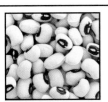

Black-Eyed Peas Small, oval, and white with black spots. Mild flavor. Many uses.

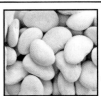

Lima Beans Small or large. Mild, buttery flavor. Many uses.

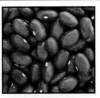

Red Beans Small. Dark red. Hearty flavor. Many uses.

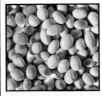

White Beans Small and white. Mild flavor. Many uses, including baked beans and soups.

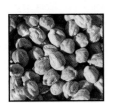

Garbanzo Beans Also known as chickpeas. Round with rough texture. Nut-like flavor. Many uses.

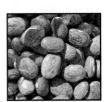

Pinto Beans Small, oval beans with pink dots. Mild flavor. Many uses, including chili and refried beans.

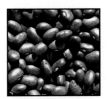

Black Beans Hearty flavor. Many uses, including rice and beans.

Buy and Store Tofu

Tofu is often sold refrigerated in the produce department. Firm tofu is dense and solid. Soft and silken tofu are creamy and blend well with other ingredients. Some tofu has added calcium.

Refrigerated tofu is perishable. Check the expiration date. Some packaging allows longer storage than others. Rinse any leftover tofu and cover it with fresh water to store. Change the water daily and use within one week. Tofu can also be frozen.

Buy and Store Nuts and Seeds

Nuts—almonds, cashews, pecans, walnuts, and more—come in cans, jars, and bags. They are sold shelled or unshelled; salted, seasoned, or unsalted; whole, ground, sliced, or chopped; and in trail mixes. Look for sunflower and pumpkin seeds, too. Peanut butter and nut butters can be spread on sandwiches, celery sticks, or apple slices.

Store nuts and seeds in a dry, cool place in airtight containers. Some nut butters need refrigerating.

✓ **Reading Check** **Identify** How should you store fresh eggs?

Eggs in Food Science

Have you eaten scrambled, fried, poached, or hard-cooked eggs? Eggs are used to:

◆ Hold ingredients together.

◆ Thicken foods such as custard and pies.

◆ Add lightness and help baked goods rise.

◆ Coat or glaze foods.

◆ Give structure to batter and dough.

What Happens When Eggs Cook?

Proteins in eggs coagulate when heated. The molecules unwind and collide with one another. As the temperature rises, they bond and gradually form a solid—the cooked egg.

When eggs are overcooked, water leaches from the eggs and tightens the bonds between proteins. This makes eggs dry or rubbery.

What Makes Egg Whites Fluffy and Firm?

Whipping makes egg whites foamy and increases their volume. Beating egg whites unwinds and lengthens their proteins so they can clump together. As proteins coagulate, they form a protective, stable coat around the air bubbles. The result is a stiff foam perfect for a soufflé, mousse, or meringue.

To beat egg whites, first separate the whites and yolks. Make sure no yolk—not even a little—mixes into the white. Fat in the yolk prevents egg whites from foaming.

Beat the egg whites with a mixer or rotary beater at high speed. Their appearance and texture will change from foamy, to soft, to stiff. Beating time makes the difference.

◆ **Foamy Whites** Beat until air starts to mix in. Bubbles and foam form. Egg whites remain transparent.

◆ **Soft Peaks** Beat until the mixture gets white, shiny, and thick. When you lift the beaters, the whites stand up in peaks that bend over.

◆ **Stiff Peaks** Beat until the peaks stand straight up, then stop. Overbeaten whites get dry and break.

Handle beaten egg whites gently so air bubbles do not break. Fold them into other ingredients.

✓ **Reading Check** **Name** What are three functions of eggs in recipes?

Cook Eggs

To keep eggs tender, tasty, and safe, cook eggs at low or medium temperatures. Fully cooked eggs have firm whites and yolks with no visible liquid egg. Runny yolks are undercooked and still may contain harmful bacteria. For egg casseroles and quiches, use a meat thermometer. The internal temperature should reach 160°F (71°C).

Ways to Cook Eggs

Eggs are cooked alone and in mixed dishes. **Quiche**, for example, is a main-dish pie with a filling of eggs, milk, and other ingredients. Eggs are ingredients in many recipes, too.

You begin most egg dishes by cracking the eggs. You may need to separate the yolk and white. Cold eggs separate more easily. An egg separator provides an easy, safe way to separate eggs.

◆ **Hard-Cooked or Soft-Cooked** Place eggs in the shell in a saucepan. Cover with cold water. Bring the water to a boil, then remove the saucepan from the heat. Cover it. Hot water continues to cook the eggs. Wait 5 minutes (soft-cooked) or 15 minutes (hard-cooked). After hard-cooking, immediately run cold water over eggs. That stops cooking and helps prevent a green ring around the yolk. You can refrigerate hard-cooked eggs for one week.

◆ **Fried** Gently break eggs into a bowl. Then, slip them into a hot nonstick skillet with a small amount of fat. Keep the yolks whole. Cook slowly at a low temperature until the yolks are firm. To finish cooking the yolks, cover the skillet or carefully turn over the eggs with a turner.

Food Prep How To

SEPARATE EGGS

1	Place a clean egg separator across the rim of a small bowl.
2	Crack the egg in the center.
3	Hold the egg over the round part of the egg separator. Gently pull the shell apart. Slip the yolk into the egg separator.
4	Let the white flow through into the bowl. Then, drop the yolk into a different bowl.

STEP 4

Food Prep How To

SCRAMBLE EGGS

1 Heat 1 Tbsp. (15 mL) butter or soft margarine in a skillet.

TIP The fat should be just hot enough so that a drop of water sizzles.

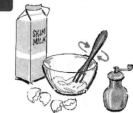
STEP 2

2 Mix two eggs in a bowl with 2 Tbsp. (30 mL) fat-free milk or water and a dash of pepper.

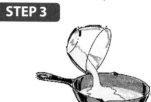
STEP 3

3 Pour the egg mixture into the hot skillet. Do not stir.

4 As the eggs begin to set, gently draw a turner or spoon completely across the bottom of the skillet. Large, soft curds will begin to form. The uncooked portion will flow to the bottom.

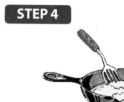
STEP 4

5 Repeat as needed until eggs are firm.

TIP Avoid constant stirring. The mixture will get mushy.

♦ **Omelet** An **omelet** is cooked like a large egg pancake. It can be folded in half with filling inside. Start by slightly beating raw eggs and pour them into a skillet. Cook until firm in a flat shape without stirring. Lift the edge of the cooked mixture with a spatula, allowing uncooked egg to flow underneath. Continue cooking until the omelet is set, but still moist on the surface. Once firm, fill it and then fold in half. Shredded cheese and chopped vegetables, meat, chicken, or seafood are good fillings.

♦ **Baked** Break eggs into a bowl. Then, slip them into a greased baking dish. Add a splash of milk, if desired. Bake at 325°F (160°C) until firm.

♦ **Microwaved** Scramble or bake eggs in the microwave oven. Check a cookbook for power level and time. Microwave only until the yolks are cooked. During standing time, the white will finish cooking. Heat and steam pressure can build up inside whole eggs and yolks. Pierce the yolks to prevent them from bursting. Do not microwave eggs in the shell. They will explode!

✓ **Reading Check** **Explain** How can you tell if an egg is fully cooked?

Prepare Legumes and Nuts

You can enjoy legumes and nuts in many ways—on their own or in mixed dishes.

Cook with Beans

Beans are great in soups, salads, baked dishes, and more! The flavors and textures of beans, peas, and lentils blend well with other foods. Dry beans take time to prepare, but canned beans are convenient. Try these quick dishes with canned beans:

◆ Add canned garbanzo, kidney, or white beans to tossed salads, soups, stews, or pasta sauce.

◆ Mash canned beans for spreads or dips.

◆ Wrap refried beans, scrambled eggs, and cheese in a flour tortilla for a breakfast burrito.

◆ Combine lima beans and corn for a complete protein.

Prepare Tofu

Tofu only needs heating. It has a mild flavor. Tofu soaks up flavors from other foods and seasonings.

◆ **Use Firm Tofu** Add tofu cubes to soups, stir-fries, stews, and salads. Add it to ground beef for tacos or spaghetti sauce.

HOT JOBS!

Recipe Developer

Recipe developers create or adapt recipes for cookbooks, media, restaurants, and the food industry. They write the recipe, then prepare it many times for the desired results.

Careers Find out more about careers. Go to this book's Online Learning Center at **glencoe.com**.

Food Prep How To

COOK DRY BEANS

STEP 1

1   After sorting and soaking dry beans for 4 hours, drain. Put drained soaked beans in a large pot with a cover. Add about 3 cups (750 mL) of fresh cold water for each cup (250 mL) of soaked beans.

2   Cover, but leave the lid slightly ajar so steam can escape. This keeps the beans from boiling over.

STEP 2

3   Simmer beans until tender. This takes one to three hours, depending on the type of beans. If needed, add more hot water to keep the beans covered. If undercooked, beans may feel gritty or hard. If overcooked, they get mushy and fall apart.

TIP   Add salt, sugar, and acidic foods, such as tomatoes and vinegar, near the end of the cooking time since they toughen beans.

◆ **Use Soft Tofu** Blend soft or silken tofu with seasonings for dips, spreads, or salad dressings.

Nuts for Flavor and Texture

Nuts taste great just as they are. They also add flavor and texture to mixed dishes such as salads and baked goods. Since nuts are high in fat, use small amounts. Chop them so they go further. Toast them to enhance their flavor.

✓ **Reading Check** **Explain** Why are canned beans more convenient than dry beans?

EASY RECIPES Everyday Favorites

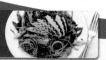

Red Beans and Rice

Customary	Ingredients	Metric
2 links	Smoked lean sausage	2 links
½ cup	Celery, chopped	125 mL
½ cup	Green bell pepper, chopped	125 mL
½ cup	Onion, chopped	125 mL
3 cloves	Garlic, minced	3 cloves
2 cans (28 oz.)	Red beans, undrained, divided	900 mL
¼ tsp.	Cayenne pepper	1 mL
4 cups	Cooked rice	1 L

Try This!
Add canned diced tomatoes. Garnish with grated cheese, parsley, or cilantro.

Yield: 6 servings, 1¼-cup (310 mL) each

❶ Cut sausage links in half lengthwise and cut in 1-inch pieces.

❷ Cook sausage in a large non-stick skillet over low heat until it is brown on all sides. Remove meat from skillet. Set aside.

❸ Using the fat left from the sausage to cook the celery, bell pepper, onion, and garlic until tender. Return sausage to the skillet.

❹ Mash one can of beans in a bowl. Mix with Cayenne pepper. Add mashed beans and the second can of beans to vegetable-sausage mixture.

❺ Let mixture simmer 20 minutes. Stir often. Serve over hot cooked rice.

Nutritional Information Per Serving: 348 calories, 7 g total fat (7 g saturated fat), 13 mg cholesterol, 730 mg sodium, 56 g total carbohydrate (11 g fiber, 1 g total sugars), 14 g protein

Percent Daily Value: vitamin A 2%, vitamin C 20%, calcium 6%, iron 20%

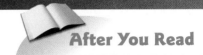

After You Read

CHAPTER SUMMARY

Eggs, beans, nuts, and seeds—part of the Meat and Beans Group—are high in protein and other nutrients. Enjoy and combine them with other foods. Buy eggs, beans, and nuts wisely and store them properly for freshness and food safety. Eggs serve many functions in recipes. Both cooking them and whipping the egg whites coagulates their proteins. Eggs can be prepared in many ways. Uncooked dry beans must be soaked for at least fours hours and take one to three hours to cook. Canned beans are already cooked. Nuts and tofu are very versatile foods and can be added to many dishes. Nuts are also often eaten alone.

Vocabulary Review

1. Use each of these vocabulary words in a sentence.

Content Vocabulary
- legume (p. 424)
- tofu (p. 425)
- egg substitute (p. 425)
- quiche (p. 429)
- omelet (p. 430)

Academic Vocabulary
- promote (p. 424)
- convenient (p. 426)

Review Key Concepts

2. Explain how eggs, beans, and nuts fit into a healthful eating plan.

3. Summarize tips for buying and storing eggs, beans, and nuts.

4. Discuss how food science applies to preparing eggs.

5. Compare the many ways to safely cook eggs.

6. Describe how to prepare beans and nuts for flavor, quality, and nutrition.

Critical Thinking

7. Design a meal in which eggs are featured, along with foods from the other four food groups.

8. Revise a recipe for a dish you have eaten by substituting tofu for a traditional ingredient. Create a nutritional analysis to show how the substitution would change the nutrients and calories in the recipe.

9. Compare and Contrast shell eggs and egg substitutes. Why might some people choose one over the other? Which would you use? Why?

Real-World Skills and Applications

Technology

10. Eggs, Beans, and Nuts Online Get your teacher's permission to use the Internet to learn 15 facts. Find five interesting facts you did not know about each of these foods: eggs, beans, and nuts. Share what you learn with the class in a creative way. List the Web sites you used to compile your information.

Problem-Solving

11. Beans on the Menu Imagine that you are planning new menu items for fundraising at the Saturday football games. They must be nutritious and low cost. What menu items with beans could you promote? Choose three appealing recipes that include beans and analyze their nutrition and cost per serving.

Interpersonal and Collaborative

12. Egg Safety Follow your teacher's instructions to form groups. Collaborate to create a pamphlet with food safety tips for buying, storing, and preparing eggs. Include both illustrations and text. Work together to first create an outline, then to assign writing and editing tasks.

Financial Literacy

13. Substitute for Savings A recipe calls for 4 cans (6 cups) of cooked beans and 1½ lbs. of ground beef. Beef is $4.99 per lb. and beans are $1.25 per can. How much will you save if you use dry beans and firm tofu instead? Tofu costs $1.39 for 12 ounces (¾ lb.). A 2-lb. package of dry beans is $2.38 and makes 12 cups of cooked beans.

14. Legumes Around the World Get your teacher's permission to use the Internet to research legumes in a country where they are a main protein source. Determine why they are popular. How are they prepared and in what types of dishes are they used? Share your findings with the class in an oral report.

15. Newer Types of Eggs Research newer types of eggs, such as organic eggs, omega-3-rich eggs, and eggs with more vitamin E or less cholesterol. For information, check egg cartons at the supermarket and use resources at the library. Compare their pros and cons in a written report.

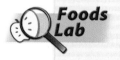

16. Compare Egg Preparation Try two of the basic egg preparation methods described in this chapter. Would you use either method again for a quick meal or snack? Why or why not? Compare the taste, color, smell, texture, and cooking time of each. Which do you prefer?

 Additional Activities For additional activities go to this book's Online Learning Center at glencoe.com.

Academic Skills

English Language Arts

17. Write an Ad Write a radio advertisement for eggs, beans, or nuts. This ad should tell your audience about healthful ways to eat these foods or the benefits of the nutrients they contain. You can also share statistics related to research about eggs, beans, or nuts. Word choice really matters. Your ad should draw attention, arouse interest, inform, and cause the listener to take action.

> **NCTE 12** Use language to accomplish individual purposes.

Social Studies

18. Eggs Around the World Egg dishes are found around the world. Research some common dishes that use eggs and tell where they originate. Describe their ingredients and methods of preparation. Use a chart or poster to show your research.

> **NCSS I A Culture** Analyze and explain the ways groups, societies, and cultures address human needs and concerns.

Mathematics

19. Dry Beans Marta must figure out how many pounds of dry beans to buy to make her favorite bean soup. One pound of dry beans makes about 12 servings of bean soup. Figure how many ounces of beans Marta will need to use if she wants to serve a group of three, four, or six people.

Math Concept When solving an equation, it is important to check your work by considering how reasonable it is. You can use front-end estimation, or you can round and estimate a reasonable answer.

Starting Hint One pound of beans is too much for a group of three, four, or six people, so divide three, four, and six into 12 to find how much of a pound is needed.

 For more math help, go to the Math Appendix

> **NCTM Number and Operations** Compute fluently and make reasonable estimates.

STANDARDIZED TEST PRACTICE

ESSAY
Read the paragraph and write an answer on a separate piece of paper.

> **Test-Taking Tip** If you do not know the answer to a question, make a note and move on to the next question. Come back to it later, after you have answered the rest of the questions.

Eggs can be served in many ways for meals and snacks. They provide complete protein, along with several important vitamins and minerals. A large egg also contains about 215 milligrams of cholesterol. The Dietary Guidelines for Americans advises eating less than 300 milligrams of cholesterol a day for heart health. All of the cholesterol in eggs comes from their yolks.

20. Based on information in the paragraph, the chapter, and your own label-reading experience, write a one-paragraph essay about the nutrition in eggs and how you could eat eggs without consuming too much cholesterol.

CHAPTER 30
Fats and Oils

Explore the Photo ▶▶
Oils, soft margarine, avocados, and salad dressing provide heart-healthy fats. Just go easy—not too much! *What foods with healthy oils are part of your meals and snacks?*

Writing Activity

Write an Expository Essay

Use What You Know Expository writing explains and informs. Think about a process, appliance, tool, or another food-related topic that you know well. Write an essay that explains your topic to your audience. Explain your position clearly and support it with facts.

Writing Tips

1. **Define** your purpose and audience.

2. **Explain** your main idea in a clear thesis statement.

3. **List** facts as supporting details.

Reading Guide

Before You Read

Understanding It is normal to have questions when you read. Write down questions while reading—many of them will be answered as you continue. If they are not, you will have a list ready for your teacher when you finish.

Read to Learn

Key Concepts

- **Summarize** the differences between oils and solid fats.
- **Suggest** ways to use healthy oils in food preparation.
- **Discuss** how food science applies to fats.
- **Explain** how to buy and store oils and solid fats.
- **Describe** the main functions of fats in food preparation.

Main Idea

Oils and solid fats make foods moist, tender, and flavorful. Different types of fats have different cooking qualities. Use mostly oils, which are healthier for you than solid fats.

Content Vocabulary

◇ oil
◇ hydrogenation
◇ rancidity
◇ oxidation
◇ antioxidant
◇ smoke point

Academic Vocabulary

You will find these words in your reading and on your tests. Use the glossary to look up their definitions if necessary.

- ■ essential
- ■ expose

Graphic Organizer

As you read, use a graphic organizer like the one below to list the qualities of liquid and solid fats.

Liquid Fats	Solid Fats

 Graphic Organizer Go to this book's Online Learning Center at glencoe.com to print out this graphic organizer.

Academic Standards

 Science
NSES Content Standard F Develop an understanding of personal and community health.

 English Language Arts
NCTE 4 Use written language to communicate effectively.
NCTE 9 Develop an understanding of diversity in language use across cultures.

 Mathematics
NCTM Measurement Understand measurable attributes of objects and the units, systems, and processes of measurement.

NCTE National Council of Teachers of English	**NSES** National Science Education Standards
NCTM National Council of Teachers of Mathematics	**NCSS** National Council for the Social Studies

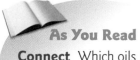

Vocabulary

You can find definitions in the glossary at the back of this book.

As You Read

Connect Which oils and solid fats do you eat on a regular basis?

Oils and Solid Fats: The Differences

Two forms of fat—oils and solid fats—give unique qualities to food. While both provide food energy, they affect your health differently.

◆ An **oil** is a fat that is liquid at room temperature. Canola, corn, cottonseed, olive, safflower, soybean, and sunflower are commonly used oils. Nuts, seeds, olives, avocados, and some fish also contain oils.

◆ **Solid fats** are fats that are firm at room temperature. Butter, stick margarine, shortening, and lard are solid fats. Meat and many milk products contain solid fats. A few plant oils, including coconut oil and palm kernel oil, have solid fats in them too.

All fats are mixtures of saturated and unsaturated fatty acids. Solid fats are more saturated and may have trans fats. That makes them solid. Oils contain more monounsaturated and polyunsaturated fats. That makes them liquid.

Health Connection

As a nutrient group, fats are **essential**, or necessary. They carry fat-soluble vitamins A, D, E, and K in food and in your body. Oils are your main vitamin E source. Some polyunsaturated fats are essential for growth and the nervous system. Both oils and solid fats provide energy—about 120 calories per tablespoon.

Because their fatty acids differ, oils and solid fats affect health differently.

◆ Vegetable oils—in moderate amounts—can be heart healthy. Eat them instead of solid fats. Unsaturated fats do not raise bad cholesterol (LDL) levels in your blood. Omega-3, an unsaturated fat in walnuts, seeds and some coldwater fish such as salmon, tuna and mackerel may have other heart health benefits.

◆ Solid fats can increase heart disease risk. Along with cholesterol, their saturated fats and any trans fats they contain tend to raise LDL cholesterol levels in blood.

Fat Choices Oils and solid fats are mixtures of saturated and unsaturated fats. Oils have mostly unsaturated fats. *How might you use these oils in food preparation?*

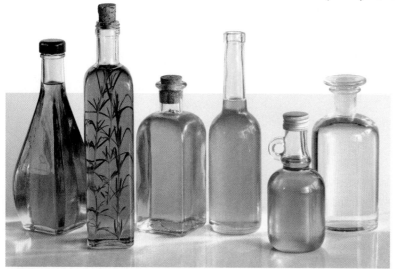

MyPyramid Advice

Go easy on fatty foods! MyPyramid advises eating lean meat and mostly low-fat and fat-free milk and milk products. It also says that most fats should be unsaturated. Make oils your main source of fat. Limit solid fats such as butter or shortening.

Consume two tablespoons or six teaspoons (30 mL) of oils daily—if you eat 2,000 calories daily. Consume slightly more or less depending on your calorie needs. That amount of healthy oils contains vitamin E and enough essential fatty acids. Limit the amount for energy balance.

Here are some foods that provide 1 tablespoon (15 mL) of healthy oil:

- 1 tablespoon (15 mL) vegetable, olive, canola, or other oil.
- About 1 tablespoon (15 mL) mayonnaise or soft (trans fat-free) margarine.
- 3 tablespoons (45 mL) Italian dressing.
- 24 large black olives.
- ½ medium avocado (avocados fit in the Fruit Group).
- 1 ounce (28 g) peanuts, most nuts, or seeds (nuts and seeds belong in the Meat and Beans Group).
- 1½ tablespoons (25 mL) peanut butter (nuts and seeds belong in the Meat and Beans Group).

✓ **Reading Check** **Explain** What are the health benefits of using oils in place of solid fats?

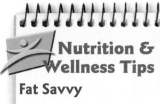

Nutrition & Wellness Tips

Fat Savvy

✓ Use butter-flavored cooking oil spray for flavor with few added calories.

✓ Try pesto or herbed olive oil on bread instead of stick margarine or butter.

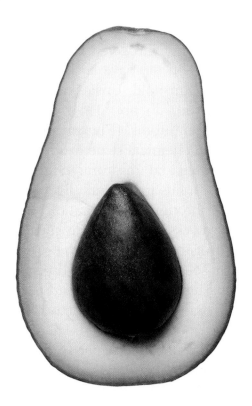

Spreads for Health Consider mashed avocado or guacamole as a spread for sandwiches. *Why are avocado spreads healthier choices than butter or stick margarine?*

Fitting In Healthy Oils

To get health benefits from oils—without consuming too much—try these strategies.

◆ Switch to oils or soft margarine. Use them instead of stick margarine or butter on bread, vegetables, potatoes, pasta, and more.

◆ Use nuts in place of other protein-rich foods on occasion. Try walnuts on salad, pine nuts in pesto sauce, or almonds in rice.

◆ Enjoy sliced avocado on salads and in sandwiches.

◆ Use sensible amounts of salad dressing. Make your own dressing with healthy oils.

◆ Eat some fatty, cold-water fish, such as salmon.

✓ **Reading Check** **List** What are three ways to use oils in food preparation?

Fats in Food Science

Fats have unique qualities. Unlike sugar, they do not dissolve in water. Solid fats soften and melt with warmth and get firm with cold. Their chemistry makes the difference.

Liquids vs. Solids

Chemistry explains why oils and solid fats, such as stick margarine, differ. All fats are made of carbon, hydrogen, and oxygen. Saturated fats, such as butter, have all the hydrogen their molecules can hold. Unsaturated fats, such as vegetable oil, do not. Their molecules lack some hydrogen atoms. (**Figure 30.1** shows the difference in chemical structure between molecules of saturated and unsaturated fats.)

Some fats are naturally liquid, but are made more solid through hydrogenation. **Hydrogenation** is the process of adding hydrogen to unsaturated fats. Hydrogenation changes the structure of oil, making it solid or semisolid. Hydrogenation also creates trans fats, which are not heart healthy.

Fats are hydrogenated for many reasons. Besides becoming more solid, they do not turn rancid as fast. Healthier, trans fat-free margarine and shortening is available.

What Makes Fat Rancid?

Have you ever smelled oils, nuts, or chips that have an unpleasant aroma? That may signal rancidity. **Rancidity** is the change in the quality of oils and solid fats when they oxidize. Their natural chemical structure breaks down when they are exposed to oxygen. To **expose** means to come in contact with. Changes caused by contact with oxygen are called **oxidation**. Oxidation is the main reason that high-fat foods spoil.

Antioxidants added to fats and oils slow oxidation. An **antioxidant** is a substance that helps prevent oxidation. Vitamin E is added to oils, for example, as an antioxidant. Oils are more likely to oxidize than solid fats.

Liquid Fats

Oils are better for healthful food preparation than most solid fats. Different oils have different functions and flavors. Most oils work well in salad dressings. Mayonnaise, certain salad dressings, and soft (tub or squeeze) margarine with no trans fats are mainly oil. Important differences among oils include:

◆ **Smoke Point** Oils for frying, stir-frying, or sautéing should have a high smoke point and tolerate heat better. The **smoke point** is the temperature when fat produces smoke. Oils with high smoke points include canola, peanut, and vegetable oils. Sesame oil and extra virgin olive oil are not good for hot frying.

◆ **Flavor** Choose mild-flavored oils for recipes when you do not want to overpower other flavors. Use stronger-flavored oils for their unique flavors.

Figure 30.1   Unsaturated vs. Saturated Fats

Hydrogen in Fats Saturated fats have more hydrogen in their molecules than unsaturated fats do. *How do fats become solid?*

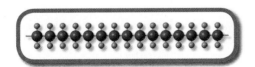

Saturated Fatty Acid

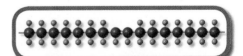

Unsaturated Fatty Acid

Solid Fats

Butter, stick margarine, and other solid fats often are used in baking. They have a lower smoke point and break down with continued frying. Popular types include:

◆ **Butter** Butter gives baked goods and other foods a pleasant flavor and smooth mouth feel. Choose butter when its flavor is important. Spreadable butter is mixed with a small amount of oil, such as canola oil. It stays softer when refrigerated than regular butter, which makes it good for spreading.

◆ **Margarine** Stick margarine, a hydrogenated fat, can substitute for butter, but has less flavor. That is fine in foods like brownies: chocolate is the main flavor. Margarine usually costs less than butter. It has no cholesterol and usually less saturated fat but has trans fat. Diet or reduced-calorie margarine contains more water. It may be a good spread, but is not the best choice for baking.

◆ **Lard** Lard is solid white fat from hogs. It has a slight meaty flavor. Lard is used mostly in baking, including savory and tender pastries. Some ethnic foods use it. Tortillas and refried beans, for example, are often made with lard.

◆ **Shortening** Shortening is hydrogenated vegetable fat. It is used like lard in baking. It stays solid at a wide temperature range. Unlike butter and margarine, which are about 80 percent fat, shortening and lard are 100 percent fat.

Which Oil? Stores sell many different kids of oils—from different sources and at different prices. *Which oil would you use for a stir fry? Which oil could you use for a homemade salad dressing?*

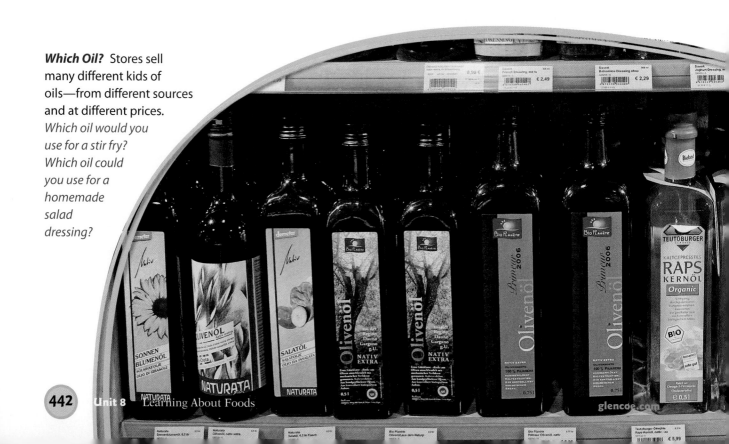

Buy and Store Oils and Solid Fats

To buy fats and oils wisely:

◆ Choose oils and solid fats to match their purpose.

◆ Check the Nutrition Facts to compare total, saturated, and trans fats. Look for trans fat-free spreads and dressings.

◆ Compare prices. Specialty oils and butter can cost more. Buy only the amount you can use before it turns rancid.

Storage for Oils and Solid Fats

Fats and oils need proper storage. Heat, light, and oxygen can change the texture and flavor, and turn them rancid.

◆ Refrigerate butter, margarine, and other solid fats or freeze them for up to six months. Keep them tightly covered.

◆ Keep oils tightly covered in a cool, dark place. They turn rancid faster than solid fats do. Olive oil does not keep well when refrigerated.

◆ Store salad dressings and mayonnaise in the refrigerator.

✓ **Reading Check** **Identify** How can you find margarine with less saturated fat as you shop?

Discover International Foods

Canada

Like the United States, Canada has a rich cuisine that reflects the diversity of its immigrants and its First Nation, or aboriginal, people. Many traditional favorites came from early British and French immigrants, made with products of Canada's different agricultural areas. British Columbia is known for fruit, nuts, and seafood. Provinces in the central plains produce beef, wheat, canola, and flaxseed. Ontario produces wild rice. Fish cakes and salmon dishes are popular in coastal regions. Quebec has French cooking traditions.

Languages Across Cultures

nanaimo bar (nə-´nī-mō bär) layered dessert of crumb, custard, and soft chocolate, originated on Vancouver Island in British Columbia

saskatoon berries (sas-kə-´tün) small red to purple berries, grown in Saskatchewan and Manitoba, made into desserts, breads, sauces, and other fruit dishes

 Recipes Find out more about International recipes on this book's Online Learning Center through glencoe.com.

NCTE 9 Develop an understanding of diversity in language use across cultures.

Cook with Oils and Solid Fats

Fats have many functions in food. The type you use affects food's color, aroma, flavor, tenderness, and structure.

◆ **Color** Because fats carry heat, they contribute to browning, or the Maillard reaction.

◆ **Flavor** Many fats have distinct flavors. Fats also carry flavors from other ingredients.

◆ **Smooth Texture** Fats give foods a smooth mouth feel.

◆ **Tenderness and Flakiness** Fats tenderize and add moisture to baked products and help make pastry flaky.

◆ **Air** Butter or margarine is creamed with sugar to make many baked goods. That brings in air, or lightness.

✓ **Reading Check** **Identify** What are six functions of fat in cooking and baking?

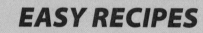

EASY RECIPES

International Flavors

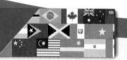

Pancakes with Maple Syrup

Customary	Ingredients	Metric
1 cup	All-purpose flour	250 mL
½ cup	Whole wheat flour	125 mL
1 Tbsp.	Baking powder	15 mL
1 tsp.	Salt	5 mL
1¼ cup	Lowfat milk	300 mL
2 Tbsp.	Canola oil	30 mL
1 cup	Maple syrup	250 mL

Try This!
Chopped nuts and sliced bananas or berries make excellent additions to pancakes.

Yield: 6 servings, 3-pancakes each

❶ Combine dry ingredients and mix. Add oil, along with the milk, to the dry ingredients.
❷ Stir to combine but do not overmix.
❸ Pour ¼ cup of batter per pancake onto hot, lightly oiled skillet or pan. Cook until top of pancake bubbles then flip and cook one minute more.
❹ Top with maple syrup.

Nutritional Information Per Serving: 295 calories, 4 g total fat (1 g saturated fat), 4 mg cholesterol, 614 mg sodium, 61 g total carbohydrate (2 g fiber, 34 g sugars), 5 g protein

Percent Daily Value: vitamin A 2%, vitamin C 0%, calcium 20%, iron 10%

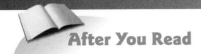

After You Read

CHAPTER SUMMARY

Oils and solid fats give unique qualities to food. Both provide food energy, but they affect health differently. Oils with mostly unsaturated fats are heart healthy. Solid fats with more saturated fats are not. Consume oils for their health benefits, but keep energy in balance. Hydrogenation changes oils to solid fats. Rancidity spoils their quality. Choose oils and solid fats to match their purpose. Check the Nutrition Facts to compare the fat content. Store fats properly to keep their quality. Fats contribute tenderness, flakiness, lightness, color, flavor and smooth texture.

Vocabulary Review

1. Use each of these vocabulary words in a sentence.

Content Vocabulary
◇ oil (p. 438)
◇ hydrogenation (p. 440)
◇ rancidity (p. 441)
◇ oxidation (p. 441)
◇ antioxidant (p. 441)
◇ smoke point (p. 441)

Academic Vocabulary
■ essential (p. 438)
■ expose (p. 441)

Review Key Concepts

2. Summarize the differences between oils and solid fats.

3. Suggest ways to use healthy oils in food preparation.

4. Discuss how food science applies to fats.

5. Explain how to buy and store oils and solid fats.

6. Describe the main functions of fats in food preparation.

Critical Thinking

7. Explain how you might tell if oil you plan to use for making salad dressing is fresh. If it is not fresh, what might have happened to it?

8. List three ways you could use vegetable oil spray in food preparation. Explain the possible benefits of using this product.

9. Analyze fat choices. Peggy has decided to use oils instead of solid fats in her diet. Instead of using one Tbsp. of butter on her vegetables, she will use 2 Tbsp. of olive oil. Is this a good plan? Why or why not?

Real-World Skills and Applications

Decision Making

10. Compare Fats Research the percentage of saturated, polyunsaturated, and mono-unsaturated fats in three oils and three solid fats. Create pie charts to compare these types of oils and fats. Write conclusions about each option. Which are the most heart-smart? Rank them accordingly.

Collaboration and Interpersonal

11. Myths About Fats Does margarine have less fat than butter? Does light olive oil have fewer calories than regular olive oil? Research oils and solid fats. Create a true or false quiz with ten myths about fats, and explanations for the answers. Swap with another student, and take the quiz created by that student.

Technology

12. Oil Production Blog Get your teacher's permission to do online research to learn more about a common oil, such as soybean, corn, canola, or olive oil. Find out about the crop used to produce it, where it is produced, and how the oil is used. Create a short blog entry with basic production facts.

Financial Literacy

13. Cost Comparison You want to make banana walnut muffins. You have all the ingredients except for oil. At the store you find walnut oil that costs $4.45 for 12 ounces (175 mL). You also find canola oil that costs $6.15 for 24 ounces (350 mL). Which oil is more cost-effective?

14. Make Butter Butter is made from cream. Design a demonstration to explain how butter is made and why it forms. Share your demonstration in your foods class. Measure how much butter is produced. Compare the flavor to store-bought butter.

15. Choose a Spread Go to a supermarket. Use food labels to compare the fat, saturated fat, trans fat, cholesterol, and calories in several spreads: butter, stick margarine, soft margarine, mayonnaise, and a reduced-fat or reduced-calorie spread. Compare prices. Make a comparison chart. Explain which spread you would buy.

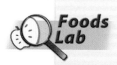

16. Taste Test for Oils Choose at least six different oils to taste test—for example, canola, light olive, extra virgin olive, peanut, walnut, sesame, or other oils. With separate spoons, put a small sample of each on a small piece of lettuce to taste. Write descriptive terms for each oil. As a class, suggest uses for each oil.

Additional Activities For additional activities go to this book's Online Learning Center at glencoe.com.

Academic Skills

English Language Arts

17. Heart-Healthy Cooking Create a brochure on cooking with fats for heart health. Research the reasons and ways to reduce saturated fat and increase unsaturated fats. Create a brochure with easy tips for teens to use.

> **NCTE 4** Use written language to communicate effectively.

Science

18. Fatty Acids Omega-3 and Omega-6 acids are heart healthy. You will find them in fatty fish such as salmon, as well as walnuts, canola oil, avocados, and flaxseed.

Procedure Research one of these foods. List the health effects of its fatty acids.

Analysis Present your answers in a two-paragraph report. List specific details.

> **NSES Content Standard F** Develop an understanding of personal and community health.

Mathematics

19. Count and Convert Fat Ryan kept track of how much fat he consumed in a day. Help him analyze the results—remember that he should have only two to four tablespoons of fat daily.

Breakfast: pancakes with 1 Tbsp. oil, plus 1 tsp. butter. Lunch: apple with 2 Tbsp. peanut butter. Dinner: taco salad with 1 Tbsp. avocado, and the shell cooked in 2 tsp. oil.

Math Concept **Customary System** The customary system is the system of weights and measures used in the United States. In the customary system, 1 Tbsp. = 3 tsp.

Starting Hint Convert teaspoons to tablespoons then add the tablespoons.

 For more math help, go to the Math Appendix.

> **NCTM Measurement** Understand measurable attributes of objects and the units, systems, and processes of measurement.

STANDARDIZED TEST PRACTICE

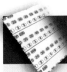

MULTIPLE CHOICE
Read the paragraph. Write your answer on a separate piece of paper.

Test-Taking Tip When taking a test, if you suspect that a question is a trick item, make sure that you do not read too much into it. Avoid imagining detailed situations in which the answer could be true.

Because trans fats are not heart-healthy companies must list them in their nutrition facts. Products can show zero trans fats if there is ½ a gram or less per serving. Words like "hydrogenated" or "partially hydrogenated" are clues to trans fats.

20. Based on the paragraph, which of the following is true?
   a. Trans fat is the healthiest kind.
   b. Hydrogenated fat is the best kind for your health.
   c. Companies can completely hide information from consumers.
   d. If you ate a food labeled as no trans fat, you still might consume some.

Discover Organic Foods

The word *organic* refers to the way farmers grow and process agricultural products. Learning the difference between organic foods and traditionally grown foods can help you make informed decisions about choosing foods that are best for you, considering nutrition, quality, taste, cost and other factors.

My Journal

If you completed the journal entry from page 348, refer to it to see if there are more things you want to learn about organic foods now that you have read the unit.

Project Assignment

In this project you will:

- Conduct research.
- Write a summary of your research.
- Write interview questions.
- Interview a person in your community who is knowledgeable about laws and regulations required for labeling food as organic.
- While interviewing, take notes, and after interviewing, transcribe your notes.
- Make a presentation to your classmates.

Academic Skills You Will Use ....
English Language Arts

NCTE 5 Use different writing process elements to communicate effectively.

NCTE 8 Use information resources to gather information and create and communicate knowledge.

STEP 1 Choose and Research a Topic

Choose an aspect of the organic food industry to research. Possible topics include history, conventional versus organic farming, government standards and certification, environmental impact, and taste and nutritional value. Write a summary of your research.

STEP 2 Plan Your Interview

Use the results of your research to develop a list of interview questions. Keep these writing skills in mind as you develop your questions.

Writing Skills
- Use complete sentences.
- Use correct spelling and grammar.
- Organize your questions in the order you want to ask them.

STEP 3 Connect with Your Community

Use the interview questions you wrote in Step 2 to interview someone in your community who is knowledgeable about organic food. This person can be a farmer, grocer, chef, or anyone else in your neighborhood who is involved in the organic food industry. Use these listening skills as you conduct your interview:

Listening Skills
- Make eye contact.
- Ask additional questions to ensure your understanding.
- Show your interest by responding appropriately.

STEP 4 Create and Present a Report

Use the Unit Thematic Project Checklist to plan and give an oral report. Use these speaking skills as you present your final report.

Speaking Skills
- Speak clearly and concisely.
- Be sensitive to the needs of your audience.
- Use standard English to communicate.

STEP 5 Evaluate Your Presentation

Your project will be evaluated based on:
- Accuracy of your time line
- Content of your presentation
- Mechanics—presentation and neatness

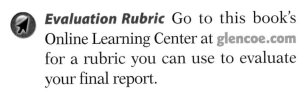 **Evaluation Rubric** Go to this book's Online Learning Center at **glencoe.com** for a rubric you can use to evaluate your final report.

Project Checklist

Plan	✓ Conduct research. ✓ Write a summary of your research. ✓ Write interview questions. ✓ Conduct an interview. ✓ Transcribe the notes from your interview. ✓ Plan your presentation.
Present	✓ Make a presentation to your class explaining the results of your research and interview. ✓ Invite the students of the class to ask any questions they may have. Answer these questions. ✓ When students ask questions, demonstrate in your answers that you respect their perspectives. ✓ Turn in your research summary, interview questions, and interview notes to your teacher.
Academic Skills	✓ Conduct research to gather information. ✓ Communicate effectively. ✓ Organize your presentation so the audience can follow along easily. ✓ Thoroughly express your ideas.

Unit 9

Combination Foods

Chapters in this Unit

Chapter 31 Salads
Chapter 32 Quick and Yeast Breads
Chapter 33 Mixed Foods and Snacks
Chapter 34 Desserts

Unit Thematic Project Preview

Explore Food Industry Careers

There are many exciting career opportunities in the food industry! In the unit thematic project at the end of this unit, you will choose a career in the food industry that interests you. You will identify a professional who works in this industry and arrange to "shadow" him or her for a few hours. Then, you will create a presentation about "a day in the life" of that person and present it to your class.

My Journal

The number of food industry careers is growing. Write a journal entry about the topics below.
- What careers in the food industry interest you?
- Has a food industry professional ever influenced the way you think about food? How?

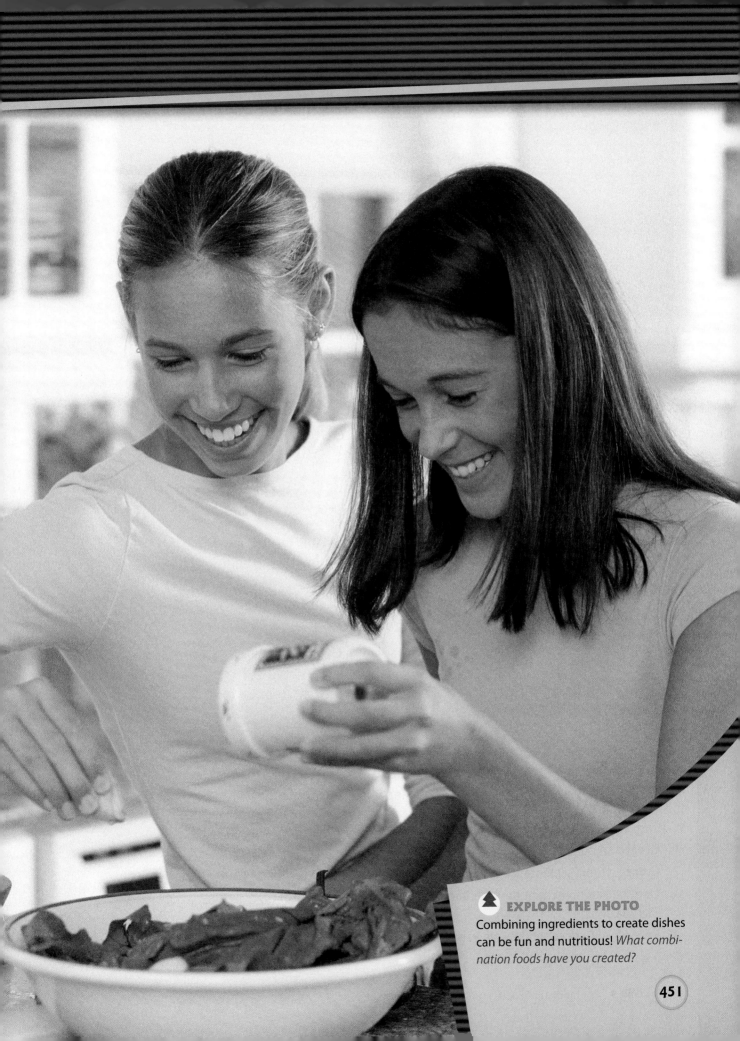

EXPLORE THE PHOTO
Combining ingredients to create dishes can be fun and nutritious! *What combination foods have you created?*

CHAPTER 31
Salads

Explore the Photo ▶▶
Salads are an easy, tasty way to include a variety of foods in your eating plan. *What ingredients do you put in your salads?*

Writing Activity
Persuasive Essay

Persuasive Essay Write an effective, persuasive essay to encourage teens to choose salads for school lunch or at a fast food restaurant. Remember to clearly state your reasons for choosing salad.

Writing Tips

1. **Create** an outline.
2. **Create** a topic sentence for each paragraph.
3. **Use** transition words at the beginning of each paragraph.
4. **Reread**, edit, correct, and rewrite as necessary.

Reading Guide

Before You Read

Look It Up As you read this chapter, keep a dictionary at hand in addition to the glossary at the back of the book. If you hear or read a word that you do not know, look it up in the glossary or the dictionary. Before long, this practice will become a habit. You will be amazed at how many new words you learn.

Read to Learn

Key Concepts
- **Explain** how salads contribute to healthful eating.
- **Discuss** selection and storage of salads and salad ingredients.
- **Describe** the types of salads and their preparation.
- **Compare** salad dressings.
- **Apply** nutrition advice to salad bar choices.

Main Idea

Salads can add flavor, variety, and nutrients to your food choices. Serve salads as snacks, appetizers, side dishes, main dishes, or even for dessert.

Content Vocabulary

◇ salad greens
◇ crouton
◇ emulsion
◇ vinaigrette
◇ emulsifier

Academic Vocabulary

You will find these words in your reading and on your tests. Use the glossary to look up their definitions if necessary.

- mixture
- process

Graphic Organizer

As you read, use a Web diagram like the one below to organize the different types of salads dresssings you can make.

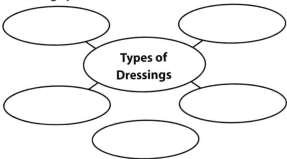

 Graphic Organizer Go to this book's Online Learning Center at **glencoe.com** to print out this graphic organizer.

Academic Standards ■

 Science
NSES Content Standard A Develop abilities necessary to do scientific inquiry.

 English Language Arts
NCTE 9 Develop an understanding of diversity in language use across cultures.

 Mathematics
NCTM Number and Operations Compute fluently and make reasonable estimates.

 Social Studies
NCSS III H Examine physical and cultural patterns and cultural transmission of customs and ideas.

NCTE National Council of Teachers of English
NCTM National Council of Teachers of Mathematics

NSES National Science Education Standards
NCSS National Council for the Social Studies

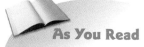

Vocabulary

You can find definitions in the glossary at the back of this book.

As You Read

Connect What ingredients can you add to your salads to make them more healthful?

What Is in Your Salad?

Salad can be much more than just lettuce. You can create a tasty salad **mixture**, or combination, using a wide variety of nutrient-dense foods.

Salads for Healthful Eating

Nutritional benefits of salads come from their ingredient mix. Ingredients can come from any or all five food groups and from healthy oils.

◆ **Grain Products** Rice, pasta, bulgur wheat, wild rice, and couscous are some grain products that add complex carbohydrates, B vitamins, and perhaps fiber to salads.

◆ **Vegetables and Fruits** A variety of vegetables and fruits—fresh, canned, and frozen—provide vitamins A and C, folate, potassium, fiber, and more. **Figure 31.1** shows key nutrients in four types of salad greens.

◆ **Dairy Foods** Cheese, cottage cheese, and yogurt supply calcium, protein, and riboflavin.

◆ **Meat, Poultry, Fish, Dry Beans, Eggs, and Nuts** Besides protein, these provide iron, zinc, and B vitamins. Beans add fiber, too!

◆ **Salad Dressings** Many salad dressings are made with healthy oil, such as olive, canola, soybean, or peanut oil. Use oil-based dressings in small amounts since they provide calories and fat.

✓ **Reading Check** **Explain** How can you make salads nutritious?

Figure 31.1	**Salad Greens Nutrition**

Rate Your Salad Greens The darker the salad greens, the more nutrients they have. *How would you compare the nutrients in these salad greens?*

Percent Daily Value per 1 cup (250 mL) shredded, or chopped fresh					
	Vitamin A	Vitamin C	Folate	Potassium	Fiber
Butterhead lettuce	36	3	10	4	2
Iceberg lettuce	7	3	5	3	4
Romaine lettuce	55	18	16	3	4
Spinach (raw)	84	21	21	7	4

How to Buy and Store Salad Ingredients

Good salads start with good ingredients. In chapters 24 through 30, you learned how to select and store foods used in salad.

Salad Greens and Dressings

A pleasing combination of **salad greens**, or edible raw leaves, makes salads interesting. Look for salad greens that are crisp, free of damage, and at their peak.

Prewashed salad greens and slaw mixes are bagged and ready to use. Check the sell-by date for freshness. You might pay extra for convenience. Keep perishable salad ingredients in separate airtight containers in your refrigerator.

You can buy many types of prepared dressings, such as Italian, and blue cheese. Many versions are made with with less or no fat. You can also buy oil and vinegar to make your own dressing.

Prepared Salads

For more convenience, buy prepared salads from the deli or salad ingredients from the salad bar. Keep these perishable foods refrigerated for freshness and safety.

✓ **Reading Check** **Explain** How should you care for fresh greens after you buy them?

Make Great Salads

Salads can be full of many colors, textures, and flavors, and cooked and raw ingredients. They can be or served cold or hot.

Most salads have these parts:

- ◆ **Base** The foundation on which other ingredients are placed—for example, the lettuce under pasta salad.
- ◆ **Body** The main part of the salad. For example, tuna, celery, and bell pepper are typical in tuna salad.
- ◆ **Dressing** The sauce in a salad. Dressing adds moisture, holds ingredients together, and enhances and blends flavor.
- ◆ **Garnish** The decoration on the salad, such as a fresh sprig of herbs or toasted nuts.

Prepare Salad Ingredients

The first step in the **process**, or method, of making a salad is to prepare the ingredients. Wash fresh salad ingredients carefully under cool running water. Drain thoroughly. Before washing iceberg lettuce, remove the core. Dry greens by blotting gently with a paper towel or using a salad spinner.

Plan salad-making ahead for convenience. Wash fruits and vegetables, then get them cut and ready. Cook chicken, fish, eggs, pasta or other grains ahead and refrigerate. Stock up on canned or frozen fruit.

Food Prep How To

MAKE A TOSSED SALAD

Choose crisp salad greens with evenly colored leaves and no wilting. Wash and dry all fresh ingredients carefully.

1 Tear rather than cut salad greens into bite-size pieces.

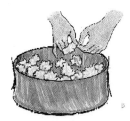

TIP Cutting greens with a knife may cause the edges to brown.

2 Cut other ingredients. For example, you may grate carrots, slice cucumbers, dice green peppers, and separate sliced onions into rings.

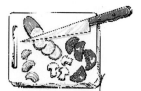

3 Toss ingredients gently by turning them over several times with utensils to mix them.

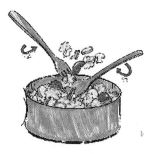

TIP If the salad will not be served right away, cover and refrigerate it without dressing so it will stay fresh and crisp.

4 Toss the salad with the dressing just before you serve it, or serve the dressing separately so the greens do not wilt.

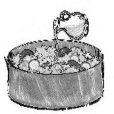

Tossed Greens Salad

A tossed greens salad is made of bite-size pieces of salad greens and dressing. You might start with two or three mild-flavored greens, such as romaine or Bibb lettuce. Add smaller amounts of zesty greens, such as arugula, for flavor. To make it more interesting—and nutritious—toss in other ingredients or add toppings such as:

- Shredded cheese
- Citrus slices, chopped apples, berries, raisins, or dried cranberries
- Sliced vegetables such as celery, tomato, or mushrooms.
- Beans, sunflower seeds, or toasted chopped nuts
- Fresh herbs, garlic, tomato, or onion slices
- **Croutons**, or crunchy dried bread cubes, plain or seasoned

Tossed greens salads can be light or hearty. Turn a light, tossed green salad into a main dish by adding protein foods like sliced meat, chicken, or turkey.

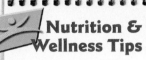

Mixed Salads

You can make a mixed salad with a variety of ingredients from one or more food groups, combined with light dressing. Potato salad, pasta salad, egg salad, carrot-raisin salad, coleslaw, and ambrosia are popular examples.

Make salads more flavorful and nutritious with interesting ingredients. These popular salads have new twists:

- **Carrot Salad** Apple slices, shredded carrot, jicama strips, and sunflower seeds, with citrus dressing.
- **Mixed Fruit Salad** Sliced strawberries, melon, peaches, and kiwifruit with lemon-poppyseed dressing and ginger.
- **Tuna or Chicken Salad** Canned tuna or cut-up chicken, diced celery, grapes, toasted walnuts, and plain low-fat yogurt.
- **Bean Salad** Several types of canned beans (rinsed and drained), chopped onion and celery, and honey-mustard dressing, served on mixed greens.

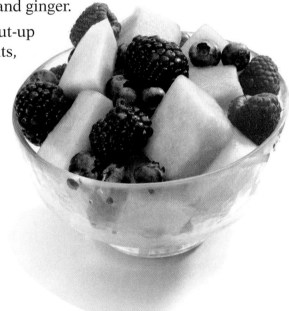

Mixed Salads: More than Just Greens
Combine many nutritious ingredients for a delicious mixed salad. *What kinds of mixed salad combinations could you make?*

Arranged Salads

Arranged salads use colorful, flavorful ingredients, artfully arranged on the plate. Arranged salads often have a base of leafy greens. The body of the salad is arranged in an attractive pattern on the base. Salad dressing may be poured on top or served alongside. You might arrange:

◆ Red and green pepper sticks, fanned around a scoop of herbed cottage cheese on greens.

◆ Antipasto salad: sliced meat, cheese cubes, olives, cherry tomatoes, chili peppers, and Italian dressing.

Arranged salads can be creative. Invent your own without a recipe. Choose ingredients with a pleasing variety of colors, shapes, and flavors that go well together.

✓ Reading Check **Recall** What should you do to prepare salad greens?

Salad Dressings

A variety of salad dressings add different flavors. You can purchase them in bottles or as mixes, or make them yourself. Store-bought dressings come in regular, low-fat, and fat-free varieties.

Many salad dressings are called emulsions by food scientists. An **emulsion** is a mixture of liquids—such as oil and water—the droplets of which do not normally blend with each other. Another ingredient helps these liquids blend.

Grain Salad: All Dressed Up
This grain salad, called tabbouleh, is made with bulgur wheat, tomato, onion, parsley, and mint, and is dressed with olive oil and lemon juice. *Besides olive oil, what other healthy oils could be used in salad dressings?*

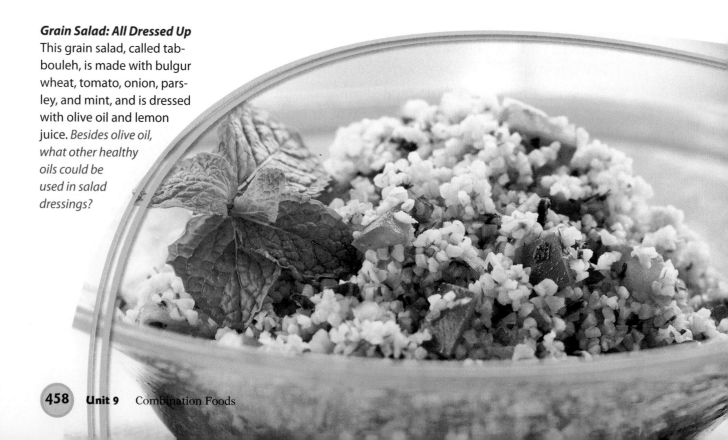

Oil-and-Vinegar Dressings

Some basic salad dressings are made from oil and vinegar. They include French, Italian, or vinaigrette dressings. **Vinaigrette** is a mixture of oil and vinegar, often with herbs and spices.

Shake oil and vinegar together in a tightly covered container. The oil will divide into many small particles distributed evenly throughout the vinegar. However, if the mixture sits for even a very short time, the oil and vinegar will separate. Adding a little mustard helps hold oil and vinegar together longer.

To make a vinaigrette, combine three parts oil and one part vinegar or citrus juice, then add herbs. Use olive, canola, or another healthy oil. For less fat and fewer calories, use less oil—perhaps two parts oil and two parts vinegar. If you use a mild balsamic vinegar, you might even skip the oil.

Mayonnaise-Type Dressings

Mayonnaise is made with oil, egg yolks, and vinegar or lemon juice. Mayonnaise does not separate. It is a permanent emulsion.

In mayonnaise, the egg works as an **emulsifier**, which means that it coats the droplets of oil so they stay evenly scattered throughout the vinegar, juice, or other liquids. In prepared foods, emulsifiers include egg yolks and whites, starches, gelatin, and fine powders such as mustard powder. Many sauces, gravies, and cream soups are permanent emulsions, too. Whole milk is a permanent emulsion that occurs naturally.

Many mayonnaise-type dressings have other ingredients for added flavor. These include herbs, cheese, and mustard. Thousand Island, creamy Italian, and blue cheese dressings are examples of flavored mayonnaise-type dressings.

Mayonnaise is used to dress many mixed salads, such as potato salad and egg salad. Mayonnaise is high in fat. Use it sparingly. For some salads, low-fat yogurt is a good substitute.

Other Salad Dressings

Salads may be dressed in other ways, too. Try these alternatives with fewer calories and less fat than other dressings:

◆ Yogurt dressing, made by blending plain or flavored yogurt with pureed fruit or herbs.

◆ Cooked dressing, made by thickening fruit or vinegar with egg, cornstarch, or flour.

◆ Juice, such as lemon juice, and a touch of salt.

✓ **Reading Check** **Compare** What is the difference between a temporary and a permanent emulsion?

HOT JOBS!

Food Photographer
Food photographers take food pictures for all kinds of media. They apply art and photographic skills to make food look delicious.

Careers Find out more about careers. Go to this book's Online Learning Center at **glencoe.com**.

Nutrition & Wellness Tips

Dress Lightly!

✓ Start with much less dressing than you think you need, then add more if needed.

✓ Serve dressing on the side so people can add only what they need.

Salad Bar Savvy

Salad bars in supermarkets, restaurants, fast-food places, and school cafeterias have many healthful food choices.

The average salad from a salad bar is not always low-fat or low-calorie. In fact, it can have more than 1,000 calories! It is up to you to make wise choices.

◆ Fill your plate with a variety of vegetables and fruits.

◆ Include cooked dry beans, hard-cooked eggs, lean meat, turkey, nuts or seeds, or shrimp or tuna for protein.

◆ Go easy on mixed salads in oil-based or mayonnaise dressings, such as pasta salad.

◆ Have just a little salad dressing, or choose a fat-free variety.

◆ Go easy on higher-fat ingredients, such as cheese.

◆ Make just one trip to the salad bar. Use a small plate.

✓ **Reading Check** **Interpret** Why might calories add up in a salad from a salad bar?

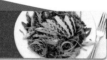

EASY RECIPES — Everyday Favorites

Sunshine Salad

Customary	Ingredients	Metric
4 cups	Spinach leaves, packed	1 L
⅓	Red onion, sliced thin	⅓
⅓	Red bell pepper, sliced	⅓
½	Whole cucumber, sliced	½
2	Oranges, peeled and chopped in bite-sized pieces	2
¼ cup	Bottled low-fat vinaigrette	60 mL

Try This!
Use different greens. Create your own vinaigrette. Top with croutons, toasted nuts, or pumpkin seeds.

Yield: 4 servings, 1 cup (250 mL) each

① Toss spinach, onion, bell pepper, cucumber, and oranges in a large bowl.
② Add dressing. Toss lightly.
③ Serve immediately.

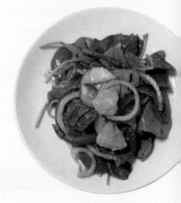

Nutritional Information Per Serving: 71 calories, 1 g total fat (0 g saturated fat), 1 mg cholesterol, 150 mg sodium, 14 g total carbohydrate (3 g fiber, 8 g sugars), 2 g protein

Percent Daily Value: vitamin A 25%, vitamin C 80%, calcium 6%, iron 6%

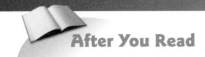
After You Read

CHAPTER SUMMARY

Salads add nutrition and flavor to your eating plan. Ingredients come from all five food groups. For freshness and safety, keep perishable salads and salad ingredients chilled. Salads may have a base, a body, dressing, and a garnish. They may be tossed, mixed, or arranged. You can eat them as a meal or as snacks. Protein-rich ingredients can turn a salad into a main dish. Salad dressings add moisture, hold ingredients together, and enhance flavor. The types include oil-and-vinegar, mayonnaise-type, cooked, and others. Salad bars provide many options. Choose wisely for good nutrition.

Vocabulary Review

1. Use each of these vocabulary words in a sentence.

Content Vocabulary
◇ salad greens (p. 455)
◇ crouton (p. 457)
◇ emulsion (p. 458)
◇ vinaigrette (p. 459)
◇ emulsifier (p. 459)

Academic Vocabulary
■ mixture (p. 454)
■ process (p. 456)

Review Key Concepts

2. Explain how salads contribute to healthful eating.

3. Discuss selection and storage of salads and salad ingredients.

4. Describe the types of salads and their preparation.

5. Compare salad dressings.

6. Apply nutrition advice to salad bar choices.

Critical Thinking

7. Analyze why a salad spinner can be useful kitchen equipment for salad-making.

8. Advise ways to cut back on fat and calories and boost nutrients in salads.

9. Create a recipe for a regular or lower-fat vinaigrette dressing with your choice of oil, vinegar, and herbs or spice.

Real-World Skills and Applications

Set Goals and Make Decisions

10. Design a Salad Imagine you are a menu planner for a fast-food restaurant. You decide to create a nutritious salad. Write the factors to consider. Describe your salad with an ingredient list.

Collaborative and Interpersonal

11. Science Teamwork Follow your teacher's instructions to form small groups. Use a permanent emulsion, such as mayonnaise to create a hypothesis about how permanent emulsions react to a change in temperature. Test your hypothesis as a group. Write a lab report. Include your hypothesis, procedure and the analysis of your results.

Technology

12. Recipe Search Get your teacher's permission to search online for salad recipes. Label the recipes and their sources. Compile them to create a class salad recipe book.

Financial Literacy

13. Salad Dressing Alternatives Instead of adding an ounce of an oily dressing to your green salad, consider adding an ounce of fruit. If salad dressing costs 20¢ per ounce, and mandarin oranges cost 89¢ for an 11-ounce can, how much can you save on each salad you prepare this way?

14. Great Greens Visit a produce department to identify unusual salad greens, such as arugula, Belgian endive, curly endive, escarole, and radicchio. Ask the produce manager about their qualities, uses, and flavors. If possible, do a taste test. Make a chart comparing at least five varieties.

15. Dressy or Droopy? Put two dry lettuce leaves in separate storage containers. Coat one with salad dressing. Refrigerate both overnight. Compare them the next day. Write observations. Draw conclusions. Explain how to prepare tossed salads ahead to keep them fresh and crisp.

NSES Content Standard A Develop abilities necessary to do scientific inquiry.

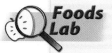
16. Make a Dressing Make a vinaigrette with three parts oil and one part vinegar. Choose the type of oil and vinegar. Add your choice of herbs. Next, prepare the same vinaigrette with less oil. Taste-test both on small salads. Compare flavors. Write your results, along with the two complete recipes.

Additional Activities For additional activities go to this book's Online Learning Center at glencoe.com.

Academic Skills

 English Language Arts

17. Language of Salads Choose a country. Find out about salads enjoyed there. Create a glossary with the native name, pronunciation, and country of each salad. Clearly describe the ingredients and preparation. With other classmates, categorize salads in a worldwide salad menu.

> **NCTE 9** Develop an understanding of diversity in language use across cultures.

 Social Studies

18. Balsamic Vinegar Balsamic vinegar is a flavored vinegar from central Italy. Made from aged grapes, it is darker, thicker, sweeter, and more expensive than other vinegars. Find a recipe other than one for salad dressing that calls for balsamic vinegar. Where does the recipe originate? Give your answers in a short oral presentation.

> **NCSS III H** Examine physical and cultural patterns and cultural transmission of customs and ideas.

 Mathematics

19. Solving Proportions Vinaigrette is made with three parts oil and one part vinegar. Lara planned to double the recipe, so she began pouring tablespoons of oil into a mixing bowl. When she had poured 5 tablespoons into the bowl, she realized that she had run out of oil. How much vinegar should she add so the proportion will match her needs?

Math Concept Equivalent ratios have the same meaning. To find an equivalent ratio, multiply or divide both sides by the same number.

Starting Hint Write a ratio that shows how to make vinaigrette. Set it equal to another ratio that shows how Lara made her vinaigrette. Use x to represent the unknown quantity. Solve for x.

 For more math help, go to the Math Appendix.

> **NCTM Number and Operations** Compute fluently and make reasonable estimates.

STANDARDIZED TEST PRACTICE

ESSAY

Read the paragraph and write an answer on a separate piece of paper.

> **Test-Taking Tip** At the beginning of a test, review it quickly to see what kinds of questions are on it. You may find multiple choice, matching, true or false, short answer, extended response, and essay questions.

For many, the word *salad* means iceberg lettuce with a few other chilled vegetables. But the word simply means a mixture of foods. Many salads do not even use lettuce as an ingredient. Some salads are desserts, and a few salads contain so many calories from fat that they are not as healthful. Appetizer, main dish, or dessert salads are on the menu to stay!

20. Based on the paragraph and the chapter, write a paragraph about an interesting way to make a salad.

CHAPTER 32

Quick and Yeast Breads

Explore the Photo ▶▶

Bread baking can be satisfying and fun. You might make a stack of hot blueberry pancakes or bake a batch of whole wheat muffins. *You probably enjoy eating many kinds of breads, but have you tried making your own? What kinds?*

Writing Activity

Describe a Viewpoint

A Toast to Bread Write a descriptive paragraph about the type of bread you enjoy the most. Think about why you like it. Is there a specific ingredient that you like? Is it part of a favorite celebration? Use adjectives to enhance your paragraph.

Writing Tips

1. **Write** a strong topic sentence.
2. **Orient** the reader by presenting details in a logical order.
3. **Select** precise transition words.

Reading Guide

Before You Read

Use Notes When you are reading, keep a notepad handy. When you come upon a section or term you are unfamiliar with, write the word or a question. After you have finished, look up the terms or try to answer your questions.

Read to Learn

Key Concepts
- **Explain** the purpose of ingredients in baking.
- **Discuss** the food science of leavening and gluten.
- **Summarize** skills for successful baking.
- **Compare** methods for making quick and yeast breads.
- **Identify** ways to store bread and baking ingredients for freshness.

Main Idea

Baking takes special cooking skills, but provides delicious homemade baked goods.

Content Vocabulary

- ◇ self-rising flour
- ◇ batter
- ◇ dough
- ◇ leavening agent
- ◇ extract
- ◇ yeast
- ◇ gluten
- ◇ yeast bread
- ◇ quick bread
- ◇ flat bread
- ◇ muffin method
- ◇ biscuit method
- ◇ knead

Academic Vocabulary

You will find these words in your reading and on your tests. Use the glossary to look up their definitions if necessary.

- ▪ enhance
- ▪ consistent

Graphic Organizer

Use a graphic organizer like the one below to categorize the various breads described in this chapter as quick, yeast, or flat breads. Note why each bread fits in its category.

Quick Breads	Yeast Breads	Flat Breads

 Graphic Organizer Go to this book's Online Learning Center at **glencoe.com** to print out this graphic organizer.

Academic Standards ▪

 English Language Arts
NCTE 12 Use language to accomplish individual purposes.

 Science
NSES Content Standard A Develop abilities necessary to do scientific inquiry.
NSES Content Standard F Develop an understanding of personal and community health.

 Social Studies
NCSS IX A Explain how cultural elements can facilitate global understanding.

 Mathematics
NCTM Number and Operations Understand the meaning of operations and how they relate to one another.

NCTE National Council of Teachers of English
NCTM National Council of Teachers of Mathematics

NSES National Science Education Standards
NCSS National Council for the Social Studies

Baking Basics

Have you ever wondered why bread has a different texture from cake, or why muffins sometimes stick to the pan? Understanding baking principles helps you prepare any baked product. Baking is cooking with dry heat, usually in an oven.

What Ingredients Do

Most baked products use the same basic ingredients for specific purposes. Together, they make products with the shape, texture, and flavor you want. Convenience mixes have most ingredients already mixed in. You add water and sometimes, milk, oil, butter, or an egg.

◤◇Vocabulary

You can find definitions in the glossary at the back of this book.

Flour

Flour is usually the main ingredient. It provides proteins and starch for structure. Wheat flour is most common. Barley, buckwheat, corn, oats, rice, and rye are milled for flour, too.

- **All-Purpose Flour** is enriched white flour from the grain's endosperm. It gives good results for most baked products.

- **Whole-Wheat Flour** is from the whole grain. It has more fiber than all-purpose flour. You can often replace two-thirds of the all-purpose flour with whole-wheat flour.

- **Self-Rising Flour** is flour with salt and baking powder mixed in. Use it only when the recipe calls for it.

- **Bread Flour** gives bread a strong structure.

Liquids

Liquids moisten dry ingredients and help bind them together. They produce steam, which helps dough rise. They also help make many chemical changes in mixtures. Water, milk, juice, yogurt, and sour cream are some liquids used in baking.

A mixture is either a batter or a dough, depending on the amount of liquid.

- **Batter** is a flour mixture that is thin enough to be poured or dropped from a spoon. Muffins, pancakes, and cakes are made from batter.

- **Dough** is a flour mixture that is stiff enough to be shaped by hand, rolled, or cut. Biscuits, some cookies, pie crust, and breads are made from dough.

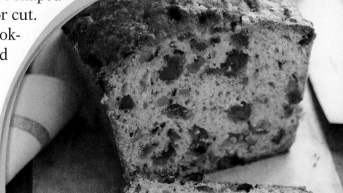

Bountiful Breads Have you ever tried apricot nut muffins, cheddar herb bagels, or pumpkin bread? *What extras might you add to a basic muffin or biscuit recipe?*

Leavening Agents

A **leavening agent** is a substance that makes baked goods rise. This includes baking soda, baking powder, and yeast. They trap air or gas in the mixture.

Fats

Fats and oils add flavor, richness, and tender texture. They also help brown the crust. Solid fat—such as butter, stick margarine, shortening, or lard—is preferred for many baked foods. Some recipes call for vegetable oil. Each fat contributes a different flavor and texture. Substituting oils for solid fats changes the results and brings down the saturated fat and trans fat content.

Sweeteners

Sweeteners contribute to the volume, flavor, tenderness, and texture. They allow yeast to work, so the dough can rise and the crust can brown. Common sweeteners include granulated, or white, sugar, brown sugar (white sugar with molasses added), powdered, or confectioners', sugar, and honey. Artificial sweeteners can be used in recipes specifically developed for them.

Salt

Besides adding flavor, salt helps control the action of yeast and tightens gluten. Too much salt slows down the rising process. Salt-free bread rises faster than regular bread.

Eggs

Many baked products need eggs to make them tender and add color, flavor, and richness. Eggs also help bind mixtures together. Beaten eggs help bread rise.

Other Ingredients

Many ingredients **enhance**, or improve, the flavor and appearance and boost fiber and nutrients. Nuts, dried fruits, onions, cheese, herbs, and spices are often used in baked goods. Other flavorings include chocolate, coconut, and extracts. An **extract** is concentrated flavoring from food or plants.

✓ **Reading Check**) **Recall** What kind of flour could you use for most baked goods?

The Science of Baking

To bake yeast bread, you mix the ingredients, knead the dough, and let it rise. As it bakes, dough rises and expands more. The result is a light, tasty loaf. This happens because of physical and chemical changes.

Nutrition & Wellness Tips

Bake with Less Fat

✓ Substitute a little applesauce, mashed bananas, or mashed beans for up to half of the butter or oil—for a somewhat different result.

✓ Use buttermilk or low-fat or fat-free yogurt in place of sour cream, butter, or margarine in some breads.

Why Do Baked Goods Rise?

Leavening is the process that makes baked goods rise and become light and porous. As batter or dough bakes, gas expands and makes tiny holes as it escapes.

All baked goods are leavened partly by air and steam. When you sift flour, or cream fat and sugar together, air gets trapped in the mixture. Air also gets trapped when you beat egg whites. Oven heat turns water to steam, which takes up more room than water. Trapped steam expands the batter or dough, making it rise.

Leavening agents—baking soda, baking powder, and yeast—also produce carbon dioxide gas.

How Baking Soda and Baking Powder Leaven

Baking soda forms carbon dioxide and leavens when combined with an acid and heat. It is used in recipes with acidic ingredients, such as buttermilk, yogurt, molasses, vinegar, or citrus juice.

Baking powder is baking soda plus powdered acid (cream of tartar) and cornstarch. It is used in recipes with no acidic ingredient. Carbon dioxide forms when baking powder mixes with liquid.

Double acting baking powder is baking soda, cornstarch, and two other compounds. It reacts twice—when batter gets moist and when batter heats in the oven. That ensures a consistent release of leavening bubbles as the dough or batter bakes. **Consistent** means even. Some recipes use both baking powder and baking soda.

How Yeast Leavens

Yeast is a simple fungus that produces gas as it grows. Warmth, food (sugars), and moisture make it grow quickly.

Yeast breaks down sugars in flour, giving off carbon dioxide and alcohol. (The alcohol evaporates during baking.) Proteins in flour trap the carbon dioxide bubbles in the dough. As that happens, dough rises and becomes lighter. Yeast also gives bread its distinctive aroma and flavor.

Sourdough breads are leavened by yeast and by bacteria that produce carbon dioxide. Friendly bacteria produce flavorful acidic byproducts that give a sour taste.

What Does Gluten Do?

When wheat flour mixes with water, it forms gluten. **Gluten** is a stretchy, elastic protein. Gluten holds dough together. The more dough gets mixed or kneaded, the stronger and stretchier gluten gets.

Leavening agents work with gluten. When yeast produces carbon dioxide, gluten stretches and dough rises. Gluten traps carbon dioxide, forming tiny pockets in the dough. As baking continues, heat causes protein and starch to coagulate. The result? A baked product with a firm shape.

Without gluten, yeast bread could not be made. It would expand from steam and carbon dioxide, then collapse. Wheat flour is good for bread baking because it has enough gluten-forming proteins. Other flours do not. Corn, barley, millet, oats, rice, and rye flours have few proteins that form gluten, if any.

✓ **Reading Check**   **Compare**   What are the differences between baking soda, baking powder, and yeast?

Successful Baking

Successful baking depends on following the recipe exactly.

◆ Use the exact ingredients. A different ingredient, such as honey in place of sugar, gives a different flavor and texture.

◆ Measure accurately.

◆ Follow the recipe's mixing directions—no shortcuts.

◆ Use the correct size pan. If a pan is too small, the mixture may overflow as it rises. If a pan is too large, the product will be thin and may dry out.

◆ Use the correct oven temperature. A temperature that is too high causes overbrowning, poor volume, and a tough texture. A temperature that is too low causes a pale color, soggy texture, uneven grain, and a sunken center.

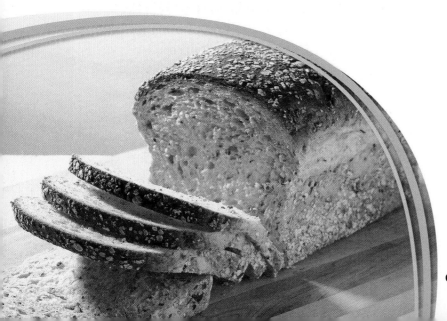

Bubbles in Bread Carbon dioxide in wheat dough causes gluten to rise and expand. Small holes remain after the bread is baked. *How would you describe the texture of this bread?*

Baker

Bakers mix ingredients for baking breads, pastry, and other baked goods. They work in grocery and specialty stores and for large food producers.

Careers Find out more about careers. Go to this book's Online Learning Center at glencoe.com.

Prepare Pans for Baking

Prepare pans before baking to easily remove baked goods later. A recipe may call for a greased, greased and floured, or ungreased pan. Use unsalted butter or margarine. Salt could cause the crust to overbrown and stick to the pan. Flour makes the product easier to remove and absorbs extra fat.

Set the Oven Temperature

The right oven temperature may depend on the type of pan. Some pans retain more heat than others. Most recipes are designed for shiny metal pans. For dull metal pans, lower the temperature about 10°F (1°C). For glass pans, lower the temperature about 25°F (4°C).

Preheat the oven for about 10 minutes before baking. This will ensure the right temperature for proper baking and rising.

When You Place Pans in the Oven

Place pans in the oven so air circulates freely for even baking. Leave at least 1 inch (2.5 cm) of space between each pan and between the pans and oven walls. Pans that touch each other or the oven door create hot spots that overbrown food.

◆ **One Pan** Place the pan in the oven's center.

◆ **Two Pans** Place each pan on a separate rack in diagonally opposite corners.

Discover International Foods

Germany

Bread, or *brot* in German made with rye, whole wheat, barley, oats, and other types of flour—is a staple in German meals. Most German breads are made with sourdough. Other breads include pumpernickel, a steamed bread. Dinner meals feature pork, as well as poultry, beef or game, often served as sausages. Side dishes may include root vegetables, such as carrots or turnips, spinach, peas, beans, or cabbage (perhaps as sauerkraut). Potatoes, noodles, or dumplings may fill out a meal.

Languages Across Cultures

muesli (*'myüs-lē*) means mixture in German; a popular breakfast cereal made of raw or toasted grains (barley, millet, oats, etc.) dried fruit, and nuts and served with milk, yogurt, or fruit juice.

spaetzle (*'shpet-slə*) means "little sparrow" in German; small dumplings or tiny noodles, boiled and often served with a sauce or in soups or other dishes.

 Recipes Find out more about international recipes at this book's Online Learning Center at glencoe.com.

- **Three Pans** Place two pans on one rack in diagonally opposite corners. Place the third pan on another rack in a different corner.

- **Four Pans** Place two pans on one rack in diagonally opposite corners. Place the other two pans on another rack in the other diagonal corners.

✓ **Reading Check** **Predict** What might happen to a baked product if you did not preheat the oven?

Bread Basics

Why is pita bread flat, but bagels are not? Understanding baking can help you appreciate all kinds of breads!

Types of Bread

Breads fit in three categories, depending on their leavening agent.

- A **yeast bread** is a bread in which the leavening agent is yeast. Bread, bagels, and breadsticks are yeast breads.

- A **quick bread** is a bread in which the leavening agent is baking powder or baking soda. They mix and rise faster than yeast breads. Pancakes, muffins, and some loaf breads are quick breads.

- A **flat bread** is a bread made with little or no leavening agent. Naan, pita bread, and tortillas are flat breads.

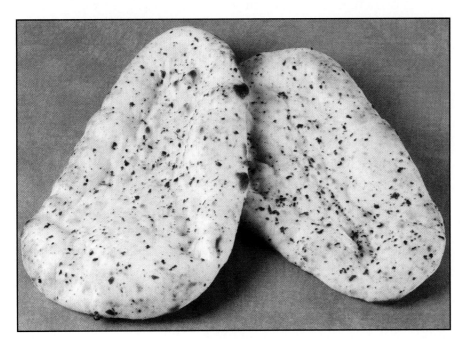

Flat Bread Naan is a popular flat bread in India. It is often served with meals. *What type of bread do you eat with meals?*

Making Quick Breads

Most quick breads are mixed by the muffin method or the biscuit method.

Muffins and More

Muffins, banana bread, cornbread, waffles, and pancakes are prepared with the muffin method. In the **muffin method**, the liquids and dry ingredients are mixed separately and then stirred together until just combined.

The muffin method has three steps:

♦ Sift together all dry ingredients to combine them evenly.

♦ Blend liquid ingredients separately.

♦ Add liquid ingredients to dry ingredients. Stir just until the dry ingredients are moistened, leaving some lumps.

Spoon the batter into a loaf pan or divide the batter evenly among the muffin cups. Bake according to recipe directions.

Check the crust of muffins and quick bread loaves for doneness. It should be golden brown, slightly rough, and shiny. The sides should pull away slightly from the sides of the pan. When the top is tapped gently, it should feel firm. A toothpick inserted in the center will come out clean.

Before removing muffins and loaves from the pan, loosen them by running a spatula around the edges.

For pancakes, pour about ¼ cup (60 mL) batter onto a lightly greased hot skillet or griddle. Turn with a turner when the tops are bubbly and the edges appear dry. The cooked side should be golden brown. Cook briefly on the other side.

Biscuits

The biscuit method of mixing gives biscuits a flaky texture. In the **biscuit method**, fat is cut into dry ingredients, liquid is added, and the dough is kneaded. To make biscuit dough:

♦ Sift the dry ingredients together in a mixing bowl.

♦ Cut the shortening into dry ingredients using a pastry blender, two table knives, or a fork. Stop when the mixture looks like coarse crumbs.

♦ Mix in the liquid ingredients with a fork just until blended. Gently knead dough when the mixture comes away from the side of the bowl.

Kneading the dough helps develop the gluten. To **knead** means to work dough by repeatedly folding, pressing, and turning it.

Roll and cut biscuits after kneading and bake. Biscuits are done when lightly browned on top and lighter, creamy color on the sides. They should double in size and have straight sides.

Food Prep How To

KNEAD BISCUIT DOUGH

Turn the dough out onto a clean, lightly floured surface.

STEP 1

1 Gently fold the dough in half.

2 Push down on the dough with the heels of both hands.

STEP 2

3 Fold the dough over, give it a quarter turn, and press it again. Continue to knead by repeating the folding and pushing process.

STEP 3

TIP Knead biscuit dough for only about 30 seconds. If you knead too long, the biscuits will be tough.

Food Prep How To

ROLL AND CUT BISCUITS

1 Using light, gentle strokes, roll the dough out to an even thickness, in a circle ½-inch (1.2 cm) thick.

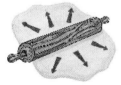

2 Dip the cutter in flour. Cut the biscuits, pushing straight down.

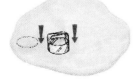

TIP Flour keeps the dough from sticking to the cutter. Cutting straight down will give you evenly shaped biscuits.

3 Use a spatula or turner to put the biscuits onto the baking sheet. Leave about 1 inch (2.5 cm) space between the biscuits.

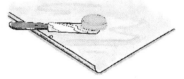

4 Push the leftover dough together. Do not knead it.

TIP Kneading the dough again would make the gluten too strong. The biscuits would be tough.

5 Roll and cut more biscuits.

Making Yeast Breads

Making yeast bread from scratch takes several hours. For most of the time, the dough is sitting and rising. The typical steps for making yeast bread from scratch are shown in **Figure 32-1**.

✓ Reading Check) **Suggest** What could happen if you did not take enough time to knead your dough?

| **Figure 32.1** | **Steps in Making Yeast Bread** |

Homemade Yeast Bread Mixing, kneading, and baking yeast bread can be a cozy way to spend a rainy Saturday afternoon. *What happens as you knead dough?*

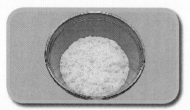
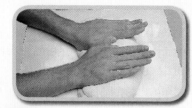
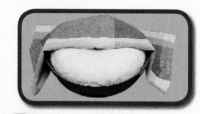

1 Combine the ingredients as directed in the recipe. The ingredients should be at room temperature. Add dry yeast to warm water. Always use a thermometer to measure liquid temperature before adding yeast. Yeast dies at temperatures above 140°F (60°C). When the mixture bubbles, it is ready to use.

2 Knead the dough for several minutes. It will become satiny and elastic with little bubbles under the surface.

3 Let the dough rise. Cover it with a cloth. Set it in a warm place. It will double in size as gas bubbles form and grow (about 1 to 2 hours).

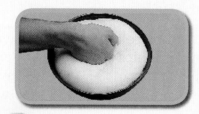
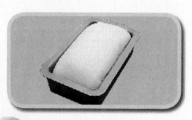

4 Punch down the dough. Gently press your fist in the center. Pull the dough from the sides of the bowl and press down again. This works out the large air bubbles.

5 Shape the dough into loaves or rolls. Place the dough into a pan or onto a baking sheet. Let the dough rise again.

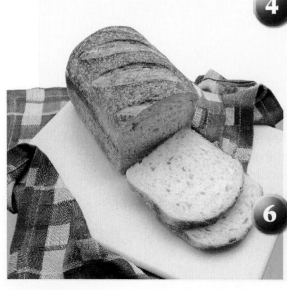

6 Bake according to the recipe directions. Bread is done if it sounds hollow when you tap it. An instant-read thermometer will read 210°F (100°C).

Faster Bread Making

You can speed up the process of baking bread with convenience products and even microwaving.

Baking with Convenience

Convenience products make bread baking easy.

◆ **Dry Mixes** Use a boxed mix. You usually just need to stir in liquid, then finish the preparation.

◆ **Refrigerated Batter or Dough** Refrigerated dough is ready to bake. Frozen dough is usually placed on a greased pan to thaw and rise before baking.

◆ **Brown-and-Serve** These rolls and breads just need to be heated to brown them.

Speed up your bread baking with appliances, too. A bread machine will mix, knead, and bake bread dough. Some electric mixers have a dough hook for kneading.

Microwaving Hints

A microwave oven can be helpful, use it to warm ingredients, thaw frozen bread dough, or warm baked yeast breads.

Microwaving works for muffins and other quick breads. They are more moist, rise higher, and bake faster than in a conventional oven. They do not brown, however. The basic steps:

◆ Fill containers half full. If you do not have a microwave-safe muffin pan, arrange custard cups on a plate.

◆ Put containers on a rack or inverted saucer to let the air circulate underneath.

◆ Rotate containers during cooking for even baking.

◆ Since baked goods do not brown, use batters with color— pumpkin bread, for example—or add a topping.

✓ Reading Check) **Suggest** What convenience products could you use to make homemade bread quickly?

Store Bread and Ingredients

Get the best results by buying and storing ingredients properly.

◆ **Flour** If the recipe does not specify a type, use all-purpose flour. Store all flour in a cool, dry place.

◆ **Sweeteners** Choose the sweetener called for in the recipe. Store in a tightly closed container in a cool, dry place.

◆ **Leavening Agents** Active dry yeast comes in packages that do not need refrigeration until they are opened. Store baking soda and baking powder covered in a cool, dry place.

Store Homemade Bread

Breads stay freshest in airtight containers, aluminum foil, or plastic bags at room temperature in a dry place. In hot, humid weather, yeast bread should be refrigerated to prevent it from molding. Enjoy home-prepared breads within a few days of baking. For longer storage, freeze them.

✓ Reading Check **Explain** How would you store bread?

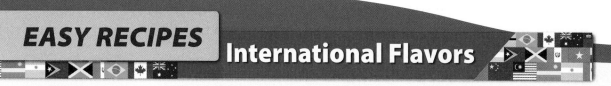

EASY RECIPES — International Flavors

Soft Pretzels

Customary	Ingredients	Metric
1½ cups	Warm water	375 mL
1⅛ tsp.	Dry active yeast	6 mL
2 Tbsp.	Brown sugar	30 mL
1¼ tsp.	Salt	6 mL
3 cups	All-purpose flour	750 mL
1 cup	Whole wheat flour	250 mL
1	Egg, lightly beaten	1

Try This!

Top pretzels with sea salt or cinnamon and sugar just before you put them in the oven. Or serve baked pretzels with mustard.

Yield: 8 pretzels

1. Line 2 large baking sheets with parchment paper and set aside. Pour the warm water into a large mixing bowl. Sprinkle the yeast on top and stir to dissolve and let stand until mixture is foamy.

2. Stir in sugar and salt. Add flours to bowl and mix well. Turn dough out onto a lightly floured surface and knead until satiny and smooth. Set dough in a greased bowl and allow to rise until double in size, for at least 30 minutes.

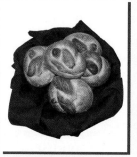

3. When the dough has risen, punch it down and divide it into eight equal pieces. Roll each piece into a 16-inch-long rope. Twist each rope into a pretzel shape. (To form pretzels, shape each rope into a U; cross the two sides of the U over each other, twist and press the ends down on the pretzel.) Place pretzels on the prepared baking sheet and cover lightly with a cloth. Allow to rise again in a warm place for at least 15 minutes. Preheat oven to 425°F (218°C).

4. Brush the tops of the pretzels generously with lightly beaten egg. Bake the pretzels until golden brown, about 10 minutes.

Nutritional Information Per Serving: 201 calories, 1 g total fat (0 g saturated fat), 26 mg cholesterol, 462 mg sodium, 43 g total carbohydrate (2 g fiber, 7 g sugars), 6 g protein

Percent Daily Value: vitamin A 0%, vitamin C 0%, calcium 2%, iron 15%

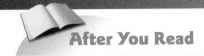

After You Read

CHAPTER SUMMARY

Flour, liquid, fat, sugar, salt, eggs, and leavening agents are the basic ingredients in baked goods. Understanding leavening agents and gluten helps make baking successful. Follow recipe instructions for combining ingredients, preparing pans, and baking. Breads fit into three categories: quick breads, yeast breads, and flat breads. Convenience products can save time for homemade bread. Bread and baking ingredients need to be purchased wisely and stored properly.

Vocabulary Review

1. **Use each of these vocabulary words in a sentence.**

Content Vocabulary
- self-rising flour (p. 466)
- batter (p. 466)
- dough (p. 466)
- leavening agent (p. 467)
- extract (p. 467)
- yeast (p. 468)
- gluten (p. 469)
- yeast bread (p. 471)
- quick bread (p. 471)
- flat bread (p. 471)
- muffin method (p. 472)
- biscuit method (p. 472)
- knead (p. 472)

Academic Vocabulary
- enhance (p. 467)
- consistent (p. 468)

Review Key Concepts

2. **Explain** the purpose of the ingredients in baking.
3. **Discuss** the food science of leavening and gluten.
4. **Summarize** skills for successful baking.
5. **Compare** methods for making quick and yeast breads.
6. **Identify** ways to store bread and baking ingredients for freshness.

Critical Thinking

7. **Revise** a bread recipe that uses all-purpose flour. What might happen to its nutritional value, color, and texture if you substituted whole-wheat flour?
8. **Explain** how you might reply if your friend says, I've never seen my grandmother measure anything, and her baked goods turn out great. Why should I measure accurately?"
9. **Predict** what might happen to dry yeast if the water you add is too hot or too cold.

Real-World Skills and Applications

Problem Solving

10. Plan a Bake Sale Imagine that you are helping organize a bake sale as a school fundraiser. Write a plan for where you could go for advice, what events you could organize, and how you could boost the nutritional value of foods at the bake sale.

Collaborative and Interpersonal

11. Breads Around the World Follow your teacher's instructions to form small groups. Create a bulletin board or poster showing the many different types of bread eaten around the world: quick breads, yeast breads, and flat breads. Show a picture of the breads and a map of the country or region they come from.

Technology

12. Home Baking Show Write the script for a PowerPoint presentation. Show how to use storebought dough in creative ways. Create an outline or storyboard, then develop the presentaton. Show it in class. Have other students take notes and share their ideas.

Financial Literacy

13. Wraps—A Sandwich Alternative Instead of making sandwiches with two pieces of bread, consider instead making a wrap with a tortilla. If a loaf of bread costs $2.49 and will make 9 sandwiches, and a pack of 12 tortillas costs $1.30, would buying tortillas instead of bread be cost-effective?

14. Share with a Child Find a children's book about bread. Read it with a child and talk together about how bread is made. What information will you share? How can you keep the child's attention? Write a brief summary about the book and the experience.

15. Kitchen Test Pour ¼ cup (60 mL) water into each of two glasses and ¼ cup (60 mL) lemon juice into a third. Add ½ teaspoon (2 mL) baking powder to one glass of water. Add ¼ teaspoon (1 mL) baking soda to the other glass of water. Add ¼ teaspoon (1 mL) baking soda to the lemon juice. Write your observations, explanation, and conclusions.

> **NSES A** Develop abilities necessary to do scientific inquiry.

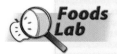

16. Muffin Experiment Prepare two batches of muffins, one by mixing muffin batter just until the flour is moistened and the other by mixing the batter until it has a smooth consistency. Bake both batches. Compare your results in appearance, texture, and flavor. Write your conclusions.

Additional Activities For additional activities go to this book's Online Learning Center at glencoe.com.

Academic Skills

 English Language Arts

17. Essay on Baking Many people consider bread-making a hobby. Others call it an art, a science, or a creative experience. Write an essay that explains how it can be all four. Use examples to make your points. In your essay, include an opening, body, and closing.

> **NCTE 12** Use language to accomplish individual purposes.

 Social Studies

18. Real Bagels Bagels are made by first boiling them, then baking them. This gives them the crusty outside with the doughy inside. Conduct research to find out what other bread products have crusty exteriors with doughy insides. Find out what they taste like and where they were developed. Write a report on your findings.

> **NCSS IX A** Explain how cultural elements can facilitate global understanding.

 Mathematics

19. Serving Sizes When you read the nutrition label for a loaf of bread, values will often be listed for a serving size of one slice. What if you eat two slices? What if you eat half of one slice? If a serving of whole wheat bread has 70 calories, 12 g of carbohydrates, and 4 g of protein, how many calories, carbohydrates, and protein will be in two slices and ½ of a slice?

Math Concept Multiply and divide numbers to increase or decrease proportions.

Starting Hint If 1 slice is a serving, multiply the calories, carbohydrates, and protein by 2 for 2 servings. Divide the calories, carbohydrates, and protein by 2 for ½ serving.

 For more math help, go to the Math Appendix

> **NCTM Number and Operations** Understand the meaning of operations and how they relate to one another.

STANDARDIZED TEST PRACTICE

MULTIPLE CHOICE
Read the paragraph and write an answer on a separate piece of paper:

Reading bread and bread products labels is important. Even some loaves labeled as all-natural have high fructose corn syrup or other chemicals in the ingredients list. Another thing to check is the expiration or sell-by date. Keep an eye out for mold as this date approaches. You may wish to store bread in the freezer to keep it past the expiration date, although bread does not taste quite as good when defrosted.

20. Based on the paragraph, which of the following is true?
   a. There is no such thing as all-natural bread anymore.
   b. Bread is no longer good after its expiration date.
   c. You can keep breads longer by freezing them.
   d. Defrosted bread has lost important nutrients.

> **Test-Taking Tip** Try to avoid talking about a test with other students right before taking it. Test anxiety can be contagious.

CHAPTER 33
Mixed Foods and Snacks

Explore the Photo ▶▶
Chances are, some of your favorite foods include sandwiches, pizza, and snack foods. *What are your favorites?*

Writing Activity

Step-by-Step Guide

Soups, Stews, and Casseroles, Oh My!
Mixed dishes are prepared in steps that a cook must follow. Write a step-by-step guide for a mixed dish that you enjoy. It can be a soup, stew, casserole, or another type of dish that requires multiple steps. Be clear and concise. Follow the standard recipe format.

Writing Tips

1. **Explain** terms the reader may not know.

2. **Write** the steps in chronological order.

3. **Use** appropriate transition words and precise verbs.

Reading Guide

Before You Read

Pace Yourself Short blocks of concentrated reading are more effective than one long session. Focus on reading for ten minutes. Take a short break. Then, read for another 10 minutes.

Read to Learn

Key Concepts

- **Explain** how to prepare sandwiches for nutrition and flavor.
- **List** guidelines for preparing a nourishing pizza.
- **Describe** five nourishing snacks you could make.
- **Describe** how to make nutritious, flavorful soups and stews
- **List** nourishing and easy casseroles, skillet dinners, and stir-fries.
- **Explain** three ways to thicken soups, stews, and other food mixtures.

Main Idea

Combination foods—sandwiches, pizza, stews, casseroles, and others—are nourishing and flavorful. Make these dishes from scratch or with convenience foods.

Content Vocabulary

◇ spread
◇ open-face sandwich
◇ bisque
◇ stock
◇ chowder
◇ stew
◇ gelatinization

Academic Vocabulary

You will find these words in your reading and on your tests. Use the glossary to look up their definitions if necessary.

■ specified
■ original

Graphic Organizer

How To Thicken Soups and Stews	Problems that May Occur	Solutions

 Graphic Organizer Go to this book's Online Learning Center at glencoe.com to print out this graphic organizer.

Academic Standards ▪

 English Language Arts
NCTE 7 Conduct research and gather, evaluate, and synthesize data to communicate discoveries.
NCTE 9 Develop an understanding of diversity in language use across cultures.

 Science
NSES Content Standard A Develop abilities necessary to do scientific inquiry.

 Social Studies
NCSS IX A Explain how cultural elements can facilitate global understanding.

 Mathematics
NCTM Number and Operations Compute fluently and make reasonable estimates.

NCTE National Council of Teachers of English
NCTM National Council of Teachers of Mathematics

NSES National Science Education Standards
NCSS National Council for the Social Studies

Super Sandwiches

Sandwiches are convenient and easy anytime—for any meal or snack. Depending on the fillings, a sandwich can be a complete meal!

Each ingredient in a sandwich provides, or supplies, nutrients. A sandwich can provide complex carbohydrates and B vitamins from bread (fiber, too, if whole grain); calcium and protein from cheese; vitamins A and C and fiber from vegetables and fruit; and protein and iron from foods such as lean meat, turkey, tuna, eggs, or beans.

Stock Up for Sandwich Making

You can put almost anything in a sandwich. Keep a variety of ingredients handy. Sandwiches have four main components.

♦ **Bread** Sliced bread, rolls, pita bread, bagels, tortillas, and English muffins are just a few of your options.

♦ **Spreads** A **spread** is used on bread to add flavor and moisture. Mayonnaise, butter, margarine, and pesto are spreads with more fat and calories; spread them on thinly. Try lower-fat or fat-free alternatives. Try chutney, fruit spread, relish, mustard, or hummus on sandwiches.

♦ **Main Fillings** Fill sandwiches with sliced lean deli meats, cheese, tuna, chicken, peanut butter, or tofu. Hard cook eggs for egg salad sandwiches, or cook hamburger or salmon patties for burgers. Shop for lean and low-fat choices.

♦ **Extra Fillings** Sliced tomatoes, green or red peppers, onions and lettuce are common favorites. Try sliced zucchini, chopped avocado, shredded carrots, drained sauerkraut, or spinach leaves. Add fruit, perhaps apple or banana slices.

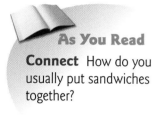

▷Vocabulary

You can find definitions in the glossary at the back of this book.

As You Read

Connect How do you usually put sandwiches together?

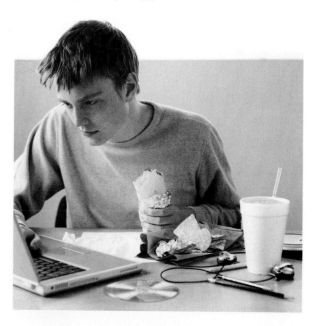

A Taco Is a Sandwich! Sandwiches can go beyond deli meat and two slices of bread. *What sandwiches from different ethnic cuisines have you tried?*

Build Great Sandwiches

You do not need a recipe for most sandwiches. Just add spread to bread, stack or stuff it with fillings, and perhaps add a top slice of bread. An **open-face sandwich** has only a bottom slice of bread.

Other sandwiches, especially hot ones such as burgers, take more cooking skills. Hot or cold, light or hearty—be creative!

Cold Sandwiches

◆ **Stack** a hero, sub, hoagie, grinder, or poor boy. Layer these long sandwiches with meat, cheese, and sliced veggies.

◆ **Pack** pitas. Fill them with salad mixtures. Hummus, tahini, and falafel make a filling vegetarian pita. Try mashed avocado topped with lettuce, red onion and tomato slices.

◆ **Wrap** it up. A wrap is flat bread rolled around filling. Try lean turkey, Monterey Jack cheese, shredded lettuce and carrots, and salsa in a corn tortilla.

Hot Sandwiches

◆ **Grill** a sandwich. Lightly coat the outside surfaces of bread with vegetable oil spray, margarine, or butter. Cook one side in a skillet until golden brown, then cook the other side. Add sliced tomato to grilled cheese sandwiches for more nutrients.

◆ **Spoon** sloppy joe filling or barbecued meat onto whole wheat buns. Brown lean ground beef, turkey, or soy crumbles, drain, then simmer in sauce.

◆ **Broil** open-face tuna melts. Spread tuna salad on English muffin halves and top with green bell peppers and low-fat cheese. Then broil until the cheese melts.

◆ **Pan broil** a lean burger. Cook to an internal temperature of 160°F (71°C). Serve on a bun with vegetables.

Sandwiches—By Other Names

Burritos, quesadillas, and spring rolls are sandwiches. A sandwich is any filling put in or on bread or another wrapper.

◆ **Gyros** are Greek. The filling is seasoned, cooked lamb, chopped tomato, and cucumber-yogurt dressing, stuffed in a pita pocket.

◆ **Calzones** are hand-held pizza variations with Italian origins. Dough is folded over the filling, sealed, then baked.

◆ **Spring rolls** (egg rolls) from Asia are chopped vegetables, meat, poultry, or fish rolled in pastry wrappers, then fried or steamed.

Restaurant Manager

Restaurant managers may run a sandwich or pizza place, or a full-service restaurant. They coordinate all activities in a restaurant.

Careers Find out more about careers. Go to this book's Online Learning Center at glencoe.com.

◆ **Empanadas** from Spain and South America are single-serving turnovers. Meat or vegetable filling is folded inside pastry crust, then baked. A similar British food is called a Cornish pasty.

Sandwiches on the Go

Sandwiches are portable! Pack ingredients such as lettuce and tomato separately to keep them fresh. Tuck them into sandwiches just before eating. That also keeps sandwiches from getting soggy. Keep sandwiches chilled for freshness and safety—especially in warm weather.

Most cold sandwiches can be made ahead of time. Wrap them in plastic or foil or put them in zippered plastic bags so they do not dry out. Refrigerate them for up to a day, or freeze for up to a week.

Egg salad, mayonnaise, lettuce and other uncooked vegetables lose quality when frozen. Use these ingredients only in refrigerated sandwiches.

✓ **Reading Check** **Recall** What are three ways to add food-group foods to your sandwiches?

Pizza for Meals and Snacks

You can enjoy pizza for any meal or as a snack. You can buy frozen pizzas, order pizza at a restaraunt, or have one delivered to your door. You can also make your own pizza at home, or add extra vegetables to a frozen pizza for added nutrition.

Pizza Packed with Nutrients

Pizza can pack a lot of nutrition into one slice. It can also be high in calories. The nutrients and calories in pizza depend on its ingredients. To make your pizza more healthful, try the following strategies:

◆ Choose whole-grain crust for more fiber, and thin crust for fewer calories.

◆ Pile on vegetable or fruit toppings for vitamins A and C, folate, potassium, and fiber.

◆ Select mostly lean, high-protein Meat and Beans Group options such as ham, lean ground beef, chicken, fish, or grilled tofu for toppings.

◆ Cheese is a good source of calcium and protein. Consider using part-skim mozzarella or other low-fat cheeses to reduce fat and calories.

Make Your Own Pizza

Pizza is simple to make. You need a crust or base, sauce, and your choice of toppings.

◆ **Base** The crust is usually made of yeast dough, rolled or patted. It can be thick or thin. You can buy a refrigerated or frozen crust. Follow the package directions for preparing it. Some types are already rolled in a circle. Others are folded and need to be pressed into a pan. Use a flat, round pizza pan or a shallow, rectangular baking pan. You can also use English muffins, bagel halves, sliced French bread, or pita bread.

◆ **Sauce** Spread sauce evenly over the crust. Try canned pasta sauce, taco sauce, ketchup, barbecue sauce, salsa, pesto sauce, hoisin sauce, or just oil and herbs. You can make your own pizza sauce by mixing canned tomato puree with dried herbs such as oregano, basil, and thyme. On fruit pizza, use pureed fruit or cranberry sauce for the sauce.

◆ **Seasonings** Add flavor with fresh or dry herbs, such as oregano, basil, rosemary, sage, garlic, or chili flakes; spices such as cinnamon or nutmeg on fruit pizzas; or sun-dried tomatoes or chile peppers.

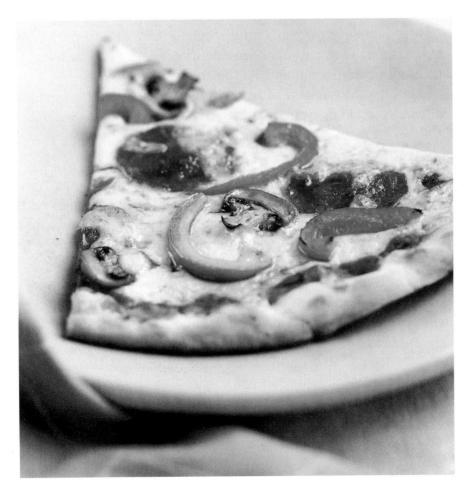

Create a Pizza! When you have an urge for a special pizza, try making it. Ready-made crusts and canned sauce cut down on preparation time. *What pizza combination would provide foods from all food groups?*

◆ **Toppings** Add any toppings you like. Be creative! Add vegetables like tomatoes, broccoli, eggplant, bell pepper, zucchini, or carrot; and leafy greens such as spinach or arugula. Fruit might include sliced pears, apples, pineapple, mandarin orange segments, or dried fruit. Protein-rich foods like ground beef, sausage, ham, chicken, shrimp, salmon, tofu, tempeh, or canned drained beans add nutrition and taste. Top your pizza with grated or shredded mozzarella, cheddar, Swiss, feta, gouda, and soy cheese. Choose two cheeses for variety. Consider using low-fat cheese.

Bake your pizza in a conventional oven until lightly brown. Baking time depends on the ingredients. This generally takes about 20 minutes at 425°F (218°C) for an unbaked crust. English muffin pizzas with pre-cooked toppings need to be heated in a microwave or toaster oven only until the cheese melts.

Pizza freezes well and reheats easily in a conventional, microwave, or toaster oven. Lay pizza on a paper towel in a microwave oven so the crust does not get soggy.

✓ **Reading Check** **Identify** What are some quick ways to make pizza at home?

Great Snacks

Most people enjoy snacking. Snacks can satisfy between-meal hunger. They can also provide food energy and nutrients. The health benefits depend on the snacks you choose.

Snack foods are sold almost anywhere. Use your nutrition knowledge and consumer skills to make smart choices.

Snack Nutrition

Snacks can be light or filling, depending on your needs. Wise snacks provide nutrient-dense foods from MyPyramid's five food groups. Well-chosen snacks supply food-group foods that you miss at mealtime. For example, for more whole grains, you can snack on crunchy whole-wheat crackers.

All kinds of whole grains, fruits, vegetables, and yogurt make excellent snacks. These foods provide important nutrients, yet usually have fewer calories, less fat, and less added sugar than processed foods. Keep some on hand at home.

What about chips, candy bars, and soft drinks? They usually are high in calories, fat, added sugar, or sodium—with few if any other nutrients. Enjoy them in small amounts occasionally, not daily. Avoid impulse snacking by keeping nutritious, low-fat snacks on hand to eat instead.

Easy Snacks

Many nutrient-rich snacks come ready to eat: fresh fruit, raw vegetables, low-fat yogurt and cheese, rice cakes, whole-grain crackers, hard-cooked eggs, peanut butter, and nuts. Other tasty snacks require a few simple steps. Try these healthy snacks:

- **Spread for Crackers or Celery Sticks** Try cottage cheese mixed with chopped fruits, vegetables, or herbs. Make a hearty spread of mashed cooked beans, cilantro or parsley, and other seasonings.

- **Yogurt Dip** Mix plain yogurt or low-fat cottage cheese with minced onion, garlic powder, chopped parsley, dill, chopped chives, or chili powder.

- **Fruit Dip** Blend ½ cup (125 mL) mashed fruit with 1 cup (250 mL) vanilla low-fat yogurt. Mix in 1 tablespoon (15 mL) honey. Serve with fruit chunks or small whole fruit.

- **Tortilla Points** Spray a corn tortilla lightly with vegetable oil spray. Sprinkle on 1 tablespoon (15 mL) Parmesan cheese and 1 teaspoon (5 mL) sesame seeds. Cut the tortilla in triangles. Bake at 350°F (180°C) until the cheese melts and the tortilla triangles are crisp.

- **Popcorn** Buy already-popped corn or ready-pop corn for the microwave oven. For the least fat, pop your own in a hot-air popper or a microwave oven popper. For more flavor, season plain popcorn with herbs or spices.

- **Trail Mix** Trail mix is a dry snack mix. Combine any of these: nuts, seeds, dried fruit, pretzels, mini-crackers, coconut, and dry cereal.

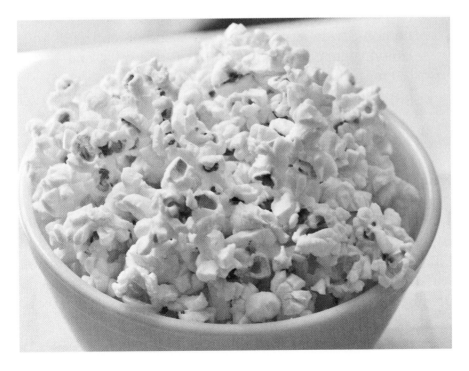

Snack Smart! Make your own snack food shopping list. Include nutrient-dense food-group foods not too high in fat, sugar, or sodium. *What are the advantages of planning ahead for snacking?*

More Snack Ideas

◆ Make a small salad, or have a cup of soup.

◆ Make a mini-sandwich.

◆ Have a small serving of leftovers, such as a pizza slice.

◆ Add fresh or canned fruit to yogurt or cottage cheese.

✓ **Reading Check** **Review** What nutritional benefits can snacks offer?

Snack Beverages

Beverages make great snacks. They help fulfill your body's need for water. Beverages with fruit or vegetable juices, milk, or yogurt provide many nutrients. (See **Figure 33.1.**)

Coffee drinks, tea, and soft drinks such as cola supply few or no vitamins and minerals. Instead, they may supply a lot of added sugar. Many also contain caffeine, a substance that stimulates the nervous system. Too much caffeine or sugar can make some people anxious or unable to sleep. For this reason, you should avoid foods and drinks with caffeine late in the day.

Creating fruit juice combinations is fun. A mixture of fruit juices is called fruit punch. Add chilled seltzer water to make it sparkle. For garnish, float lemon or orange slices in the punch.

Blender Shakes

Make delicious and nutritious shakes. Combine fruit, fruit juice, milk, and yogurt. Blend on high speed in a blender or food processor until smooth. Try these:

◆ **Banana Shake** Cut a ripe banana in chunks; freeze. Blend frozen banana with ⅔ cup (150 mL) fat-free milk.

◆ **Lemon-Strawberry Smoothie** Blend ½ cup (125 mL) lemon yogurt, ½ cup (125 mL) fat-free milk, and ¼ cup (60 mL) sliced strawberries.

◆ **Sunshine Shake** Blend ¾ cup (175 mL) chilled pineapple or orange juice, ¼ cup (60 mL) plain fat-free or low-fat yogurt, 2 teaspoons (10 mL) honey, and 3 crushed ice cubes.

Hot Beverages

A hot beverage on a cold day helps warm you up. You can heat apple cider or drink hot tea with milk. Cocoa made with milk is popular, too. Follow the guidelines for cooking with milk in Chapter 27. If spices such as cinnamon or cloves are simmered with the beverage, it is called a mulled drink. To mull, simmer a mixture for at least 10 minutes to blend the flavors. Serve hot in mugs. Garnish with a cinnamon stick or citrus slice.

Figure 33.1 | **Beverage Snack Nutrition**

Beverage Choices Compare the calories in an 8-ounce (250 mL) drink. *Which beverages do you choose most often? What beverages may be the best choices for nutrition?*

Beverage	Calories	Nutrients
Yogurt Fruit Smoothie	180	Protein calcium, vitamins C and D, riboflavin
Cola, Regular	100	
Unsweetened Tea or Black Coffee	0	
Tomato Juice	40	Vitamins A and C, folate
Flavored Calorie-Free Water	0	
Vitamin C-Fortified Grape Drink	130	Vitamin C
Hot Cocoa with Milk	190	Protein, calcium, vitamins C and D, riboflavin
Orange Juice	110	Vitamin C, potassium
Thick Vanilla Shake	294	Protein, fat, calcium

Microwave Beverages Pay careful attention when microwaving beverages, especially those with milk. Some develop, or create, a surface film, which lets steam build up underneath. Hot liquid may spurt from the container, causing burns. Stir before microwaving to prevent this. Stir again after microwaving to blend hotter and cooler parts of the liquid.

◆ Use 100% power when heating a beverage unless the recipe specifies a different power level.

◆ Reheat hot beverages. One serving takes about 1½ minutes at 100% power. Two servings may take about 3 minutes.

✓ Reading Check **Explain** How could snack beverages contribute to a healthful eating plan?

Soup or Stew—For Variety

Nutritious and flavorful, soups and stews are also very versatile.

◆ **Bisque** is a thick, rich soup made with finely mashed or ground seafood, poultry, or vegetables. Bisques are traditionally made with butter and cream.

◆ **Stock**, or broth is seasoned liquid from cooking meat, fish, or vegetables. Bouillon and consommé are like broth, but clarified, or cleared of food solids.

◆ **Chowder** is a thick, chunky soup made with vegetables, fish, or seafood.

◆ **Stew** is a thick, hearty mixture of chunky vegetables and perhaps meat, poultry, or fish cooked slowly in liquid.

◆ **Chilled fruit** soups are sweet and refreshing. Strawberries, peaches, and melons make delicate soups.

What Is in the Bowl?

Many soups and stews include nutrient-dense foods from two or more food groups:

- ◆ **Grain Products** Rice, barley, pasta, and other grain products are hearty additions. They add B vitamins, iron, fiber, and complex carbohydrates. The starch acts as a thickener.

- ◆ **Vegetables and Fruits** Vegetables and fruits provide flavor, color, vitamins, minerals, fiber, and interesting textures.

- ◆ **Dairy Foods** Creamy soups, such as bisques and chowders, are made with milk, yogurt, or cheese, and provide calcium and protein.

- ◆ **Meat, Beans, and More** Meat, poultry, fish, cooked dry beans, or tofu turn simple soups into protein-rich meals.

Create Soups or Stews

Go beyond using a can opener! Try making soups and stews from scratch. Some take time, so plan ahead. Others can be prepared quickly.

Make Stock and Broth-Based Soups and Stews

You can buy canned broth, or stock, or make your own. Here is how: Cook meat or poultry—such as a whole stewing chicken, or pork or beef shoulder—slowly in a covered pot of liquid. Add onion, celery, carrots, herbs, and spices for flavor. Bring it to a boil. Lower the heat, and simmer gently until the meat is tender or the chicken falls off the bones. Let the broth cool, strain it, and skim fat off the top. You can use some of the meat or poultry in the stew or soup and save some for a salad or casserole.

As You Read

Connect What type of soup or stew do you eat most often?

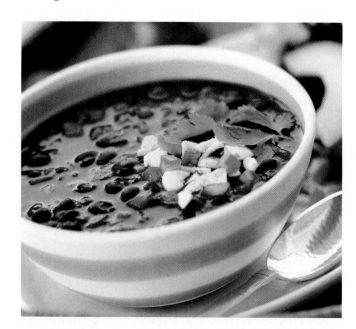

Soups and Stews Around the World People in cultures all over the world make great-tasting, nutrient-rich soups and stews. *What soups or stews can you name from another region of the United States, or from another country or culture?*

Make Milk-Based Soups

Creamy soups, such as chowder and bisque, are made with milk or cream, or with a white sauce. Take special care when you cook with milk so it does not scorch or curdle. Heat milk-based soups over low heat. Add acidic ingredients such as tomato sauce very slowly to hot milk while stirring to avoid curdling.

Try Chilled Soup

To make chilled fruit soup, start with fresh, canned, or frozen fruit. Use a blender or food processor to puree one or more types of fruit. Blend in juice, yogurt, or milk, plus spices such as cinnamon, nutmeg, or cloves. Refrigerate. You can also make chilled pumpkin, squash, or other vegetable soups.

Time-Saving Tips for Homemade Soups and Stews

Manage time by making a large batch of soup or stew. Freeze what you do not eat for later. To save preparation time:

◆ Use canned broth or bouillon cubes in place of homemade stock.

◆ Use canned, frozen, or leftover cooked vegetables or fruit.

◆ Add leftover meat or poultry to soup or stew.

◆ Cook part or all of the recipe in a microwave oven.

Keep Nutrition High

Soups and stews provide nutrients from their flavorful ingredients. To add nutrients and variety, yet keep fat and sodium low:

◆ Use fat-free evaporated milk or buttermilk instead of cream in creamed soups.

◆ Stir nonfat dry milk or low-fat or fat-free yogurt into creamed soup for more calcium.

◆ Dilute condensed soups with low-fat or fat-free milk instead of water.

◆ Thicken soups with pureed vegetables or other starchy foods such as legumes, potatoes, pasta, barley, or rice.

◆ Use herbs and spices to add flavor.

Convenience Soups and Stews

For quick meals, keep convenience soups and stews on hand. Check labels for directions. Many canned and frozen soups and stews just need heating. Condensed soup, however, has some of the water removed in processing. To prepare it, add water or milk before heating. Dehydrated soup has all natural moisture removed. Add liquid, then heat.

Prepared soups and stews can be high in fat and sodium. Check the Nutrition Facts panel on food labels.

To add your own touch to convenience soups or stews:

◆ **Combine Several Canned Soups** Choose flavors that go together—perhaps vegetable soup with chicken soup. Add the amount of liquid **specified**, or listed, on each can.

◆ **Add Ingredients** Mix in leftover cooked meat, poultry, fish, vegetables, rice, or pasta. Add herbs and spices.

Storing Soups and Stews

Cover and refrigerate cooked soups and use them in two to three days. You can also freeze small batches of soup or stew in covered plastic bowls or freezer bags for up to three months.

Store canned soups and packaged mixes in a cool, dry place. Keep frozen soups in the freezer until you are ready to prepare them.

✓ **Reading Check** **Recall** If you were in a hurry, what type of soup could you make?

Mixed Main Dishes

A mixed main dish combines a variety of ingredients for a hearty meal. Mixed dishes have several benefits:

◆ **Economical** These meals may need only small amounts of costly ingredients, such as meat.

◆ **Time-Saving** With some mixtures, you need only one pan or skillet for the whole meal. That saves on cleanup time!

◆ **Nutritious and Appealing** You can make mixed dishes with foods from any and all food groups.

Casserole Creations

A casserole is a type of baking dish. A casserole is also a mixture of foods baked in a casserole dish. You can create a great casserole without a recipe. Use **Figure 34.1** (on page 494) as an ingredient guide.

In a conventional oven, a 1½ quart (1.5 L) casserole usually bakes for about 30 minutes at 350°F (180°C) if the ingredients are precooked. Cover the casserole until the last 15 minutes. Then remove the cover for browning.

To microwave casseroles, spread the mixture evenly in the dish. Stir or turn the dish halfway through the cooking time and again at the end. Cover it to hold in moisture.

Quick and Simple Skillet Meals

Simply combine ingredients in a skillet, as a one-dish meal.

◆ Stir cooked broccoli, sweet red peppers, or other vegetables into macaroni and cheese as the cheese melts.

◆ Prepare a packaged mix of seasoned rice, noodles, or couscous. Stir in leftover cooked vegetables, meat, or poultry.

◆ Simmer browned, drained ground turkey, instant rice, tomato sauce, vegetables, and seasonings.

Super Stir-Fries

Stir-frying is a cooking method. Small pieces of food cook quickly in a small amount of oil over high heat. Food is stirred as it cooks. A dish prepared by stir-frying is called a stir-fry.

You can stir-fry in a skillet, or a wok. A wok is a stir-fry pan with a narrow, round bottom and a wide top.

✓ **Reading Check** **Analyze** How might a mixed main dish simplify meal preparation?

Discover International Foods

India

India's varied geography grows many crops including wheat, rice, legumes, spices, and tropical fruits. Religion significantly influences its cuisine. Hindus do not eat beef; many are vegetarian. Muslims do not eat pork. A typical meal may be a main dish, such as pilau (cooked meat, fish, or vegetables over rice), biryani (seasoned meat, rice, nuts, and raisins), and kababs (skewered meat). Vegetable side dishes, chutney, and rice or bread such as naan or chapatis, often are served, too. Bread is the eating utensil.

Languages Across Cultures

curry (ˈkər-ē) general term that refers to many hot, spicy stews from India. Curry powder, a mixture of spices, is a common ingredient.

dal (ˈdäl) Hindi term for dried peas, beans, and lentils; a dish made with lentils, tomato, onion, and or spices.

 Recipes Find out more about international recipes on this book's Online Learning Center through glencoe.com.

NCTE 9 Develop an understanding of diversity in language use across cultures.

Figure 34.1   **Create Nutritious Casseroles**

Casserole Mix and Match Choose one or more ingredients from each row to create a casserole. The suggested amounts are for a 1½ quart (1.5 L) casserole dish. *What ingredients—and how much—would you mix and match to make a great casserole to fill a 1½ quart casserole dish?*

Type of Ingredient	Total Amount to Use	Examples
Cooked Grain Products These give the casserole its body and help thicken it. They also add flavor, texture, and nutrients: complex carbohydrates, B vitamins, and perhaps fiber.	2-4 cups (500 mL-1 L)	Cooked spaghetti, egg noodles, macaroni, couscous or other pasta, brown or white rice, barley, grits
Vegetables These contribute variety, flavor, texture, appearance, and nutrients: vitamins A and C, and fiber. Starchy vegetables, such as potatoes, can also help thicken it.	1-2 cups (250-500 mL)	Any cooked, canned, or frozen vegetables, such as corn, green beans, peas, carrots, zucchini or yellow squash, broccoli, eggplant, mushrooms, onions, and bell peppers
Lean Meats, Fish, Poultry, Beans, Tofu, Eggs, or Cheese These add protein as well as other nutrients. They also contribute to the casserole's body and appeal.	1-1½ cups (250-350 mL)	Cut-up leftover meat, poultry, or fish; cooked, drained ground beef; canned tuna or salmon; cubed, sliced, or shredded cheese; firm tofu cubes; canned kidney, pinto, or other beans; diced, hard-cooked eggs
Liquid This helps bind, or hold, the ingredients together and adds flavor and nutrients. Different liquids supply different nutrients.	1-1½ cups (250-350 mL)	Broth; fruit or vegetable juice; milk; spaghetti sauce; canned soup such as asparagus, celery, chicken, mushroom, shrimp, tomato, or pea, or white sauce
Toppings These enhance flavor, appearance, and texture. They keep the protein ingredients from drying out.	To taste	Fresh or dry bread crumbs; cracker crumbs; crispy, canned noodles; crushed flake cereal; chopped, toasted nuts; Parmesan cheese; grated cheese
Seasonings and Other Ingredients These add flavor and texture.	¼-½ tsp. (1-3 mL) herbs or spices	Seasonings: Dried or fresh chopped herbs such as oregano, parsley, basil, thyme, or marjoram; ground ginger, mace, cinnamon, chili powder, cayenne or black pepper
	¼-½ cup (60-120 mL) other ingredients	Other Ingredients: Chopped celery, green pepper, onions, nuts, or seeds.

Food Science of Thickening

Many soups, stews and mixed dishes are thickened in these ways:

♦ **Water Evaporation** As liquid boils, water evaporates, producing a thicker stock or sauce. Chefs call this a reduction. Liquid is reduced to less than its **original**, or beginning, volume.

♦ **Pureed Foods** Pureed or mashed vegetables or cooked dry beans thicken food mixtures.

♦ **Starchy Ingredients** Starch in cereal grains (corn, wheat, rice), dry beans, and potatoes is a thickener. Heat flour or cornstarch with liquid to thicken.

Food Prep How To

PREPARE A STIR-FRY

1 Cut vegetables in small, uniform pieces for quick, even cooking. On a separate cutting board, cut meat, poultry, or fish into thin strips.

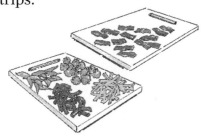

2 Put only a small amount of oil in the wok or skillet. Heat it before adding other ingredients.

3 Cook the pieces of meat, poultry, or fish using high heat, stirring constantly. When done, remove them to a clean plate.

TIP If you use precooked meat, poultry, or fish, skip this step.

4 Begin cooking the vegetable pieces. Cook and stir over high heat until the vegetables begin to wilt.

TIP Start with the tougher vegetables, like carrots. They take longer to cook. Add tender vegetables, like tomatoes, toward the end of this step.

5 When the vegetables are done, add the cooked meat, poultry, or fish, or the firm tofu .

6 Add liquid and seasonings last. Cover the pan and allow the vegetables to steam until tender-crisp.

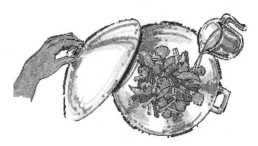

Gelatinization

Starches thicken liquids in a process called **gelatinization**. Starch molecules are too large to dissolve in water. Instead starch clusters, or granules, absorb water and swell as starch molecules loosen. With less liquid outside the granules, the mixture thickens. Once starch mixtures thicken, or gelatinize, and cool, starch becomes firm and rigid if not stirred. It forms a gel and holds its shape.

Starch forms lumps as liquids thicken if starch granules are not evenly dispersed. Granules around the outside swell and form a waterproof gel around the lump. To avoid lumps, first put the starch in a small amount of cold water. Mix it completely. Then pour the starch mixture into hot soup, sauce, or gravy, and blend.

✓ **Reading Check** **Describe** What process allows starch to be used as a thickener?

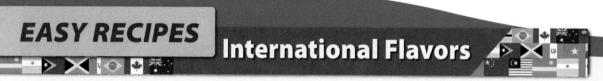

EASY RECIPES — International Flavors

Mulligatawny

Customary	Ingredients	Metric
2 Tbsp.	Vegetable oil	30 mL
2 cup	Onion, finely chopped	500 mL
1 cup	Cooked chicken breast	250 mL
1 tsp.	Coriander	5 mL
1 tsp.	Cumin	5 mL
1½ tsp.	Curry powder	7 mL
4 cups	Low-sodium chicken broth	1 mL
4 cloves	Garlic, minced	4 cloves
1 cup	Dried lentils	250 mL
½ tsp.	Turmeric	2 mL
2 cups	Cooked rice	500 mL

Try This!
This dish is often served with lamb shoulder instead of, or in addition to, the lentils.

Yield: 6 servings, 1½-cups (375 mL) each

❶ In a large stock pot, cook onions in the oil until tender.
❷ Cut chicken into small cubes and add to pot. Add remaining ingredients except rice and simmer, uncovered, for 45 minutes.
❸ Serve in soup bowls over rice.

Nutritional Information Per Serving: 204 calories, 8 g total fat (1 g saturated fat), 9 mg cholesterol, 308 mg sodium, 24 g total carbohydrate (2 g fiber, 3 g sugars), 9 g protein

Percent Daily Value: vitamin A 0%, vitamin 6%, calcium 4%, iron 6%

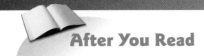

After You Read

CHAPTER SUMMARY

Mixed dishes can provide a variety of nutrients depending on the ingredients you use. For a quick meal or snack, keep a variety of nutrient-dense sandwich ingredients on hand. Whether you buy pizza or make it, boost its nutrition with whole-grain crust and food-group toppings. You can prepare healthful snacks and snack drinks with nourishing ingredients, using little effort. Soups and stews fit in any meal. Prepare them with foods from two or more food groups. Make broth-based soups or stews, milk-based soups and stews, and fruit soups. You can create a tasty, nutritious casserole. Skillet meals and stir-fries are other quick mixed dishes.

Vocabulary Review

1. Use each of these vocabulary words in a sentence.

Content Vocabulary
- spread (p. 482)
- open-face sandwich (p. 483)
- bisque (p. 489)
- stock (p. 489)
- chowder (p. 489)
- stew (p. 489)
- gelatinization (p. 496)

Academic Vocabulary
- specified (p. 492)
- original (p. 495)

Review Key Concepts

2. Explain how to prepare sandwiches and pizza for nutrition and flavor.

3. List guidelines for preparing a nourishing pizza.

4. Describe five nourishing snacks you can make.

5. Describe how to make nutritious, flavorable soups and stews.

6. List nourishing and easy casseroles, skillet dinners, and stir-fries.

7. Explain three ways to thicken soups, stews, and other food mixtures.

Critical Thinking

8. Analyze the pros and cons of choosing diet soft drinks as snack beverages.

9. Create a skillet meal by starting with packages cous cous mix or with uncooked rice and broth.

Real-World Skills and Applications

Goal Setting and Decision Making

10. Sandwich Savvy Adriana tracked her daily meals. She sees that does not eat enough from the Milk, Vegetable, and Fruit Groups. She decided to make changes in her sandwich choices to eat more of these foods. Write descriptions of five sandwiches that could each provide at least two of these food groups.

Collaborative and Interpersonal

11. Reinvent School Pizza Imagine that your school wants to make its popular pepperoni pizza lower in fat and more nutrient-dense. With your teacher's permission, form into groups of three. With your team, create a survey to identify toppings that are nutritious and appeal to students.

Technology

12. Nutrition Database Design a nutrition database using a spreadsheet or database program, for at least ten soups and stews. Make sure to include at least two soups with meat, and two without meat. Show how the ingredients in two cups (500 mL) of each contribute toward MyPyramid food groups, and/or identify significant nutrient contributions.

Financial Literacy

13. Casserole Meat Costs You can save money and satisfy even the pickiest eaters by making a casserole with ground beef at $2.30 per pound, instead of top sirloin steak at $9.99 per pound. Compare the difference in cost of each in one pound and two pound portions.

14. Child Development Plan a sandwich or pizza to make with a young child. Why would it be a good choice? Describe fun learning activities to do with the child as you prepare and eat the food. Why are these activities appropriate for the child's developmental level?

15. Homemade or Convenience? Find a recipe for a popular mixed dish, such as lasagna, tuna casserole, or chicken curry. Then, find a frozen version of the same dish at the store. Compare the ingredients, nutrition, cost per serving, and preparation times. Why might you make or buy this dish? Give your answers in an oral report.

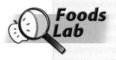
16. Skillful Stir-Frying Prepare two samples of stir-fry vegetables. For one sample, cut vegetables into uniform sizes. For the other, cut vegetables into varying sizes and shapes. Stir-fry both samples for the same amount of time. Compare the texture, flavor, and appearance. Write a report with your conclusions.

Additional Activities For additional activities go to this book's Online Learning Center at **glencoe.com**.

Academic Skills

 English Language Arts

17. A Slice of History Do research to learn about the history of pizza. Learn about its origins and how it became popular in the United States. Compare the Italian and American versions. Write an essay with an opening, body, and close.

> **NCTE 7** Conduct research and gather, evaluate, and synthesize data to communicate discoveries.

 Social Studies

18. Paella Jambalaya was inspired by Spanish paella (pä-'ā-yə). Traditionally this rice dish includes shellfish, chicken, and vegetables cooked with rice. Find and write down two or more versions of this recipe. Note their major differences in preparation and/or ingredients.

> **NCSS IX A** Explain how cultural elements can facilitate global understanding.

 Mathematics

19. Flavored Spreads Go Farther Imagine that you would use 30% less spread if it had more flavor. How much less of each of the following spreads would you need for several people if you added herbs for extra flavor?

- ◆ 4 Tbsp. butter
- ◆ 8 oz. cream cheese

Math Concept To find a percentage without a calculator, convert the percentage to a decimal and multiuply.

Starting Hint Convert 30% to a decimal and multiply by the amount of each ingredient

 For more math help, go to the Math Appendix at the back of the book

> **NCTM Number and Operations** Compute fluently and make reasonable estimates.

STANDARDIZED TEST PRACTICE

MULTIPLE CHOICE
Read the paragraph. Write your answer on a separate piece of paper.

Test-Taking Tip Real learning occurs through studying that takes place over a period of time. Relate the information you are learning to what you already know and you will understand and retain it better. Review more than once.

Fiber in your snacks helps you feel full. Toss some sliced almonds or chopped celery into your tuna sandwich or add chopped vegetables on your pizza. You will be surprized how much more satisfied you will feel when you do!

20. Based on the paragraph, which of the following statements is true?
- **a.** Fiber alone will not fill you up.
- **b.** Snacks are always full of calories.
- **c.** Add less fiber to snacks to make them lower in calories.
- **d.** Adding fiber can be more filling.

Explore the Photo ▶▶
A dessert ends a meal with a sweet flavor. *How can dessert end a meal with both flavor and healthful eating?*

Writing Activity

Practice Expository Writing

Desert Dessert? Some people avoid desserts because they think they will gain weight. Write an essay that explains whether this idea is true or false. Support your statements with MyPyramid and the Dietary Guidelines recommendations.

Writing Tips

1. **Explain** your main idea in a clear thesis statement.

2. **List** nutrition facts and advice as supporting details.

3. **Focus** on cause-effect relationships between facts.

Reading Guide

Before You Read

Study with a Buddy It can be difficult to review your own notes and quiz yourself on what you have just read. According to research, studying with a partner for just twelve minutes can help you study better.

Read to Learn

Key Concepts

- **Analyze** how desserts fit into a healthful eating plan.
- **Distinguish** among different types of refrigerated desserts.
- **Explain** the differences among cookies, cakes, and pies.
- **Describe** how to store desserts for quality and food safety.

Main Idea

Desserts make a sweet or tart, sometimes nutritious ending to many meals! Enjoy simple desserts such as fruit, pudding, or ice cream. Buy or make baked cookies, cakes, and pies.

Content Vocabulary

◇ pudding
◇ custard
◇ shortened cake
◇ foam cake
◇ chiffon cake
◇ pastry
◇ cobbler
◇ crisp
◇ meringue

Academic Vocabulary

You will find these words in your reading and on your tests. Use the glossary to look up their definitions if necessary.

- principle
- adhere

Graphic Organizer

As you read, use a graphic organizer like the one below to write solutions to these situations.

Situation	Solution
Shaping Cookies	
Cooling a Foam Cake	
Storing an Egg-Based Dessert	

 Graphic Organizer Go to this book's Online Learning Center at **glencoe.com** to print out this graphic organizer.

Academic Standards

 English Language Arts
NCTE 8 Use information resources to gather information and create and communicate knowledge.

 Mathematics
NCTM Data Analysis and Probability Formulate questions that can be addressed with data, and collect, organize, and display relevant data to answer them.

NCTM Geometry Use visualization, spatial reasoning, and geometric modeling to solve problems.

 Social Studies
NCSS I A Analyze and explain the ways groups, societies, and cultures address human needs and concerns.

NCTE National Council of Teachers of English
NCTM National Council of Teachers of Mathematics
NSES National Science Education Standards
NCSS National Council for the Social Studies

Desserts: Nutritious and Delicious

Desserts, usually sweet, are the last course in a meal. They can offer another way to fit nourishing foods into a meal.

Some desserts are healthful, but many are high in fat, added sugars, and calories. Eat them only occasionally and in small amounts—if you have enough discretionary calories to spend. On physically active days, you may need the extra calories.

To make smart dessert choices:

◆ Choose desserts that provide food-group foods.

◆ Eat a small portion, or share it with someone.

◆ Choose or make desserts with less fat and added sugar. For example, gingersnaps and fig bars are low in fat.

◆ Use Nutrition Facts on food labels to choose cookies and other desserts wisely. Fat-free does not mean calorie-free!

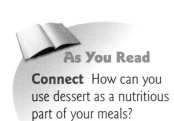

As You Read

Connect How can you use dessert as a nutritious part of your meals?

Light and Easy Desserts

Do you want a light dessert? These easy desserts have fewer calories and less fat.

◆ **Fresh fruit** is sweet and nutritious. Try serving it with cheese. Combine mixed fruits with mint, grated citrus rind or ginger, chopped nuts, a splash of fruit juice, and a little cinnamon or nutmeg.

◆ **Gelatin dessert,** mixed with chopped fruit and chopped nuts, is a make-ahead dessert.

◆ **Angel food cake** is fat-free. You can buy it ready-made. Top it with fruit, or drizzle on a little chocolate sauce.

◆ **Frozen fruit tidbits** are cold and crunchy. Freeze peeled, sliced bananas or washed grapes!

Dessert Makeovers

Some common desserts can be made with less fat or sugar. If you adjust a baked recipe, expect the new version to be a little different from the original in flavor, texture, and volume.

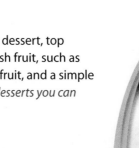

Create a 5-Minute Dessert For a quick dessert, top sorbet or frozen low-fat yogurt with fresh fruit, such as berries, peaches, kiwifruit, and tropical fruit, and a simple garnish. *What are two quick, healthful desserts you can suggest?*

For Less Fat and Cholesterol

- ◆ Use half the amount of fat (butter, margarine, shortening, or oil) in a cake or cookie recipe. Substitute an equal amount of applesauce, mashed ripe banana, or canned pumpkin. (This may slightly alter the final result.)

- ◆ Use ¼ cup (50 mL) egg substitute or two egg whites instead of one whole egg.

- ◆ Use mini chocolate chips instead of regular ones. That spreads the flavor with fewer chocolate chips.

For Less Added Sugar

Experiment to reduce sugar. In a pie, use sliced fresh or drained canned fruit rather than canned fruit filling. Try using spices like cinnamon, ginger, and nutmeg that give a sense of sweetness. Try vanilla or peppermint extracts, too. Consider recipes that call for sugar substitutes.

For More Nutrients

Some baked desserts have ingredients that add vitamins, minerals, and fiber.

- ◆ Prepare or buy desserts with nutrient-rich ingredients, like oatmeal cookies or banana-nut cake.

- ◆ Use 100 percent fruit juice as the liquid in some recipes.

- ◆ Sweeten with dried or chopped fresh fruits.

- ◆ Substitute whole-wheat flour for part of the refined flour.

✓ **Reading Check** **Explain** How can desserts fit into a healthful eating plan?

Nutrition & Wellness Tips

Give a Gift of Health

✓ Bring a plate of oatmeal cookies to a child when you babysit.

✓ Make a dessert pizza, topped with sliced apples, peaches, and other fruit.

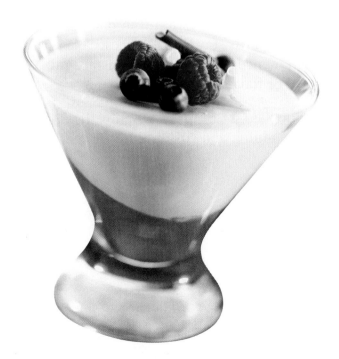

Dessert Toppings Pudding can be topped with cinnamon, raisins, berries, or almost any garnish for a chilled dessert at the end of a meal. *What other ingredients could you use to garnish pudding?*

Chilled Desserts

Chilled desserts need freezing or refrigeration. They are a nice contrast to a hot meal, especially on a hot summer day!

Frozen Desserts

Frozen desserts are served in cones and bowls, as toppings on fruit or baked foods, or in a frozen pie.

- **Ice cream** is made with cream or milk, sugar, and sometimes eggs. They range from higher butterfat to fat-free.
- **Frozen yogurt** is like ice cream with yogurt cultures. It is often low-fat or fat-free.
- **Sherbet** is a frozen mixture of sweetened fruit juice, water, and often milk.
- **Sorbet** (sȯr-ˈbā) is similar to sherbet, but without milk.

◆**Vocabulary**

You can find definitions in the glossary at the back of this book.

Puddings

Pudding is a smooth, creamy dessert made with milk, sugar, and sometimes egg and other flavorings. Most puddings are thickened with cornstarch. As the mixture gently cooks, starch absorbs water and gelatinizes. It gets firm as it chills.

For convenience, make packaged instant pudding mixes. Just add milk to the mix, beat, and chill.

Custards

Custard is a cooked, sweetened mixture of milk and eggs. It can be baked or stirred on the cooktop. Eggs thicken custard as their proteins coagulate, and give it a rich flavor.

Creamy, stirred custards are thin enough to use as a sauce. Oven-baked custards stay firm. A cheesecake is a baked custard.

For convenience, use a packaged custard mix. Drizzle puréed fruit on top for flavor and nutrition.

✓ **Reading Check** **Compare** What is the difference between homemade pudding and custard?

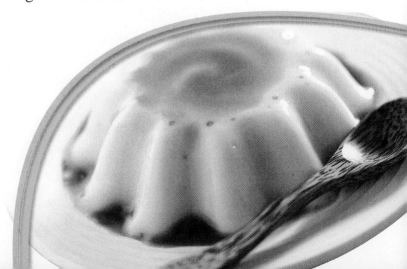

What's for Dessert? Custard with caramel sauce is a dessert with flair. In France, this dessert is called créme caramel. In Spain, the Philippines, and Latin American countries, it is called flan. *What other desserts can you name that originated in other countries?*

Baked Desserts

Making cookies, cakes, and pies can be fun. Make them from scratch, or save time with convenience products and your own touches. Follow the recipe or package directions carefully. Remember each baking **principle**, or rule, from chapter 32.

Cookies, cakes, and pies can be made from the same basic ingredients as other baked goods. Use the specific type of product that the recipe calls for. For example, some cake recipes require cake flour.

Cookies

There are hundreds of types of cookies.

Cookie dough is made with flour, fat, sugar, and sometimes eggs or a leavening agent for volume. Ingredients such as oatmeal, nuts, dried fruits, and puréed pumpkin contribute nutrients and flavor.

Cookie Types

Most cookies are a variation of six types. The main difference is how they are shaped.

- ◆ **Drop cookies** are made by dropping spoonfuls of dough onto a baking sheet. Example: oatmeal cookies.

- ◆ **Molded cookies** are made from a stiff dough and shaped by hand. They are spaced on a baking sheet and may be flattened with a fork or the bottom of a glass. Example: some peanut butter cookies.

- ◆ **Rolled cookies** are made by rolling out a stiff dough and using cookie cutters to cut shapes. Example: sugar cookies.

- ◆ **Refrigerator cookies** are sliced from a long roll of chilled dough, then baked.

- ◆ **Pressed cookies** are shaped by pushing dough through a cookie press onto a baking sheet. Dough must be stiff to keep the shape. Example: spritz cookies.

- ◆ **Bar cookies** are baked in a square or rectangular pan like a cake. After baking, they are cut in bars or squares. Example: brownies.

Tips for Cookie Making

For good-looking, good-tasting cookies, follow the recipe or package directions for mixing, shaping, and baking the dough. Check the recipe for spacing cookies on the baking sheet. Make all cookies the same shape and thickness. Test bar and drop cookies for doneness by pressing lightly with your finger. The imprint should show slightly. Follow recipe directions for cooling cookies, and let the baking sheet cool before using it again.

To save time, use refrigerated cookie dough or mixes. Add your own touches. Roll refrigerated dough in chopped nuts before you slice and bake it or stir in chopped dried fruit.

✓ **Reading Check**) **Compare** How do bar cookies differ from other types of cookies?

Cakes

Cakes belong in three categories. The differences are the ingredients beyond these basics: flour, sugar, and liquid.

◆ A **shortened cake** contains fat—shortening, margarine, or oil. Baking powder or baking soda are leveners. Eggs—yolks and whites—also are mixed into the batter. Shortened cakes are baked in round, square, rectangular, or specially shaped pans.

◆ A **foam cake** is leavened with air that comes from stiffly beating egg whites. Most foam cakes are baked in a tube pan—a deep, round pan with a center tube. The tube helps heat get to the center quickly so the cake bakes evenly. The ungreased pan lets the cake cling to the sides. That helps it rise. Angel food cake and sponge cake are foam cakes. Sponge cake has egg yolks.

◆ A **chiffon cake** is a cross between shortened and foam cakes. It has oil or another fat, plus egg yolks. It is leavened with beaten egg whites and baking powder.

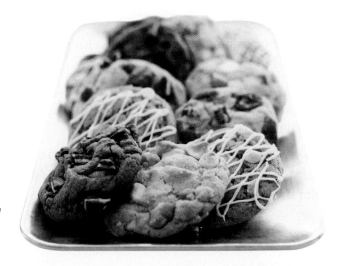

Handle with Care Warm cookies are fragile. Use a wide turner to remove them from the baking sheet. *Why are some cookies removed from the baking sheet right away, and then cooled on a wire rack?*

Tips for Mixing and Baking Cakes

A quality cake is smooth and slightly rounded. The inside is finely textured without tunnels or air bubbles. It is moist and tender with a pleasing flavor. To make your cake:

◆ **Adhere** to, or follow, recipe or package directions carefully.

◆ Grease the pan for shortened cakes, but not for foam cakes.

◆ Preheat the oven. Bake for the time shown in the recipe.

◆ Test for doneness. The top should be evenly browned. When you tap the top gently, it will spring back. A shortened cake pulls away from the sides of the pan. A foam cake continues to cling to the sides of the pan.

After Baking a Cake

Once the cake is baked, cool it properly:

◆ Shortened cakes are cooled for five to ten minutes, then removed from the pan(s) and cooled on a wire rack.

◆ Foam cakes are cooled in the pan. Turn the pan upside down so the cake will not fall.

After the cake cools, you can dust it with confectioners' sugar, frost it, or top it with fruit or berries.

✓ **Reading Check** **Compare** What makes the three general categories of cakes unique?

Pies

A pie is a crust with a flavorful filling. A two-crust pie has a top and bottom crust with filling between. A one-crust pie has a bottom crust only. A tart is a shallow crust with a filling.

A well-prepared pie has a delicate, flaky, and tender crust that is nicely browned. The filling is thick, not sticky.

Pies provide nutrients. The filling might have fruit such as apples, berries, or peaches. Or the filling could be vegetables such as pumpkin or sweet potato. Some fillings are milk-based, as in pudding or custard. Some pies have nuts in their filling.

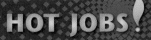

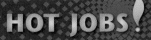HOT JOBS!

Pastry Chef
Pastry chefs have special skills for making cakes, pastries, frozen desserts, and other sweet foods. Their artistic abilities are important for decorating desserts.

Careers Find out more about careers. Go to this book's Online Learning Center at **glencoe.com**.

Check for Doneness Shortened cakes are done baking when a toothpick stuck in the center comes out clean. *What should you do if the toothpick does not come out clean?*

Pie Crusts

A pie crust is made from pastry. **Pastry** is a mixture of flour, fat, cold water, and salt. It should be mixed just to cut in the fat. (See **Figure 34.1**.) Pastry forms flaky layers as it bakes.

For a one-crust pie with a filling that does not need baking, you can use a crumb crust. Finely crushed graham cracker, gingersnap, or vanilla wafer crumbs are mixed with melted butter or margarine and a little sugar. The mixture is pressed into a pie pan, baked, and cooled. Then the filling is added.

Pie crust has most of the fat in a pie. For less fat:

◆ Make a one-crust pie, or make a deep-dish pie, made in a deep baking dish with only a top crust.

◆ Use less butter or margarine in crumb crusts—just enough to make the crust moist.

Food Prep How To

REMOVE A CAKE FROM THE PAN

1 Run a spatula between the cake and the pan.

2 Place a wire rack over the top of the cake. Hold the cake and the rack securely with pot holders.

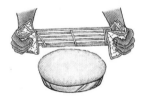

3 Turn the cake and rack upside down. Place the wire rack on a level surface, such as a counter.

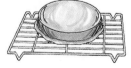

4 Lift off the cake pan. It should come off easily.

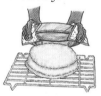

5 The cake is now upside down. Place another wire rack on the cake. Grasp both wire racks with both hands. Quickly turn them so the cake is right side up.

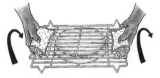

6 Remove the top wire rack. Allow the cake to cool on the bottom wire rack.

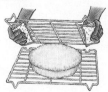

Pie Fillings

You can make pie fillings from scratch or use convenience products.

◆ Fruit is a popular pie filling. Fresh, frozen, or canned fruit work well. Canned fruit pie filling is ready to use.

◆ Cream pies have a pudding-type filling. You pour the mixture into a baked pie shell.

◆ Custard pie fillings contain eggs and milk. They are baked with the crust.

◆ Chiffon pies are made with beaten egg whites and perhaps gelatin. They are put into a baked crust, then chilled.

Convenience with Pies

For convenience, you can use packaged pie crust mix, frozen dough sticks, rolled-out pastry dough, or frozen pie shells. Instant pudding, custard mix, and canned fruit are easy fillings. You can also fill a store bought crumb crust with frozen yogurt and sliced fruit and freeze.

Cobblers and Crisps

A **cobbler** is a fruit dessert with a sweet biscuit-dough topping. Fruit is heated with sugar and other flavorings. Then poured into a baking dish, topped with biscuit dough, and baked.

Fruit **crisp** is like a cobbler, but is topped with a crumbly sweet pastry mixture. Then it is baked until crisp.

✓ **Reading Check** **Compare** How do a fruit pie, a cobbler, and a crisp differ?

Figure 34.1 | **Pie Crust**

Form the Perfect Pie Crust Making a pie crust can be very delicate work. *Why would you lightly flour the surface and the rolling pin before rolling pastry dough?*

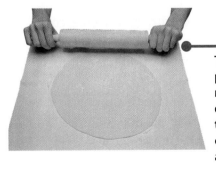

To make a pastry crust, roll the dough from the center out to make a circular shape. Use short, gentle strokes.

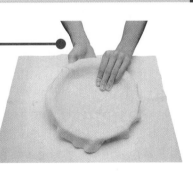

Gently roll the dough onto the rolling pin. Then, gradually unroll it into the pie pan without stretching it. Start unrolling at the edge of the pie pan.

Keep Desserts Fresh

Proper storage keeps desserts appealing and safe.

◆ **Milk- and egg-based desserts** should be refrigerated. That includes custards, cream pies, and pumpkin pies.

◆ **Fruit pies** keep better when refrigerated, too.

◆ **Cakes** with cream fillings need refrigeration. Other cakes can be stored in tightly closed containers at room temperature for several days, or frozen.

◆ **Cookies** are stored differently. Store crisp cookies with a loose-fitting cover. Soft cookies need a tight cover to stay moist. Most cookies also freeze well.

✓ **Reading Check** **Recall** Which desserts should be refrigerated?

EASY RECIPES

Everyday Favorites

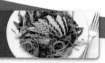

Apple Cobbler

Customary	Ingredients	Metric
5	Apples	5
¼ tsp.	Salt, divided	1 mL
1 Tbsp.	Lemon juice	15 mL
1 Tbsp.	Corn starch	15 mL
1 cup	All-purpose flour	250 mL
3 Tbsp.	Brown sugar	45 mL
¼ cup	Butter or margarine	60 mL

Try This!
You can make cobbler with any fresh, frozen, or canned fruit.

Yield: Eight ¾ cup (180 g) servings

❶ Preheat oven to 400°F (204°C).

❷ Peel and core apples. Slice thinly lengthwise and mix in a bowl with lemon juice, corn starch, sugar and ⅛ tsp. salt.

❸ Use a little of the butter to coat a 9-inch pie tin and evenly spread the apple mixture in the pan.

❹ Combine remaining salt with flour and sugar and cut the butter into the mixture with a fork or your hands until a sand-like powder is achieved. Sprinkle the flour mixture evenly over the top of the apples and bake until the top is brown, about 35 minutes.

Nutritional Information Per Serving: 169 calories, 6 g total fat (4 g saturated fat), 15 mg cholesterol, 74 mg sodium, 28 g total carbohydrate (2 g fiber, 13 g sugars), 2 g protein

Percent Daily Value: vitamin A 4%, vitamin C 60%, calcium 0%, iron 4%

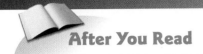

After You Read

CHAPTER SUMMARY

Desserts are the sweet end to many meals. Some desserts are nutrient dense. Others are high in fat, added sugars, and calories. With careful planning, any dessert can fit in a healthful eating plan. Many desserts are low in fat and calories and simple to prepare. Some desserts are chilled or frozen, while others are baked. Baked desserts can be baked from scratch or with convenience products. By following baking principles and recipe directions, you are more likely to create a successful dessert. Store desserts properly to keep them fresh, appealing, and safe.

Vocabulary Review

1. Use each of these vocabulary words in a sentence.

Content Vocabulary
◇ pudding (p. 504)
◇ custard (p. 504)
◇ shortened cake (p. 506)
◇ foam cake (p. 506)
◇ chiffon cake (p. 506)
◇ pastry (p. 508)
◇ cobbler (p. 509)
◇ crisp (p. 509)

Academic Vocabulary
■ principle (p. 505)
■ adhere (p. 507)

Review Key Concepts

2. Analyze how desserts fit into a healthful eating plan.

3. Distinguish among different types of refrigerated desserts.

4. Explain the differences among cookies, cakes, and pies.

5. Describe how to store desserts for quality and food safety.

Critical Thinking

6. Analyze a recipe for cake or cookies. Find a common recipe, then devise ways to add more nutrients and to trim fat, added sugar, and calories.

7. Defend the role of desserts as part of a healthful eating plan. Role-play with another student who pretends to be a person who thinks he or she needs to avoid desserts.

8. Suggest some cookies you could make with a child while babysitting. Consider recipes that are fairly easy, will not take too long, and will not dirty too many utensils.

9. Suggest ways to make or serve a cake that tastes great, but has fewer calories than most cakes.

Real-World Skills and Applications

Collaborative and Interpersonal

10. Cookie Exchange Follow your teacher's instructions to form groups. Each student in your group will find a recipe for a different cookie type. The recipes will be shared by the members of the group. Discuss the benefits of a recipe exchange.

Problem Solving and Decision Making

11. Consumer Research Research the nutrition, cost, and preparation time for three different types of convenience pie crust products. How do they compare to homemade pie crust? Would you make your own crust or buy one ready made? How would you decide which product to buy? Summarize your findings and conclusions in a written report.

Technology

12. Record a Job Interview Imagine that you are a restaurant owner who needs to hire a pastry chef. Write interview questions. With a partner, take turns as the employer and job candidate. Videotape the interviews to use in a class discussion of good interviewing skills.

Financial Literacy

13. Healthier and Cheaper You are making desserts for eight. You could buy a cookie sheet for $9.99 and frozen cookie dough for $3.00 and make cookies, or you could make yogurt parfaits. One 32-oz container of vanilla yogurt is $2.70. A small box of granola cereal is $3.00. Sixteen ounces of berries is $3.99. Add the costs and compare.

 14. Mixing Methods Investigate at least two ways to mix cake batter—for example, the conventional and the quick-mix methods. Describe and compare the methods. Find a recipe for each method. Share with the class what you learned.

 15. Visit a Local Bakery Visit a supermarket or bakery. Find out how the bakers decide what desserts to sell and what ingredients to use. Look for desserts made with whole grains, fruit, shredded or puréed vegetables, dairy, eggs, and nuts. Write a summary of your trip.

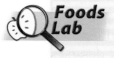 **16. Pudding: From Scratch or Convenience?** Prepare, serve, and compare three puddings: made from scratch, made from a convenience product, and ready-made. Compare their texture, appearance, and flavor. Compare the cost and time required to prepare them. Write your comparisons, observations, and conclusions.

 Additional Activities For additional activities go to this book's Online Learning Center at **glencoe.com**.

Academic Skills

 English Language Arts

17. Desserts Around the World Do research to learn about a type of cookie, cake, or pie linked to an international cultural celebration. Write a newspaper feature article with photos.

> **NCTE 8** Use information resources to gather information and create and communicate knowledge.

 Social Studies

18. Dessert Drinks Many cultures are known for their flavorful sweet drinks, such as Mexican horchata—spiced rice milk—and Chinese tea. Find and write down an interesting dessert drink recipe. Conduct research about the dessert beverage and write a paragraph to describe it.

> **NCSS I A** Analyze and explain the ways groups, societies, and cultures address human needs and concerns.

 Mathematics

19. Fruit Dip for All Make a simple fruit dip by combining 8 ounces of vanilla yogurt with 4 tablespoons of pureed peaches. This is enough for about 1 cup of fresh fruit. Create a table to show how much of each ingredient is needed for ½ cup, 1, 2, 3, and 4 cups of fruit. What is the pattern?

Math Concept Determine a pattern and generate a table based on the pattern.

Starting Hint Multiply or divide to determine how much of each ingredient you will need based on the original recipe. Place the results in a table, adding a row for each ingredient. Then, find the pattern.

 For more math help, go to the Math Appendix

> **NCTM Data Analysis and Probability** Formulate questions that can be addressed with data and collect, organize, and display relevant data to answer them.

STANDARDIZED TEST PRACTICE

MULTIPLE CHOICE
Read the paragraph and write an answer. Write your answer on a separate piece of paper:

Chocolate may have some unique health benefits. Phytonutrients in chocolate called flavonoids may be heart healthy.

> **Test-Taking Tip** Real learning occurs through studying that takes place over a period of time. Relate the information you are learning to what you already know and you will be better able to understand and retain it.

Dark chocolate has more flavonoids than lighter chocolate. Either way, chocolates are made with high fat and sugary ingredients. White chocolate does not have flavonoids because it is not really chocolate. Since they all have sugar, fat, and calories, eat small quantities.

20. Based on the paragraph, which of the following statements is true?
   a. Everyone should eat dark chocolate.
   b. Eating dark chocolate will keep you from getting sick.
   c. You can eat chocolate instead of exercising to get healthy.
   d. Dark chocolate has health benefits.

Food Industry Careers

While studying this textbook, you have learned how developing health-ful eating habits and living an active life can help you maintain good health. Many people who work in the food industry help people achieve their healthy eating goals. In this project, you will choose a career in the food industry that interests you, "shadow" someone who works in this job, and create a presentation about a "day in the life" of that person.

My Journal

If you completed the journal entry from page 450, refer to it to see if you have become interested in any other careers in the food industry while studying this unit.

Project Assignment

In this project you will:

- Select and research a food service industry career that interests you.
- Write a summary of your research.
- Find a person in your community who works in the career that you researched.
- Arrange to "shadow" this person as he or she works.
- Interview this person about his or her typical day.
- While interviewing, take notes, and after interviewing, transcribe your notes.
- Plan and make a presentation.

Academic Skills You Will Use . . . .
English Language Arts

NCTE 7 Conduct research and gather, evaluate, and syn-thesize data to communicate discoveries.

NCTE 8 Use information resources to gather information and create and communicate knowledge.

STEP 1 Choose and Research a Career

Select a career in the food industry that interests you and conduct research about it. Examples of careers include chef, food server, nutritionist, farmer, food critic, or food council employee. Write a summary of your research.

- Summarize the details of the career you have chosen.
- Explain why this career is interesting.
- Include the training and education needed to pursue this career.

STEP 2 Prepare Interview Questions

Prepare questions to interview some-one who works in your chosen career. Write questions about job responsibilities, rewards and challenges, and what a typi-cal day is like. Keep these writing skills in mind while you develop the questions.

Writing Skills

- Write open-ended questions.
- Use correct spelling and grammar.
- Organize your questions in the order you want to ask them.

STEP 3 Connect with Your Community

Identify a person in your community who works in the career you have chosen. Arrange to "shadow" this person at his or her job for an hour or two after school. Interview the person using the questions you have created in Step 2.

Interviewing Skills
- Make eye contact.
- Take clear notes so you can understand them later.
- If necessary, ask additional questions to ensure your understanding.

STEP 4 Create and Present a Report

Use the Unit Thematic Project Checklist to make oral report and give your presentation about a typical day. Use these speaking skills as you present your final report.

Speaking Skills
- Speak clearly and concisely.
- Be sensitive to the needs of your audience.
- Use standard English to communicate.

STEP 5 Evaluate Your Presentation

Your project will be reviewed and evaluated based on:
- Completeness of your research
- Content of your presentation
- Mechanics—presentation and neatness

Evaluation Rubric Go to this book's Online Learning Center at glencoe.com for a rubric you can use to evaluate your final report.

Project Checklist	
Plan	✓ Select and research a career. ✓ Summarize your research. ✓ Write interview questions. ✓ Shadow a professional who works in your chosen career. ✓ Conduct an interview. ✓ Transcribe the notes from your interview. ✓ Write an outline for an oral presentation.
Present	✓ Give an oral report to your class to describe the results of your research and interview, and a typical day in the career. ✓ Invite the students of the class to ask any questions they may have. Answer these questions. ✓ When students ask questions, demonstrate in your answers that you respect their perspectives. ✓ Turn in your research summary, interview questions, and interview notes to your teacher.
Academic Skills	✓ Conduct research to gather information. ✓ Communicate effectively. ✓ Organize your presentation so the audience can follow along easily. ✓ Thoroughly express your ideas.

MyPyramid Serving Amounts: Food Group Equivalencies

GRAIN GROUP
One ounce (28 g) equals:
1 regular slice enriched or whole grain bread
1 6-inch (15-cm) tortilla
½ burger bun, mini bagel, pita, or English muffin
1 cup (250 mL) ready-to-eat cereal (flakes or rounds)
½ cup (125 mL) cooked cereal, pasta, rice or other cooked grain
1 4½-inch (11-cm) pancake or waffle
5 whole wheat crackers
1 ounce (28 g) pretzels
3 cups (750 mL) popped corn

VEGETABLE GROUP
One cup (250 mL) equals:
2 cups (500 mL) raw leafy greens
1 cup (250 mL) cooked or chopped raw vegetables
1 cup (250 mL) cooked dry beans, peas, or lentils*
1 medium potato
1 cup (250 mL) vegetable juice

FRUIT GROUP
One cup (250 mL) equals:
1 small whole apple
1 medium grapefruit
1 cup (250 mL) berries or cut-up canned, frozen, or cooked fruit
1 large banana, orange or peach
1 cup (250 mL) fruit juice
½ cup (125 mL) dried fruit

MILK GROUP
One cup (250 mL) equals:
1 cup (250 mL) milk, buttermilk, yogurt, or pudding made with milk
1½ ounces (42 g) hard cheese, such as cheddar, Swiss, Monterey Jack, or mozzarella
2 ounces (56 g) process cheese, such as American
⅓ cup (75 mL) shredded cheese
2 cups (500 mL) cottage cheese
1 cup (250 mL) frozen yogurt
1½ cups (375 mL) ice cream

MEAT & BEANS GROUP
One ounce (28 g) equals:
1 ounce (28 g) cooked lean meat, poultry or fish
¼ cup (50 mL) cooked dry beans, peas, or lentils*
1 egg
1 tablespoon (15 mL) peanut butter
¼ cup (50 mL) egg substitute
½ ounce (14 g) nuts
¼ cup (50 mL) tofu
2 tablespoons (30 mL) hummus

* Count dry beans, peas, or lentils toward either the Vegetable Group or the Meat & Beans Group but not both.

Daily Values and DRIs for Teens

The Daily Values are standard values developed by the Food and Drug Administration (FDA) for use on food labels. Dietary Reference Intakes (DRIs) are used by nutrition professionals. They give nutrient reference amounts for specific ages and genders. Only the amounts for teens are included here. You may find it interesting to compare the DRIs for your age and gender to the Daily Values.

The DRIs include four types of nutrient reference values. Most of the values listed below are Recommended Dietary Allowances (RDAs). An RDA is the daily amount of a nutrient that will meet the needs of nearly all healthy people. For some nutrients, there is not yet enough data to establish an RDA. In that case, the value listed is an Adequate Intake (AI), an amount believed to be adequate.

Nutrient	Daily Value	Dietary Reference Intake (RDA or AI)			
		Males 9–13	Males 14–18	Females 9–13	Females 14–18
Protein	50 g	34 g	52 g	34 g	46 g
Carbohydrate (total)	300 g	130 g	130 g	130 g	130 g
Fiber	25 g	31 g	38 g	26 g	26 g
Fat (total)	65 g	**	**	**	**
Saturated fat	20 g	**	**	**	**
Cholesterol	300 mg	**	**	**	**
Vitamin A	5,000 IU (875 µg RE)	600 µg RAE	900 µg RAE	600 µg RAE	700 µg RAE
Thiamin	1.5 mg	0.9 mg	1.2 mg	0.9 mg	1.0 mg
Riboflavin	1.7 mg	0.9 mg	1.3 mg	0.9 mg	1.0 mg
Niacin	20 mg NE	12 mg NE	16 mg NE	12 mg NE	14 mg NE
Vitamin B6	2 mg	1.0 mg	1.3 mg	1.0 mg	1.2 mg
Vitamin B12	6 µg	1.8 µg	2.4 µg	1.8 µg	2.4 µg
Folate	400 µg	300 µg DFE	400 µg DFE	300 µg DFE	400 µg DFE
Biotin	300 µg	20 µg	25 µg	20 µg	25 µg
Pantothenic acid	10 mg	4 mg	5 mg	4 mg	5 mg
Vitamin C	60 mg	45 mg	75 mg	45 mg	65 mg
Vitamin D	400 IU (6.5 µg)	5 µg	5 µg	5 µg	5 µg
Vitamin E	30 IU (9 mg α-TE)	11 mg α-TE	15 mg α-TE	11 mg α-TE	15 mg α-TE
Vitamin K	80 mg	60 µg	75 µg	60 µg	75 µg
Calcium	1,000 mg	1,300 mg	1,300 mg	1,300 mg	1,300 mg
Chloride	3,400 mg	2,300 mg	2,300 mg	2,300 mg	2,300 mg
Copper	2 mg	700 µg	890 µg	700 µg	890 µg
Iodine	150 µg	120 µg	150 µg	120 µg	150 µg
Iron	18 mg	8 mg	11 mg	8 mg	15 mg
Magnesium	400 mg	240 mg	410 mg	240 mg	360 mg
Phosphorus	1,000 mg	1,250 mg	1,250 mg	1,250 mg	1,250 mg
Potassium	3,500 mg	4,500 mg	4,700 mg	4,500 mg	4,700 mg
Selenium	70 µg	40 µg	55 µg	45 µg	55 µg
Sodium	2,400 mg	1,500 mg	1,500 mg	1,500 mg	1,500 mg
Zinc	15 mg	8 mg	11 mg	8 mg	9 mg
Water	**	2.4 L	3.3 L	2.1 L	2.3 L

*Based on a diet of 2,000 calories per day   **No value established

Key to nutrient measures
g   gram
mg   milligram (1000 mg = 1 g)
µg   microgram (1000 µg = 1 mg; 1,000,000 µg = 1 g)
IU   International Unit (an old measurement of vitamin activity)

RAE   retinol activity equivalents (a measure of Vitamin A activity)
NE   niacin equivalents (a measure of niacin activity)
DFE   dietary folate equivalents (a measure of folate activity)
α-TE   alpha-tocopherol equivalents (a measure of Vitamin E activity)
L   liter

Source: USDA Home and Garden Bulletin No. 72, "Nutritive Value of Foods"

Nutritive Value of Foods Appendix

Nutrients in Indicated Quantity

Item No.	Food Description	Approximate Measure	Weight (Grams)	Food energy (Calories)	Protein (Grams)	Fat (Grams)	Cholesterol (Milligrams)	Calcium (Milligrams)	Iron (Milligrams)	Sodium (Milligrams)	Vitamin A value* Retinol equivalents	Vitamin C (Milligrams)
Beverages												
9	Club soda	12 fl oz	355	0	0	0	0	18	Tr	75	0	0
10	Regular cola	12 fl oz	369	137	Tr	Tr	0	7	0.4	15	0	0
11	Diet, artificially sweetened cola	12 fl oz	355	7	Tr	Tr	0	11	0.4	28	0	0
20	Fruit punch drink	8 fl oz	248	119	0	0	0	20	0.2	25	0	1
Dairy Product **Natural Cheese**												
32	Cheddar, cut pieces	1 oz	28	114	7	9	30	205	0.2	176	75	0
38	Cottage cheese, lowfat (2%)	1 cup	226	163	28	2	9	138	0.3	918	25	0
43	Mozzarella, part skim milk	1 oz	28	86	7	6	15	208	Tr	150	39	0
46	Parmesan, grated	1 tbsp	5	22	2	1	4	55	Tr	76	6	0
52	Pasteurized process American cheese	1 oz	28	105	6	9	26	155	Tr	417	71	0
Milk, fluid:												
78	Whole (3.3% fat)	1 cup	244	146	8	8	24	276	Tr	98	68	0
79	Reduced fat (2%)	1 cup	244	122	8	5	20	285	Tr	100	134	1
83	Nonfat (skim)	1 cup	247	86	8	Tr	5	504	0.1	128	338	3
85	Buttermilk	1 cup	245	98	8	2	10	284	0.1	257	17	2
88	Evaporated skim milk	1 cup	245	100	10	Tr	5	372	0.4	149	149	2
91	Dried, nonfat, instantized	1 cup	245	81	8	Tr	5	284	Tr	130	162	1
Milk beverages:												
94	Chocolate milk, low-fat (1%)	1 cup	250	158	8	3	8	288	0.6	152	145	2
105	Shakes, thick; Vanilla	10 oz	283	379	8	13	48	275	0.3	133	133	8
Milk desserts, frozen:												
	Ice cream, vanilla, regular (about 11% fat):											
107	Hardened	1 cup	133	267	5	14	53	168	0.2	98	146	1
109	Frozen yogurt	1 cup	200	214	9	3	10	318	0.5	120	24	1
	Ice cream, vanilla, low-fat:											
113	Hardened (about 4% fat)	1 cup	131	216	6	6	35	211	0.3	97	168	2
116	Sherbet (about 2% fat)	1 cup	193	278	2	4	0	104	0.3	89	19	11
	Yogurt, made with low-fat milk:											
117	Fruit-flavored	8 oz	245	250	11	3	10	372	0.2	142	24	2
118	Plain	8 oz	245	154	13	4	15	448	0.2	172	34	2

Tr = Trace amount
*1 RE = 3.33 IU from animal foods or 1 mcg retinol
1 RE = 10 IU from plant foods or 6 mcg beta carotene.

Nutritive Value of Foods Appendix

#	Food	Measure	Weight (g)	Calories	Protein (g)	Fat (g)	Cholesterol (mg)	Calcium (mg)	Iron (mg)	Sodium (mg)	Vitamin A (RE)	Vitamin C (mg)
Eggs												
	Eggs, large (24 oz. per dozen):											
124	Fried in margarine	1 egg	46	89	6	7	210	26	0.9	238	88	0
125	Hard-cooked, shell removed	1 egg	50	77	6	5	211	25	0.6	139	84	0
Fats and Oils												
129	Butter (4 sticks per lb) (⅛ stick)	1 tbsp	14	102	Tr	12	31	3	0.0	82	97	0
138	Margarine (⅛ stick)	1 tbsp	14	100	Tr	11	0	0	Tr	93	116	0
147	Corn oil	1 cup	218	1,927	0	218	0	0	0.0	0	0	0
	Salad dressings, commercial:											
162	French, Regular	1 tbsp	16	60	Tr	6	0	3	Tr	197	2	0
163	French, Low calorie	1 tbsp	16	24	Tr	2	0	3	0.1	179	2	0
Fish and Shellfish												
177	Fish sticks, frozen, reheated (stock, 4 by 1 by ½ in.)	1 fish stick	28	70	3	4	9	7	0.3	118	9	0
181	Haddock, breaded, fried	3 oz	85	151	16	7	57	44	1.2	105	14	0
182	halibut, broiled, with butter and lemon juice	3 oz	85	113	19	4	48	19	0.4	354	34	3
195	Tuna, canned, oil packed, chunk light	3 oz	85	168	25	7	15	11	1.2	301	20	0
196	Tuna, canned, water-pack, solid white	3 oz	85	99	22	1	26	9	1.3	287	14	0
Fruits and Fruit Juices												
198	Apples, raw, unpeeled, 2¾-in. diam.	1 apple	138	72	Tr	Tr	0	8	0.2	1	4	6
202	Apple juice, bottled or canned	1 cup	248	117	Tr	Tr	0	17	0.9	7	0	28
204	Applesauce, canned, unsweetened	1 cup	244	105	Tr	Tr	0	7	0.3	5	2	3
215	Bananas, raw, without peel, whole	1 banana	118	105	1	1	0	6	0.3	1	4	10
229	Fruit cocktail, canned, juice pack	1 cup	237	109	1	Tr	0	19	0.5	9	36	6
230	Grapefruit, raw, without peel, 3¾-in. diam.	½ grapefruit	128	41	1	Tr	0	15	0.1	0	59	44
233	Grapefruit juice, canned, unsweetened	1 cup	247	94	1	Tr	0	17	0.5	2	0	72
237	Grapes, Thompson Seedless	10 grapes	50	30	Tr	Tr	0	0	Tr	0	0	15
239	Grape juice, canned or bottled	1 cup	253	154	1	Tr	0	23	0.6	8	0	Tr
242	Kiwi fruit, raw, without skin	1 kiwifruit	76	46	1	1	0	26	0.2	4	3	71
250	Mangos, raw, without skin and seed	1 mango	207	135	1	1	0	21	0.3	4	79	57
251	Cantaloupe	1 melon	814	277	7	2	0	73	1.7	130	1,376	300
253	Nectarines, raw, without pits	1 nectarine	136	60	1	1	0	8	0.4	0	23	7
254	Oranges, raw, whole	1 orange	131	62	1	Tr	0	52	0.1	0	14	70
260	Orange juice, frozen concentrate, diluted	1 cup	249	112	2	Tr	0	27	0.3	5	12	98
262	Papayas, raw, ½-in. cubes	1 cup	140	55	1	Tr	0	34	0.1	4	77	87
263	Peaches, raw, whole, 2½-in.diam.	1 peach	98	38	1	Tr	0	6	0.2	0	16	7
273	Pears, raw, with skin, cored, Bartlett, 2½-in. diam.	1 pear	166	96	1	1	0	15	0.3	2	2	7
283	Pineapple, chunks or tidbits, juice pack	1 cup	249	149	1	Tr	0	35	0.7	2	5	24

Source: USDA Home and Garden Bulletin No. 72, "Nutritive Value of Foods"

Nutritive Value of Foods Appendix

Nutrients in Indicated Quantity

Item No.	Food Description	Approximate Measure	Weight (Grams)	Food energy (Calories)	Protein (Grams)	Fat (Grams)	Cholesterol (Milligrams)	Calcium (Milligrams)	Iron (Milligrams)	Sodium (Milligrams)	Vitamin A value* Retinol equivalents	Vitamin C (Milligrams)
287	Plantains, without peel, cooked, boiled, sliced	1 cup	190	220	2	Tr	0	4	1.1	10	86	21
288	Plums, raw, 2⅛-in. diam.	1 plum	66	30	Tr	Tr	0	4	0.1	0	11	6
297	Raisins, seedless, cup, not pressed down	1 cup	145	434	5	Tr	0	72	2.7	16	0	3
303	Strawberries, raw, capped, whole	1 cup	144	46	1	Tr	0	23	0.6	1	1	85
309	Watermelon, 4 by 8 in. wedge	1 piece	286	86	2	Tr	0	20	0.7	3	80	23
Grain Products												
311	Bagels, plain or water, enriched	1 bagel	69	177	7	1	0	61	4.1	309	0	1
314	Biscuits, from mix, 2 in. diameter	1 biscuit	30	97	2	4	2	54	0.6	274	7	Tr
Breads:												
319	Cracked-wheat bread (18 per loaf)	1 slice	26	68	2	1	0	27	0.9	138	0	0
332	Pita bread, enriched, white, 6½-in. diam.	1 pita	85	234	8	1	0	73	2.2	456	0	0
346	White bread, enriched (18 per loaf)	1 slice	26	69	2	1	0	39	0.9	177	0	0
353	Whole-wheat bread (16 per loaf)	1 slice	29	80	3	1	0	23	1.1	172	0	0
355	Bread stuffing, dry type, from mix	1 cup	140	246	4	12	0	41	1.5	720	109	0
Breakfast cereals:												
359	Cream of Wheat®, cooked	1 cup	241	106	3	Tr	0	94	8.0	431	0	0
367	Cheerios®	1 oz	30	111	4	2	0	122	10.3	213	150	6
368	Kellogg's® Corn Flakes	1 oz	25	90	2	Tr	0	15	6.7	197	136	5
383	Shredded Wheat	1 oz	25	84	3	1	0	12	0.7	2	0	3
386	Sugar Frosted Flakes, Kellogg's®	1 oz	31	114	1	Tr	0	2	4.5	148	160	6
390	Wheaties®	1 oz	30	106	3	1	0	0	8.1	218	150	6
Cakes prepared from cake mixes:												
394	Angelfood, 1/12 of cake	1 piece	57	143	3	Tr	0	47	0.1	283	0	0
396	Coffeecake, crumb, 1/2 of 8" cake	1 piece	42	136	3	4	40	47	0.7	181	15	0
398	Devil's food with chocolate frosting, 1/12 of cake	1 piece	109	405	4	16	31	102	2.7	289	61	0
Cookies, commercial:												
424	Brownies with nuts and frosting	1 brownie	34	129	2	5	12	11	1.1	50	2	0
426	Chocolate chip, 2¼ in. diam.	4 cookies	30	147	2	7	0	10	1.1	89	0	0
429	Fig bars, square, 1⅝-in. square	4 cookies	64	224	2	2	0	40	1.8	224	0	4
430	Oatmeal with raisins, 2⅝-in. diam.	4 cookies	30	135	2	5	0	11	0.7	115	2	Tr
437	Corn chips	1-oz pkg.	28	145	2	8	0	46	0.4	172	0	0
Crackers:												

Tr = Trace amount
*1 RE = 3.33 IU from animal foods or 1 mcg retinol
1 RE = 10 IU from plant foods or 6 mcg beta carotene.

No.	Food	Amount										
444	Graham, plain, 2½-in. square	2 crackers	14	59	1	1	0	3	0.5	85	0	0
448	Snack-type, standard	1 cracker	3	15	Tr	1	0	4	0.1	25	0	0
449	Wheat, thin	4 crackers	8	36	1	2	0	4	Tr	64	0	0
	Doughnuts, made with enriched flour:											
456	Cake type, plain, 3¼-in. diam.	1 doughnut	25	105	1	6	9	11	0.5	136	10	0
457	Yeast-leavened, glazed, 3¾-in. diam.	1 doughnut	60	242	4	14	4	26	1.2	205	2	Tr
458	English muffins, plain, enriched	1 muffin	58	132	5	1	0	95	2.3	246	0	1
461	Macaroni, enriched, cooked	1 cup	140	220	8	1	0	10	1.9	325	0	0
	Muffins, 2½-in. diam., commercial mix:											
467	Blueberry	1 muffin	66	183	4	4	20	38	1.1	295	15	1
468	Bran	1 muffin	58	127	5	1	0	54	3.1	183	39	0
470	Noodles (egg noodles), enriched, cooked	1 cup	160	219	7	3	46	19	2.3	378	10	0
	Pancakes, 4-in. diam.:											
474	Plain mix (with enriched flour), egg, milk, oil added	1 pancake	29	65	2	2	5	21	0.6	146	19	Tr
	Pies, 9-in. diam.:											
478	Apple, ⅛ of pie	1 piece	150	356	3	17	0	16	0.7	399	48	5
488	Lemon meringue, ⅛ of pie	1 piece	137	367	2	12	62	77	0.8	200	70	4
494	Pumpkin, ⅛ of pie	1 piece	155	316	2	14	65	146	1.9	349	660	3
	Popcorn, popped:											
497	Air-popped, unsalted	1 cup	8	31	1	Tr	0	1	0.3	1	1	0
498	Popped in vegetable oil, salted	1 cup	11	55	1	3	0	1	0.3	97	0	0
499	Sugar syrup coated	1 cup	35	135	2	1	0	2	0.5	Tr	3	0
500	Pretzels	10 twists	60	229	5	2	0	22	1.0	1,029	0	0
	Rice:											
503	Brown, cooked, served hot	1 cup	195	214	5	2	0	20	0.8	587	0	0
505	White, enriched, cooked, served hot	1 cup	158	204	4	Tr	0	16	1.9	577	0	0
	Rolls, enriched, commercial:											
509	Dinner, 2½-in.diam.	1 roll	28	87	3	2	1	50	1.0	150	0	Tr
510	Frankfurter and hamburger	1 roll	43	120	4	2	0	59	1.4	206	0	0
514	Spaghetti, enriched, cooked	1 cup	140	220	8	1	0	10	1.9	325	0	0

Legumes, Nuts, and Seeds

No.	Food	Amount										
526	Almonds, shelled, whole	1 oz	28	162	6	14	0	69	1.2	0	0	0
	Beans, dry, cooked, drained:											
527	Black	1 cup	177	312	12	15	0	64	2.3	414	0	0
528	Great Northern	1 cup	180	356	16	15	0	149	6.1	356	0	0
531	Pinto	1 cup	178	313	12	15	0	57	2.4	352	0	2
536	Black-eyed peas, dry, cooked (with cooking liquid)	1 cup	224	419	11	20	20	36	3.6	844	0	Tr

Nutritive Value of Foods Appendix

Source: USDA Home and Garden Bulletin No. 72, "Nutritive Value of Foods"

Nutrients in Indicated Quantity

Item No.	Food Description	Approximate Measure	Weight (Grams)	Food energy (Calories)	Protein (Grams)	Fat (Grams)	Cholesterol (Milligrams)	Calcium (Milligrams)	Iron (Milligrams)	Sodium (Milligrams)	Vitamin A value* Retinol equivalents	Vitamin C (Milligrams)
544	Chickpeas, cooked, drained	1 cup	169	399	15	18	0	74	3.8	409	2	2
550	Lentils, dry, cooked, with peanuts	1 cup	196	323	16	13	0	35	6.1	431	0	3
553	Mixed nuts, dry roasted, salted	1 oz	28	173	5	16	0	30	0.9	111	0	1
555	Peanuts, roasted in oil, salted	1 cup	144	863	40	76	0	88	2.2	461	0	1
557	Peanut butter	1 tbsp	16	94	4	8	0	7	0.3	73	0	0
564	Refried beans, canned	1 cup	253	367	16	13	15	96	4.2	711	0	10
Soy Products:												
567	Miso	1 cup	275	547	32	17	0	157	6.9	10,252	11	0
568	Tofu, piece 2¼ by 2¾ by 1 in.	1 piece	124	76	8	5	0	138	1.4	10	0	Tr
569	Sunflower seeds, dry, hulled	1 oz	28	162	7	14	0	33	1.9	1	1	Tr
570	Tahini	1 tbsp	15	89	3	8	0	64	1.3	17	0	0
Meat and Meat Products												
Beef, cooked:												
Braised or pot roasted:												
575	Chuck blade. lean and fat, piece	3 oz	85	258	24	17	80	10	2.5	189	0	0
577	Round, bottom, lean and fat piece	3 oz	85	190	29	8	84	7	2.3	37	0	0
578	Lean only from item 577	3 oz	85	144	24	5	61	5	2.0	32	0	0
580	Ground beef, regular, broiled, patty	4 oz	85	235	22	16	75	26	2.0	340	0	0
585	Round, eye of, lean and fat, roasted	3 oz	85	143	25	4	46	6	2.0	32	0	0
587	Sirloin, steak, broiled, lean and fat	3 oz	85	214	23	13	70	14	1.6	317	0	0
590	Beef, dried, chipped	2.5 oz	71	109	22	1	56	4	2.1	1,981	0	0
Lamb:												
593	Chops, loin, broiled, lean and fat	4 oz	72	226	16	18	68	14	1.4	281	0	0
Pork, cured, cooked:												
599	Bacon, regular	3 slices	16	87	6	7	18	2	0.2	370	2	0
601	Ham, light cure, roasted, lean and fat	3 oz	85	137	17	7	54	7	0.6	936	9	0
Luncheon meat:												
605	Chopped ham (8 slices per 6-oz pkg.)	1 slice	28	45	5	2	15	2	0.3	358	0	0
Pork, fresh, cooked:												
610	Chop, loin, pan fried, lean and fat	3 oz	44	123	12	8	35	10	0.4	169	1	Tr
614	Ribs, roasted, lean and fat	3 oz	85	279	20	22	78	21	0.9	44	3	Tr
Sausages:												

Tr = Trace amount
*1 RE = 3.33 IU from animal foods or 1 mcg retinol
1 RE = 10 IU from plant foods or 6 mcg beta carotene.

No.	Food	Measure	g	cal									
618	Bologna, slice (8 per 8-oz pkg.)	1 slice	28	86	4	7	17	24	0.3	206	7	Tr
620	Brown and serve, browned	1 link	13	44	2	4	7	2	0.2	150	0	0
621	Frankfurter, cooked (reheated)	1	57	176	8	15	43	28	1.0	712	5	0
Mixed Dishes												
629	Beef and vegetable stew, home recipe	1 cup	249	182	25	5	42	47	2.5	817	271	7
631	Chicken a la king, home recipe	1 cup	241	460	25	33	190	142	1.9	952	323	5
642	Spaghetti in tomato sauce with cheese, home recipe	1 cup	248	293	10	4	0	40	2.7	563	32	4
Fast Foods												
645	Cheeseburger, regular	1 sandwich	107	317	17	15	46	164	2.8	547	29	0
648	English muffin, egg, cheese, bacon	1 sandwich	135	382	21	19	247	258	3.7	932	140	1
649	Fish sandwich, regular, with cheese	1 sandwich	207	596	27	30	72	286	4.2	1,176	43	Tr
651	Hamburger, regular	1 sandwich	93	270	15	11	34	86	2.7	369	0	0
653	Pizza, cheese, 1/8 of 12-in. diam.	1 slice	86	237	11	10	21	181	1.6	462	68	Tr
654	Roast beef sandwich	1 sandwich	136	341	27	14	67	86	4.3	602	0	0
655	Taco	1 taco	76	98	7	3	50	64	0.9	306	9	3
Poultry and Poultry Products												
Chicken:												
Fried, flesh, with skin and bones:												
656	Breast, ½ breast, batter dipped	4.9 oz	140	365	34	19	102	27	1.9	396	35	0
657	Drumstick, batter dipped	2.5 oz	112	280	31	17	133	16	1.5	473	47	0
Roasted, flesh only:												
660	Breast, ½ breast	3.0 oz	86	162	25	6	76	13	1.0	351	14	0
662	Stewed, flesh only, light and dark meat	1 cup	140	332	43	17	116	18	2.0	109	48	0
Turkey, roasted, flesh only:												
665	Dark meat, piece, 2½ by 1⅝ by ½ in.	4 pieces	78	145	22	6	66	25	1.8	188	0	0
666	Light meat, piece, 4 by 2 by ¼ in.	2 pieces	75	117	22	2	52	14	1.0	170	0	0
667	Chopped or diced	1 cup	135	279	38	13	111	35	2.4	310	0	0
Soups, Sauces, and Gravies												
Soups, condensed:												
Canned, prepared with milk:												
679	Cream of mushroom	1 cup	248	169	6	10	10	159	1.4	861	67	0
680	Tomato	1 cup	248	136	6	3	10	159	1.4	742	82	16
Canned, prepared with water:												
681	Bean with bacon	1 cup	253	172	8	6	3	83	2.0	954	46	2
682	Beef broth, bouillon, consomme	1 cup	240	17	3	1	0	14	0.4	782	0	0
684	Chicken noodle	1 cup	241	65	3	2	14	14	1.7	868	51	0
693	Vegetarian	1 cup	241	72	2	2	0	24	1.1	827	174	1

Source: USDA Home and Garden Bulletin No. 72, "Nutritive Value of Foods"

Nutritive Value of Foods Appendix

Nutrients in Indicated Quantity

Item No.	Food Description	Approximate Measure	Weight (Grams)	Food energy (Calories)	Protein (Grams)	Fat (Grams)	Cholesterol (Milligrams)	Calcium (Milligrams)	Iron (Milligrams)	Sodium (Milligrams)	Vitamin A value* Retinol equivalents	Vitamin C (Milligrams)
	Dehydrated, prepared with water:											
697	Onion	1 pkt	100	349	9	Tr	0	257	1.6	21	1	75
	Sauces, ready to serve:											
703	Barbecue	2 tbsp	35	52	0	Tr	0	4	0.1	392	4	Tr
704	Soy	1 tbsp	16	8	1	Tr	0	3	0.3	902	0	0
	Gravies:											
708	Brown, from dry mix	1 cup	233	123	9	6	7	14	1.6	1,305	2	0
709	Chicken, from dry mix	1 serving	8	30	1	1	2	12	0.1	332	3	0
	Sugars and Sweets											
	Candy:											
711	Chocolate, milk, plain	1 oz	28	150	2	8	6	53	0.7	22	14	0
712	Chocolate, milk, with almonds	1 oz	41	216	4	14	8	92	0.7	30	18	Tr
717	Fondant, uncoated (mints, other)	1 oz	22	82	0	0	0	0	0.0	4	0	0
720	Hard candy	1 oz	28	112	0	Tr	0	1	Tr	11	0	0
723	Custard, baked	1 cup	244	232	12	9	198	271	0.9	215	159	0
724	Gelatin dessert	½ cup	120	74	1	0	0	4	Tr	90	0	0
726	Honey, strained or extracted	1 tbsp	21	64	Tr	0	0	1	0.1	1	0	Tr
727	Jams and preserves	1 tbsp	21	55	Tr	Tr	0	4	0.1	8	2	2
739	Pudding, vanilla, instant	1 cup	267	358	7	10	13	238	0.9	352	21	2
	Sugars:											
741	Brown, pressed down	1 cup	220	829	0	0	0	187	4.2	86	0	0
742	White, granulated	1 tsp	4.2	16	0	0	0	0	0.0	0	0	0
745	White, powdered, sifted	1 cup	120	467	0	Tr	0	1	Tr	1	0	0
	Syrups:											
748	Molasses, cane, blackstrap	2 tbsp	40	116	0	Tr	0	82	1.9	15	0	0
749	Table syrup (corn and maple)	2 tbsp	41	106	0	Tr	0	3	Tr	34	0	0
	Vegetables and Vegetable Products											
750	Alfalfa sprouts, raw	1 cup	33	10	1	Tr	0	11	0.3	2	3	3
761	Beans, string, cooked, drained, from frozen (cut)	1 cup	140	83	3	4	0	59	0.9	433	88	13
771	Broccoli, raw	1 spear	31	11	1	Tr	0	15	0.2	10	10	28
772	Broccoli, cooked	1 spear	38	21	1	1	0	15	0.3	110	37	24
778	Cabbage, common variety, raw, coarsely shredded	1 cup	89	21	1	Tr	0	42	0.5	16	8	29

Tr = Trace amount
*1 RE = 3.33 IU from animal foods or 1 mcg retinol
 1 RE = 10 IU from plant foods or 6 mcg beta carotene.

Nutritive Value of Foods Appendix

No.	Food	Amount										
780	Cabbage, Chinese, Pak-choi, cooked, drained	1 cup	175	66	2	5	0	145	1.4	612	304	41
784	Carrots, whole, 7½ by 1⅛ in.	1 carrot	72	30	1	Tr	0	24	0.2	50	606	4
786	Carrots, cooked, sliced, drained, from raw	1 cup	151	82	1	4	0	44	0.5	462	1,290	5
792	Celery, pascal type, raw, stalk, lrg. outer, 8 by 1½ in.	1 stalk	40	6	Tr	Tr	0	16	Tr	32	9	1
795	Collards, cooked, drained, from frozen (chopped)	1 cup	175	94	5	4	0	355	1.9	486	1,012	45
796	Corn, sweet, cooked, drained, raw ear 5 by 1¾ in.	1 ear	89	110	3	3	0	2	0.5	226	31	5
798	Corn, sweet, cooked, drained, from frozen kernels	1 cup	164	133	4	1	0	5	0.8	372	16	6
799	Corn, sweet, canned, cream style	1 cup	256	184	5	1	0	8	0.9	730	0	12
800	Corn, sweet, canned, whole kernel, vacuum pack	½ cup	128	82	3	1	0	5	0.5	273	0	7
801	Cucumber, with peel, slices	½ cup	52	8	Tr	Tr	0	8	0.2	1	3	2
806	Kale, cooked, drained, from raw	1 cup	135	119	3	4	0	93	1.2	339	921	53
813	Lettuce, raw, crisp head, as iceberg, chopped	1 cup	55	8	1	Tr	0	10	0.2	6	14	2
814	Lettuce, raw, loose leaf, chopped or shredded	1 cup	55	7	1	Tr	0	19	0.7	3	91	2
830	Peas, green, frozen, cooked, drained	1 cup	165	157	8	4	0	38	2.4	516	206	16
832	Peppers, green, raw	1 pepper	74	15	1	Tr	0	7	0.2	2	13	60
834	Potatoes, baked, with skin	1 potato	178	194	4	4	0	27	1.9	418	41	17
838	Potatoes, french fried, strip, frozen, oven heated	10 strips	50	70	1	3	0	6	0.4	194	0	7
839	Potatoes, french fried, strip, frozen, fried in veg. oil	10 strips	50	160	2	9	0	6	0.7	96	0	1
849	Potato chips	1 oz	28	155	2	11	0	7	0.5	149	0	5
852	Radishes, raw	½ cup	58	9	Tr	Tr	0	14	0.2	23	0	9
856	Spinach, raw, chopped	1 cup	30	7	1	Tr	0	30	0.8	24	141	8
858	Spinach, cooked, drained, from frozen (leaf)	1 cup	210	101	8	5	0	313	4.0	630	1,270	4
861	Squash, summer, sliced, cooked, drained	1 cup	185	68	2	4	0	48	0.7	496	57	10
862	Squash, winter, cubes, baked	1 cup	210	151	2	4	0	52	1.0	384	538	19
863	Sweet potatoes, baked in skin, peeled	1 potato	119	134	2	4	0	44	0.8	441	1,128	22
868	Tomatoes, raw, 2⅗-in. diam.	1 tomato	123	22	1	Tr	0	12	0.3	6	52	16
869	Tomatoes, canned, solids and liquid	1 cup	240	46	2	Tr	0	72	1.3	24	17	34
870	Tomato juice, canned	1 cup	243	41	2	Tr	0	24	1.0	654	56	45
877	Vegetable juice cocktail, canned	1 cup	242	44	2	Tr	0	24	1.0	653	121	56
Miscellaneous Items												
885	Catsup	1 cup	240	233	4	1	0	43	1.2	2,674	113	36
894	Mustard, prepared, yellow	1 tsp	5	3	Tr	Tr	0	4	0.1	56	0	Tr
895	Olives, canned, green, medium	4 olives	13	19	Tr	1	0	7	Tr	202	3	0
Pickles, cucumber:												
901	Dill, medium, whole, 3¾ in.	1 cup	65	12	Tr	Tr	0	6	0.3	833	6	1
903	Sweet, small, whole, 2½ in. long	1 cup	37	7	Tr	Tr	0	3	0.2	474	3	Tr

NOTE: Nutritive values of most packaged foods may be obtained from the "Nutrition Facts" panel on the container.

Nutritive Value of Foods Appendix

First aid at the scene of an emergency makes a difference. If you have been taught first aid, you can follow those steps to give care that is specific to the injury. Proceed with first aid only if you know what to do.

Always call 9-1-1 in an emergency. Report what has happened, and let the 9-1-1 operator end the call when all information has been reported.

In addition to the first aid guidelines in this appendix, you can take a first aid course from the American Red Cross or your local fire department. Be prepared to recognize and respond in a medical emergency. You might save a life!

Choking

Choking occurs when a person's airway for breathing is blocked. People, especially children, choke on bites of food or small objects, such as toy parts. What does choking look like?

- No breathing in or out
- The person cannot speak and usually grabs the throat
- Bluish color to the lips and face

1. To know if a person's airway is blocked, ask, "Are you O.K.?" or "Can you speak?" If there is no response or only a high pitch squeal, the person is choking.

2. Begin a cycle of five back blows followed by five stomach thrusts. Perform the back blows with the heel of your hand in the middle of the victim's back, in the direction of the head. Give five back blows in quick succession.

3. The stomach thrusts are given with your arms around the victim's abdomen. Grasp your hands in front above the belly button. Thrust inward and upward five times in quick succession. Continue the cycle of back blows and stomach thrusts until the choking is relieved or help arrives.

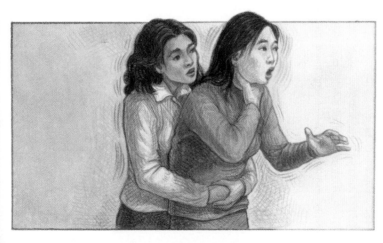

◀ Use stomach thrusts to unblock the victim's airway.

CPR

CPR is cardio (heart) pulmonary (lungs) resuscitation (restart.) If someone has a heart attack causing breathing and heartbeat to stop, immediate CPR is necessary to save their life. Act quickly and decisively. Look for:

- Not conscious
- Will not respond when you call out.
- No breathing

1. Firmly tap the shoulder and ask, "Are you O.K.?" This is to know if the victim is conscious. If no response, check for breathing.

2. Lean over the victim to feel for breath from the nose or mouth, listen for breath, and watch for the chest to rise and fall. If not breathing, give two normal size breaths into the victim's mouth. Use a barrier over the victim's mouth if one is available.

3. Check for heartbeat by placing two fingers along the side of the neck. If there is no heartbeat, overlap your hands on the victim's chest between the nipples. With arms straight, compress the chest 1-1/2 to 2 inches at a rate of 100 compressions per minute. Give 30 compressions. Repeat the cycle of two breaths and 30 compressions until help arrives.

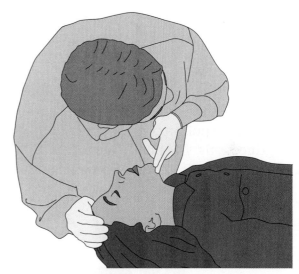

▲ Use the head tilt-chin lift method to open the airway.

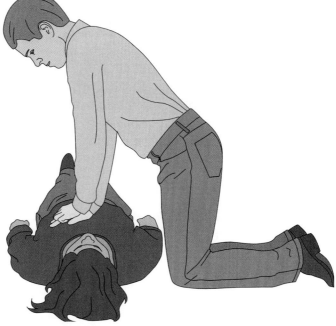

▶ Lean forward so that your shoulders are over the victim. Keep your arms straight.

Poisoning

Poisoning is caused by eating or drinking a harmful substance. These can include medicines, detergents, lawn chemicals, bug spray, cosmetics, house plants or anything that can make you sick. Suspect poisoning if you notice:

- Odd odor on the breath
- Stains or odors on clothes
- Redness or a strange substance around the mouth
- A bottle or container nearby
- The person is sleepy, confused or unconsciousness

1. If conscious, a poison victim may be able to tell you what he/she took. If not conscious, you will have to observe for signs that poisoning has occurred.

2. Call the poison control center immediately and follow their directions. The phone number is 800-222-1222 from anywhere in the U.S. If there is a container of suspect poison, have it in your hand when you make the call.

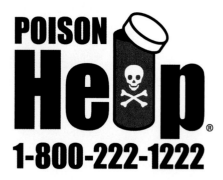

3. The poison control center may tell you to give water, give liquid charcoal or cause the victim to vomit. Only do one of these if the victim is awake and you are told to do so.

Eye Rinse

If something gets into the eyes, they can become irritated. Irritated eyes are red and watery, have the feeling of burning and may cause blurry vision. Dust, sand, dirty water, liquid chemicals or an eyelash are examples of what can irritate the eyes.

1. You can recognize irritated eyes by redness and tears. Irritated eyes are very uncomfortable. Moving the eye or even blinking can make the irritation worse.

2. Pour a gentle stream of clean water from a bottle, pitcher or faucet. You may also use an eyewash station if you have one available to you. Continue to flush the eyes for up to 15 minutes. Stop every five minutes and check to see if the eyes are cleared.

3. If a particle does not flush out of the eye, it is embedded. Cover the eye with a small paper cup taped in place and see a doctor. Keep pressure off the eyeball.

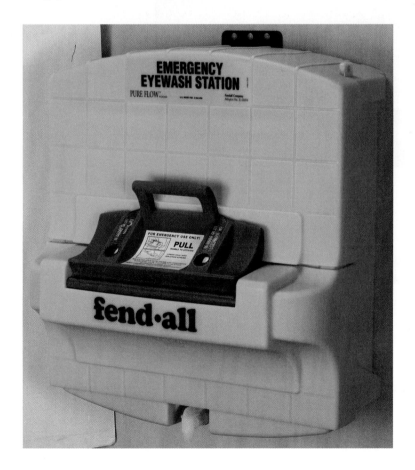

Falls

Slips, trips and falls are part of everyday life. They occur in purposeful activities like sports as well as by accident. While most falls cause little or no injury, some cause sprains and broken bones.

- When the ligaments that hold bones together in a joint are overstretched, this is called a sprain. Commonly, the ankle is sprained when it is twisted in a fall. A sprained joint will be swollen, tender to touch, painful and limited in movement.

- A broken or cracked bone is a fracture. Any strong force can break a bone. Some fractured bones remain under the skin, and the limb may look misshapen. Other more serious fractures break through the skin.

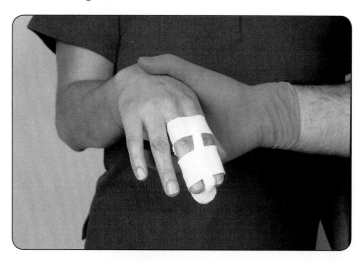

◀ This is a self-splint for fingers or toes.

- First aid for sprains and broken bones is the same because on the scene you might not be able to tell the difference. Follows the reminder RICE:
    - **R**est—keep the person still
    - **I**mmobilize—stabilize the limb in its injured position
    - **C**old—apply ice or other cold pack
    - **E**levate—if not uncomfortable, raise the injured part.

Minor Wounds

A wound is any break in the skin. Wounds are caused by forceful contact with just about anything, such as a knife, a tool, glass or the ground. Even with a minor wound there will be bleeding.

- Some examples of minor wounds are:
  - A puncture wound from stepping on a nail
  - An abrasion from scraping a knee on concrete
  - An incision from a sharp object such as broken glass or a knife
- Rinse the wound with clean water, and apply a bandage or clean cloth. Apply mild pressure to control bleeding. If blood soaks through, apply another bandage over the one already on the wound. Elevating the wounded body part to the level of the heart may reduce bleeding. Keep the wound clean, dry and protected.
- Many minor wounds will heal completely with first aid only. However, contact a doctor if the wound:
  - is on the lip and/or face
  - bleeds even after applying pressure for a while
  - is from a bite (animal or human)
  - doesn't heal and becomes infected

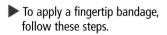
▶ To apply a fingertip bandage, follow these steps.

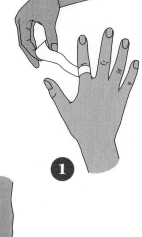
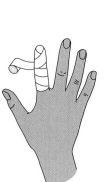
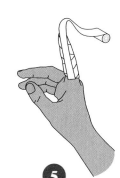

Major Wounds

Major wounds are caused by car collisions, violent fights or contact with machinery. Major wounds are dangerous because they can bleed a lot. With a major wound, an artery may be cut. This causes a forceful spurting of blood. The most important step in first aid for major wounds is to control bleeding.

- Partial or complete tearing of a body part is a major wound that can bleed generously.

  1. Place a thick bandage or cloth over the wound and apply direct pressure. Add bandages on top of the one already applied if they soak through. Continue to apply pressure. Do not attempt to apply a tourniquet.

  2. As a first aid provider, wear gloves any time you may be in contact with blood. If gloves are not available, find something that can be used as a barrier between you and another person's blood, such as newspaper or a plastic bag.

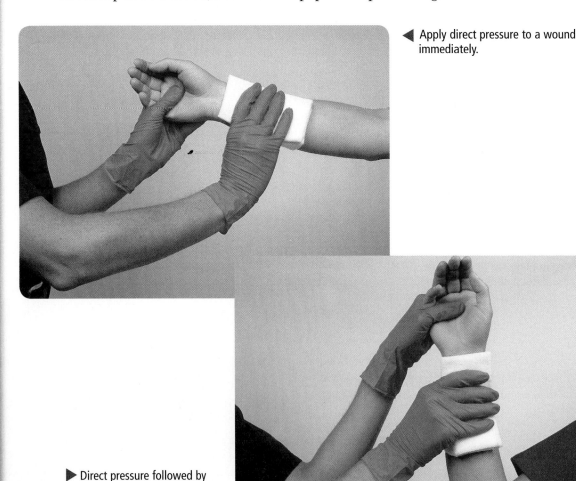

◀ Apply direct pressure to a wound immediately.

▶ Direct pressure followed by elevation is the most effective method of controlling bleeding.

Minor Burns

Exposure to the sun, hot water, a flame or a hot surface can cause a burn to the skin. Burns are classified by degree. Minor burns are called first degree or second degree.

- A first degree burn is when there is damage only to the outer layer of skin, causing redness, pain and mild swelling. Second degree burns are more severe, causing blisters to form on the skin.

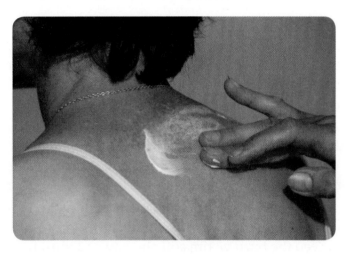

▶ This is a first-degree burn.

- A second degree burn has blisters. A second degree burn over a small or non-critical part of the body is considered a minor burn. Soothe the burn with cool water and apply a dry bandage. Do not break the blisters. Blisters bathe the burned skin with soothing fluid.

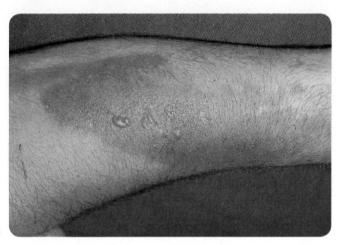

▶ This is a second-degree burn.

- It was once thought that applying butter to a minor burn was helpful. This is no longer done. While cooling a minor burn with water is a good practice, never apply ice or a cold pack directly to burned skin.

Major Burns

Major burns occur from electrocution, immersion in boiling water or fire on clothing or skin. They are life-threatening conditions that require immediate first aid and a doctor's care. Major burns include second degree burns over large areas of the body or over critical areas such as the face or hands. The most severe burn is third degree. Third degree burns destroy all layers of skin.

- A second degree burn on the hands or face is serious because of the effects of scars. Appearance and using the burned body part after healing are important. Second degree burns can be very painful.

- With a third degree burn, the skin may be white or black and leathery. The will be little pain directly on the burn, but be very painful around it. The burn victim may not be conscious. Check for breathing and heartbeat.

- Remove clothing only if it is causing more burning and not if it sticks to the skin. Apply moist, clean cloths loosely over the burn. Keep the burn victim still and covered until help arrives.

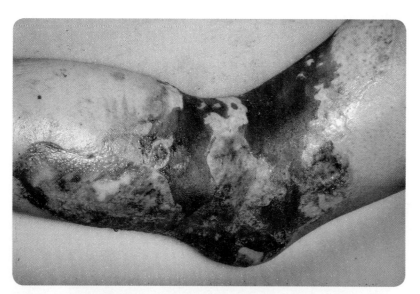

▲ This is a third-degree burn.

Number and Operations

▶ *Understand numbers, ways of representing numbers, relationships among numbers, and number systems*

Fraction, Decimal, and Percent

A percent is a ratio that compares a number to 100. To write a percent as a fraction, drop the percent sign, and use the number as the numerator in a fraction with a denominator of 100. Simplify, if possiblet. For example, 76% $= \frac{76}{100}$, or $\frac{19}{25}$. To write a fraction as a percent, convert it to an equivalent fraction with a denominator of 100. For example, $\frac{3}{4} = \frac{75}{100}$, or 75%. A fraction can be expressed as a percent by first converting the fraction to a decimal (divide the numerator by the denominator) and then converting the decimal to a percent by moving the decimal point two places to the right.

Comparing Numbers on a Number Line

In order to compare and understand the relationship between real numbers in various forms, it is helpful to use a number line. The zero point on a number line is called the origin; the points to the left of the origin are negative, and those to the right are positive. The number line below shows how numbers in fraction, decimal, percent, and integer form can be compared.

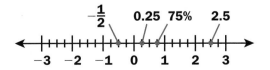

Percents Greater Than 100 and Less Than 1

Percents greater than 100% represent values greater than 1. For example, if the weight of an object is 250% of another, it is 2.5, or $2\frac{1}{2}$, times the weight.

Percents less than 1 represent values less than $\frac{1}{100}$. In other words, 0.1% is one tenth of one percent, which can also be represented in decimal form as 0.001, or in fraction form as $\frac{1}{1,000}$. Similarly, 0.01% is one hundredth of one percent or 0.0001 or $\frac{1}{10,000}$.

Ratio, Rate, and Proportion

A ratio is a comparison of two numbers using division. If a basketball player makes 8 out of 10 free throws, the ratio is written as 8 to 10, 8:10, or $\frac{8}{10}$. Ratios are usually written in simplest form. In simplest form, the ratio "8 out of 10" is 4 to 5, 4:5, or $\frac{4}{5}$. A rate is a ratio of two measurements having different kinds of units—cups per gallon, or miles per hour, for example. When a rate is simplified so that it has a denominator of 1, it is called a unit rate. An example of a unit rate is 9 miles per hour. A proportion is an equation stating that two ratios are equal. $\frac{3}{18} = \frac{13}{78}$ is an example of a proportion. The cross products of a proportion are also equal. $\frac{3}{18} = \frac{13}{78}$ and $3 \times 78 = 18 \times 13$.

Representing Large and Small Numbers

In order to represent large and small numbers, it is important to understand the number system. Our number system is based on 10, and the value of each place is 10 times the value of the place to its right.

Math Appendix

The value of a digit is the product of a digit and its place value. For instance, in the number 6,400, the 6 has a value of six thousands and the 4 has a value of four hundreds. A place value chart can help you read numbers. In the chart, each group of three digits is called a period. Commas separate the periods: the ones period, the thousands period, the millions period, and so on. Values to the right of the ones period are decimals. By understanding place value you can write very large numbers like 5 billion and more, and very small numbers that are less than 1, like one-tenth.

Scientific Notation
When dealing with very large numbers like 1,500,000, or very small numbers like 0.000015, it is helpful to keep track of their value by writing the numbers in scientific notation. Powers of 10 with positive exponents are used with a decimal between 1 and 10 to express large numbers. The exponent represents the number of places the decimal point is moved to the right. So, 528,000 is written in scientific notation as 5.28×10^5. Powers of 10 with negative exponents are used with a decimal between 1 and 10 to express small numbers. The exponent represents the number of places the decimal point is moved to the left. The number 0.00047 is expressed as 4.7×10^{-4}.

Factor, Multiple, and Prime Factorization
Two or more numbers that are multiplied to form a product are called factors. Divisibility rules can be used to determine whether 2, 3, 4, 5, 6, 8, 9, or 10 are factors of a given number. Multiples are the products of a given number and various integers.

For example, 8 is a multiple of 4 because $4 \times 2 = 8$. A prime number is a whole number that has exactly two factors: 1 and itself. A composite number is a whole number that has more than two factors. Zero and 1 are neither prime nor composite. A composite number can be expressed as the product of its prime factors. The prime factorization of 40 is $2 \times 2 \times 2 \times 5$, or $2^3 \times 5$. The numbers 2 and 5 are prime numbers.

Integers
A negative number is a number less than zero. Negative numbers like -8, positive numbers like $+6$, and zero are members of the set of integers. Integers can be represented as points on a number line. A set of integers can be written $\{\ldots, -3, -2, -1, 0, 1, 2, 3, \ldots\}$ where ... means "continues indefinitely."

Real, Rational, and Irrational Numbers
The real number system is made up of the sets of rational and irrational numbers. Rational numbers are numbers that can be written in the form a/b where a and b are integers and $b \neq 0$. Examples are 0.45, $\frac{1}{2}$, and $\sqrt{36}$. Irrational numbers are non-repeating, non-terminating decimals. Examples are $\sqrt{71}$, π, and $0.020020002\ldots$.

Complex and Imaginary Numbers
A complex number is a mathematical expression with a real number element and an imaginary number element. Imaginary numbers are multiples of i, the "imaginary" square root of -1. Complex numbers are represented by $a + bi$, where a and b are real numbers and i represents the imaginary element. When a quadratic equation does not

have a real number solution, the solution can be represented by a complex number. Like real numbers, complex numbers can be added, subtracted, multiplied, and divided.

Vectors and Matrices

A matrix is a set of numbers or elements arranged in rows and columns to form a rectangle. The number of rows is represented by m and the number of columns is represented by n. To describe the number of rows and columns in a matrix, list the number of rows first using the format $m \times n$. Matrix A below is a 3×3 matrix because it has 3 rows and 3 columns. To name an element of a matrix, the letter i is used to denote the row and j is used to denote the column, and the element is labeled in the form $a_{i,j}$. In matrix A below, $a_{3,2}$ is 4.

$$\text{Matrix A} = \begin{pmatrix} 1 & 3 & 5 \\ 0 & 6 & 8 \\ 3 & 4 & 5 \end{pmatrix}$$

A vector is a matrix with only one column or row of elements. A transposed column vector, or a column vector turned on its side, is a row vector. In the example below, row vector b' is the transpose of column vector b.

$$b = \begin{pmatrix} 1 \\ 2 \\ 3 \\ 4 \end{pmatrix}$$

$$b' = (1 \quad 2 \quad 3 \quad 4)$$

▶ Understand meanings of operations and how they relate to one another

Properties of Addition and Multiplication

Properties are statements that are true for any numbers. For example, $3 + 8$ is the same as $8 + 3$ because each expression equals 11. This illustrates the Commutative Property of Addition. Likewise, $3 \times 8 = 8 \times 3$ illustrates the Commutative Property of Multiplication.

When evaluating expressions, it is often helpful to group or associate the numbers. The Associative Property says that the way in which numbers are grouped when added or multiplied does not change the sum or product. The following properties are also true:

- **Additive Identity Property:** When 0 is added to any number, the sum is the number.

- **Multiplicative Identity Property:** When any number is multiplied by 1, the product is the number.

- **Multiplicative Property of Zero:** When any number is multiplied by 0, the product is 0.

Rational Numbers

A number that can be written as a fraction is called a rational number. Terminating and repeating decimals are rational numbers because both can be written as fractions.

Math Appendix

Decimals that are neither terminating nor repeating are called irrational numbers because they cannot be written as fractions. Terminating decimals can be converted to fractions by placing the number (without the decimal point) in the numerator. Count the number of places to the right of the decimal point, and in the denominator, place a 1 followed by a number of zeros equal to the number of places that you counted. The fraction can then be reduced to its simplest form.

Writing a Fraction as a Decimal

Any fraction $\frac{a}{b}$, where $b \neq 0$, can be written as a decimal by dividing the numerator by the denominator. So, $\frac{a}{b} = a \div b$. If the division ends, or terminates, when the remainder is zero, the decimal is a terminating decimal. Not all fractions can be written as terminating decimals. Some have a repeating decimal. A bar indicates that the decimal repeats forever. For example, the fraction $\frac{4}{9}$ can be converted to a repeating decimal, $0.\overline{4}$

Adding and Subtracting Like Fractions

Fractions with the same denominator are called like fractions. To add like fractions, add the numerators and write the sum over the denominator. To add mixed numbers with like fractions, add the whole numbers and fractions separately, adding the numerators of the fractions, then simplifying if necessary. The rule for subtracting fractions with like denominators is similar to the rule

for adding. The numerators can be subtracted and the difference written over the denominator. Mixed numbers are written as improper fractions before subtracting. These same rules apply to adding or subtracting like algebraic fractions. An algebraic fraction is a fraction that contains one or more variables in the numerator or denominator.

Adding and Subtracting Unlike Fractions

Fractions with different denominators are called unlike fractions. The least common multiple of the denominators is used to rename the fractions with a common denominator. After a common denominator is found, the numerators can then be added or subtracted. To add mixed numbers with unlike fractions, rename the mixed numbers as improper fractions. Then find a common denominator, add the numerators, and simplify the answer.

Multiplying Rational Numbers

To multiply fractions, multiply the numerators and multiply the denominators. If the numerators and denominators have common factors, they can be simplified before multiplication. If the fractions have different signs, then the product will be negative. Mixed numbers can be multiplied in the same manner, after first renaming them as improper fractions. Algebraic fractions may be multiplied using the same method described above.

538 Math Appendix

Dividing Rational Numbers

To divide a number by a rational number (a fraction, for example), multiply the first number by the multiplicative inverse of the second. Two numbers whose product is 1 are called multiplicative inverses, or reciprocals. $\frac{7}{4} \times \frac{4}{7} = 1$. When dividing by a mixed number, first rename it as an improper fraction, and then multiply by its multiplicative inverse. This process of multiplying by a number's reciprocal can also be used when dividing algebraic fractions.

Adding Integers

To add integers with the same sign, add their absolute values. The sum takes the same sign as the addends. An addend is a number that is added to another number (the augend). The equation $-5 + (-2) = -7$ is an example of adding two integers with the same sign. To add integers with different signs, subtract their absolute values. The sum takes the same sign as the addend with the greater absolute value.

Subtracting Integers

The rules for adding integers are extended to the subtraction of integers. To subtract an integer, add its additive inverse. For example, to find the difference $2 - 5$, add the additive inverse of 5 to 2: $2 + (-5) = -3$. The rule for subtracting integers can be used to solve real-world problems and to evaluate algebraic expressions.

Additive Inverse Property

Two numbers with the same absolute value but different signs are called opposites. For example, -4 and 4 are opposites. An integer and its opposite are also called additive inverses. The Additive Inverse Property says that the sum of any number and its additive inverse is zero. The Commutative, Associative, and Identity Properties also apply to integers. These properties help when adding more than two integers.

Absolute Value

In mathematics, when two integers on a number line are on opposite sides of zero, and they are the same distance from zero, they have the same absolute value. The symbol for absolute value is two vertical bars on either side of the number. For example, $|-5| = 5$.

Multiplying Integers

Since multiplication is repeated addition, $3(-7)$ means that -7 is used as an addend 3 times. By the Commutative Property of Multiplication, $3(-7) = -7(3)$. The product of two integers with different signs is always negative. The product of two integers with the same sign is always positive.

Dividing Integers

The quotient of two integers can be found by dividing the numbers using their absolute values. The quotient of two integers with the same sign is positive, and the quotient of two integers with a different sign is negative. $-12 \div (-4) = 3$ and $12 \div (-4) = -3$. The division of integers is used in statistics to find the average, or mean, of a set of data. When finding the mean of a set of numbers, find the sum of the numbers, and then divide by the number in the set.

Math Appendix

Adding and Multiplying Vectors and Matrices

In order to add two matrices together, they must have the same number of rows and columns. In matrix addition, the corresponding elements are added to each other. In other words $(a + b)_{ij} = a_{ij} + b_{ij}$. For example,

$$\begin{pmatrix} 1 & 2 \\ 2 & 1 \end{pmatrix} + \begin{pmatrix} 3 & 6 \\ 0 & 1 \end{pmatrix} = \begin{pmatrix} 1+3 & 2+6 \\ 2+0 & 1+1 \end{pmatrix} = \begin{pmatrix} 4 & 8 \\ 2 & 2 \end{pmatrix}$$

Matrix multiplication requires that the number of elements in each row in the first matrix is equal to the number of elements in each column in the second. The elements of the first row of the first matrix are multiplied by the corresponding elements of the first column of the second matrix and then added together to get the first element of the product matrix. To get the second element, the elements in the first row of the first matrix are multiplied by the corresponding elements in the second column of the second matrix then added, and so on, until every row of the first matrix is multiplied by every column of the second. See the example below.

$$\begin{pmatrix} 1 & 2 \\ 3 & 4 \end{pmatrix} \times \begin{pmatrix} 3 & 6 \\ 0 & 1 \end{pmatrix} = \begin{pmatrix} (1\times3)+(2\times0) & (1\times6)+(2\times1) \\ (3\times3)+(4\times0) & (3\times6)+(4\times1) \end{pmatrix} = \begin{pmatrix} 3 & 8 \\ 9 & 22 \end{pmatrix}$$

Vector addition and multiplication are performed in the same way, but there is only one column and one row.

Permutations and Combinations

Permutations and combinations are used to determine the number of possible outcomes in different situations. An arrangement, listing, or pattern in which order is important is called a permutation. The symbol P(6, 3) represents the number of permutations of 6 things taken 3 at a time. For P(6, 3), there are $6 \times 5 \times 4$ or 120 possible outcomes. An arrangement or listing where order is not important is called a combination. The symbol C(10, 5) represents the number of combinations of 10 things taken 5 at a time. For C(10, 5), there are $(10 \times 9 \times 8 \times 7 \times 6) \div (5 \times 4 \times 3 \times 2 \times 1)$ or 252 possible outcomes.

Powers and Exponents

An expression such as $3 \times 3 \times 3 \times 3$ can be written as a power. A power has two parts, a base and an exponent. $3 \times 3 \times 3 \times 3 = 3^4$. The base is the number that is multiplied (3). The exponent tells how many times the base is used as a factor (4 times). Numbers and variables can be written using exponents. For example, $8 \times 8 \times 8 \times m \times m \times m \times m \times m$ can be expressed $8^3 m^5$. Exponents also can be used with place value to express numbers in expanded form. Using this method, 1,462 can be written as $(1 \times 10^3) + (4 \times 10^2) + (6 \times 10^1) + (2 \times 10^0)$.

Squares and Square Roots

The square root of a number is one of two equal factors of a number. Every positive number has both a positive and a negative square root. For example, since $8 \times 8 = 64$, 8 is a square root of 64. Since $(-8) \times (-8) = 64$, −8 is also a square root of 64. The notation $\sqrt{}$ indicates the positive square root, $-\sqrt{}$ indicates the negative square root, and $\pm\sqrt{}$ indicates both square roots. For example, $\sqrt{81} = 9$, $-\sqrt{49} = -7$, and $\pm\sqrt{4} = \pm2$. The square root of a negative number is an imaginary number because any two factors of a negative number must have different signs, and are therefore not equivalent.

Logarithm

A logarithm is the inverse of exponentiation. The logarithm of a number x in base b is equal to the number n. Therefore, $b^n = x$ and $\log_b x = n$. For example, $\log_4(64) = 3$ because $4^3 = 64$. The most commonly used bases for logarithms are 10, the common logarithm; 2, the binary logarithm; and the constant e, the natural logarithm (also called $ln(x)$ instead of $\log_e(x)$). Below is a list of some of the rules of logarithms that are important to understand if you are going to use them.

$$\log_b(xy) = \log_b(x) + \log_b(y)$$
$$\log_b(x/y) = \log_b(x) - \log_b(y)$$
$$\log_b(1/x) = -\log_b(x)$$
$$\log_b(x)y = y\log_b(x)$$

▶ *Compute fluently and make reasonable estimates*

Estimation by Rounding

When rounding numbers, look at the digit to the right of the place to which you are rounding. If the digit is 5 or greater, round up. If it is less than 5, round down. For example, to round 65,137 to the nearest hundred, look at the number in the tens place. Since 3 is less than 5, round down to 65,100. To round the same number to the nearest ten thousandth, look at the number in the thousandths place. Since it is 5, round up to 70,000.

Finding Equivalent Ratios

Equivalent ratios have the same meaning. Just like finding equivalent fractions, to find an equivalent ratio, multiply or divide both sides by the same number. For example, you can multiply 7 by

both sides of the ratio 6:8 to get 42:56. Instead, you can also divide both sides of the same ratio by 2 to get 3:4. Find the simplest form of a ratio by dividing to find equivalent ratios until you can't go any further without going into decimals. So, 160:240 in simplest form is 2:3. To write a ratio in the form 1:n, divide both sides by the left-hand number. In other words, to change 8:20 to 1:n, divide both sides by 8 to get 1:2.5.

Front-End Estimation

Front-end estimation can be used to quickly estimate sums and differences before adding or subtracting. To use this technique, add or subtract just the digits of the two highest place values, and replace the other place values with zero. This will give you an estimation of the solution of a problem. For example, $93,471 - 22,825$ can be changed to $93,000 - 22,000$ or $71,000$. This estimate can be compared to your final answer to judge its correctness.

Judging Reasonableness

When solving an equation, it is important to check your work by considering how reasonable your answer is. For example, consider the equation $9\frac{3}{4} \times 4\frac{1}{3}$. Since $9\frac{3}{4}$ is between 9 and 10 and $4\frac{1}{3}$ is between 4 and 5, only values that are between 9×4 or 36 and 10×5 or 50 will be reasonable. You can also use front-end estimation, or you can round and estimate a reasonable answer. In the equation 73×25, you can round and solve to estimate a reasonable answer to be near 70×30 or 2,100.

Math Appendix

Algebra

▶ Understand patterns, relations, and functions

Relation
A relation is a generalization comparing sets of ordered pairs for an equation or inequality such as $x = y + 1$ or $x > y$. The first element in each pair, the x values, forms the domain. The second element in each pair, the y values, forms the range.

Function
A function is a special relation in which each member of the domain is paired with exactly one member in the range. Functions may be represented using ordered pairs, tables, or graphs. One way to determine whether a relation is a function is to use the vertical line test. Using an object to represent a vertical line, move the object from left to right across the graph. If, for each value of x in the domain, the object passes through no more than one point on the graph, then the graph represents a function.

Linear and Nonlinear Functions
Linear functions have graphs that are straight lines. These graphs represent constant rates of change. In other words, the slope between any two pairs of points on the graph is the same. Nonlinear functions do not have constant rates of change. The slope changes along these graphs. Therefore, the graphs of non-linear functions are *not* straight lines. Graphs of curves represent nonlinear functions. The equation for a linear function can be written in the form

$y = mx + b$, where m represents the constant rate of change, or the slope. Therefore, you can determine whether a function is linear by looking at the equation. For example, the equation $y = \frac{3}{x}$ is nonlinear because x is in the denominator and the equation cannot be written in the form $y = mx + b$. A nonlinear function does not increase or decrease at a constant rate. You can check this by using a table and finding the increase or decrease in y for each regular increase in x. For example, if for each increase in x by 2, y does not increase or decrease the same amount each time, the function is nonlinear.

Linear Equations in Two Variables
In a linear equation with two variables, such as $y = x - 3$, the variables appear in separate terms and neither variable contains an exponent other than 1. The graphs of all linear equations are straight lines. All points on a line are solutions of the equation that is graphed.

Quadratic and Cubic Functions
A quadratic function is a polynomial equation of the second degree, generally expressed as $ax^2 + bx + c = 0$, where a, b, and c are real numbers and a is not equal to zero. Similarly, a cubic function is a polynomial equation of the third degree, usually expressed as $ax^3 + bx^2 + cx + d = 0$. Quadratic functions can be graphed using an equation or a table of values. For example, to graph $y = 3x^2 + 1$, substitute the values −1, −0.5, 0, 0.5, and 1 for x to yield the point coordinates (−1, 4), (−0.5, 1.75), (0, 1), (0.5, 1.75), and (1, 4). Plot these points on a coordinate

grid and connect the points in the form of a parabola. Cubic functions also can be graphed by making a table of values. The points of a cubic function from a curve. There is one point at which the curve changes from opening upward to opening downward, or vice versa, called the point of inflection.

Slope
Slope is the ratio of the rise, or vertical change, to the run, or horizontal change of a line: slope = rise/run. Slope (m) is the same for any two points on a straight line and can be found by using the coordinates of any two points on the line:

$$m = \frac{y_2 - y_1}{x_2 - x_1}, \text{ where } x_2 \neq x_1$$

Asymptotes
An asymptote is a straight line that a curve approaches but never actually meets or crosses. Theoretically, the asymptote meets the curve at infinity. For example, in the function $f(x) = \frac{1}{x}$, two asymptotes are being approached: the line $y = 0$ and $x = 0$. See the graph of the function below.

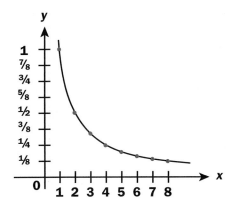

Represent and analyze mathematical situations and structures using algebraic symbols

Variables and Expressions
Algebra is a language of symbols. A variable is a placeholder for a changing value. Any letter, such as x, can be used as a variable. Expressions such as $x + 2$ and $4x$ are algebraic expressions because they represent sums and/or products of variables and numbers. Usually, mathematicians avoid the use of i and e for variables because they have other mathematical meanings ($i = \sqrt{-1}$ and e is used with natural logarithms). To evaluate an algebraic expression, replace the variable or variables with known values, and then solve using order of operations. Translate verbal phrases into algebraic expressions by first defining a variable: Choose a variable and a quantity for the variable to represent. In this way, algebraic expressions can be used to represent real-world situations.

Constant and Coefficient
A constant is a fixed value unlike a variable, which can change. Constants are usually represented by numbers, but they can also be represented by symbols. For example, π is a symbolic representation of the value 3.1415.… A coefficient is a constant by which a variable or other object is multiplied. For example, in the expression $7x^2 + 5x + 9$, the coefficient of x^2 is 7 and the coefficient of x is 5. The number 9 is a constant and not a coefficient.

Monomial and Polynomial
A monomial is a number, a variable, or a product of numbers and/or variables such as 3×4. An algebraic expression

that contains one or more monomials is called a polynomial. In a polynomial, there are no terms with variables in the denominator and no terms with variables under a radical sign. Polynomials can be classified by the number of terms contained in the expression. Therefore, a polynomial with two terms is called a binomial ($z^2 - 1$), and a polynomial with three terms is called a trinomial ($2y^3 + 4y^2 - y$). Polynomials also can be classified by their degrees. The degree of a monomial is the sum of the exponents of its variables. The degree of a nonzero constant such as 6 or 10 is 0. The constant 0 has no degree. For example, the monomial $4b^5c^2$ had a degree of 7. The degree of a polynomial is the same as that of the term with the greatest degree. For example, the polynomial $3x^4 - 2y^3 + 4y^2 - y$ has a degree of 4.

Equation

An equation is a mathematical sentence that states that two expressions are equal. The two expressions in an equation are always separated by an equal sign. When solving for a variable in an equation, you must perform the same operations on both sides of the equation in order for the mathematical sentence to remain true.

Solving Equations with Variables

To solve equations with variables on both sides, use the Addition or Subtraction Property of Equality to write an equivalent equation with the variables on the same side. For example, to solve $5x - 8 = 3x$, subtract $3x$ from each side to get $2x - 8 = 0$. Then add 8 to each side to get $2x = 8$. Finally, divide each side by 2 to find that $x = 4$.

Solving Equations with Grouping Symbols

Equations often contain grouping symbols such as parentheses or brackets. The first step in solving these equations is to use the Distributive Property to remove the grouping symbols. For example $5(x + 2) = 25$ can be changed to $5x + 10 = 25$, and then solved to find that $x = 3$.

Some equations have no solution. That is, there is no value of the variable that results in a true sentence. For such an equation, the solution set is called the null or empty set, and is represented by the symbol $\varnothing$ or {}. Other equations may have every number as the solution. An equation that is true for every value of the variable is called the identity.

Inequality

A mathematical sentence that contains the symbols < (less than), > (greater than), ≤ (less than or equal to), or ≥ (greater than or equal to) is called an inequality. For example, the statement that it is legal to drive 55 miles per hour or slower on a stretch of the highway can be shown by the sentence $s \le 55$. Inequalities with variables are called open sentences. When a variable is replaced with a number, the inequality may be true or false.

Solving Inequalities

Solving an inequality means finding values for the variable that make the inequality true. Just as with equations, when you add or subtract the same number from each side of an inequality, the inequality remains true. For example, if you add 5 to each side of the inequality $3x < 6$, the resulting inequality $3x + 5 < 11$ is also true. Adding or subtracting the same number from each side of an inequality does not affect the inequality sign. When multiplying or dividing each side of an inequality by the same positive number, the inequality remains true. In such cases, the inequality symbol does not change. When multiplying or dividing each side of an inequality by a negative number, the inequality symbol must be reversed. For example, when dividing each side of the inequality $-4x \geq -8$ by -2, the inequality sign must be changed to $\leq$ for the resulting inequality, $2x \leq 4$, to be true. Since the solutions to an inequality include all rational numbers satisfying it, inequalities have an infinite number of solutions.

Representing Inequalities on a Number Line

The solutions of inequalities can be graphed on a number line. For example, if the solution of an inequality is $x < 5$, start an arrow at 5 on the number line, and continue the arrow to the left to show all values less than 5 as the solution. Put an open circle at 5 to show that the point 5 is *not* included in the graph. Use a closed circle when graphing solutions that are greater than or equal to, or less than or equal to, a number.

Order of Operations

Solving a problem may involve using more than one operation. The answer can depend on the order in which you do the operations. To make sure that there is just one answer to a series of computations, mathematicians have agreed upon an order in which to do the operations. First simplify within the parentheses, often called graphing symbols, and then evaluate any exponents. Then multiply and divide from left to right, and finally add and subtract from left to right.

Parametric Equations

Given an equation with more than one unknown, a statistician can draw conclusions about those unknown quantities through the use of parameters, independent variables that the statistician already knows something about. For example, you can find the velocity of an object if you make some assumptions about distance and time parameters.

Recursive Equations

In recursive equations, every value is determined by the previous value. You must first plug an initial value into the equation to get the first value, and then you can use the first value to determine the next one, and so on. For example, in order to determine what the population of pigeons will be in New York City in three years, you can use an equation with the birth, death, immigration, and emigration rates of the birds. Input the current population size into the equation to determine next year's population size, then repeat until you have calculated the value for which you are looking.

▶ *Use mathematical models to represent and understand quantitative relationships*

Solving Systems of Equations

Two or more equations together are called a system of equations. A system of equations can have one solution, no solution, or infinitely many solutions. One method for solving a system of equations is to graph the equations on the same coordinate plane. The coordinates of the point where the graphs intersect is the solution. In other words, the solution of a system is the ordered pair that is a solution of all equations. A more accurate way to solve a system of two equations is by using a method called substitution. Write both equations in terms of y. Replace y in the first equation with the right side of the second equation. Check the solution by graphing. You can solve a system of three equations using matrix algebra.

Graphing Inequalities

To graph an inequality, first graph the related equation, which is the boundary. All points in the shaded region are solutions of the inequality. If an inequality contains the symbol $\leq$ or $\geq$, then use a solid line to indicate that the boundary is included in the graph. If an inequality contains the symbol $<$ or $>$, then use a dashed line to indicate that the boundary is not included in the graph.

▶ Analyze change in various contexts

Rate of Change

A change in one quantity with respect to another quantity is called the rate of change. Rates of change can be described using slope:

$$\text{slope} = \frac{change\ in\ y}{change\ in\ x}$$

You can find rates of change from an equation, a table, or a graph. A special type of linear equation that describes rate of change is called a direct variation.

The graph of a direct variation always passes through the origin and represents a proportional situation. In the equation $y = kx$, k is called the constant of variation. It is the slope, or rate of change. As x increases in value, y increases or decreases at a constant rate k, or y varies directly with x. Another way to say this is that y is directly proportional to x. The direct variation $y = kx$ also can be written as $k = \frac{y}{x}$. In this form, you can see that the ratio of y to x is the same for any corresponding values of y and x.

Slope-Intercept Form

Equations written as $y = mx + b$, where m is the slope and b is the y-intercept, are linear equations in slope-intercept form. For example, the graph of $y = 5x - 6$ is a line that has a slope of 5 and crosses the y-axis at $(0, -6)$. Sometimes you must first write an equation in slope-intercept form before finding the slope and y-intercept. For example, the equation $2x + 3y = 15$ can be expressed in slope-intercept form by subtracting $2x$ from each side and then dividing by 3: $y = -\frac{2}{3}x + 5$, revealing a slope of $-\frac{2}{3}$ and a y-intercept of 5. You can use the slope-intercept form of an equation to graph a line easily. Graph the y-intercept and use the slope to find another point on the line, then connect the two points with a line.

Geometry

▶ *Analyze characteristics and properties of two- and three-dimensional geometric shapes and develop mathematical arguments about geometric relationships*

Angles

Two rays that have the same endpoint form an angle. The common endpoint is called the vertex, and the two rays that make up the angle are called the sides of the angle. The most common unit of measure for angles is the degree. Protractors can be used to measure angles or to draw an angle of a given measure. Angles can be classified by their degree measure. Acute angles have measures less than 90° but greater than 0°. Obtuse angles have measures greater than 90° but less than 180°. Right angles have measures of 90°.

Triangles

A triangle is a figure formed by three line segments that intersect only at their endpoints. The sum of the measures of the angles of a triangle is 180°. Triangles can be classified by their angles. An acute triangle contains all acute angles. An obtuse triangle has one obtuse angle. A right triangle has one right angle. Triangles can also be classified by their sides. A scalene triangle has no congruent sides. An isosceles triangle has at least two congruent sides. In an equilateral triangle all sides are congruent.

Quadrilaterals

A quadrilateral is a closed figure with four sides and four vertices. The segments of a quadrilateral intersect only at their endpoints. Quadrilaterals can be separated into two triangles. Since the sum of the interior angles of all triangles totals 180°, the measures of the interior angles of a quadrilateral equal 360°. Quadrilaterals are classified according to their characteristics, and include trapezoids, parallelograms, rectangles, squares, and rhombuses.

Two-Dimensional Figures

A two-dimensional figure exists within a plane and has only the dimensions of length and width. Examples of two-dimensional figures include circles and polygons. Polygons are figures that have three or more angles, including triangles, quadrilaterals, pentagons, hexagons, and many more. The sum of the angles of any polygon totals at least 180° (triangle), and each additional side adds 180° to the measure of the first three angles. The sum of the angles of a quadrilateral, for example, is 360°. The sum of the angles of a pentagon is 540°.

Three-Dimensional Figures

A plane is a two-dimensional flat surface that extends in all directions. Intersecting planes can form the edges and vertices of three-dimensional figures or solids. A polyhedron is a solid with flat surfaces that are polygons.

Math Appendix

Polyhedrons are composed of faces, edges, and vertices and are differentiated by their shape and by their number of bases. Skew lines are lines that lie in different planes. They are neither intersecting nor parallel.

Congruence

Figures that have the same size and shape are congruent. The parts of congruent triangles that match are called corresponding parts. Congruence statements are used to identify corresponding parts of congruent triangles. When writing a congruence statement, the letters must be written so that corresponding vertices appear in the same order. Corresponding parts can be used to find the measures of angles and sides in a figure that is congruent to a figure with known measures.

Similarity

If two figures have the same shape but not the same size they are called similar figures. For example, the triangles below are similar, so angles A, B, and C have the same measurements as angles D, E, and F, respectively. However, segments AB, BC, and CA do not have the same measurements as segments DE, EF, and FD, but the measures of the sides are proportional.

For example, $\dfrac{\overline{AB}}{\overline{DE}} = \dfrac{\overline{BC}}{\overline{EF}} = \dfrac{\overline{CA}}{\overline{FD}}$.

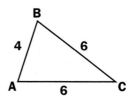
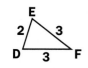

Solid figures are considered to be similar if they have the same shape and their corresponding linear measures are proportional. As with two-dimensional figures, they can be tested for similarity by comparing corresponding measures. If the compared ratios are proportional, then the figures are similar solids. Missing measures of similar solids can also be determined by using proportions.

The Pythagorean Theorem

The sides that are adjacent to a right angle are called legs. The side opposite the right angle is the hypotenuse.

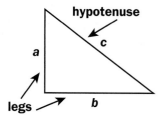

The Pythagorean Theorem describes the relationship between the lengths of the legs a and b and the hypotenuse c. It states that if a triangle is a right triangle, then the square of the length of the hypotenuse is equal to the sum of the squares of the lengths of the legs. In symbols, $c^2 = a^2 + b^2$.

Sine, Cosine, and Tangent Ratios

Trigonometry is the study of the properties of triangles. A trigonometric ratio is a ratio of the lengths of two sides of a right triangle. The most common trigonometric ratios are the sine, cosine, and tangent ratios. These ratios are abbreviated as *sin*, *cos*, and *tan*, respectively.

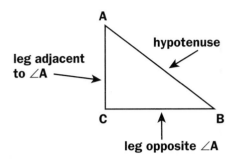

If ∠*A* is an acute angle of a right triangle, then

$$sin \angle A = \frac{\text{measure of leg opposite } \angle A}{\text{measure of hypotenuse}},$$

$$cos \angle A = \frac{\text{measure of leg adjacent to } \angle A}{\text{measure of hypotenuse}}, \text{ and}$$

$$tan \angle A = \frac{\text{measure of leg opposite } \angle A}{\text{measure of leg adjacent to } \angle A}.$$

▶ *Specify locations and describe spatial relationships using coordinate geometry and other representational systems*

Polygons
A polygon is a simple, closed figure formed by three or more line segments. The line segments meet only at their endpoints. The points of intersection are called vertices, and the line segments are called sides. Polygons are classified by the number if sides they have. The diagonals of a polygon divide the polygon into triangles. The number of triangles formed is two less than the number of sides. To find the sum of the measures of the interior angles of any polygon, multiply the number of triangles within the polygon by 180. That is, if *n* equals the number of sides, then (*n* − 2) 180 gives the sum of the measures of the polygon's interior angles.

Cartesian Coordinates
In the Cartesian coordinate system, the *y*-axis extends above and below the origin and the *x*-axis extends to the right and left of the origin, which is the point at which the *x*- and *y*-axes intersect. Numbers below and to the left of the origin are negative. A point graphed on the coordinate grid is said to have an *x*-coordinate and a *y*-coordinate. For example, the point (1,–2) has as its *x*-coordinate the number 1, and has as its *y*-coordinate the number –2. This point is graphed by locating the position on the grid that is 1 unit to the right of the origin and 2 units below the origin.

The *x*-axis and the *y*-axis separate the coordinate plane into four regions, called quadrants. The axes and points located on the axes themselves are not located in any of the quadrants. The quadrants are labeled I to IV, starting in the upper right and proceeding counterclockwise. In quadrant I, both coordinates are positive. In quadrant II, the *x*-coordinate is negative and the *y*-coordinate is positive. In quadrant III, both coordinates are negative. In quadrant IV, the *x*-coordinate is positive and the *y*-coordinate is negative. A coordinate graph can be used to show algebraic relationships among numbers.

▶ *Apply transformations and use symmetry to analyze mathematical situations*

Similar Triangles and Indirect Measurement
Triangles that have the same shape but not necessarily the same dimensions are called similar triangles. Similar triangles

have corresponding angles and corresponding sides. Arcs are used to show congruent angles. If two triangles are similar, then the corresponding angles have the same measure, and the corresponding sides are proportional. Therefore, to determine the measures of the sides of similar triangles when some measures are known, proportions can be used.

Transformations

A transformation is a movement of a geometric figure. There are several types of transformations. In a translation, also called a slide, a figure is slid from one position to another without turning it. Every point of the original figure is moved the same distance and in the same direction. In a reflection, also called a flip, a figure is flipped over a line to form a mirror image. Every point of the original figure has a corresponding point on the other side of the line of symmetry. In a rotation, also called a turn, a figure is turned around a fixed point. A figure can be rotated 0°–360° clockwise or counterclockwise. A dilation transforms each line to a parallel line whose length is a fixed multiple of the length of the original line to create a similar figure that will be either larger or smaller.

▶ *Use visualizations, spatial reasoning, and geometric modeling to solve problems*

Two-Dimensional Representations of Three-Dimensional Objects

Three-dimensional objects can be represented in a two-dimensional drawing in order to more easily determine properties such as surface area and volume. When you look at the triangular prism, you can see the orientation of its three

dimensions, length, width, and height. Using the drawing and the formulas for surface area and volume, you can easily calculate these properties.

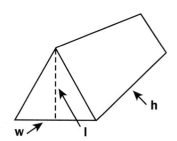

Another way to represent a three-dimensional object in a two-dimensional plane is by using a net, which is the unfolded representation. Imagine cutting the vertices of a box until it is flat then drawing an outline of it. That's a net. Most objects have more than one net, but any one can be measured to determine surface area. Below is a cube and one of its nets.

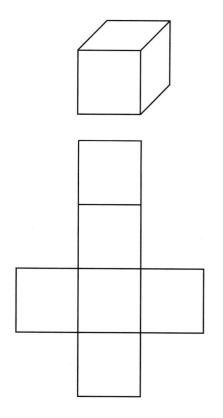

Measurement

▶ *Understand measurable attributes of objects and the units, systems, and processes of measurement*

Customary System

The customary system is the system of weights and measures used in the United States. The main units of weight are ounces, pounds (1 equal to 16 ounces), and tons (1 equal to 2,000 pounds). Length is typically measured in inches, feet (1 equal to 12 inches), yards (1 equal to 3 feet), and miles (1 equal to 5,280 feet), while area is measured in square feet and acres (1 equal to 43,560 square feet). Liquid is measured in cups, pints (1 equal to 2 cups), quarts (1 equal to 2 pints), and gallons (1 equal to 4 quarts). Finally, temperature is measured in degrees Fahrenheit.

Metric System

The metric system is a decimal system of weights and measurements in which the prefixes of the words for the units of measure indicate the relationships between the different measurements. In this system, the main units of weight, or mass, are grams and kilograms. Length is measured in millimeters, centimeters, meters, and kilometers, and the units of area are square millimeters, centimeters, meters, and kilometers. Liquid is typically measured in milliliters and liters, while temperature is in degrees Celsius.

Selecting Units of Measure

When measuring something, it is important to select the appropriate type and size of unit. For example, in the United States it would be appropriate when describing someone's height to use feet and inches. These units of height or length are good to use because they are in the customary system, and they are of appropriate size. In the customary system, use inches, feet, and miles for lengths and perimeters; square inches, feet, and miles for area and surface area; and cups, pints, quarts, gallons or cubic inches and feet (and less commonly miles) for volume. In the metric system use millimeters, centimeters, meters, and kilometers for lengths and perimeters; square units millimeters, centimeters, meters, and kilometers for area and surface area; and milliliters and liters for volume. Finally, always use degrees to measure angles.

▶ *Apply appropriate techniques, tools, and formulas to determine measurements*

Precision and Significant Digits

The precision of measurement is the exactness to which a measurement is made. Precision depends on the smallest unit of measure being used, or the precision unit. One way to record a measure is to estimate to the nearest precision unit. A more precise method is to include all of the digits that are actually measured, plus one estimated digit. The digits recorded, called significant digits, indicate the precision of the measurement. There are special rules for determining significant digits. If a number contains a decimal point, the number of significant digits is found by counting from left to right, starting with the first nonzero digit.

If the number does not contain a decimal point, the number of significant digits is found by counting the digits from left to right, starting with the first digit and ending with the last nonzero digit.

Surface Area

The amount of material needed to cover the surface of a figure is called the surface area. It can be calculated by finding the area of each face and adding them together. To find the surface area of a rectangular prism, for example, the formula $S = 2lw + 2lh + 2wh$ applies. A cylinder, on the other hand, may be unrolled to reveal two circles and a rectangle. Its surface area can be determined by finding the area of the two circles, $2\pi r^2$, and adding it to the area of the rectangle, $2\pi rh$ (the length of the rectangle is the circumference of one of the circles), or $S = 2\pi r^2 + 2\pi rh$. The surface area of a pyramid is measured in a slightly different way because the sides of a pyramid are triangles that intersect at the vertex. These sides are called lateral faces and the height of each is called the slant height. The sum of their areas is the lateral area of a pyramid. The surface area of a square pyramid is the lateral area $\frac{1}{2}bh$ (area of a lateral face) times 4 (number of lateral faces), plus the area of the base. The surface area of a cone is the area of its circular base (πr^2) plus its lateral area (πrl, where l is the slant height).

Volume

Volume is the measure of space occupied by a solid region. To find the volume of a prism, the area of the base is multiplied by the measure of the height, $V = Bh$. A solid containing several prisms can be broken down into its component prisms. Then the volume of each component can be found and the volumes added. The volume of a cylinder can be determined by finding the area of its circular base, πr^2, and then multiplying by the height of the cylinder. A pyramid has one-third the volume of a prism with the same base and height. To find the volume of a pyramid, multiply the area of the base by the pyramid's height, and then divide by 3. Simply stated, the formula for the volume of a pyramid is $V = \frac{1}{3}bh$. A cone is a three-dimensional figure with one circular base and a curved surface connecting the base and the vertex. The volume of a cone is one-third the volume of a cylinder with the same base area and height. Like a pyramid, the formula for the volume of a cone is $V = \frac{1}{3}bh$. More specifically, the formula is $V = \frac{1}{3}\pi r^2 h$.

Upper and Lower Bounds

Upper and lower bounds have to do with the accuracy of a measurement. When a measurement is given, the degree of accuracy is also stated to tell you what the upper and lower bounds of the measurement are. The upper bound is the largest possible value that a measurement could have had before being rounded down, and the lower bound is the lowest possible value it could have had before being rounded up.

Data Analysis and Probability

▶ *Formulate questions that can be addressed with data and collect, organize, and display relevant data to answer them*

Histograms

A histogram displays numerical data that have been organized into equal intervals using bars that have the same width and no space between them. While a histogram does not give exact data points, its shape shows the distribution of the data. Histograms also can be used to compare data.

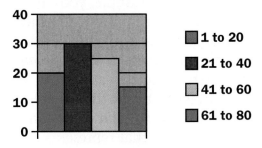

- 1 to 20
- 21 to 40
- 41 to 60
- 61 to 80

Box-and-Whisker Plot

A box-and-whisker plot displays the measures of central tendency and variation. A box is drawn around the quartile values, and whiskers extend from each quartile to the extreme data points. To make a box plot for a set of data, draw a number line that covers the range of data. Find the median, the extremes, and the upper and lower quartiles. Mark these points on the number line with bullets, then draw a box and the whiskers. The length of a whisker or box shows whether the values of the data in that part are concentrated or spread out.

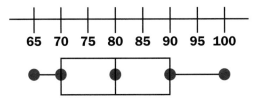

Scatter Plots

A scatter plot is a graph that shows the relationship between two sets of data. In a scatter plot, two sets of data are graphed as ordered pairs on a coordinate system. Two sets of data can have a positive correlation (as x increases, y increases), a negative correlation (as x increases, y decreases), or no correlation (no obvious pattern is shown). Scatter plots can be used to spot trends, draw conclusions, and make predictions about data.

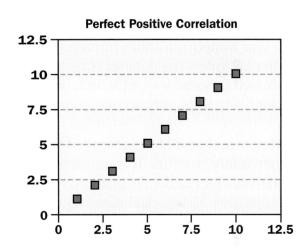

Perfect Positive Correlation

Randomization

The idea of randomization is a very important principle of statistics and the design of experiments. Data must be selected randomly to prevent bias from influencing the results. For example, you want to know the average income of people in your town but you can only use a sample of 100 individuals to make determinations about everyone. If you select 100 individuals who are all doctors, you will have a biased sample. However, if you chose a random sample of 100 people out of the phone book, you are much more likely to accurately represent average income in the town.

Statistics and Parameters

Statistics is a science that involves collecting, analyzing, and presenting data. The data can be collected in various ways—for example through a census or by making physical measurements. The data can then be analyzed by creating summary statistics, which have to do with the distribution of the data sample, including the mean, range, and standard error. They can also be illustrated in tables and graphs, like box-plots, scatter plots, and histograms. The presentation of the data typically involves describing the strength or validity of the data and what they show. For example, an analysis of ancestry of people in a city might tell you something about immigration patterns, unless the data set is very small or biased in some way, in which case it is not likely to be very accurate or useful.

Categorical and Measurement Data

When analyzing data, it is important to understand if the data is qualitative or quantitative. Categorical data is qualitative and measurement, or numerical, data is quantitative. Categorical data describes a quality of something and can be placed into different categories. For example, if you are analyzing the number of students in different grades in a school, each grade is a category. On the other hand, measurement data is continuous, like height, weight, or any other measurable variable. Measurement data can be converted into categorical data if you decide to group the data. Using height as an example, you can group the continuous data set into categories like under 5 feet, 5 feet to 5 feet 5 inches, over 5 feet five inches to 6 feet, and so on.

Univariate and Bivariate Data

In data analysis, a researcher can analyze one variable at a time or look at how multiple variables behave together. Univariate data involves only one variable, for example height in humans. You can measure the height in a population of people then plot the results in a histogram to look at how height is distributed in humans. To summarize univariate data, you can use statistics like the mean, mode, median, range, and standard deviation, which is a measure of variation. When looking at more than one variable at once, you use multivariate data. Bivariate data involves two variables. For example, you can look at height and age in humans together by gathering information on both variables from individuals in a population. You can then plot both variables in a scatter plot, look at how the variables behave in relation to each other, and create an equation that represents the relationship, also called a regression. These equations could help answer questions such as, for example, does height increase with age in humans?

▶ Select and use appropriate statistical methods to analyze data

Measures of Central Tendency

When you have a list of numerical data, it is often helpful to use one or more numbers to represent the whole set. These numbers are called measures of central tendency. Three measures of central tendency are mean, median, and mode. The mean is the sum of the data divided by the number of items in the data set. The median is the middle number of the ordered data (or the mean of the two middle numbers). The mode is the number or numbers that occur most often. These measures of central tendency allow data to be analyzed and better understood.

Measures of Spread

In statistics, measures of spread or variation are used to describe how data are distributed. The range of a set of data is the difference between the greatest and the least values of the data set. The quartiles are the values that divide the data into four equal parts. The median of data separates the set in half. Similarly, the median of the lower half of a set of data is the lower quartile. The median of the upper half of a set of data is the upper quartile. The interquartile range is the difference between the upper quartile and the lower quartile.

Line of Best Fit

When real-life data are collected, the points graphed usually do not form a straight line, but they may approximate a linear relationship. A line of best fit is a line that lies very close to most of the data points. It can be used to predict data. You also can use the equation of the best-fit line to make predictions.

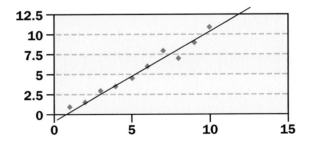

Stem and Leaf Plots

In a stem and leaf plot, numerical data are listed in ascending or descending order. The greatest place value of the data is used for the stems. The next greatest place value forms the leaves.

For example, if the least number in a set of data is 8 and the greatest number is 95, draw a vertical line and write the stems from 0 to 9 to the left of the line. Write the leaves from to the right of the line, with the corresponding stem. Next, rearrange the leaves so they are ordered from least to greatest. Then include a key or explanation, such as $1|3 = 13$. Notice that the stem-and-leaf plot below is like a histogram turned on its side.

```
0|8
1|3 6
2|5 6 9
3|0 2 7 8
4|0 1 4 7 9
5|1 4 5 8
6|1 3 7
7|5 8
8|2 6
9|5
```
Key: **1|3 = 13**

▶ Develop and evaluate inferences and predictions that are based on data

Sampling Distribution

The sampling distribution of a population is the distribution that would result if you could take an infinite number of samples from the population, average each, and then average the averages. The more normal the distribution of the population, that is, how closely the distribution follows a bell curve, the more likely the sampling distribution will also follow a normal distribution. Furthermore, the larger the sample, the more likely it will accurately represent the entire population. For instance, you are more likely to gain more representative results from a population of 1,000 with a sample of 100 than with a sample of 2.

Validity

In statistics, validity refers to acquiring results that accurately reflect that which is being measured. In other words, it is important when performing statistical analyses, to ensure that the data are valid in that the sample being analyzed represents the population to the best extent possible. Randomization of data and using appropriate sample sizes are two important aspects of making valid inferences about a population.

▶ *Understand and apply basic concepts of probability*

Complementary, Mutually Exclusive Events

To understand probability theory, it is important to know if two events are mutually exclusive, or complementary: the occurrence of one event automatically implies the non-occurrence of the other. That is, two complementary events cannot both occur. If you roll a pair of dice, the event of rolling 6 and rolling doubles have an outcome in common (3, 3), so they are not mutually exclusive. If you roll (3, 3), you also roll doubles. However, the events of rolling a 9 and rolling doubles are mutually exclusive because they have no outcomes in common. If you roll a 9, you will not also roll doubles.

Independent and Dependent Events

Determining the probability of a series of events requires that you know whether the events are independent or dependent. An independent event has no influence on the occurrence of subsequent events, whereas, a dependent event does influence subsequent events. The chances that a woman's first child will be a girl are $\frac{1}{2}$, and the chances that her second child will be a girl are also $\frac{1}{2}$ because the two events are independent of each other. However, if there are 7 red marbles in a bag of 15 marbles, the chances that the first marble you pick will be red are $\frac{7}{15}$ and if you indeed pick a red marble and remove it, you have reduced the chances of picking another red marble to $\frac{6}{14}$.

Sample Space

The sample space is the group of all possible outcomes for an event. For example, if you are tossing a single six-sided die, the sample space is {1, 2, 3, 4, 5, 6}. Similarly, you can determine the sample space for the possible outcomes of two events. If you are going to toss a coin twice, the sample space is {(heads, heads), (heads, tails), (tails, heads), (tails, tails)}.

Computing the Probability of a Compound Event

If two events are independent, the outcome of one event does not influence the outcome of the second. For example, if a bag contains 2 blue and 3 red marbles, then the probability of selecting a blue marble, replacing it, and then selecting a red marble is $P(A) \times P(B) = \frac{2}{5} \times \frac{3}{5}$ or $\frac{6}{25}$.

If two events are dependent, the outcome of one event affects the outcome of the second. For example, if a bag contains 2 blue and 3 red marbles, then the probability of selecting a blue and then a red marble without replacing the first marble is $P(A) \times P(B$ following $A) = \frac{2}{5} \times \frac{3}{4}$ or $\frac{3}{10}$. Two events that cannot happen at the same time are mutually exclusive. For example, when you roll two number cubes, you cannot roll a sum that is both 5 and even. So, $P(A$ or $B) = \frac{4}{36} + \frac{18}{36}$ or $\frac{11}{18}$.

How to Use This Glossary

- Content vocabulary terms in this glossary are words that relate to this book's content. They are **highlighted yellow** in your text.
- Words in this glossary that have an asterisk (*) are academic vocabulary terms. They help you understand your school subjects and are used on tests. They are **boldfaced blue** in your text.
- Some of the vocabulary words in this book include pronunciation symbols to help you sound out the words. Use the pronunciation key to help you pronounce the words.

Pronunciation Key		
a . . . . at	ô . . . . fork, all	th . . . thin
ā . . . . ape	oo . . . wood, put	th . . . this
ä . . . . father	ōō . . . fool	zh . . . treasure
e . . . . end	oi . . . oil	ə . . . . ago, taken, pencil, lemon, circus
ē . . . . me	ou . . . out	′ . . . . . indicates primary stress (symbol in front of and *above* letter)
i . . . . it	u . . . . up	′ . . . . . indicates secondary stress (symbol in front of and *below* letter)
ī . . . . ice	ū . . . . use	
o . . . . hot	. . . . rule	
ō . . . . hope	. . . . pull	
. . . . saw	. . . . sing	

à la carte • atherosclerosis

 A

à la carte On a menu, without side dishes; each item is priced separately. (p. 251)

* **accurate** Factual or free from error. (p. 214)

acid A chemical that tastes sour. (p. 381)

action plan A step-by-step way to reach goals. (p. 14)

additive A substance added to foods during processing to make them safer, more appealing, or more nutritious. (p. 53)

* **adhere** To follow, such as a guideline or direction. (p. 507)

aerobic activity An activity that works the heart and lungs. (p. 20)

* **affect** To shape or influence; to produce an effect or change to. (pp. 119, 224)

al dente Tender but slightly firm. (p. 359)

allergen A protein substance in food that triggers an allergic reaction. (p. 199)

anticipate To expect or predict; to look forward to. (p. 69)

antidote A substance that works against a poison. (p. 85)

antioxidant A substance that helps prevent oxidation. (p. 441)

appetite A psychological desire for food. (p. 11)

appetizer A small portion of food served at the start of the meal. (p. 229)

appropriate Suitable for a particular purpose, person, or occasion. (pp. 82, 108)

atherosclerosis The hardening of the arteries. (p. 202)

B

bacteria Microscopic living organisms. (p. 66)

bakeware Pots and pans for baking in the oven. (p. 270)

batter A flour mixture that is thin enough to be poured or dropped from a spoon. (p. 466)

biscuit method A process by which fat is cut into dry ingredients, liquid is added, and the dough is kneaded. (p. 472)

bisque A thick, rich soup made with finely mashed or ground seafood, poultry, or vegetables. Bisques are traditionally made with butter and cream. (p. 490)

body composition The measure of how much bone, muscle, fluids, and body fat a person has. (p. 149)

body image How a person views his or her body. (p. 151)

Body Mass Index (BMI) An estimate of body composition used as an indicator for obesity. (p. 149)

bran The coarse, outer layer of the grain. (p. 352)

brunch A breakfast-lunch combination. (p. 228)

buffet service Serving dishes of food are arranged on a table or counter. People serve themselves, then carry their food to an eating area. (p. 330)

C

calorie A unit of energy. (p. 21)

carbohydrate A nutrient that serves as the body's main energy source. (p. 97)

carbohydrate loading A strategy to increase the store of energy in the muscles. (p. 166)

cardiopulmonary resuscitation (CPR) A life-saving technique to restart a person's breathing and heartbeat. (p. 85)

cardiorespiratory endurance How well the heart and lungs can keep up with the body's activity. (p. 20)

carotenoid The pigment that gives vegetables deep-yellow, orange, and red colors. (p. 369)

cereal grain A seed from a grass that is processed and cooked to become edible. (p. 355)

chemical change A change in the substance of food. (p. 302)

chiffon cake A cross between shortened and foam cakes. (p. 506)

chlorophyll The pigment that makes vegetables green. (p. 368)

chowder A thick, chunky soup made with vegetables, fish, or seafood. (p. 490)

cider A beverage made by pressing juice from fruit. (p. 384)

citrus fruit A fruit that has a thick rind and juicy pulp. (p. 380)

coagulate To thicken. (p. 397)

cobbler A baked fruit dessert with a sweet biscuit-dough topping. (p. 509)

combination food A food with several ingredients from two or more food groups. (p. 132)

* **community** A group of people who live in the same area. (pp. 43, 370)

comparison shopping Comparing prices of different forms, container sizes, and brands in order to get the best value. (p. 240)

condiment A substance added in small amounts to food, often at the table, to improve, adjust, or complement the food's flavor. (p. 293)

* **conduct** A mode of personal behavior. (p. 333)

conduction Transfer of heat energy through diret contact between a heating element and the food. (p. 305)

* **conflict** A disagreement or opposition to. (p. 217)

* **consistent** Marked by eveness. (p. 468)

contaminate To make impure. (p. 66)

* **contribute** To add to something. (p. 269)

convection Heat transfers through the circulation or flow of heated molecules of either gas or liquid. (p. 305)

convection oven Cooking appliance that uses a fan to circulate hot air at a high speed. (p. 266)

convenience cooking Cooking using convenience foods or partially or fully prepared or processed foods. (p. 282)

convenience food A partly prepared or ready-to-eat food. (p. 225) *convenient* Easy to use. (p. 426)

conventional oven Cooking appliance that circulates hot air around food. (p. 266)

cooking power The amount of electricity that a microwave oven uses to generate microwaves. (p. 310)

cookware Pots and pans used mostly on the cooktop. (p. 270)

coronary heart disease A cardiovascular disease of the heart and blood vessels. (p. 202)

cover Another name for a place setting. (p. 331)

crisp A baked fruit dessert topped with a crumbly sweet pastry mixture. (p. 509)

cross-contamination Spreading harmful bacteria from one food to another. (p. 70)

crouton A crunchy, dried bread cube. (p. 457)

crucial Important; critical; essential. (p. 84)

cuisine The typical foods and ways of preparing foods associated with a cultural group. (p. 38)

cuisine Specific foods and cooking styles. (p. 251)

culture The shared beliefs, values, and behaviors of a group of people. (p. 8)

culture The shared beliefs, values, attitudes, behaviors, history, and expressions shared by a group of people. (p. 39)

cultured product A milk product made by fermenting milk with bacteria cultures. (p. 396)

curd The small solid lumps formed when milk curdles. (p. 399)

curdle To separate into many small lumps (curds) and a watery liquid (whey) as proteins coagulate. (p. 397)

cured meat A meat treated with salt, sugar, and sodium nitrate to slow spoilage and add distinctive flavors. (p. 413)

custard A cooked, sweetened mixture of milk and eggs. (p. 504)

custom The way a group of people traditionally behave. (p. 39)

customary measurement system The measurement system commonly used in the United States. (p. 285)

Daily Values (DV) The recommended amounts in an eating plan with 2,000 calories a day. (p. 239)

danger zone The temperature range in which bacteria grow fastest between 40°F and 140°F. (p. 72)

dehydration A significant loss of body fluids. (p. 163)

dehydration A serious health problem caused by lack of water. (p. 27)

denaturing The process of breaking down protein's structure. (p. 397)

determine To decide by looking at choices. (p. 149)

develop To promote the growth of; to slowly create or grow. (pp. 162, 358, 399)

diabetes A condition in which the body cannot control blood sugar properly. (p. 200)

diet Everything you eat and drink. (p. 114)

Dietary Guidelines for Americans Science-based guidelines about nutrition and physical activity for healthy Americans over the age of two. (p. 114)

differentiate To see a difference (p. 310)

discretionary calorie An extra calorie that can be consumed after eating enough from the other food groups while staying within total calorie budget. (p. 136)

diversity The variety of people of different races and cultures. (p. 38)

dough A flour mixture that is stiff enough to be shaped by hand, rolled, or cut. (p. 466)

dovetailing Doing two tasks simultaneously. (p. 320)

drupe A fruit with a large pit that grows on trees. (p. 381)

dry-heat cooking Cooking food uncovered, without adding liquid or fat. (p. 306)

eating disorder An illness that involves harmful attitudes about the body, self, and food. (p. 196)

economic A production factor; of or relating to the production, development, and management of material wealth. (p. 236)

Glossary

* **effect** To influence or bring about a result. (p. 408)

egg substitute An alternative to eggs made from egg whites. (p. 425)

electrolyte A mineral that helps maintain the body's fluid balance. (p. 164)

empty-calorie food A nutrient-poor food whose calories come from added sugars, fat, or both. (p. 133)

emulsifier Coats droplets of oil so they stay evenly scattered throughout a liquid. (p. 459)

emulsion A mixture of liquids, the droplets of which do not normally blend with each other. (p. 458)

endosperm The inner part of the grain. (p. 352)

endurance The ability to continue physical activity for a long time without becoming too tired. (p. 20)

energy balance Balance between what you eat and how much energy you expend. (p. 152)

Energy Star A label that indicates energy efficiency. (p. 264)

EnergyGuide label A label that compares energy consumption and energy cost of an appliance. (p. 264)

* **enhance** Improve in quality, or value. (p. 467)

enrich To add back nutrients to food that were lost during processing. (p. 53)

entrée A main dish. (p. 251)

environment All of the external factors influencing the life and activities of people. (p. 40)

* **environment** The circumstances or conditions by which one is surrounded. (p. 174).

enzyme A special protein that helps chemical reactions happen. (p. 369)

* **essential** Necessary or important. (p. 438)

* **establish** To set up (p. 325)

* **estimate** An inexact amount; use knowledge to guess. (pp. 126, 240)

ethnic food A food commonly enjoyed by an ethnic group. (p. 39)

etiquette Polite behavior that shows respect and consideration for others. (p. 333)

* **examine** To study closely. (p. 186)

* **exceed** To surpass or be greater than. (p. 50)

* **expose** To come in contact with or to make accessible to a particular action. (p. 441)

extract Concentrated flavoring from food or plants. (p. 467)

* **factor** An element that contributes to wellness, such as genetics or a certain life event. (p. 6)

fad diet A weight loss plan that is popular for a short time, often based on misinformation. (p. 155)

family style Type of meal service where food is placed in serving dishes on the table. People help themselves and pass serving dishes to each other. (p. 330)

fermentation A chemical reaction that slowly splits complex compounds into similar substances. (p. 396)

fetus An unborn baby that has acquired its basic form and is no longer an embryo. (p. 172)

fiber Plant material that cannot be digested. (p. 97)

fillet A sides of fish cut from the bones and backbone. (p. 413)

finfish Fish with fins, backbones, and gills. (p. 413)

first aid Immediate care that prevents more injury and relieves pain. (p. 85)

flammable Burns easily. (p. 84)

flat bread A bread made with little or no leavening agent. (p. 471)

flatware Knives, forks, and spoons for eating. (p. 331)

flavonoid The pigment that gives vegetables red, purple, and blue colors. (p. 369)

flavor The combination of a food's taste, smell, and texture. (p. 12)

flexibility The ability to move muscles and joints through their full range of motion. (p. 20)

foam cake A cake made with stiffly beaten egg whites, which makes them light and airy. They are lower in fat than shortened cakes. (p. 506)

food A form of matter made of many different chemicals that can be ingested and used by an organism as a source of nutrition and energy. (p. 302)

food allergy An allergic reaction to a substance in food. (p. 199)

food budget An amount of money the family plans to spend on food. (p. 236)

food jag Wanting just one food for a while. (p. 176)

food processing Preparing and handling food for safety, nutrition, convenience, and appeal. (p. 52)

food science The study of the nature of foods and the changes that occur in them. (p. 302)

foodborne illness An acute gastrointestinal infection caused by food that contains harmful bacteria. (p. 66)

fortify To add nutrients to food that are not naturally present. (p. 53)

freezer burn Unappealing dried-up white areas on food caused by improper or inadequate packaging before freezing. (p. 72)

fruit juice concentrate Juice with most of the water removed. (p. 384)

fruit nectar A thick, sugar-sweetened beverage of fruit juice and pulp, which contains fiber. (p. 383)

frying Cooking in small or large amounts of fat. (p. 308)

garnish An edible decoration that adds a contrasting color, texture, flavor, temperature, or shape to food. (p. 336)

gelatinization Using starch to thicken a liquid. (p. 496)

generic brand A brand that usually has a plain label and no brand name. (p. 240)

germ The small base of the seed. (p. 352)

giblet The edible internal organ of poultry, such as the heart, liver, or gizzard. (p. 412)

gluten A stretchy, elastic protein. (p. 469)

gluten intolerance The inability to digest gluten, a protein found in wheat, rye, barley, and sometimes oats. (p. 198)

health claim A statement that a food provides certain health benefits. (p. 239)

health fraud False and possibly harmful approaches to health care. (p. 216)

health risk The likelihood of developing health problems. (p. 114)

healthy weight A person's appropriate weight based on age, height, growth pattern, and body type. (p. 149)

heaping A measurement that is above the top of the cup or spoon. (p. 286)

Heimlich maneuver A life-saving technique for choking. (p. 85)

herb A fragrant, edible leaf, used to season food. (p. 292)

herbal supplement A substance that comes from plants. (p. 217)

high blood pressure A condition of too much pressure on the heart and arteries as the heart beats. (p. 202)

high-density lipoprotein A type of protein that removes cholesterol from blood and artery walls to the liver. (p. 202)

homogenized Processed to break fat globules into tiny drops and mix them permanently and evenly in milk. (p. 397)

hunger A physical need for food. (p. 11)

hydrogenation The process of adding hydrogen to unsaturated fats. (p. 440)

impulse buying Buying something you do not need because it appeals to you. (p. 236)

in season Fruits and vegetables harvested at the time of year when they are ripe. (p. 370)

* **indicate** To show or point out. (p. 264)

* **influence** To affect or sway. (p. 127)

ingredient One of the items of food needed to create a recipe. (p. 282)

intensity How hard the body works during an activity. (p. 25)

irradiation Passing food through radiant energy to kill some disease-carrying bacteria. (p. 53)

Glossary

Glossary

knead To work dough by repeatedly folding, pressing, and turning it. (p. 472)

lactate To produce milk. (p. 173)

lacto-ovo-vegetarian A person who eats dairy food and eggs in addition to foods from plant sources. (p. 186)

lactose intolerance The inability to digest lactose, the sugar found in milk products. (p. 198)

lactose The natural sugar in milk. (p. 394)

lacto-vegetarian A person who eats dairy foods and foods from plant sources, but not eggs. (p. 186)

lean meat Meat that has less fat, saturated fat, and cholesterol. (p. 406)

leavening agent A substance that makes baked goods rise. (p. 467)

legume An edible seed grown in a pod. (p. 424)

level off To scrape any extra off the top of the measuring cup, using a straight edge. (p. 286)

life cycle The time from conception through adulthood. (p. 172)

lifestyle The way a person lives their life. (p. 6)

lipid A fat that circulates in your bloodstream. (p. 202)

* logical Sensible. (p. 407)

low birth weight A birth weight less than 5½ pounds (2.5 kg). (p. 172)

low-density lipoprotein A type of protein that deposits blood cholesterol on artery walls, causing atherosclerosis. (p. 202)

Maillard reaction A chemical reaction in meat that causes browning. (p. 409)

major appliance A large appliance. (p. 264)

malnutrition Poor nutrition caused by nutrient deficiencies, food shortages, or poverty. (p. 107)

marbling Flecks of fat throughout meat. (p. 406)

marinade A mixture of an acidic food, like citrus juice or vinegar, and seasonings. (p. 409)

meat cut A slice or portion from a specific part of the animal. (p. 409)

media literacy The ability to know how to find reliable information sources, evaluate how accurate the information is, and apply what you learn. (p. 214)

menu A list of foods to be served. (p. 224)

meringue A stiffly beaten mixture of egg whites and sugar. (p. 509)

metric system A system of weights and measures based on multiples of ten. (p. 285)

microwave An appliance that cooks food using electromagnetic radiation. (p. 309)

microwave oven Cooking appliance that cooks with waves of energy that produce heat inside food. (p. 266)

mineral An inorganic nutrient that is essential for health and growth. (p. 102)

* minimize To lower or play down; to reduce or lessen. (pp. 119, 380)

* mixture A combination of items or ingredients. (p. 454)

moist-heat cooking Cooking food using hot liquid, steam, or both. (p. 307)

muffin method A process by which liquids and dry ingredients are mixed separately and then stirred together until just combined. (p. 471)

MyPyramid A food guidance system from the U.S. Department of Agriculture. (p. 126)

national brand A brand sold by major food companies. (p. 240)

nutrient A chemical that performs a specific job in the body. (p. 96)

nutrient content claim A statement that a food has more or less of a nutrient or food substance. (p. 239)

nutrient-dense food A food that provides high amounts of vitamins and minerals for relatively few calories. (p. 115)

Nutrition Fact Specific information about the nutrition in one serving of food. (p. 239)

nutrition The processes by which the body uses nutrients in food for growth and maintenance. (p. 6)

obesity A condition of having a significant or measurably large amount of excess body fat. (p. 151)

* **obtain** To receive or attain by planned effort or action. (p. 187)

oil A fat that is liquid at room temperature. (p. 438)

omelet A dish cooked like a large egg pancake. (p. 430)

open dating The packages are marked with dates that tell how long the product will be fresh. (p. 243)

open-face sandwich A sandwich that has only the bottom slice of bread. (p. 483)

organ meat Liver, heart, kidney, and tongue meats. (p. 406)

organic farming Growing foods without synthetic fertilizers or pesticides. (p. 50)

* **original** Related to a beginning. (p. 495)

overweight A condition of having too much body fat. (p. 151)

ovo-vegetarian A person who eats eggs and foods from plant sources, but not dairy foods. (p. 186)

oxidation Changes caused by contact with oxygen. (p. 441)

papillae Tiny bumps on the tongue that contain taste buds. (p. 12)

pasteurized Heat-treated to kill bacteria that could cause disease or spoiled milk. (p. 397)

pastry A mixture of flour, fat, cold water, and salt. (p. 508)

* **perceive** To see or attain awareness. (p. 197)

* **percentage** A portion of a whole. (p. 21)

perishable Easily spoiled. (p. 72)

pesticide A poison that kills insects or other pests. (p. 84)

physical activity Using muscles to move the body. (p. 20)

physical change A change in the shape or size, but not the chemical structure. (p. 302)

physical fitness Having the energy and ability to do everything you want and need to do in your daily life. (p. 20)

place setting The arrangement of tableware for one person. (p. 331)

plate service Type of meal service where food is served on each person's plate, then plates are brought to the table. (p. 330)

poison control center A medical facility that gives free advice about handling poison emergencies. (p. 85)

pome A fruit with a core and seeds that grows on trees. (p. 381)

* **potential** The possibility for growth and development. (p. 23)

poultry Chicken, turkey, or other birds raised as food. (p. 406)

prenatal The time between conception and birth. (p. 172)

pre-preparation step A step to get food and equipment ready. (p. 320)

* **principle** A rule set to govern action. (p. 505)

* **process** A function or continuing natural activity. (p. 96)

* **process** An action or series of actions, changes, or functions bringing about a result. (p. 352)

produce Fresh vegetables, fruits, and herbs. (p. 370)

* **project** To estimate or plan ahead. (p. 289)

* **promote** To help or further. (p. 424)

protein A substance the body uses to build new cells and repair injured ones. (p. 99)

pudding A smooth, creamy dessert made with milk, sugar, egg, and other flavorings. (p. 504)

quiche A main dish with a filling of eggs, milk, and other ingredients. (p. 429)

quick bread A bread in which the leavening agent is baking powder or baking soda. (p. 471)

Glossary

R

R.S.V.P. An acronym for a French phrase that means "Please Reply." (p. 336)

radiation Energy that is transmitted through airwaves. (p. 305)

rancidity The change in the quality of oils and solid fats when they oxidize. (p. 441)

range A large cooking stove. (p. 266)

recipe Ingredients and instructions for preparing a dish. (p. 282)

Recommended Dietary Allowances (RDAs) Governmental advice about daily nutrient needs for most healthy people. (p. 107)

recycling Sorting and disposing of reusable items so their materials can be made into new products . (p. 325)

refined grain A grain that is milled to remove the bran and the germ. (p. 352)

regional food A food that is special in one geographical area. (p. 42)

* **regulation** A rule or order. (p. 250)

* **relate** To be connected to. (p. 306)

* **require** To need or ask for by right or authority. (p. 50)

* **resource** Something one uses to get what they want, meet goals, and complete tasks. (p. 8)

resource The time, money, or energy needed to complete a task. (p. 224)

ripe Fully developed; mature. (p. 382)

risk factor A condition that increases your chances of developing a problem. (p. 115)

rub An herb or spice mixture applied to meat, poultry, or fish before cooking. (p. 293)

S

salad green An edible raw leaf. (p. 455)

sanitation Maintaining cleanliness. (p. 69)

score To make shallow cuts. (p. 409)

scratch cooking Preparing a dish from unprepared foods. (p. 282)

sedentary Physically inactive. (p. 25)

self-rising flour Flour with salt and baking powder mixed in. (p. 466)

* **sequence** An order or connected series. (p. 331)

* **sequence** A specific order. (p. 251)

shelf life The length of time foods stay safe and appealing to eat. (p. 53)

shellfish Fish that have shells instead of bones and fins. (p. 413)

shortened cake Cakes made with butter or other solid fat, so they are richer and heavier than foam cakes. (p. 506)

* **signal** Show signs or indicate. (p. 68)

* **significant** Of a noticeably or measurably large amount; important. (pp. 151, 372)

* **simultaneous** At the same time. (p. 320)

small appliance A piece of portable electric equipment. (p. 268)

smoke point The temperature when fat produces smoke. (p. 441)

* **specific** Restricted to a particular thing. (p. 172)

* **specified** Listed or name in detail. (p. 492)

spice A seasoning from the bark, buds, seeds, roots, or stems of plants and trees. (p. 292)

spread A food used on bread to add flavor and moisture. (p. 482)

standing time A period of time when food continues to cook after microwaving. (p. 311)

staple A basic food item kept on hand. (p. 236)

starch Many sugar units attached together; a complex carbohydrate. (pp. 97, 352)

stemware A glass with a stem between the flat bottom of the glass and its bowl. (p. 331)

steroid A drug that acts like male hormones. (p. 165)

stew A thick, hearty mixture of chunky vegetables and perhaps meat, poultry, or fish cooked slowly in liquid. (p. 490)

stock Seasoned liquid, or broth, from cooking meat, fish, or vegetables. (p. 490)

store brand A supermarket's own products. (p. 240)

* **strategy** A plan for achieving goals. (p. 164)

strength The power to work muscles against resistance. (p. 20)

stress Mental, emotional, or physical strain. (p. 7)

sugar A simple carbohydrate that is digested quickly. (p. 97)

supplement A dietary substance that contains nutrients and other food substances that add to your diet. (p. 108)

surimi Minced processed fish with other ingredients for flavor that is shaped and colored to look like shellfish. (p. 413)

sustainable agriculture The responsible use of resources to produce food without damaging the environment (p. 50)

tender-crisp Tender, but still firm and slightly crisp. (p. 373)

tofu A cheeselike curd made from soybeans. (p. 425)

trade-off Giving something up in order to have something else. (p. 225)

* **trait** A distinguishing feature or characteristic. (p. 44)

* **transfer** To move to another place. (p. 288)

tumbler A glass without a stem. (p. 331)

underweight A condition of having too little body fat. (p. 151)

unit price How much an ounce, pound, or other unit of the item costs. (p. 240)

* **valid** Good or well- grounded and justifiable. (p. 226)

vegan A person who eats only foods from plant sources. (p. 186)

vegetarian A person who avoids eating meat, poultry, and fish. (p. 186)

vinaigrette A mixture of oil and vinegar. (p. 459)

vitamin A nutrient that regulates body processes and helps other nutrients do their work. (p. 100)

volume How much space the ingredient takes up. (p. 286)

weight How heavy or light the ingredient is. (p. 286)

wellness A person's best level of health. (p. 6)

whey The watery liquid that separates from the curds when milk curdles. (p. 399)

whole grain A grain that has the entire grain kernel. (p. 352)

work center An area devoted to a certain type of task (p. 318)

work plan A list of all steps for preparing a recipe or meal. (p. 318)

work triangle The imaginary line conncecting the three types of work centers. (p. 318)

yeast A simple plant (fungus) that produces gas as it grows. (p. 463)

yeast bread A bread in which the leavening agent is yeast. (p. 471)

yield How much food a farm produces per acre or area; how much a recipe makes, or the number of servings. (pp. 50, 283)

Index

A

À la carte, 251
Accidents
    handling, 85, 86
    preventing, 82–85
Acids, 369, 381, 409
Action plans, 14
    for kitchen emergencies, 85
    for sports nutrition, 164
    for wellness, 14
Active living. *See* Physical
    activity
Activity Pyramid, 26
Adapting/adjusting recipes
    converting ingredient
      amounts, 128
    doubling, 41
    for healthier desserts, 503
    increasing or decreasing
      yield, 11, 289, 290
    for nutritional makeover,
      296
    for vegetarians, 188–189
Additives, 53, 54
Adjusting recipes. *See* Adapting/
    adjusting recipes
Adolescence. *See* Teen years
Adulthood, 178–179
Advertising, 215
Aerobic activities, 20
After-school activities, 24
Age, as meal planning issue, 224
Agricultural managers, 53
Agricultural scientists, 372
Agriculture, 50, 52
Air, in baked goods, 444
Al dente, 359
Alcoholic beverages, guidelines
    for, 119
Allergens, 199, 238
All-liquid diets, 156
All-purpose flour, 466
Altitude, in cooking, 306
Amino acids, 99, 100, 353
Amounts, in recipes, 282. *See
    also* Adapting/adjusting
    recipes
Anemia, 103
Angel food cake, 502
Animal food sources, 99. *See
    also* Meat(s); Poultry
Anorexia nervosa, 196, 197
Antidotes, poison, 85
Anti-oxidants, 441
Appearance, of food
    for appealing meals, 229,
      339–340

    food choices influenced by,
      11
Appearance, personal, 6
Appetite, 11
Appetizers, 229
Appliances, 264. *See also* Tools,
    kitchen
    major, 264–267
    for moist-heat cooking, 307
    preventing accidents with,
      82–84
    recipe instructions for, 282
    small, 268–269
Aquaculture, 52
Argentina, foods from, 407
Arroz con gandules, 382
Arroz con pollo, 227
Aseptic packaging, 54
Atherosclerosis, 202

B

B vitamins, 101, 353, 406. *See
    also* specific B vitamins
Baba ghanoush, 289
Back injuries, preventing, 83
Bacteria, 66
    avoiding spread of, 69
    contamination by, 66
    cross-contamination by, 70
    illnesses caused by, 67
    spoilage caused by, 73
Baguette, 153
Baked apples, 503
Bakers, 470
Bakeware, 270, 505
Baking, 306, 466–471
    breads, 466–471
    desserts, 505–510
    eggs, 430
    ingredient amounts for, 290
    ingredient functions in,
      466–467
    with oils/fats, 444
    science of, 467–469
    success tips for, 469–471
    tools for, 275
    vegetables, 373
Baking pans, 270
Baking powder, 468
Baking soda, 468
Balance, activity for, 20, 22
Banquet managers, 337
Bar cookies, 505
Barley, 354
Basal metabolic rate (BMR),
    106, 178
Bases, 369
Basting, 309

Basting spoons, 275
Batter, 466
Beans, 424–427
    cooking, 431
    in meal plans, 117, 425
    in salads, 454
    in soups and stews, 490
Beaters, 274
Beating (in general), 291
Beating egg whites, 293
Beef, 410, 411
Berries, 381
Beverages, 229
    fruit, 383–384
    for snacks, 488–489
Binge eating disorder, 196, 197
Biotechnology, 52
Biscuit method (quick breads),
    472
Biscuits, 472, 473
Bisque, 490
Blanching, 309
Blender shakes, 488
Blenders, 268
Blini, 354
Blood, nutrients for health of,
    103
Blood sugar, 201
BMI. *See* Body Mass Index
BMR. *See* Basal metabolic rate
Body composition, 21, 149
Body fat, 98
    in body composition, 149
    calorie equivalent for, 152
    functions of, 149
    and risk factors of over-
      weight, 115
    and weight, 151
Body image, 151
Body Mass Index (BMI), 149,
    150
Body processes
    energy for, 105–106
    nutrients for regulating, 96
    during sleep, 176
Body types, 148, 149, 151
Boiling, 308
Boiling point, altitude and, 306
Bones
    in body composition, 149
    milk product nutrients for,
      392
    minerals for, 102, 103
    strengthening, 22
    and weight-lifting, 165
Boning knives, 274
Borscht, 354
Bottle-feeding, 174
Braising, 309, 416, 417

Brands, 240, 352
Bread flour, 466
Bread knives, 274
Breads, 464–476
    baking, 466–471
    faster methods for, 475
    quick breads, 471–473
    shopping for, 356
    storing, 476
    storing ingredients for,
        475–476
    types of, 471
    yeast breads, 474, 475
Breakfast, planning, 226–227
Breast cancer, soy intake and,
    187
Breast-feeding, 173
British Isles, foods from, 119
Broiling, 306–307
    meat, 417
    sandwiches, 483
Broth, 490
Browning, 309
Bruises, preventing, 83
Brunch, 228
Buckwheat, 354
Budget
    calorie, 136, 172, 175
    food, 9, 236
Buffet service, 334, 341
Bulgur, 354
Bulimia nervosa, 196, 197
Burns, preventing, 83, 84
Butter, 442
Buying foods. See Shopping for
    foods

C

Cafeteria cooks, 84
Caffeinated drinks, 164
Cakes, 506–508, 510
Calcium
    in bones and teeth, 102, 103
    foods for, 133
    functions and sources of,
        104
    in meal plans, 117
    from milk foods, 129
    during pregnancy, 172
    soda and loss of, 225
    for teens, 115, 177
    for vegetarians, 187
Calorie budget, 136
    for children, 175
    during pregnancy, 172
Calories, 21, 103
    for active living, 162
    from added sugars and fats,
        133
    balancing numbers of, 115
    balancing sources of, 105
    body fat equivalent in, 152

burned from activity, 21
    in carbohydrates, 105
    discretionary, 136, 138
    and energy balance, 152
    extra, 97
    in fat-free foods, 237
    in fats, 105, 117
    on food labels, 238, 239
    for losing weight, 154
    from nutrient-dense foods,
        115, 133
    percentage of fats in, 117,
        118
    in proteins, 105
    recipe information on, 283
    recommended daily number
        of, 106
    in vegetables, 366
    for vegetarians, 187
Calzones, 483
Campylobacter jejuni, 67
Can openers, 274
Canada, foods from, 41, 443
Cancer
    breast, 187
    colon, 22
    eating plan for, 203
    and obesity, 151
Canned foods, 242
Canning, 53
Carbohydrate loading, 166
Carbohydrates, 97–98
    for active living, 162
    calories in, 105
    chemical makeup of, 303
    dietary guidelines for, 118
    in eggs, beans, and nuts, 424
    energy from, 97, 105
    in fruits, 129
    in grains, 129, 352
    in milk products, 392
    during physical activity, 163
    in pre-activity meals, 163
    in vegetables, 129, 366
Carbonated drinks, 164, 225
Cardiopulmonary resuscitation
    (CPR), 85
Cardiorespiratory endurance, 20
Careers
    agricultural manager, 53
    agricultural scientist, 372
    baker, 470
    banquet manager, 337
    cafeteria cook, 84
    caterer, 227
    chef, 442
    community health nurse,
        197
    consultant dietitian, 165
    cook, 415
    cookbook author, 291
    dietitian, 133

family and consumer
    sciences teacher, 13
fitness trainer, 22
food and nutrition writer,
    216
food editor, 491
food historian, 43
food photographer, 459
food processing occupations,
    393
food scientist, 99
food service manager, 69
food stylist, 383
food technologist, 188
grocery store worker, 240
kitchen designer, 266
party planner, 325
pastry chef, 507
product demonstrator, 311
public health educator, 115
recipe developer, 431
restaurant manager, 484
restaurant server, 253
restaurant-supply salesper-
    son, 355
social and human services
    assistant, 173
weight-loss counselor, 151
Caribbean, foods from, 382
Carotenoids, 369, 381
Casserole dishes, 270
Casseroles, 493, 494
Caterers, 227
Celebrations, foods linked with,
    39
Celiac disease, 198, 468
Cells, nutrients for building/
    repairing, 96
Cereal grains, 355
Cereals
    cooking, 360
    salt in, 198
    shopping for, 356–357
Ceviche, 55
CFCS, 214
Challenging yourself, 25
Cheese, 397–398, 492
    cooking with, 400
    in meal plans, 117
    in Milk Group, 131
Chefs, 442
Chef's knives, 274
Chemical changes to food, 302
Chemicals
    contamination of food by, 68
    safety with, 84
Chewing food, 152, 203
Chiffon cakes, 507
Chiffon pies, 509
Childhood, nutrition during,
    175–176
Chimichurri, 407
China, foods from, 85

Chloride, 104
Chlorophyll, 368, 381
Cholesterol, 99, 440
    blood, 202
    in eggs, beans, and nuts, 424
    and fats, 98
    guidelines for, 117–118
    HDL and LDL, 202, 440
    in meat, poultry, and fish,
        406
    in teen diets, 115
Chopping, 291
Chowder, 490
Chutney, 293
Citrus fruits, 380, 381
Cleaning kitchen, 323
Climate, traditional foods and,
    40
Clostridium botulinum, 67
Clostridium perfringens, 67
Coagulation, 395
Cobblers, 510
Colanders, 276
Cold-pack cheeses, 398
Collagen, 408
Colon cancer, 22
Color of foods
    for appealing meals, 229
    and cooking with oils/fats,
        444
    fruits, 381
    meats, 409
    vegetables, 368–369
    when spoiled, 74
Combination foods, 132. See
    also Mixed foods
Combining skills, 291–292
Community, healthful food in,
    179–180
Community health nurses, 197
Community information
    sources, 215
Community kitchens, 180
Comparison shopping, 240
Complete proteins, 100, 187
Complex carbohydrates, 97
Computers, in agriculture, 52
Condiments, 294
Conduction, 304, 305
Conservation, 325–328
Consultant dietitians, 165
Consumerism, 212–218
    and advertising, 215
    and health fraud, 216, 217
    media literacy for, 214–215
    and news reports about
        food/nutrition, 217
Containers for food, 72, 74
Contamination
    cross-contamination, 70
    sources of, 66, 68
Convection ovens, 266, 304, 305
Convenience cooking, 282, 509

Convenience foods, 54, 225
    cost of, 242
    meat, poultry, and fish, 413
    prepared salads, 455
    soups and stews, 492
    vegetables, 371
Convenience stores, 237
Conventional ovens, 266
Converting measurements, 11,
    128
Cookbook authors, 291
Cookies, 505–506, 510
Cooking, 300–312
    changes to food during, 302
    combination methods of,
        309
    common terms in, 309
    dry-heat, 306–307
    effect of altitude on, 306
    effects of heat in, 304
    eggs, 429–430
    with fats and oils, 444
    fruits, 386
    frying, 308–309
    grains, 355, 359–360
    guidelines for doneness,
        74–75
    heat transfer in, 304–305
    ingredient functions in, 302
    legumes, 431
    meat, poultry, and fish, 409,
        410, 415–418
    methods for, 306–309
    microwave, 309–311
    with milk products, 400
    moist-heat, 307–308
    for nutrition and flavor, 312
    pizza, 486
    science of, 302
    soups and stews, 491
    vegetables, 368, 373–374
Cooks, 415
Cookware, 270–271
Cool downs, 25
Cooling racks, 275
Co-ops, 237
Coordination, physical activity
    and, 20, 22, 23
Coronary heart disease, 202
Courtesy, 243–244, 253. See also
    Manners
Couscous, 326
Covers, 335
CPR (cardiopulmonary
    resuscitation), 85
Cream, 398
Cream cheese, 395
Cream pies, 509
Creaming, 291
Crisps, 510
Critical thinking skills, in
    evaluating health news, 218

Cross-contamination, avoiding,
    70
Cuisines, 38, 40, 42, 251. See
    also International foods
Culture, 8, 36–44
    benefits of ethnic/regional
        foods, 43
    food choices influenced
        by, 8. See also Interna-
        tional foods
    and food customs, 38–40, 44
Cultured milk products, 394
Cups and saucers, 335, 336
Curd (cheese), 397
Curdling, 395
Cured meats, 413
Curing foods, 53
Curry, 190, 493
Custard pies, 509
Custards, 504
Customary measurement
    system, 285
Customs, 39
Cuts, preventing, 82
Cutting boards, 274
Cutting foods, 82
Cutting in, 291
Cutting skills, 291
Cutting tools, 274

D
Daily calorie budget, 115
Daily meal plans, 136, 137
Daily Values, 239
Dairy products. See Milk (dairy)
    products
Dal, 493
Danger zone (temperature), 72,
    73
Decision making, 13, 14
Decorations, table, 336
Deep-fat frying (french frying),
    309
Dehydration, 27, 163
Denaturing, 395
Desserts, 229, 500–510
    adjusting recipes for, 503
    baked, 505–510
    chilled, 504
    choosing, 502
    storing, 410
Diabetes, 151, 200–201
Dicing, 291
Diet(s), 114. See also Meal plans
    energy balance in, 152–153
    fad, 155–156
    for healthy weight, 153
    of teens, 115
    vegetarian, 186
    for weight loss. See Losing
        weight
Diet pills, 156

Dietary Guidelines for Americans, 112–120, 172
    for alcoholic beverages, 119
    for carbohydrates, 118
    for fats and cholesterol, 117–118
    for food choices, 117
    for food safety, 119
    for lowering health risks, 196
    for nutrients, 115
    for physical activity, 116
    recommendations from, 114
    for sodium and potassium, 119
    for weight, 115
Dietary Reference Intakes (DRIs), 107
Dietary supplements. See Supplements
Dietitians, 133
Digestion, 96–97, 152
Dim sum, 85
Directions, in recipes, 282
Discount stores, 237
Discretionary calories, 136, 138
Diseases. See also Health problems
    atherosclerosis, 202
    cancer, 22, 151, 187, 203
    diabetes, 200–201
    heart disease, 22, 99, 117, 151, 202
    HIV/AIDS, 203
    osteoporosis, 22, 103
Dishes, 335
Dishwashers, 267
Distribution costs, 50
Diversity, 38, 44
Double boilers, 270
Dough, 466
Dovetailing tasks, 320
Draining, 292
Draining tools, 276
DRIs (Dietary Reference Intakes), 107
Drop cookies, 505
Drupes, 381
Dry ingredients, measuring, 272, 286–287
Dry measuring cups, 272
Dry storage, 73
Dry-heat cooking, 306–307
Drying of foods, 53
Duration (time) of activity, 165

E

E. coli, 67
Eating disorders, 196–197
Eating habits, of children, 176
Efficiency, 322
Egg substitute, 425

Eggs, 424–430
    in baking, 467
    cross-contamination from, 70
    functions in recipes, 302
    in Meat Group, 131
    safe-handling instructions for, 71
    in salads, 454
    for vegetarians, 186
Egypt, foods from, 289
Elastin, 408
Electric skillets, 268
Electrical shocks, preventing, 83
Electricity rates, 269
Electrolytes, 164
Emergencies, handling, 85, 86
Emotional health, 7–8, 197
Emotions, 9, 22
Empanadas, 407, 484
Empty-calorie foods, 133, 138
Emulsifiers, 459
Emulsions, 458
Endosperm, 352
Endurance, building, 20
Energy
    activity and improvement in, 22
    and activity level, 154
    for adults, 178
    for body processes, 105–106
    from breakfast, 226
    from carbohydrates, 97, 105
    conserving, 326
    daily needs for, 105, 106
    from fats, 98, 105
    in food, 104, 105
    food choices influenced by, 9
    from fruits, 380
    as meal-planning resource, 225
    measured in calories, 103
    nutrients and, 103, 105–106
    for physical activities, 27
    from proteins, 99, 105
    using calories for, 21
    for vegetarians, 187
Energy balance, 106, 115, 152
Energy Star logo, 264
EnergyGuide label, 264
Enriched foods, 53
Entertaining, 340–342
Entrées, 251
Environment, 40
Environmental protection, 50
Enzymes, 369, 382, 409
Equipment. See Kitchen equipment
Equivalent measures, 285
Escherichia coli (E. coli), 67
Esophagus, in digestive process, 97

Essential amino acids, 99, 100, 187
Essential fats, 438
Estimation, 243
Ethnic foods, 38–43. See also International foods
Etiquette, 337. See also Manners
Evaporated milk, 396
Events, foods linked with, 39
Exercise. See also Physical activity
    for fitness. See Physical fitness
    with friends and family, 22
    for healthy weight, 153
    with weight machines, 23
Extracts, 467

F

Factors
    in food customs, 42
    in wellness, 6
Fad diets, 155–156
Falls, preventing, 83
Family, food choices and, 9, 225
Family and consumer sciences teachers, 13
Family meals, 10, 179, 224
Family style service, 334
Farmers' markets, 237
Farming, 50, 52
Fasting, 39, 156
Fats, 98–99. See also Oils
    added to food, 133
    buying, 443
    calories in, 105
    carbohydrates with, 97
    chemical makeup of, 303
    and cholesterol, 440
    cooking with, 444
    in eggs, beans, and nuts, 424
    energy from, 98, 105
    in food science, 440–442
    functions in recipes, 302
    guidelines for, 117–118
    and health problems, 438
    in meat, poultry, and fish, 406
    in milk products, 392
    in MyPyramid, 439
    in pie crusts, 509
    storing, 443
Fat-soluble vitamins, 102, 107
FDA. See Food and Drug Administration
Federal Trade Commission, 216
Fermentation, 394
Fertilizers, 50
Fetus, 172
Fiber, 97
    in fruits, 380
    in grains, 98, 129, 352

in teen diets, 115
in vegetables, 366
Field trip snacks, 178
Fillets, fish, 413
Finfish, 413
Fires, 83
  preventing, 84
  putting out, 86
First aid, 85
Fish, 413–415, 418
  cross-contamination from, 70
  in Meat Group, 131
  in MyPyramid, 407
  nutrients in, 406
  in salads, 454
  in soups and stews, 490
F.I.T. (frequency, intensity, time), 165
Fitness. See Physical fitness
Fitness log, 27
Fitness trainers, 22
Flakiness of foods, 444
Flammable materials, 84
Flat breads, 471
Flatware, 335, 336
Flavonoids, 369, 381
Flavor of food
  for appealing meals, 229
  boosting, 294
  cooking for, 312, 444
  diversity of, 38
  ethnic, 43
  herbs and spices for, 293, 295
  oils, 441
  sensing, 12
  vegetables, 374
Flavorings, in recipes, 302
Flexibility, activity for, 20, 22
Flour, 466
  functions in recipes, 302
  measuring, 287
  storing, 475
Fluids, 100
  in body composition, 149
  and vigorous physical activity, 163–164
Fluoride, 104
Foam cakes, 507
Folate (folic acid), 101
  during pregnancy, 172
  from vegetable and fruit groups, 129
Folding in, 292
Food, 302
  chemical makeup of, 302, 303. See also Nutrients
  conserving, 328
  as meal-planning resource, 225
Food additives, 53, 54

Food and Drug Administration (FDA), 53, 69, 215, 216, 238
Food and nutrition writers, 216
Food assistance programs, 179
Food banks, 180
Food budget, 9, 236
Food choices. See also Meal plans
  for babies, 174
  for breakfast, 226
  for children, 175
  for dessert, 502
  for gaining weight, 155
  guidelines for, 117
  and health in adulthood, 179
  for healthy weight, 153
  and hunger vs. appetite, 11
  identifying, 13
  influences on, 8–10
  for losing weight, 154
  for lunches, 227
  from menus, 251–252
  from MyPyramid, 133
  for snacks, 230
  for social activities, 178
  for sports performance, 166
  during teen years, 176–177
  for vegetarians, 187
Food cooperatives, 237
Food customs, 38–40, 44
Food editors, 491
Food exchanges, 238
Food groups. See also specific groups
  amounts from, 136
  discretionary calories from, 138
  in eating plans, 134
  in MyPyramid, 129–131
  portion sizes for, 135
Food heritage, 41
Food historians, 43
Food industry, 48–56
  food supply chain in, 50–51
  safety issues in, 55
  technology in, 52–54
  and world hunger, 55, 56
Food jags, 176
Food labels, 238
  additives on, 54
  allergens on, 199
  calories on, 154, 155
  fats on, 117
  food processing/growing information on, 240
  for meat, poultry, and fish, 412
  nutrient amounts on, 107
  nutrient content claims on, 241
  nutrition information on, 239

safe-handling instructions on, 71
Food packaging, 54
Food photographers, 459
Food preferences, 224, 225
Food preparation equipment. See Appliances; Tools, kitchen
Food prices
  comparing, 240
  for convenience foods vs. whole foods, 54
  economic factors in, 236
  influences on, 50
  at restaurants, 250
Food processing, 52
Food processing occupations, 393
Food processors, 268
Food quality, shopping tips for, 71, 242, 243
Food safety, 64–76
  avoiding cross-contamination, 70
  controlling food temperature, 74–76
  in Dietary Guidelines for Americans, 119
  with eggs, 71
  food label instructions for, 71
  food storage for, 71–74
  foodborne illness, 66–68
  government agencies for, 69
  with meat, poultry, and fish, 71, 415, 417
  with milk, 399
  for packed lunches, 228
  sanitation for, 69–70
  in serving food, 75
  shopping tips for, 242, 243
  with vegetables, 372
Food science, 302
  baking, 467–469
  eggs in, 428
  fats and oils in, 440–442
  fruits in, 381–382
  milk products in, 394–395
  of protein, 408–410
  thickening foods, 495–496
  vegetables in, 368–371
Food scientists, 99
Food sensitivities, 198–199
Food service managers, 69
Food shortages, 55, 56
Food spoilage, 73–74
Food Stamp Program, 180
Food storage. See Storing food
Food stylists, 383
Food supplies
  local, 40
  safety of, 55
  sustainability of, 186
Food supply chain, 50–51

Index

Food technologists, 53, 188
Food temperature. *See* Temperature of food
Foodborne illness, 66–68
Foods lab, 324, 325
Fortified foods, 53
France, foods from, 153
Fraudulent information, 216
Freezer, storing foods in, 72
Freezer burn, 72
Frequency of activity, 165
Fresh foods, 240, 242
Freshness dates, 238
Friends, food choices and, 9
Frozen foods, 242
    desserts, 502, 504
    fruit tidbits, 502
    milk products, 398
    yogurt, 504
Fruit dip, 487
Fruit Group, 129, 130, 135
Fruit juice, 383–384
Fruit nectar, 383
Fruit pies, 509, 510
Fruit sauce, 385
Fruits, 378–386
    buying, 382–384
    classifying, 381
    colors of, 381
    convenience options for, 384
    cooking, 386
    as desserts, 502
    enzymes in, 382
    in food science, 381–382
    forms of, 242
    health benefits of, 380
    in meal plans, 117
    in MyPyramid, 380
    nutrient density of, 133
    during pregnancy, 172
    preparation of, 386
    in salads, 454
    seasonal, 384
    in soups and stews, 490, 491
    storing, 385
    types of, 381
    washing, 66
Frying, 308–309, 430
Ful, 289
Fungi, contamination by, 68

G

Gaining weight, 152–155
    by building muscle, 165
    during pregnancy, 172
Garbage disposals, 268
Garnishing, 292, 340, 456
Gazpacho, 21
Gelatin, 408
Gelatin desserts, 502
Gelatinization, 496
Generic brands, 240

Geography, influence of, 40
Germ (grains), 352, 356
Germany, foods from, 470
Germs (microorganisms), 356
Giblets, 412
Glasses, 335, 336
Gluten, 469
Gluten intolerance, 198
Gluten-free baking, 468
Goals
    for fitness, 23, 27
    mini-, 25
    for physical activity, 24
    setting, 14
    for weight, 154–156
Goi cuon, 253
Government agencies. *See also* specific agencies
    for food safety, 69
    web sites of, 215
Government food and nutrition assistance programs, 180
Government safety regulations, 50, 55
Grain Group, 129, 130, 135, 353
Grains, 350–360
    cereal, 355
    cooking, 355, 359–360
    as fiber source, 98
    and gluten intolerance, 198
    kinds of, 354
    in meal planning, 117, 353–354
    in MyPyramid, 353
    nutrients in, 352, 353
    oatmeal, 355
    pasta, 355
    during pregnancy, 172
    refined, 352
    in salads, 448, 454
    shopping for, 356–357
    in soups and stews, 490
    storing, 358–359
    whole, 98, 117, 129, 133, 352
Graters, 274
Greece, foods from, 177
Green methods, 324
Grilling, 373, 483
Grocery store workers, 240
Growth and development, 148–152
    and carbohydrate loading, 166
    during teen years, 176–177
    and weight lifting, 165
Gyros, 483

H

HACCP (Hazard Analysis and Critical Control Points), 68
Hand washing, 69

Hazard Analysis and Critical Control Points (HACCP), 68
HDL (high-density lipoprotein), 202, 440
Headnotes, 282
Health benefits
    of ethnic/regional foods, 43
    of fruits, 380
    of milk products, 392
    of oils, 438
    of physical activity, 21–22, 116
    of salads, 454
    of vegetables, 366
Health claims, 239
Health fraud, 216, 217
Health problems. *See also* Illness
    avoiding, 196
    cholesterol, 202
    eating disorders, 196–197
    eating plans for, 200–203
    from fat consumption, 438
    food allergies, 199
    food sensitivities, 198–199
    high blood pressure, 202
    pre-diabetes, 200
    from steroid use, 165
    weight risk factors for, 115
Health risks, 114, 196
Healthful lifestyle, 6. *See also* Wellness
Healthy weight, 115, 149–155, 165
Heart, 20, 22
Heart disease
    and active lifestyle, 22
    coronary heart disease, 202
    eating plan to prevent, 202
    and fat consumption, 117
    and fat intake, 99
    and obesity, 151
Hearty meals, planning, 228, 229
Heat, effects of, 304
Heat transfer, 304–305
Heimlich maneuver, 85
Herbal supplements, 217
Herbs, 293, 295
HHS (United States Department of Health and Human Services), 114
High blood pressure, 202
High-density lipoprotein (HDL), 202, 440
HIV/AIDS, 203
Holidays, foods linked with, 39
Home-delivered meals, 180
Hominy, 354
Homogenized milk, 395
Hors d'oeuvre, 153
Hunger, 11, 55, 56
Hydration, 100, 164

Hydrogenated oils, 98
Hydrogenation, 440
Hydroponics, 52
Hygiene, 69

I

Ice cream, 504
Illness, 203. See also Health
  problems
    bacterial, 67
    foodborne, 66–68
    phytonutrients for preven-
      tion of, 107
    risk factors for, 115
Immigration, food choices and,
  40
Impulse buying, 236
Incomplete proteins, 100
India, foods from, 493
Indoor recreation, 24
Infancy, nutrition during,
  173–174
Infant formula, 173
Information. See also Food
  labels
    collecting, 13
    evaluating. See Consumer-
      ism
    on how to take medicines,
      204
    reliable sources of, 214, 215
    standards for, 55
Ingredients
    for baking, 292, 466–467
    for casseroles, 494
    on food labels, 238
    functions in cooking, 302
    measuring, 286–288
    in recipes, 282
    for salads, 455
    for sandwiches, 482
    substitutions, 284–285
Institute of Medicine, 107
Intensity of activity, 25, 165
International foods. See also
  Ethnic foods
    from Argentina, 407
    from British Isles, 119
    from Canada, 443
    from the Caribbean, 382
    from China, 85
    from Egypt, 289
    from France, 153
    from Germany, 470
    from Greece, 177
    from India, 493
    from Italy, 201
    from Mexico, 227
    from North Africa, 326
    from Peru, 55
    from Russia, 354
    from Spain, 21

    for vegetarians, 190
    from Vietnam, 253
Iron
    foods for, 133
    functions and sources of,
      104
    from grains, 129, 353
    for healthy blood, 103
    from meat and beans, 129
    pairing vitamin C with, 188
    during pregnancy, 172
    for teens, 177
    for vegetarians, 187
Irradiation, 53
Italy, foods from, 201

J

Jerk, 382
Jobs, active, 24. See also Careers
Juice, 164

K

Kippers, 119
Kitchen
    cleanliness of, 70
    organizing. See Organizing
      the kitchen
Kitchen designers, 266
Kitchen equipment, 262–276
    cookware and bakeware,
      270–271
    major appliances, 264–267
    as meal-planning resource,
      225
    small appliances, 268–269
    tools, 272–276
Kitchen fires, 83
Kitchen safety, 80–86
    for accident prevention,
      82–85
    handling emergencies, 85, 86
Kitchen scales, 272
Kitchen shears, 274
Kneading, 292, 472
Knife safety, 82
Knife skills, 291
Knowledge, food choices and, 9

L

La Leche League, 173
Lactation, 173
Lacto-ovo-vegetarians, 186, 187
Lactose intolerance, 198, 392
Lacto-vegetarians, 186, 187
Ladles, 275
Lamb, 410
Lard, 442
Large intestine, 97
LDL (low-density lipoprotein),
  202, 440
Lean meat, 406

Leavening agents, 302, 467–469,
  476
Leftovers, 74, 76
Legumes, 426–427. See also
  Beans
    cooking, 431
    as fiber source, 98
    in Meat Group, 131
Length, measuring, 288
Life cycle, 172
Life stage nutrition, 170–180
    adulthood, 178–179
    childhood, 175–176
    family and community
      support for, 179–180
    infancy, 173–174
    planning meals for, 224
    pregnancy, 172
    teen years, 176–177
Lifestyle
    changes in, 179
    food choices influenced by, 9
    physically active, 21
    for wellness, 6
Lifestyle activities, 24
Light meals, planning, 228
Linens, 335, 336
Lipids, 202
Lipoproteins, 202
Liquid measuring cups, 272
Liquids
    in baking, 466
    functions in recipes, 302
    measuring, 287
Listeria monocytogenes, 67
Liver, digestion in, 97
Local food supplies, 40
Longevity, impact of wellness
  on, 6
Losing weight
    guidelines for, 152–153
    risk in, 152
    strategies for, 154
Low birth weight, 172
Low-density lipoprotein (LDL),
  202, 440
Lunches, planning, 227, 228
Lungs, 20

M

Macronutrients, 96
    carbohydrates, 97–98
    fats, 98–99
    proteins, 99–100
Magnesium, 103, 104, 115
Maillard reaction, 409
Main dishes, 229
Maintaining weight, guidelines
  for, 152–153
Major appliances, 264–267
Mall foods, 178
Malnutrition, 107

Manners
  at meals, 337–339
  at restaurants, 252–253
  when shopping, 243–244
  at work, 338
Marbling (in meats), 406
Margarine, 442
Marinades, 409
Marinating, 292
Meal patterns, 224
Meal plans, 222–230. *See also*
  Food choices; Menus
  for appealing meals, 229
  for breakfast, 226–227
  for cancer, 203
  for chewing problems, 203
  daily, 136, 137
  for diabetes, 201
  eggs, beans, and nuts in, 425
  for family meals, 224
  food groups in, 134
  food preferences in, 225
  grains in, 353–354
  guidelines for, 118
  for health problems, 200
  for hearty meals, 228, 229
  for HIV/AIDS, 203
  for light meals, 228
  for lunches, 227, 228
  milk products in, 394
  nutrient balance in, 117–118
  oils in, 440
  to prevent heart disease, 202
  resources management in,
    225
  for snacks, 230
  vegetables in, 367, 368
  for vegetarians, 188, 189
Meal service, types of, 334, 341
Measurements, converting, 11,
  128. *See also* Adapting/adjust-
  ing recipes
Measuring, 285–288
Measuring spoons, 272
Measuring tools, 272
Meat(s)
  buying, 411–412
  composition of, 408
  cooking, 409, 410, 415–417
  cross-contamination from,
    70
  food labels for, 238
  in MyPyramid, 407
  nutrients in, 406
  religious practices involv-
    ing, 39
  safe-handling instructions
    for, 71
  in salads, 454
  shopping for, 410–412, 414
  in soups and stews, 490
  storing, 415

Meat and Beans Group, 129,
  131
  dry beans and peas in, 367
  portion sizes for, 135
  during pregnancy, 172
  vegetarian choices from, 188
Meat cuts, 409, 411
Meat thermometers, 75, 275
Meatless meals, 99
Media, food choices and, 9
Media literacy, 214–215
Medical nutrition therapy, 203
Medications, 204
Melons, 381
Mental health, 7–8, 151
Mental math, 243
Mental performance, wellness
  and, 6
Menus, 224. *See also* Meal plans
  making choices from,
    251–252
  using foods on hand, 225
Meringues, 510
Metabolism, 105–106, 178
Metal spatulas, 275
Metric measurement system,
  285
Mexico, foods from, 227
Micronutrients, 96
  minerals, 102–104
  vitamins, 100–102
Microwave cooking, 309–311
  beverages, 489
  breads, 475
  eggs, 430
  fruits, 386
  vegetables, 373
Microwave ovens, 266, 309–310
  cookware for, 271
  thawing foods in, 74
Microwave-safe packaging, 54
Milk, 395–396
  cooking with, 400
  in meal plans, 117
  nutrient density of, 133
  during physical activity, 164
Milk Group, 129, 131
  portion sizes for, 135
  during pregnancy, 172
  vegetarian choices from, 188
Milk (dairy) products, 390–400.
  See also Milk Group
  cheese, 117, 397–398, 400,
    492
  cream and sour cream, 398
  in food science, 394–395
  frozen, 398
  health benefits of, 392
  and lactose intolerance, 198
  in meal plans, 394
  milk, 117, 164, 395–396, 400
  in MyPyramid, 393
  nutrient density of, 133

  nutrients in, 392
  during pregnancy, 172
  preparation of, 398–400
  in salads, 454
  shopping for, 396–398
  in soups and stews, 490
  storage of, 398–399
  for vegetarians, 186
  yogurt, 38, 117, 133, 394,
    397
Mincing, 291
Minerals, 102–104
  for active living, 162
  in eggs, beans, and nuts, 424
  in fruits, 380
  in grains, 353
  in meat, poultry, and fish,
    406
  in milk products, 392
  in Nutrition Facts, 239
  for teens, 177
  in vegetables, 366, 367
Mirepoix, 153
Mixed foods, 132, 480–486,
  490–496
  main dishes, 493–495
  pizza, 484–486
  sandwiches, 482–484
  soups and stews, 490–492
Mixers, 268
Mixing bowls, 274, 292
Mixing spoons, 274
Mixing tools, 274
Moist-heat cooking, 307–308
Molded cookies, 505
Moldy food, 74
Money
  for food budget, 236
  as meal-planning resource,
    225
Mood, activity and, 22
Moussaka, 177
Mouth, digestion in, 97, 152
Muesli, 470
Muffin method (quick breads),
  471–472
Mugs, 335
Mujudarah, 190
Muscle
  in body composition, 21, 149
  building, 99, 155, 165
  lost with fad diets, 155
Muscular strength and endur-
  ance, 20
MyPyramid, 124–138, 172
  choosing foods from, 133
  combination foods in, 132
  eggs, beans, and nuts in, 425
  fats and oils in, 439
  food groups in, 129–131
  food plan levels from, 134,
    136–138
  fruits in, 380

grains in, 353
guidelines for using, 128
interpreting, 126–127
meat, poultry, and fish in, 407
milk products in, 393
oils in, 129, 131
in planning sports nutrition, 162
and portion sizes, 134, 135
for preventing deficiencies, 196
vegetables in, 367
for vegetarians, 188

N

Nanaimo bars, 443
National brands, 240
National information sources, 215
Natural foods, 240
Neufchâtel cheese, 395
News reports about food/nutrition, 217
Niacin, 101
Nonfat dry milk, 396
North Africa, foods from, 326
Nutrient content claims, 239, 241
Nutrient deficiencies, 107
Nutrient density, 133
Nutrient-dense foods, 115
  for family meals, 224
  for gaining weight, 155
  guidelines for selecting, 133
  for losing weight, 154
  for snacks, 230
Nutrients, 94–108. See also individual nutrients
  amounts needed, 107–108
  in beverages, 488, 489
  carbohydrates, 97–98
  dietary guidelines for, 115
  digestion of, 96–97
  in eggs, beans, and nuts, 424
  and energy, 103, 105–106
  fats, 98–99
  on food labels, 107, 238
  functions of, 96
  loss of, 304
  in meat, poultry, and fish, 406
  in milk products, 392
  minerals, 102–104
  in mother's milk, 173
  in MyPyramid food groups, 129–131
  in Nutrition Facts, 239
  in pizza, 484
  proteins, 99–100
  recipe information on, 283
  in salads, 454

in sandwiches, 482
in snacks, 486
in soups and stews, 492
in vegetables, 366
for vegetarians, 186–187
vitamins, 100–102
water, 100
Nutrition, 6
  for active lifestyle, 27
  during adulthood, 178–179
  during childhood, 175–176
  cooking for, 312
  guidelines for. See Dietary Guidelines for Americans; MyPyramid
  in healthful lifestyle, 6
  during infancy, 173–174
  in infant formula, 173
  for lowering health risks, 196
  in meal planning, 224
  for older adults, 179
  for pregnancy, 172
  programs providing assistance with, 179
  recipe makeovers for improving, 296
  during teen years, 115, 176–177
Nutrition Facts, 237–239
Nuts, 424–425, 427, 431
  in Meat Group, 131
  in salads, 454

O

Oatmeal, 355
Obesity, 151
Oils, 438–444. See also Fats
  functions in recipes, 302
  hydrogenated, 98
  in MyPyramid, 129, 131
  unsaturated, 98
Omega-3 fatty acids, 98
Omelets, 430
Online stores, 237
Open dating, 243
Oranges, 38
Organ meat, 406
Organic farming, 50
Organic foods, 240
Organizing the kitchen, 316–328
  to conserve and recycle, 325–328
  for efficiency, 322
  and evaluation of foods lab, 325
  finishing and cleaning up, 323
  identifying preparation tasks, 320
  making a schedule, 321–322
  for physical challenges, 318

for teamwork, 324
work centers, 318, 319
work plans, 319
work triangle, 318
Osteoporosis, 22, 103
Outdoor recreation, 24
Ovens, 266
Overweight, 115, 151
Ovo-vegetarians, 186
Oxidation, 441

Packaging, 54, 327
Paella, 21
Pan-broiling, 307, 417
Pan-frying, 308
Papillae, 12
Parasites, 68
Paring knives, 274
Party foods, 178
Party planners, 325
Pasta, 355, 357, 359
Pasteurized milk, 395
Pastry blenders, 274
Pastry brushes, 275
Pastry chefs, 507
Patterns, determining, 369
Peak performance, guidelines for, 163–164
Peas, 117
Peelers, 274
Peeling, 291
Percent Daily Values, 239
Percentage, 21, 107
Perishable foods
  amounts to buy of, 241
  serving times for, 75
  storage of, 72
Peru, foods from, 55
Pesticides, 50, 84
Pesto, 293
Pho, 253
Phosphorus, 102–104
Physical activity, 18–27
  and Activity Pyramid, 26
  during adulthood, 178
  aerobic, 20
  benefits of, 21–22, 116
  and body composition, 21
  for cardiorespiratory endurance, 20
  for coordination and balance, 20
  energy for, 106, 154
  excuses for avoiding, 23
  for flexibility, 20
  for gaining weight, 155
  goals for, 24
  guidelines for, 116
  in healthful lifestyle, 6
  for healthy weight, 153
  identifying choices for, 13

Index

level of, 24
  for muscular strength and
    endurance, 20
  MyPyramid recommenda-
    tion for, 127
  nutrition for. *See* Sports
    nutrition
  safety in, 25, 27
  types of, 24–25
Physical challenges
  and kitchen safety, 84
  and organization of kitchen,
    318
Physical changes to food, 302
Physical fitness, 20, 27, 116
Physical health, 7
Physical performance, wellness
    and, 6
Phytonutrients, 107
  in eggs, beans, and nuts, 424
  in fruits, 380
  in vegetables, 366
Pie crust, 508, 509
Pies, 507–509
Pizza, 484–486
Place settings, 335, 336
Plant food sources
  cholesterol in, 99
  in international foods, 190
  phytonutrients from, 107
  protein in, 100
  for vegetarians, 186, 187
Plate service, 334
Plates, 335, 336
Poison control center, 85
Poisoning
  getting help for, 85
  preventing, 84
Poisons, contamination by, 68
Polenta, 201
Pomes, 381
Popcorn, 487
Pork, 410
Portion sizes, 134, 135
  for appealing meals, 229
  for gaining weight, 155
  for losing weight, 154
  for meat, poultry, and fish,
    407
  for oils, 429
  at restaurants, 252
Potassium, 104, 115, 119, 129
Potential, 23
Pots, 270
Poultry, 406
  buying, 412
  cooking, 409, 417
  cross-contamination from,
    70
  food labels for, 238
  in Meat Group, 131
  in MyPyramid, 407
  nutrients in, 406

safe-handling instructions
    for, 71
  in salads, 454
  shopping for, 412, 414
  storing, 415
Pre-diabetes, 200
Pregnancy, nutrition during, 172
Preheating, 309
Prenatal period, 172
Preparing food, 280–296
  adjusting recipe yield, 289,
    290
  calories added when, 133
  combining skills in, 291–292
  condiment use in, 294
  with convenience cooking,
    282
  cutting skills in, 291
  fruits, 386
  herb and spice use in, 293,
    295
  identifying tasks for, 320
  measuring, 285–288
  milk products, 398–400
  nutritional recipe make-
    overs, 296
  recipe use, 282–285
  salads, 456
  with scratch cooking, 282
Pre-preparation steps, 282, 320
Preservation of foods, 53
Pressed cookies, 505
Preventive nutrition, 196
Prices of food. *See* Food prices
Priorities, food choices and, 9
Process cheeses, 398
Processed foods, 52, 98
Produce, 370. *See also* Fruits;
    Herbs; Vegetables
Product demonstrators, 311
Production costs, 50
Protective gear, 27
Proteins, 99–100
  for active living, 162
  and bacteria growth, 66
  calories in, 105
  carbohydrates with, 97
  chemical makeup of, 303
  in eggs, beans, and nuts,
    129, 424
  energy from, 99, 105
  enzymes, 369, 382
  excess, 166
  food science of, 408–410
  in meat, poultry, and fish,
    129, 406
  in milk products, 129, 392
  nutrient density of, 133
  for vegetarians, 187
Public health educators, 115
Public health regulations, 250
Puddings, 504

Q
Quality of foods, 71, 242, 243
Queso blanco, 227
Quiche, 429
Quick breads, 471–473
Quinoa, 55, 190, 354

R
Radiation, 304, 305
Rancidity, 440, 441
Ranges, 266–267
Rational numbers, 163
Ratios, 41
RDAs. *See* Recommended
    Dietary Allowances
RDs (registered dietitians), 214
Recipe developers, 431
Recipes, 282–285. *See also*
    Adapting/adjusting recipes
  Apple Cobbler, 510
  Asian Stir-Fried Vegetables,
    86
  Balsamic Vinaigrette, 138
  Beans and Vegetables on
    Toast, 120
  Blini, 360
  Chicken Quesadillas, 230
  Chimichurri Sauce, 429
  Cinnamon Baked Apples,
    218
  Egg Cream, 400
  Fruit, Granola, and Yogurt
    Parfait, 14
  Fruit Salad, 244
  Ful Mesdames, 296
  Gazpacho, 28
  Hummus, 44
  Italian-Style Chicken Strips,
    108
  Lime Quinoa with
    Vegetables, 56
  Mulligatawny, 496
  New England Clam
    Chowder, 276
  Orange-Mint Couscous, 328
  Pancakes with Maple Syrup,
    444
  Party Guacamole, 342
  Pasta Salad, 76
  Quick and Hearty Chili, 312
  Quick Marinara Sauce, 204
  Ratatouille, 156
  Red Beans and Rice, 432
  Roasted Pineapple, 386
  Soft Pretzels, 476
  Southwest Salad, 190
  Sunshine Salad, 460
  Trail Mix, 166
  Tzatziki, 180
  Vegetable Cole Slaw, 374

Index

Vietnamese Spring Rolls, 254
Recommended Dietary Allowances (RDAs), 107, 172
Recyclable packaging, 54
Recycling, 325, 327
Reducing, 309
Refined grains, 129, 352
Refrigerator cookies, 505
Refrigerator-freezers, 265
    storing foods in, 72
    thawing foods in, 74
Regional foods, 38, 42, 43
Registered dietitians (RDs), 214
Religion
    and food choices, 9
    foods used in practice of, 39
Research, 217
Resources, 8, 224
    food choices influenced by, 8
    identifying, 13
    managing, 225
    as meal planning issue, 224
    saved with shopping plan, 236
Restaurant managers, 484
Restaurant meals, 248–254
    choice of restaurant, 250
    manners, 252–253
    menu choices, 251–252
    paying bills, 253, 254
Restaurant-supply salespeople, 355
Riboflavin, 101
Rice, 38, 358, 360
Ripened cheeses, 398
Risk factors, 115
    lowering, 196
    with obesity, 151
Risotto, 201
Roasting, 306
    meat, 416, 417
    poultry, 417
    vegetables, 373
Roasting pans, 270
Rolled cookies, 505
Rolling pin and cover, 275
Rounding, 243
Rubber scrapers, 274, 275
Rubs, 293
Russia, foods from, 354

S

Safe-handling instructions, 71
Safety
    of food. See Food safety
    in food industry, 55
    in kitchen, 80–86
    with knives, 82
    with microwave ovens, 311
    in physical activity, 25, 27
    with ranges and ovens, 267

Safety regulations, 50, 55
Salad bars, 460
Salad dressings, 454, 456, 458–459
Salad greens, 454, 455
Salads, 452–460
    arranged, 45
    buying ingredients for, 455
    dressings for, 454, 456, 458–459
    ingredients for, 454
    making, 456
    mixed, 457
    nutrients in, 454
    parts of, 455
    salad bars, 460
    storing ingredients, 455
    of tossed greens, 457
Salmon, 38
Salmonella, 67
Salsa, 293
Salt. See also Sodium
    in baking, 467
    in cereal, 198
    in teen diets, 115
Sandwiches, 482–484
Sanitation
    for bottle-feeding babies, 174
    for food safety, 69–70
Saskatoon berries, 443
Saturated fats, 98, 99, 105, 115, 441
Saucepans, 270
Sautéing, 308
Schedules, 224, 321–322
School information sources, 215
Scientific studies, 217
Scones, 119
Scratch cooking, 282
Searing, 309
Seasonal produce, 370, 384
Seasoning(s), 292, 293, 295
    ethnic, 43
    functions in recipes, 302
Seasoning blends, 293
Sedentary routine, 25
Seeds, 131, 427
Self-esteem, 6, 22, 151
Self-rising flour, 466
Servers, restaurant, 253
Serving meals, 332–342
    in appealing way, 339–340
    buffet style, 341
    for enjoyable eating, 337
    for entertaining, 340–342
    safety in, 75
    and table manners, 337–339
    table setting, 334–336
    types of meal service, 334
Serving size, 239. See also Portion sizes
Shapes of foods, 229

Shelf life, 53, 72
Shellfish, 413
Sherbet, 504
Shocks, electrical, 83
Shopping for foods, 234–244
    amounts to buy, 241
    breads, 356
    choosing right form of food, 242
    comparing prices, 240
    creating plan for, 236–237
    customer courtesy in, 243–244
    eggs, beans, and nuts, 426–427
    fats and oils, 443
    food budget for, 236
    and food label information, 238–241
    fruits, 382–384
    grains, 356–357
    list for, 236
    meat, poultry, and fish, 410–414
    milk products, 396–398
    for safety and quality, 71, 242, 243
    salad ingredients, 455
    times for, 237
    types of places for, 237
    vegetables, 370–371
Shortened cakes, 507
Shortening, 442
Side dishes, 229, 251
Sifters, 274
Signals of illness, 68
Simmering, 308, 373
Simple carbohydrates, 97
Simultaneous tasks, 320
Skillet meals, 493
Skillets, 270
Skills, as meal-planning resource, 225
Sleep, body processes during, 176
Slicing knives, 274
Slotted spoons, 276
Slow cookers, 268
Small appliances, 268–269
Small intestine, 97
Smell, taste of food and, 12
Smoke point (oils), 441
Snacks, 486–489
    beverages for, 488–489
    for children, 175
    pizza, 484–486
    planning, 230
    sandwiches, 482–484
    for teens, 177
Social activities, food choices for, 178
Social and human services assistants, 173

Social health, 8, 151
Soda, calcium loss and, 225
Sodium, 104, 115, 119
Solid fats, 288, 438, 439, 442–444. *See also* Fats
Sorbet, 504
Soups, 490–492
Sour cream, 398
Sourdough breads, 468
Souvlaki, 177
Soy
    healthy amounts of, 187
    for vegetarians, 188, 189
Soy milk, 393
Spaetzle, 470
Spain, foods from, 21
Special food needs, planning menus for, 224
Special health concerns, 194–204
    coronary heart disease, 202–203
    diabetes, 200–201
    disease prevention, 196
    eating disorders, 196–197
    food sensitivities, 198–199
    illness, 203
    medications, 204
Specialty stores, 237
Spices, 293, 295
Spoilage of food, 73–74
Sports drinks, 164
Sports nutrition, 160–166
    choices for peak performance, 163–164
    guidelines for, 165–166
    using MyPyramid in planning, 162
Spreads, 487
Spring rolls, 483
Standards, 55
Standing time, 311
Staphylococcus aureus (Staph), 67
Staples, 236
Starches, 97, 352
    for active living, 162
    in cooking grains, 355
    in grain group foods, 129
Steamer baskets, 270
Steaming, 308, 373
Stemware, 335
Steroids, 165
Stews, 490–492
Stir-frying, 309, 373, 495
Stirring, 292
Stock, 490
Stomach, 97
Storage of kitchen tools, 272
Store brands, 240
Storing food
    bread ingredients, 475–476
    breads, 476

desserts, 410
eggs, beans, and nuts, 424–425
fats and oils, 443
for food safety, 71–74
fruits, 385
grains, 358–359
herbs and spices, 293
ingredients for breads, 475–476
leftovers, 76
meat, poultry, and fish, 415
milk products, 398–399
salad ingredients, 455
soups and stews, 492
vegetables, 370, 371
Strainers, 276
Strength, activity and, 20, 22
Stress, 7–8, 22
Stress management, 6, 8, 155
Stretching, for flexibility, 20
Substitutions, 284–285
Sugars, 97, 99
    added to food, 133
    guidelines for using, 118
    measuring, 287
    in teen diets, 115
Sugary drinks, 164
Supermarkets, 237
Supplements, 108
    evaluating information about, 216
    herbal, 217
Supply and demand, 50
Support, for wellness plan, 14
Surface area, 428
Surimi, 413
Sustainable agriculture, 50
Sweating, 23, 162
Sweetened condensed milk, 396
Sweeteners. *See also* Sugars
    in baking, 467
    functions in recipes, 302

T

Tabbouleh, 448
Table manners, 337–339
Table setting, 334–336
Tableware, 335
Tagines, 326
Talk-sing test, 25
Taste buds, 12
Taste of food, sensing, 12
Teamwork, 324
Technology
    food choices influenced by, 9
    in food industry, 52–54
Teen years
    body composition during, 149
    nutrition during, 115, 176–177

Tempeh, 425
Temperature, for baking, 469, 470
Temperature of food
    for appealing meals, 229
    controlling, 74–76
    in freezer, 72
    measuring, 288
    in recipes, 283
    in refrigerator, 72
    sensing, 12
    when completely cooked, 74–75
    when serving, 75
Temperature zones (food storage), 72, 73
Tender-crisp vegetables, 373
Tenderizing meats and poultry, 409
Tenderness of foods, 444
Testing food products, 53
Texture of food
    for appealing meals, 229
    and cooking with oils/fats, 444
    sensing, 12
    when spoiled, 74
Thawing foods, 73, 74
Thiamin, 101
Thickening foods, 495–496
Time
    as meal-planning resource, 225. *See also* Schedules
    in recipes, 283
Toaster ovens, 268
Toasters, 268
Toasting, 309
Tofu, 85, 425, 427, 431–432, 490
Tongs, 275
Tongue, 12
Tools, kitchen, 272–276, 282
Tortilla points, 487
Trade-offs, in resource use, 225
Trail mix, 487
Traits, cultural, 44
Trans fats, 98, 99, 105, 115
Travel, food choices and, 40
Trends, food choices and, 9
Tropical fruits, 381
Tumblers, 335
Turkey, thawing, 73
Turners, 275
Type 1 diabetes, 201
Type 2 diabetes, 22, 201

U

UHT milk, 396
Umami, 12
Underweight, 115, 151
Unit price, 240
United States, food traditions of, 41–42

Index

United States Department of Agriculture (USDA), 69, 114, 238
United States Department of Health and Human Services (HHS), 114
Units of measure, 285–286
Universal product code (UPC), 238
Unripened cheeses, 398
Unsaturated fats, 98, 441
UPC (universal product code), 238
USDA. *See* United States Department of Agriculture
Utility forks, 275
Utility knives, 274

V

Veal, 410
Vegans, 186, 187
Vegetable Group, 129, 130
   dry beans and peas in, 367
   portion sizes for, 135
Vegetable oils, 98, 99
Vegetables, 364–374
   baking, 373
   buying, 370–371
   cleaning, 372
   colors of, 368–369
   cooking, 368, 373–374
   as fiber source, 98
   food safety for, 372
   in food science, 368–371
   forms of, 242
   as fruits, roots, and flowers, 368
   health benefits of, 366
   in meal plans, 117, 367, 368
   in MyPyramid, 367
   nutrient density of, 133
   nutrients in, 366
   during pregnancy, 172
   preparing, 372
   in salads, 454
   in soups and stews, 490
   storing, 370, 371
   subgroups of, 367
   washing, 66
Vegetarians, 184–191
   adapting traditional recipes for, 188–189
   international foods for, 190
   meal plans for, 188, 189
   MyPyramid for, 188
   nutrients for, 186–187
   types of, 186
Vietnam, foods from, 253
Vinaigrettes, 458
Vinegar, 293
Viruses, contamination by, 68
Vitamin A, 102, 107

Vitamin B6, 101
Vitamin B12, 101, 187
Vitamin C, 101, 107, 188, 215
Vitamin D, 187
Vitamin E, 115
Vitamins, 100–102
   for active living, 162
   in eggs, beans, and nuts, 129, 424
   in fruits, 129, 380
   in grains, 129, 353
   in meat, poultry, and fish, 129, 406
   in milk products, 392
   in Nutrition Facts, 239
   for teens, 177
   too much of, 107
   in vegetables, 129, 366, 367
Volume, 286

W

Warehouse stores, 237
Warming up, 25
Washing
   of fruits and vegetables, 66
   of hands, 69
Water
   chemical makeup of, 303
   conserving, 327
   daily allowance of, 163
   as nutrient, 100
   and vigorous physical activity, 27, 162–164
Water content of foods, 116, 392
Water-soluble vitamins, 101, 107
Weight, body, 146–156
   and body image, 151
   and energy balance, 106
   and growth rate, 148
   healthy, 115, 149–150, 152–153
   issues with, 151
   management of, 21, 115
   in morning vs. evening, 176
   reaching goals for, 154–156
Weight, of recipe ingredients, 286
Weight machines, 23
Weight management
   energy balance for, 115
   physical activity for, 21
Weight-loss counselors, 151
Wellbeing, sense of, 22
Wellness, 4–14
   benefits of, 6
   choosing, 13
   eating for, 11–12
   and influences on food choices, 8–10
   lifestyle for, 6
   mental and emotional health, 7–8

   physical health, 7
   social health, 8
   taking action for, 14
Whey (cheese), 397
Whipping, 292
Whole grains, 129, 352
   as fiber source, 98
   in meal plans, 117
   nutrient density of, 133
Whole-wheat flour, 466
WIC (Women, Infants, and Children) Program, 180
Wire whisks, 274
Woks, 270
Women, Infants, and Children (WIC) Program, 180
Work centers, 318, 319
Work plans, 319
Work triangle, 318
World hunger, 55, 56

Y

Yeast, 468, 469
Yeast breads, 471, 474, 475
Yield (of farm acreage), 50
Yield (of recipes), 283
   adjusting, 11
   doubling, 41
   increasing or decreasing, 289, 290
Yogurt, 38, 394, 397
   in meal plans, 117
   in Milk Group, 131
   nutrient density of, 133
Yogurt cheese, 399
Yogurt dip, 487

Z

Zinc, 104, 129, 177, 187

Index